The Collected Works of D. W. Winnicott

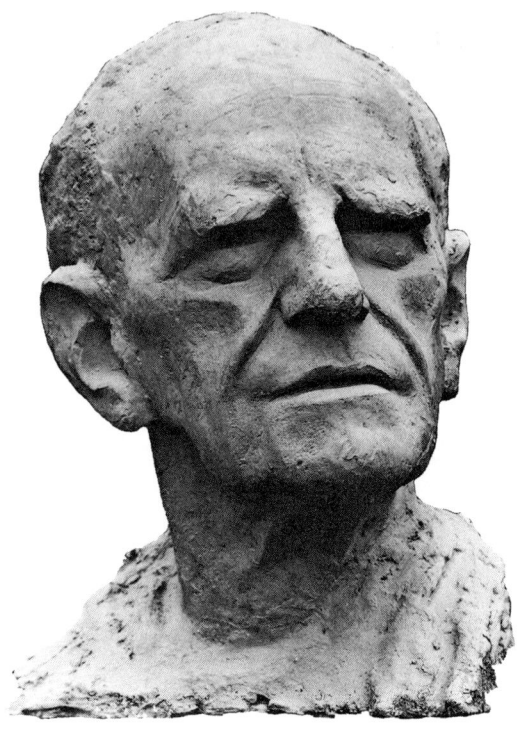

Oscar Nemon's bust of D. W. Winnicott, plaster cast, 1971

Reproduced courtesy of the Oscar Nemon Estate

The Collected Works of D. W. Winnicott

Volume 12, Appendices and Bibliographies

General Editors
Lesley Caldwell and Helen Taylor Robinson

Volume Editor
Robert Adès

Managing Editor
Amal Treacher Kabesh

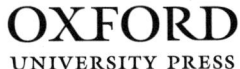

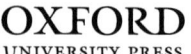

Oxford University Press is a department of the University of Oxford. It furthers the University's objective of excellence in research, scholarship, and education by publishing worldwide. Oxford is a registered trade mark of Oxford University Press in the UK and certain other countries.

Published in the United States of America by Oxford University Press
198 Madison Avenue, New York, NY 10016, United States of America.

© Oxford University Press 2017

All rights reserved. No part of this publication may be reproduced, stored in a retrieval system, or transmitted, in any form or by any means, without the prior permission in writing of Oxford University Press, or as expressly permitted by law, by license, or under terms agreed with the appropriate reproduction rights organization. Inquiries concerning reproduction outside the scope of the above should be sent to the Rights Department, Oxford University Press, at the address above.

You must not circulate this work in any other form
and you must impose this same condition on any acquirer.

Library of Congress Cataloging-in-Publication Data
Names: Winnicott, D. W. (Donald Woods), 1896–1971, author. |
Caldwell, Lesley, editor. | Taylor Robinson, Helen, editor.
Title: The collected works of D. W. Winnicott / edited by Lesley Caldwell and
Helen Taylor Robinson.
Description: Oxford; New York: Oxford University Press, [2017] |
Includes bibliographical references and index.
Identifiers: LCCN 2016026458 (print) | LCCN 2016039667 (ebook) |
ISBN 9780199399338 (set) | ISBN 9780190271336 (v. 1) | ISBN 9780190271343 (v. 2) |
ISBN 9780190271350 (v. 3) | ISBN 9780190271367 (v. 4) |
ISBN 9780190271374 (v. 5) | ISBN 9780190271381 (v. 6) | ISBN 9780190271398 (v. 7) |
ISBN 9780190271404 (v. 8) | ISBN 9780190271411 (v. 9) |
ISBN 9780190271428 (v. 10) | ISBN 9780190271435 (v. 11) |
ISBN 9780190271442 (v. 12)
Subjects: LCSH: Child psychiatry. | Child psychology. |
Psychoanalysis. | Psychotherapy.
Classification: LCC RJ499 .W479 2017 (print) | LCC RJ499 (ebook) | DDC
618.92/8914—dc23
LC record available at https://lccn.loc.gov/2016026458

1 3 5 7 9 8 6 4 2
Printed by Sheridan Books, Inc., United States of America

COMPLETE CONTENTS OF
THE *COLLECTED WORKS OF D. W. WINNICOTT*

VOLUME 1: 1911–1938

Foreword by Christopher Bollas	xlvii
Acknowledgements	li
Editors' Note	lv
General Introduction to the *Collected Works*	lvii
LESLEY CALDWELL AND HELEN TAYLOR ROBINSON	
Introduction to Volume 1	3
KEN ROBINSON	

PART 1 School to Medical Training, 1911–1920s

1. Letter to His Mother, Elizabeth, ca. 2 September 1911–1913	27
2. Letter to Stanley Ede, ca. 1912–1913	29
3. Smith, 1913	31
4. Letter to His Family, 3 November 1913	35
5. Letter to His Family, ca. 23 December 1913	37
6. The Night Attack, 1914	39
7. Letter to His Family, 9 May 1914	43
8. The Best Remedy, 1914	45
9. Letter to His Mother, Elizabeth, n.d., late 1916	49
10. Letter to His Family, 9 December 1916	51
11. Letter to His Sister, Violet, 15 November 1919	53
12. A Shropshire Surgeon, 1920	57
13. St Bartholomew's Hospital Amateur Dramatic Club, 1920	59
14. A Reminder to the Binder, 1921	63

15. The Snag, 1921 — 65

16. What Is Worthwhile in Medicine, ca. 1917–1923 — 67

PART 2 First Contributions to Medicine, 1926–1930

1. Varicella Encephalitis and Vaccinia Encephalitis, with Nancy Gibbs, 1926 — 75

2. Case for Diagnosis (? Poliomyelitis with Some Spasticity), 1926 — 91

3. Case for Diagnosis (? Infantile Hemiplegia), 1926 — 93

4. Two Cases of Post-Encephalitic Hypernoea, 1926 — 95

5. Case of Stunted Growth, 1927 — 99

6. The Only Child, 1928 — 101

7. Facial Nerve Paralysis, 1928 — 111

8. Facial Nerve Paralysis, Associated with Fits, 1928 — 113

9. Encephalitis After Measles and Chicken-pox, 1928 — 115

10. Muscle Weakness, Altered Gait and Absent Deep Reflexes after Measles, 1928 — 117

11. Abscess in Frontal Lobe: Post-Mortem Findings in a Case Shown at a Previous Meeting of the Section, with Elisabeth O'Flynn, 1928 — 119

12. Rheumatism in Children, 1929 — 123

13. Hemiplegia Noticed After Diphtheria, 1929 — 127

14. Measles Encephalitis, 1930 — 129

15. Symptoms Suggesting Post-Encephalitis, 1929 — 131

16. The Diagnosis of Chorea, 1929 — 133

17. Enuresis (abstract), 1929 — 141

18. Short Communication on Enuresis, 1930 — 143

19. Pathological Sleeping, 1930 — 149

20. Hæmoptysis: Case for Diagnosis, 1931 — 151

21. Pre-systolic Murmur, Possibly Not Due to Mitral Stenosis, 1931 — 153

22. A Clinical Example of Symptomatology Following
    the Birth of a Sibling, ca. 1931 — 155

23. Child Psychiatry: The Body as Affected by Psychological
    Factors, ca. 1931 — 159

24. On In-Patient Treatment for Rheumatic Fever
    and Chorea, ca. 1923–1931 — 161

PART 3 *Clinical Notes on Disorders of Childhood*, 1931

Preface — 167
Introduction — 169

1. History-Taking — 173
2. Physical Examination — 187
3. A Note on Temperature and the Importance of Charts — 195
4. The Nose and Throat — 203
5. The Heart, with Special Reference to Rheumatic Carditis — 207
6. Rheumatic Fever — 219
7. The Rheumatic Clinic — 225
8. Active Heart Disease — 229
9. Growing Pains — 235
10. Arthritis Associated with Emotional Disturbance — 239
11. Fidgetiness — 245
12. A Note on Normality and Anxiety — 255
13. Anxiety (*continued*) — 275
14. Disease of the Nervous System — 281
15. Walking — 291
16. Mental Defect — 299
17. Convulsions, Fits — 303
18. Micturition Disturbances — 315
19. Masturbation — 323
20. Speech Disorders — 329

PART 4 Further Writings, 1932–1939

1. Abstract: Psychoanalysis and Medicine, by F. Alexander, 1933 — 339
2. Abstract: Repression and Rationalisation, by H. Lundholm, 1934 — 341
3. Papular Urticaria and the Dynamics of Skin Sensation, 1934 — 343
4. Discussion: The Difficult Child by G. A. Auden, 1934 — 353
5. Abstract: A Contribution to the Problem of Psycho-physical Relations with Special Reference to Dermatology, by M. Barinbaum, 1935 — 357
6. The Manic Defence, 1935 — 359
7. The Teacher, the Parent and the Doctor, 1936 — 375
8. Letter to Robina Addis, April 1936 — 389
9. Contribution to a Discussion on Enuresis, 1936 — 391
10. Mental Hygiene of the Pre-School Child, 1936 — 397
11. Appetite and Emotional Disorder, 1936 — 413
12. Review: *Wayward Youth* by August Aichhorn, 1936 — 433
13. Review: *On the Bringing Up of Children* by Five Psycho-analysts, 1936 — 437
14. Review: *Child Psychiatry* by Leo Kanner, 1937 — 439
15. Letter to Roger Money-Kyrle, 13 May 1937 — 441
16. Notes on a Little Boy, 1938 — 443
17. Shyness and Nervous Disorders in Children, 1938 — 445
18. Skin Changes in Relation to Emotional Disorder, 1938 — 449
19. Letter to Mrs Neville Chamberlain, 10 November 1938 — 463
20. Letter to John Bowlby, 6 December 1938 — 465

Chronology — 467
References — 473
Contributors — 479
Credits — 481
Index — 487

VOLUME 2: 1939–1945

Editors' Note	xlvii
Introduction to Volume 2	3
CHRISTOPHER REEVES	

PART 1 1939

1. Letter to the *British Medical Journal*, Circumcision, 14 January	25
2. Letter to the *British Medical Journal*, Pruritus and Psychology, 22 April	29
3. The Delinquent and Habitual Offender	31
4. The Deprived Mother	35
5. Early Disillusion	43
6. Letter to the *British Medical Journal*, Evacuation of Small Children, 16 December	47
7. The Psychology of Juvenile Rheumatism	49
8. Aggression, ca. 1939	65
9. Delinquency: Continued, ca. 1930s	73

PART 2 1940

1. Letter to Kate Friedlander, 8 January	79
2. Children and Their Mothers	81
3. Discussion of War Aims	87
4. Children in the War	95

PART 3 1941

1. Report on Q Camps	103
2. Letter to the *British Medical Journal*, Communal Feeding in Schools, 6 September	107
3. On Influencing and Being Influenced	109
4. Review: *The Moral Paradox of Peace and War* by Prof J. C. Flügel	115

5. Review: *The Cambridge Evacuation Survey* edited by Susan Isaacs   117

6. The Observation of Infants in a Set Situation   121

7. Meet to be Stolen From   141

PART 4 1942

1. Resolution K: On Scientific Aims in Psychoanalysis   145

2. Child Department Consultations   149

3. Letter to the *British Medical Journal*, Loneliness in Infancy, 17 October   165

4. Why Children Play   167

5. Review: *The Nursing Couple* by Merell P. Middlemore   171

PART 5 1943

1. A Doctor Looks at the Psychiatric Social Worker   177

2. Delinquency Research   195

3. Memorandum on 'The Relationship Between Clinical Paediatrics and Child Psychology'   201

4. Letter to the *Lancet*, Prefrontal Leucotomy, 10 April   207

5. Letter to the *Lancet*, Prefrontal Leucotomy, 15 May   209

6. Treatment of Mental Disease by Induction of Fits   211

7. Letter to the *British Medical Journal*, Responsibility and Freedom, 21 August   217

8. Getting to Know Your Baby   221

9. The Wearing of Masks in the Nursing of Premature and Older Infants   227

10. Letter to the *British Medical Journal*, Shock Treatment of Mental Disorder, 25 December   229

PART 6 1944

1. Letter to Roger North   233

2. Why Do Babies Cry?   237

Complete Contents of the Collected Works of D. W. Winnicott   xi

3. Psychological Aspects of Birching   247

4. Letter to the *British Medical Journal*, Shock Therapy, 12 February   251

5. A Tendency in Therapeutics   255

6. Introduction to a Symposium on the Psycho-Analytic Contribution to the Theory of Shock Therapy   261

7. Kinds of Psychological Effect of Shock Therapy   265

8. What About Father?   271

9. Their Standards and Yours   277

10. What Do We Mean by a Normal Child?   281

11. Support for Normal Parents   287

12. Letter to Dr Marjorie Franklin, 19 October   291

13. Infant Feeding   293

14. The Problem of Homeless Children, with Clare Britton   299

15. Ocular Psychoneuroses of Childhood   313

PART 7 1945

1. The Only Child   323

2. The Evacuated Child   329

3. The Return of the Evacuated Child   335

4. Thinking and the Unconscious   341

5. Twins   343

6. Memorandum on Corporal Punishment   349

7. Home Again   353

8. Primitive Emotional Development   357

9. Evidence Given to the Home Office Committee on Children's Homes   369

10. Letter to the *British Medical Journal*, Physical Therapy in Mental Disorder, 22 December   379

11. Towards an Objective Study of Human Nature	381
12. Breast Feeding	389

Chronology	397
References	403
Contributors	407
Credits	409
Index	413

VOLUME 3: 1946–1951

Editors' Note	xlvii
Introduction to Volume 3 VINCENZO BONAMINIO AND PAOLO FABOZZI	3

PART 1 1946

1. Children's Hostels in War and Peace	23
2. Educational Diagnosis	29
3. Letter to the *British Medical Journal,* Psychology in the Child's Education, 29 June	35
4. Letter to Lord Beveridge, 15 October	37
5. Letter to *The Times*, 6 November	39
6. Letter to Ella Sharpe, 13 November	41
7. Some Psychological Aspects of Juvenile Delinquency	43
8. Psychological Aspects of Juvenile Delinquency (n.d., ca. late 1940s)	49

PART 2 1947

1. Hate in the Countertransference	59
2. Physical Therapy of Mental Disorder	69
3. Residential Management as Treatment for Difficult Children	77
4. Further Thoughts on Babies as Persons	95
5. The Child and Sex	101
6. Letter to the *British Medical Journal,* Battle Neurosis Treated with Leucotomy, 13 December	113

PART 3 1948

1. Reparation in Respect of Mother's Organized Defence Against Depression — 117
2. Paediatrics and Psychiatry — 123
3. Letter to the *British Medical Journal*, 'Pathies in a State Service, 14 February — 141
4. The Gwrw Tree — 143
5. Letter to Anna Freud, 6 July — 147
6. Review: *The Psychology of the Unwanted Child* by Agatha H. Bowley — 149
7. Review: *Parents' Questions* by The Child Study Association of America — 151
8. Disorders of Childhood — 153
9. Review: *The Psychoanalytic Study of the Child, Volume 2* edited by Anna Freud, Willie Hoffer, Edward Glover, *et al.* — 157
10. Review: *The Personality of the Pre-School Child* by Professor Werner Wolff — 159
11. Obituary: Susan Isaacs — 161
12. Primary Introduction to External Reality: The Early Stages — 165
13. Environmental Needs; the Early Stages; Total Dependence and Essential Independence — 171

PART 4 1949

1. Letter to Paul Federn, 3 January — 179
2. Letter to the *British Medical Journal*, Taking Children's Temperatures, 6 January — 181
3. Letter to Marjorie Stone, 14 February — 183
4. The Infancy of Juliet — 185
5. Letter to Roger Money-Kyrle, 22 March — 195
6. Letter to Roger Money-Kyrle, 31 March — 197
7. Letter to Roger Money-Kyrle, 2 May — 199

8. Birth Memories, Birth Trauma, and Anxiety	201
9. Letter to Joan Riviere, 19 May	221
10. Letter to Roger Money-Kyrle, 13 June	223
11. Notes on the Discussion Held on Dr Winnicott's Paper 'The Birth Trauma'	225
12. Letter to Roger Money-Kyrle, 22 June	229
13. Letter to Roger Money-Kyrle, 24 June	231
14. Letter to Joan Riviere, 24 June	233
15. Review: *Handbook of Child Guidance* by Ernest Harms	235
16. Letter to *The Times*, Punishment and Crime: A Psychologist's View, 10 August	237
17. Letter to R. S. Hazlehurst, 1 September	239
18. Letter to S. H. Hodge, 1 September	241
19. Letter to the *British Medical Journal*, Paddington Green's Children's Hospital, 24 September	243
20. Mind and Its Relation to the Psyche-Soma	245
21. Leucotomy	259
22. Review: *Art Versus Illness* by Adrian Hill	265
23. A Man Looks at Motherhood	269
24. The Baby as a Going Concern	273
25. Where the Food Goes	277
26. The End of the Digestive Process	281
27. The Baby as a Person	285
28. Close-up of Mother Feeding Baby	289
29. The World in Small Doses	293
30. The Innate Morality of the Baby	299
31. Weaning	303
32. Young Children and Other People	307
33. Stealing and Telling Lies	313

34. The Impulse to Steal	319
35. Sex Education in Schools	323
36. Enuresis: Notes for a lecture to the Tavistock Children's Department (n.d., ca. 1949)	327

PART 5 1950

1. Letter to Clare Britton [Excerpt], early 1950	331
2. Aggression in Relation to Emotional Development	333
3. Letter to *The Times*, Neglected Children, 31 January	349
4. Letter to Otho W. S. Fitzgerald, 3 March	351
5. Childhood Psychosis	353
6. Letter to P. D. Scott, 11 May	357
7. Letter to *The Times*, Maladjusted Children: Damaging Effect of Delay, May 13	361
8. Review: *Infancy of Speech and Speech of Infancy* by Leopold Stein	363
9. Letter to Roger Money-Kyrle, 10 July	365
10. The Deprived Child and How He Can Be Compensated for Loss of Family Life	367
11. Letter to Roger Money-Kyrle, 8 August	381
12. Letter to Hannah 'Queen' Henry, 31 October	383
13. Letter to Roger Money-Kyrle, 16 November	385
14. Knowing and Learning	387
15. Instincts and Normal Difficulties	393
16. Growth and Development in Immaturity	397
17. Some Thoughts on the Meaning of the Word Democracy	407
18. 'Yes, But How Do We Know It's True?'	423

PART 6 1951

1. Review: *The Child and the Magistrate* by J. A. F. Watson	431
2. Letter to W. R. Bion, 22 January	433

3. Letter to James Strachey, 1 May — 435
4. The Foundation of Mental Health — 437
5. Visiting Children in Hospital — 441
6. Transitional Objects and Transitional Phenomena — 447
7. Review: *The Inner World of Man: with Psychological Drawings and Paintings* by Frances G. Wickes — 463
8. Letter to the *Lancet*, Leucotomy in Psychosomatic Disorders, 18 August — 465
9. Letter to the *British Medical Journal*, Ethics of Prefrontal Leucotomy, 25 August — 467
10. Review: *Jealousy in Children* by Edmund Ziman, M.D. — 469
11. Letter to *The Times*, Nursery Schools: A Definition of Functions, 8 September — 471
12. Review: *The Psychoanalytic Study of the Child*, Volumes 3–4 and Volume 5 edited by Anna Freud, Willie Hoffer, and Edward Glover — 473
13. Letter to Edward Glover, 23 October — 475
14. Notes on the General Implications of Leucotomy — 477
15. Review: *On Not Being Able to Paint* by Marion Milner — 483
16. Review: *Problems of Infancy and Childhood* — 487
17. Review: *Papers on Psycho-Analysis* by Ernest Jones — 489
18. Review: *Infant Feeding and Feeding Difficulties* by Philip Rainsforth Evans and Ronald Mackeith — 491

Chronology — 495
References — 501
Contributors — 507
Credits — 509
Index — 515

VOLUME 4: 1952–1955

Editors' Note	xlvii
Introduction to Volume 4	3
DOMINIQUE SCARFONE	

PART 1 1952

1. The Ordinary Devoted Mother and Her Baby: The First Week	21
2. The Ordinary Devoted Mother and Her Baby: Baby Bites	25
3. Letter to Hanna Segal, 21 February	29
4. Letter to The *Lancet*, Frontal Lobes of the Human Brain, 8 March	33
5. Psychoses and Child Care	35
6. Letter to Augusta Bonnard, 3 April	45
7. Letter to Willi Hoffer, 4 April	47
8. Letter to S. S. Davidson, 5 May	49
9. Letter to H. Ezriel, 20 June	51
10. Letter to Ernest Jones, 22 July	53
11. Anxiety Associated with Insecurity	55
12. Letter to Melanie Klein, 17 November	59
13. Letter to Roger Money-Kyrle, 27 November	63

PART 2 1953

1. Letter to Hanna Segal, 22 January	71
2. Letter to Herbert Rosenfeld, 22 January	73
3. Letter to Herbert Rosenfeld, 17 February	77
4. Symptom Tolerance in Paediatrics: A Case History	79
5. Letter to W. Clifford M. Scott, 19 March	97
6. Review in *British Medical Journal*: Twins: A Study of Three Pairs of Identical Twins by Dorothy Burlingham	101
7. Review in *New Era*: A Study of Three Pairs of Identical Twins by Dorothy Burlingham	103

8. The Unconscious — 107

9. Letter to Esther Bick, 11 June — 109

10. Review: *Maternal Care and Mental Health* by John Bowlby — 111

11. Review: *Psycho-Analysis and Child Psychiatry* by Edward Glover — 115

12. Review: *Problems of Infancy and Childhood* edited by Milton Senn — 117

13. Letter to Sylvia Payne, 7 October — 119

14. Letter to David Rapaport, 9 October — 121

15. Letter to Hannah Ries, 27 November — 123

16. Review: *Childhood and Society* by Erik H. Erikson — 125

17. Review: *Direct Analysis: Selected Papers* by John N. Rosen — 127

18. Review: *Psychoanalytic Studies of the Personality* by W. R. D. Fairbairn, with Masud Khan — 129

19. Two Adopted Children — 139

20. Mother, Teacher, and the Child's Needs — 151

21. Transitional Objects and Transitional Phenomena — 159

PART 3 1954

1. Letter to W. Clifford M. Scott, 27 January — 177

2. Letter to Charles Rycroft, 5 February — 179

3. Letter to *The Spectator*, A Psychiatrist's Choice, 12 February — 181

4. Letter to W. Clifford M. Scott, 26 February — 183

5. The Depressive Position in Normal Emotional Development — 185

6. Metapsychological and Clinical Aspects of Regression Within the Psycho-Analytical Set-Up — 201

7. Letter to Anna Freud, 18 March — 219

8. Letter to Betty Joseph, 13 April — 221

9. Letter to W. Clifford M. Scott, 13 April — 223

10. Letter to Sir David K. Henderson, 10 May — 227

11. Letter to John Bowlby, 11 May — 231

12. Review: *Child Psychotherapy* by S. R. Slavson — 233

13. Letter to Klara Frank, 20 May	235
14. Letter to Sir David K. Henderson, 20 May	237
15. Letter to Anna Freud and Melanie Klein, 3 June	241
16. Letter to Michael Fordham, 11 June	245
17. Review: *Aggression and Its Interpretation* by Lydia Jackson	247
18. Needs of the Under-Fives	249
19. Letter to Harry Guntrip, 20 July	257
20. Letter to *The Times*, Sponsored Television, 21 July	259
21. Letter to Harry Guntrip, 13 August	261
22. Review: *Clinical Management of Behavior Disorders in Children* by Harry Bakwin and Ruth Morris Bakwin	265
23. Letter to Thomas Stapleton, 20 September	267
24. Letter to Roger Money-Kyrle, 23 September	269
25. Letter to D. Chaplin, 18 October	271
26. Character Types: The Foolhardy and the Cautious: On *Funfairs, Thrills and Regressions* by Michael Balint	273
27. Letter to *The Times*, 'Pin-up' Pictures at Approved School, 1 November,	279
28. Play in the Analytic Situation	281
29. Withdrawal and Regression	283
30. Pitfalls in Adoption	291
31. Preface to *The First Treasured Possession* by Olive Stevenson	297

PART 4 1955

1. Holding and Interpretation: Fragment of an Analysis	303
Chronology	475
References	481
Contributors	485
Credits	487
Index	491

VOLUME 5: 1955–1959

Editors' Note	xlvii
Introduction to Volume 5	3
JENNIFER JOHNS AND MARCUS JOHNS	

PART 1 1955

1. Letter to Roger Money-Kyrle, 10 February	19
2. On Adoption	21
3. Letter to Thomas Stapleton, 3 March	25
4. Memorandum from Paddington Green Children's Hospital Psychology Department on Homosexuality and the Law	27
5. Letter to Emilio Rodrigue, 17 March	31
6. Letter to Roger Money-Kyrle, 17 March	33
7. Private Practice	35
8. Letter to Charles Rycroft, 21 April	43
9. Group Influences and the Maladjusted Child: The School Aspect	45
10. For Stepparents	55
11. Clinical Varieties of Transference	61
12. Adopted Children in Adolescence	67
13. Letter to the *British Medical Journal*, Comforters, 13 August	77
14. Letter to Michael Fordham, 26 September	79
15. Letter to Hanna Segal, 6 October	81
16. Letter to Wilfred R. Bion, 7 October	83
17. Letter to Anna Freud, 18 November	87
18. A Case Managed at Home	89
19. Foreword to *Any Wife, Any Husband* by Dr Joan Graham	99
20. First Experiments in Independence	101
21. A Note on Regression and Reassurance	107
22. Letter to Charles M. Schulz, 1955	109

23. The Toddler, the Second Adoption, Telling Children About Adoption, undated, ca. mid-1950s. ... 111

PART 2 1956

1. What Do We Know About Babies as Cloth Suckers? ... 115
2. Letter to the *British Medical Journal*, Prefrontal Leucotomy, 28 January ... 119
3. Letter to Joan Riviere, 3 February ... 121
4. Fragments Concerning Varieties of Clinical Confusion ... 125
5. On 'A Study of Envy and Gratitude' by Melanie Klein ... 129
6. Letter to Enid Balint, 22 March ... 133
7. Psycho-Analysis and the Sense of Guilt ... 135
8. The Antisocial Tendency ... 149
9. Letter to Gabriel Casuso, 4 July ... 159
10. Letter to Oliver H. Lowry, 5 July ... 161
11. Paediatrics and Childhood Neurosis ... 165
12. Letter to Charles Rycroft, 7 October ... 171
13. Letter to Charles Rycroft, 17 October ... 173
14. Letter to J. Peter M. Tizard, 23 October ... 175
15. Letter to Barbara Lantos, 8 November ... 179
16. Primary Maternal Preoccupation ... 183
17. Notes on Adolescence, ca. 1956 ... 189

PART 3 1957

1. Letter to Anna M. Kulka, 15 January ... 197
2. Letter to Charles Rycroft, 17 January ... 199
3. Letter to Thomas Main, 24 January ... 201
4. Address Introducing Margaret Mead, VIIIth Ernest Jones Lecture ... 203
5. Letter to Margaret Mead, 31 January ... 205

6. Letter to Thomas Main, 25 February	207
7. Letter to Melanie Klein, 7 March	209
8. Remarks on a Discussion of Balint's Paper on Technique	211
9. Letter to Michael Balint, 27 March	213
10. Letter to Michael Balint, 4 April	215
11. Letter to Tsuicheu Cheu, 4 April	217
12. Letter to *The Times*, I Qant Stand It, 11 April	219
13. Letter to Martin James, 17 April	221
14. Review: *Six Children* by Estelle J. Foote	223
15. The Contribution of Psycho-Analysis to Midwifery	225
16. Letter to Mary Applebey, 27 May	233
17. Foreword to *The Case as the Patient Sees It: Psychoanalysis*	235
18. Letter to Joan Riviere, 21 June	237
19. Letter to Prunella Briance, 15 July	239
20. The Capacity to Be Alone	241
21. On the Contribution of Direct Child Observation to Psycho-Analysis	249
22. Letter to Augusta Bonnard, 1 October	255
23. Hallucination and Dehallucination	257
24. Letter to Michael Balint, 3 October	261
25. Letter to Francesca Bion, 3 October	263
26. Integrative and Disruptive Factors in Family Life	265
27. Advising Parents	277
28. Letter to Augusta Bonnard, 7 November	285
29. Excitement in the Aetiology of Coronary Thrombosis	287
30. The Mother's Contribution to Society	293
31. Health Education Through Broadcasting	297
32. Preface to *Collected Papers: Through Paediatrics to Psychoanalysis*	301

PART 4 1958

1. Letter to Grantly Dick-Read, 15 January	305
2. Letter to Marianne Baumann, 20 January	307
3. Funeral Address for Ernest Jones	309
4. Psychogenesis of a Beating Fantasy	313
5. Review: *The Psychoanalytic Study of the Child, Volume 11* edited by Ruth S. Eissler, Anna Freud, Heinz Hartmann, and Ernst Kris	317
6. The First Year of Life: Modern Views on the Emotional Development	319
7. The Psychology of Separation	333
8. Letter to Anna Freud, 14 May	337
9. Where Angels Fear to Tread, or A Comment on Generic Teaching	339
10. Letter to Marianne Baumann, 5 June	345
11. Letter to Anna Freud, 8 June	347
12. Letter to Joan Riviere, 13 June	349
13. Child Analysis in the Latency Period	351
14. Letter to R. D. Laing, 18 July	361
15. Review: *The Psychoanalytic Study of the Child, Volume 12* edited by Ruth S. Eissler, Anna Freud, Heinz Hartmann, and Ernst Kris	363
16. Letter to Herbert Rosenfeld, 16 October	365
17. The Family Affected by Depressive Illness in One or Both Parents	367
18. On 'Separation Anxiety' by John Bowlby	379
19. Letter to Anna Freud, 7 November	383
20. Letter to Victor Smirnoff, 19 November	385
21. Obituary: Ernest Jones	389
22. Obituary: Dr Ambrose Cyril Wilson	399
23. Review: *The Doctor, His Patients, and the Illness* by M. Balint	401

24. Transitional Objects and Transitional Phenomena — 405

25. Theoretical Statement of the Field of Child Psychiatry — 421

PART 5 1959

1. Review: *Envy and Gratitude* by Melanie Klein — 433
2. Letter to Reginald Lightwood, 10 February — 437
3. Letter to Miss Maw, 16 February — 439
4. Memorandum on Gisburne House — 441
5. Classification: Is There a Psycho-Analytic Contribution to Psychiatric Classification? — 445
6. Letter to *The Times*, Nursery Schools Essential, 25 March — 461
7. Letter to Donald Meltzer, 21 May — 463
8. Letter to Kenneth Soddy, 9 June — 465
9. Letter to Paul Halmos, 12 June — 467
10. Nothing at the Centre — 469
11. Letter to Dorothy E. M. Gardner, 13 July — 473
12. Letter to Arthur J. Metcalfe, 14 July — 475
13. Letter to Herman Gijsbert van der Waals, 23 July — 477
14. Letter to A. Tommy M. Wilson, 23 September — 479
15. Casework with Mentally Ill Children — 481
16. Letter to Elliot Jaques, 13 October — 493
17. Discussion of 'Grief and Mourning in Infancy' by John Bowlby — 495
18. Letter to Paula Heimann, 5 November — 501
19. Letter to Thomas Szasz, 19 November — 503
20. Counter-Transference — 505
21. The Effect of Psychotic Parents on the Emotional Development of the Child — 516
22. The Fate of the Transitional Object — 523
23. Review (film): *Going to Hospital with Mother* by James Robertson — 529

24. Foreword to *Childbirth with Confidence* by Prunella Briance	533
25. Obituary: Oscar Friedmann	535
26. Clinical Material on the Theme of a Male Patient's Exploitation of His Female Self	539
27. A Clinical Approach to Family Problems: The Family	543
Chronology	547
References	553
Contributors	561
Credits	563
Index	567

VOLUME 6: 1960–1963

Editors' Note	xlvii
Introduction to Volume 6	3
ANGELA JOYCE	

PART 1 1960

1. Saying 'No'	31
2. Letter to Michael Balint, 5 February	43
3. Letter to Jacques Lacan, 11 February	45
4. Jealousy	47
5. Letter to Merton J. Kahne, 19 February	63
6. The Effect of Psychosis on Family Life	65
7. What Irks?	73
8. The Relationship of a Mother to Her Baby at the Beginning	87
9. On Security	93
10. Aggression, Guilt and Reparation	97
11. Letter to Alexander Luria, 7 July	105
12. Letter to Ilse Hellman, 21 July	107
13. Letter to John Harvard-Watts, 28 July	109
14. Letter to Mr and Mrs Young, 28 July	111

15. Obituary: Melanie Klein	113
16. Letter to Serge Lebovici, 8 November	115
17. The Family and Emotional Maturity	117
18. Letter to Wilfred Bion, 17 November	125
19. Comments on Joseph Sandler's 'On the Concept of the Superego'	127
20. String: A Technique of Communication	135
21. The Theory of the Parent-Infant Relationship	141
22. Ego Distortion in Terms of True and False Self	159

PART 2 1961

1. Letter to Lydia James, 20 January	175
2. Letter to Sir Aubrey Lewis, 26 January	177
3. Memorandum on Organizational Aspects of Child Care at Paddington Green Children's Hospital	179
4. Adolescence: Struggling Through the Doldrums	187
5. Varieties of Psychotherapy	197
6. Feeling Guilty	205
7. Letter to Dr Joan FitzHerbert, 25 April	211
8. Review: *The Concept of Love in Childcare* by T. S. Simey	213
9. Psychoanalysis and Science: Friends or Relations?	217
10. Review: *Clinical Child Psychiatry* by Kenneth Soddy	223
11. Notes on the Time Factor in Treatment	225
12. Comments on 'Problems of Research in Psycho-Analysis' by Joseph Sandler	229
13. Letter to Masud Khan, 26 June	233
14. Letter to Pearl King, 18 July	235
15. Matti, *aet* 12½ Years: A Therapeutic Consultation	237
16. Sakari: A Therapeutic Consultation	241
17. Psycho-Neurosis in Childhood	253

18. Letter to Harry Guntrip, 15 September — 261

19. The Paediatric Department of Psychology — 263

20. Letter to Sir Aubrey Lewis, 13 October — 267

21. Envy: A Male Patient Near the End of His Analysis — 269

22. Comments on the Report of the Committee on Punishment in Prisons and Borstals — 273

23. Letter to Wilfred Bion, 16 November — 279

PART 3 1962

1. Review: *The Psychoanalytic Study of the Child, Volume 15* edited by Ruth S. Eissler, Anna Freud, Heinz Hartmann, and Marianne Kris — 283

2. The Aims of Psycho-Analytical Treatment — 285

3. Letter to Benjamin Spock, 9 April — 289

4. The Development of a Child's Sense of Right and Wrong — 295

5. Training for Child Psychiatry — 299

6. The Five-Year-Old — 309

7. The Beginnings of a Formulation of an Appreciation and Criticism of Klein's Envy Statement — 315

8. A Personal View of the Kleinian Contribution — 325

9. Dependence in Infant-Care, in Child-Care and in the Psycho-Analytic Setting — 333

10. Providing for the Child in Health and Crisis — 343

11. The Development of the Capacity for Concern — 351

12. The Psycho-Analyst and Child Psychiatry: A Matter of Economics — 357

13. The Theory of the Parent-Infant Relationship: Further Remarks — 359

14. The Theory of the Parent-Infant Relationship: Contributions to Discussion — 363

15. Review: *Letters of Sigmund Freud, 1873–1939* edited by Ernest Jones — 367

16. Review: *Psychologie du Premier Âge* by Marcel Bergeron   371

17. Review: *Un Cas de Psychose Infantile* by S. Lebovici and J. McDougall   373

18. Morals and Education   377

19. Ego Integration in Child Development   389

PART 4 1963

1. Review: *The Psychoanalytic Study of the Child, Volume 16* edited by Ruth S. Eissler, Anna Freud, Heinz Hartmann, and Marianne Kris   399

2. Letter to Ronald MacKeith, 31 January   401

3. A Note on a Case Involving Envy   403

4. Considerations in the Study of Homosexuality   407

5. The Mentally Ill in Your Caseload   409

6. Letter to Timothy Raison, 9 April   421

7. Struggling Through the Doldrums   423

8. Communicating and Not Communicating Leading to a Study of Certain Opposites   433

9. The Psychotherapy of Character Disorders   447

10. The Value of Depression   461

11. From Dependence Towards Independence in the Development of the Individual   469

12. Psychiatric Disorder in Terms of Infantile Maturational Processes   479

13. Hospital Care Supplementing Intensive Psychotherapy in Adolescence   491

14. The Tree   499

15. D. W. W.'s Dream Related to Reviewing Jung   501

16. Review: *The Non-Human Environment in Normal Development and in Schizophrenia* by Harold F. Searles   505

17. Review: *Childhood Schizophrenia* by William Goldfarb   509

18. Perversions and Pregenital Fantasy   511

19. Two Notes on the Use of Silence	513
20. Further Clinical Material on the Theme of a Male Patient's Exploitation of His Female Self	519
21. Fear of Breakdown	523
Chronology	533
References	539
Contributors	545
Credits	547
Index	551

VOLUME 7: 1964–1966

Editors' Note	xlvii
Introduction to Volume 7 ANNA FERRUTA	3

PART 1 1964

1. The Concept of the False Self	27
2. Review: *Heal the Hurt Child* by Hertha Riese	33
3. Letter to *New Society*, Love or Skill?, 23 March	37
4. The Neonate and His Mother	41
5. Deductions Drawn from a Psychotherapeutic Interview with an Adolescent	51
6. Psycho-Somatic Illness in Its Positive and Negative Aspects	67
7. Youth Will Not Sleep	79
8. Letter to Renata Gaddini, 26 June	83
9. The Importance of the Setting in Meeting Regression in Psycho-Analysis	85
10. Letter to *The Observer*, All of Mother, 25 October	91
11. Letter to John O. Wisdom, 26 October	95
12. Foreword to *The Widow's Child* by Margaret Torrie	99
13. Letter to *The Observer*, All of Mother, 8 November	101
14. This Feminism	103

15. Letter to Mrs B. J. Knopf, 26 November ... 113
16. Review: *Memories, Dreams, Reflections* by C. G. Jung ... 115
17. Introduction to the *Child, the Family, and the Outside World* ... 125
18. Roots of Aggression ... 129

PART 2 1965

1. New Light on Children's Thinking ... 139
2. Letter to Michael Fordham, 2 February ... 145
3. Letter to Humberto Nagera, 15 February ... 147
4. The Price of Disregarding Psychoanalytic Research ... 149
5. Do Progressive Schools Give Too Much Freedom to the Child? ... 157
6. Notes Made in the Train ... 163
7. The Concept of Trauma in Relation to the Development of the Individual Within the Family ... 169
8. Letter to Michael Fordham, 24 June ... 189
9. Letter to Michael Fordham, 15 July ... 191
10. Comment on Obsessional Neurosis and 'Frankie' ... 193
11. Further Comments on Obsessional Neurosis and Frankie ... 197
12. The Child, the Family and the Offender ... 203
13. Clinical Material: Theme of 'Two', also theme of 'Black' ... 207
14. Review: *Childhood and Society* by Erik H. Erikson ... 213
15. Letter to Charles Anthony Storr, 30 September ... 215
16. Review: *Normality and Pathology in Childhood* by Anna Freud ... 217
17. Letter to Martin James, 7 October ... 227
18. The Psychology of Madness ... 229
19. Case Notes for a Psychoanalytic Seminar: Withdrawal, Regression, Male Identification ... 239
20. A 70th Birthday Present ... 243

21. Dissociation Revealed in a Therapeutic Consultation	245
22. The Value of the Therapeutic Consultation	273
23. A Child Psychiatry Case Illustrating Delayed Reaction to Loss	279
24. Introduction to *The Maturational Processes and the Facilitating Environment*	305
25. Preface to *The Family and Individual Development*	309
26. Review: *Shared Fate* by H. David Kirk	311

PART 3 1966

1. Letter to *The Times*, George III, 17 January	315
2. The Split-off Male and Female Elements to Be Found in Men and Women	317
3. The Ordinary Devoted Mother	331
4. Letter to *The Times*, Psychiatric Care, 3 March	339
5. Letter to Hans Thorner, 17 March	341
6. Letter to Herbert Rosenfeld, 17 March	343
7. Social Aspects of Autism	345
8. Autism	349
9. Letter to *The Times*, Why Courts Must Act Swiftly, 26 March	365
10. Review: *Dibs: In Search of Self* by Virginia M. Axline	367
11. Letter to *The Times*, 'Blood-Tie' Child, 4 April	369
12. Letter to a Confidant, 15 April	371
13. Letter to Lili E. Peller, 15 April	373
14. Review: *The Psychoanalytic Study of the Child*, Volume 20 edited by Ruth S. Eissler, Anna Freud, Heinz Hartmann, and Marianne Kris	375
15. Letter to Sylvia Payne, 26 May	377
16. On Cardiac Neurosis in Children	379
17. The Child in the Family Group	387
18. Review: *Infantile Autism* by Bernard Rimland	397

19. Letter to Renata Gaddini, 13 September ... 399

20. Review: *Adolescents and Morality* by E. M. Eppel and M. Eppel ... 401

21. Letter to William Gillespie, 29 September ... 403

22. Review: *Absent: School Refusal as an Expression of Disturbed Family Relationships* by Max B. Clyne ... 405

23. On the Occasion of the Publication of the *Standard Edition* of Freud ... 407

24. Letter to Donald Meltzer, 25 October ... 411

25. Review: *Your Child Is a Person* by S. Chess, A. Thomas, and H. G. Birch ... 415

26. Review: *Asthma: Attitude and Milieu* by Aaron Lask ... 417

27. Preface to Renata Gaddini's Italian Translation of *The Family and Individual Development* ... 419

28. Letter to Renata Gaddini, 21 November ... 423

29. The Unconscious ... 425

30. Review: *Adoption Policy and Practice* by Iris Goodacre ... 427

31. The Location of Cultural Experience ... 429

32. The Absence of a Sense of Guilt ... 437

33. Letter to a Patient, 13 December ... 447

34. The Beginning of the Individual ... 449

35. Letter to D. N. Parfitt, 22 December ... 455

36. Discussion of 'The Clinical Handling of the Analyst's Response' by Ian Alger ... 457

37. An Allotted Spanner in the Works ... 459

Chronology ... 461
References ... 467
Contributors ... 473
Credits ... 475
Index ... 479

VOLUME 8: 1967–1968

Editors' Note	xlvii
Introduction to Volume 8	3
ANN HORNE	

PART 1 1967

1.	Letter to Mrs P. Aitken, 13 January	33
2.	D. W. W. on D. W. W.	35
3.	The Association for Child Psychology and Psychiatry Observed as a Group Phenomenon	49
4.	The Concept of a Healthy Individual	65
5.	Letter to Renata Gaddini, 9 March	79
6.	Environmental Health in Infancy	81
7.	Review: *The Successful Step-Parent* by Helen Thomson	89
8.	Delinquency as a Sign of Hope	91
9.	The Non-Pharmacological Treatment of Psychosis in Childhood	99
10.	Review: *A Home from Home* by Sheila Stewart	105
11.	A Tribute on the Occasion of Willi Hoffer's Seventieth Birthday	107
12.	Foreword to *The Hands of the Living God* by Marion Milner	115
13.	Winnicott's Wisdom: The Meaning of Mother Love	117
14.	Obituary: James Strachey	123
15.	Review: *Absent: School Refusal as an Expression of Disturbed Family Relationships* by Max B. Clyne	129
16.	Winnicott's Wisdom: How a Baby Begins to Feel Sorry and to Make Amends	131
17.	Winnicott's Wisdom: Why Do Babies Cry?	137
18.	Letter to a Colleague, 4 September	143
19.	Letter to Renata Gaddini, 4 September	145
20.	Letter to Margaret Torrie, 4 September	147

21. Letter to Margaret Torrie, 5 September	149
22. Winnicott's Wisdom: Hobgoblins and Good Habits	151
23. Letter to Wilfred R. Bion, 5 October	157
24. Letter to Gillian Nelson, 6 October	159
25. The Aetiology of Infantile Schizophrenia in Terms of Adaptive Failure	161
26. Letter to Charles Clay Dahlberg, 24 October	167
27. Playing: Creative Activity and the Search for the Self	169
28. Review: *How to Survive Parenthood* by Eda J. LeShan	181
29. The Concept of Clinical Regression Compared with that of Defence Organization	183
30. Trips into Partisanship	191
31. Letter to Arthur Miller, 13 November	195
32. Letter to Renata Gaddini, 21 November	197
33. Letter to Marjorie Spence, 23 November	199
34. Letter to Marjorie Spence, 27 November	201
35. Review: A Collection of Children's Books by Multiple Authors	203
36. Letter to R. S. W. Dowling, 8 December	205
37. Addendum to 'The Location of Cultural Experience'	207
38. Mirror-Role of Mother and Family in Child Development	211

PART 2 1968

1. The Place Where We Live	221
2. Communication Between Infant and Mother, and Mother and Infant, Compared and Contrasted	227
3. Physical and Emotional Disturbances in an Adolescent Girl	239
4. Chards Pil...	245
5. The Use of the Word 'Use'	249
6. Interpretation in Psycho-Analysis	253

Complete Contents of the Collected Works of D. W. Winnicott

7. Letter to Donald Gough, 6 March	259
8. Foreword to *Disturbed Children* by Robert J. N. Tod	261
9. Playing and Culture	263
10. *Sum*, I Am	267
11. Review: *Vulnerable Children: Three Studies of Children in Conflict* by Lindy Burton	275
12. The Effect of Loss on the Young	277
13. Review: *The Psychoanalytic Study of the Child, Volume 22* edited by Ruth S. Eissler, Anna Freud, Heinz Hartmann, and Marianne Kris	279
14. A Link Between Paediatrics and Child Psychology: Clinical Observations	283
15. Playing: A Theoretical Statement	299
16. Children Learning	313
17. Letter to L. Joseph Stone, 18 June	319
18. Review: *Human Aggression* by Anthony Storr	321
19. Sleep Refusal in Children	323
20. Letter to Mrs T., 6 September	327
21. Roots of Aggression	329
22. Foreword to *Susan Isaacs* by D. E. M. Gardener	333
23. Letter to Adam Limentani, 27 September	335
24. Letter to Renata Gaddini, 21 October	337
25. Review: *Children in Distress* by Alec Clegg and Barbara Megson	339
26. Breast-feeding as Communication	341
27. First Interview with Child May Start Resumption of Maturation	349
28. The Use of an Object and Relating Through Identifications	355
29. Clinical Illustration of 'The Use of an Object'	365
30. Further Clinical Illustration of 'The Use of an Object'	369
31. Letter to Joyce Coles, 22? November	379
32. Letter to Joyce Coles, 25? November	381

33. Letter to Karl and Sheila Britton, 25 November — 383

34. Letter to Joyce Coles, 26? November — 385

35. Letter to Joyce Coles, 29 November — 387

36. Letter to Joyce Coles, 1? December — 389

37. Letter to Joyce Coles, 4 December — 391

38. Comments on My Paper 'The Use of an Object' — 393

39. Letter to Karl Britton, 7? December — 397

40. Letter to Joyce Coles, 8 December — 399

41. Letter to Renata Gaddini, 9? December — 401

42. Letter to Joyce Coles, 10? December — 403

43. Letter to Joyce Coles, 14 December — 405

44. Letter to Karl and Sheila Britton, 14 December — 407

45. Foreword to *Therapy in Child Care* by Barbara Dockar-Drysdale — 409

46. Review: *The Psychology of Childhood and Adolescence* by C. I. Sandström — 411

47. The Squiggle Game — 413

48. Thinking and Symbol-Formation — 441

Chronology — 445
References — 451
Contributors — 457
Credits — 459
Index — 463

VOLUME 9: 1969–1971

Editors' Note — xlvii
Introduction to Volume 9 — 3
ARNE JEMSTEDT

PART 1 1969

1. Letter to Michael Rosenbluth, 3 January — 23

2. Letter to F. Robert Rodman, 10 January — 25

3. Letter to an American Correspondent, 14 January	29
4. The Use of an Object in the Context of *Moses and Monotheism*	33
5. Letter to Renata Gaddini, 19 January	39
6. Letter to Anna Freud, 20 January	41
7. Letter to Michael P. Collinson, 10 March	43
8. Contribution to a Symposium on Envy and Jealousy	47
9. Some Principles of Child Analysis	51
10. Letter to Michael B. Conran, 8 May	53
11. Letter to Agnes Wilkinson, 9 June	57
12. Letter to William W. Sargant, 24 June	59
13. Letter to *Child Care News*, Behaviour Therapy, June	63
14. Physiotherapy and Human Relations	67
15. Development of the Theme of the Mother's Unconscious as Discovered in Psycho-Analytic Practice	75
16. Freedom	79
17. The Threat to Freedom	83
18. Moon Landing	89
19. Letter to Helm Stierlin, 31 July	91
20. Review: *Indications for Child Analysis and Other Papers* by Anna Freud	93
21. Additional Note on Psycho-Somatic Disorder	95
22. Letter to Robert Tod, 6 November	99
23. The Pill	101
24. Letter to Renata Gaddini and Her Family, 15 November	111
25. Berlin Walls	115
26. The Building Up of Trust	121
27. Preface to *Dialogue with Sammy* by S. Lebovici and J. McDougall	129
28. The Mother-Infant Experience of Mutuality	131

29. Mother's Madness Appearing in the Clinical Material as an Ego-Alien Factor — 141

30. Answers to Comments on 'The Split-Off Male and Female Elements' — 149

31. Psychologists as a Group — 155

32. Commentary on *Play Therapy* by Virginia Axline — 159

PART 2 1970

1. Letter to Peter Giovacchini, 5 March — 167
2. Letter to Michael Fordham, 10 March — 169
3. Child Psychiatry, Social Work and Alternative Care — 171
4. A Personal Statement on Child Psychiatry — 175
5. Contribution to the Final Number of *Case Conference* — 179
6. The Place of the Monarchy — 181
7. Letter to Renata Gaddini, 31 August — 189
8. Cure — 191
9. Residential Care as Therapy — 199
10. Individuation — 207
11. Living Creatively — 213
12. Basis for Self in Body — 225
13. Two Further Clinical Examples — 235
14. Day Dreaming — 247
15. Dependence in Child Care — 249

PART 3 1971

1. Letter to John Davis, 1 January — 255
2. Letter to Jeannine Kalmanovitch, 7 January — 257
3. Letter to Jeannine Kalmanovitch, 19 January — 259
4. Introduction to *Playing and Reality* — 261
5. Transitional Objects and Transitional Phenomena — 265

6. Dreaming, Fantasying and Living: A Case-History
   Describing a Primary Dissociation   289

7. Creativity and Its Origins   299

8. Interrelating Apart from Instinctual Drive and in Terms of
   Cross-Identifications   319

9. Contemporary Concepts of Adolescent Development and Their
   Implications for Higher Education   337

10. Tailpiece to *Playing and Reality*   349

11. Not Less Than Everything (Extracts), ca. 1968–71   351

12. Notes for the Vienna Congress   355

PART 4 Undated Work and Winnicott's 'Ideas' File

1. Ideas and Definitions   359

2. The Day-Dreamer   361

3. Notes for a Discussion on Technique in Analysis
   of Psychotics   365

4. Knowing and Not Knowing: A Clinical Example   367

5. A Point in Technique   369

6. Note on Infant Observation   371

7. Found Objects and Waifs   373

8. Notes on Play   375

9. Cleopatra Anamnesis Imphiccough   381

10. The Niffle   383

11. A Note on the Mother-Foetus Relationship   389

12. Outline for a Study in the Sociology of Knowledge   391

13. Ditty on Enoch Powell   395

    Chronology   397
    References   403
    Contributors   409
    Credits   411
    Index   415

VOLUME 10: *Therapeutic Consultations in Child Psychiatry*

Editors' Note	xlvii
Introduction to Volume 10	3
MARCO ARMELLINI	
Acknowledgements	23

Therapeutic Consultations in Child Psychiatry

PART 1

Introduction	27
1. 'Iiro' *aet* 9 Years 9 Months	37
2. 'Robin' *aet* 5 Years	57
3. 'Eliza' *aet* 7½ Years	83
4. 'Bob' *aet* 6 Years	113
5. 'Robert' *aet* 9 Years	141
6. 'Rosemary' *aet* 10 Years	157
7. 'Alfred' *aet* 10 Years	165

PART 2

Introduction	189
8. 'Charles' *aet* 9 Years	191
9. 'Ashton' *aet* 12 Years	215
10. 'Albert' *aet* 7 Years 9 Months	235
11. 'Hesta' *aet* 16 Years	255
12. 'Milton' *aet* 8 Years	277

PART 3

Introduction	305
13. 'Ada' *aet* 8 Years	309
14. 'Cecil' *aet* 21 Months at First Consultation	337
15. 'Mark' *aet* 12 Years	371
16. 'Peter' *aet* 13 Years	405
17. 'Ruth' *aet* 8 Years	421

18. 'Mrs X' aet 30 Years	443
19. 'Lily' aet 5 Years	453
20. 'Jason' aet 8 Years 9 Months	455
21. 'George' aet 13 Years	497
Appendices	517
Chronology	537
References	543
Contributors	545
Credits	547
Index	549

VOLUME 11: *Human Nature* and *The Piggle*

Editors' Note	xlvii
Introduction to Volume 11	3
STEVEN GROARKE	

PART 1 *Human Nature*

Preface	25
Editorial note	27
Acknowledgements	29
Introduction	31

PART I The Human Child Examined: Soma, Psyche, Mind

Introduction	35
1. The Psyche-Soma and the Mind	39
Somatic Health	39
Psyche Health	40
Intellect and Health	40
2. Ill-Health	43
Somatic Ill-Health	43
Psyche Ill-Health	44
3. Inter-Relationship of Body Disease and Psychological Disorder	47
The Effect of the Body and Its Health on the Psyche	47
Heredity	47
Congenital Disorder	48
Deficiencies of Intake	49
Elimination Defects	50

Accidents	50
A Category for the Not-Yet-Known	50
Allergy	51
The Effect of the Psyche on the Body and Its Functioning	51

4. **The Psycho-Somatic Field**   53

PART II The Emotional Development of the Human Being

Introduction	59

1. **Interpersonal Relationships**   63

First Part of the Statement	63
The Family	65
Instinct	65
Love Relationships	72

2. **The Concept of Health Using Instinct Theory**   75

Imaginative Elaboration of Function	75
The Psyche	76
The Soul	76
Excited and Quiet States	77
The Oedipus Complex	78
Restatement	79
Infantile Sexuality	80
Reality and Fantasy	81
The Unconscious	82
Summary	83
Chart Showing Psychology of Small Boy in Terms of Instinct Theory	84
Defences Against Anxiety—Castration Threat	84
Breakdown of Defences	85

PART III Establishment of Unit Status

Introduction: Emotional Development Characteristic of Infancy	89

1. **The Depressive Position**   91

Concern, Guilt and Inner Personal Psychic Reality	91
The Depressive Position: Recapitulation	97
Repression Reconsidered	99
The Management of Bad Forces and Objects	99
Inner Richness and Complexity	101

2. **Development of the Theme of the Inner World**   103

Introduction	103
Paranoid Way of Life	103
Depression and the 'Depressive Position'	104
The Manic Defence	105

Complete Contents of the Collected Works of D. W. Winnicott   xliii

3. Various Types of Psycho-Therapy Material   107

4. Hypochondriacal Anxiety   113

PART IV From Instinct Theory to Ego Theory

Introduction: Primitive Emotional Development   117

1. Establishment of Relationship with External Reality   119
    Excited and Quiet Relationships   119
    The Value of Illusion and Transitional States   123
    Failure in Initial Contact   125
    Primary Creativity   126
    The Mother's Importance   128
    The Baby at Birth   129
    The Philosophy of 'Real'   130

2. Integration   133

3. Dwelling of Psyche in Body   139
    Body Experience   139
    Paranoia and Naiveté   141

4. The Earliest States   143
    Diagram of the Environment-Individual Set-Up   143
    Action of Gravity   147

5. A Primary State of Being: Pre-Primitive Stages   149

6. Chaos   153

7. The Intellectual Function   157

8. Withdrawal and Regression   159

9. The Birth Experience   161

10. Environment   169

11. Psycho-Somatic Disorder Reconsidered   175
    Asthma   175
    Gastric Ulcer   177

Appendix   179
    Synopsis I   179
    Synopsis II   182

PART 2 *The Piggle: An Account of the Psychoanalytic Treatment of a Little Girl*
EDITED BY ISHAK RAMZY

Preface by Clare Winnicott and R. D. Shepherd	187
Editor's Foreword by Ishak Ramzy	189
Introduction by D. W. Winnicott	193
1. The Patient	197
2. First Consultation	199
3. Second Consultation	207
4. Third Consultation	217
5. Fourth Consultation	227
6. Fifth Consultation	235
7. Sixth Consultation	241
8. Seventh Consultation	249
9. Eighth Consultation	255
10. Ninth Consultation	263
11. Tenth Consultation	271
12. Eleventh Consultation	279
13. Twelfth Consultation	287
14. Thirteenth Consultation	297
15. Fourteenth Consultation	305
16. Fifteenth Consultation	309
17. Sixteenth Consultation	315
Afterword: By the Parents of the Piggle	317
Chronology	319
References	325
Contributors	327
Index	329

VOLUME 12: Appendices and Bibliographies

Note on the Compilation, Structure, and Contents
of the *Collected Works*   liii
   ROBERT ADÈS
Introduction to Volume 12: Appendices and Bibliographies   3
   ROBERT ADÈS

PART 1 Winnicott's Publications

1. Chronological Bibliography of Works by D. W. Winnicott   25
2. Alphabetical Bibliography of Works by D. W. Winnicott   81
3. Complete Back Catalogue of the Published Books of D. W. Winnicott   123
4. Winnicott's Plans for Books   151
5. Reference Lists from Books in Winnicott's Back Catalogue: 159
   a. *Collected Papers: Through Paediatrics to Psychoanalysis* (1958)   159
   b. *Holding and Interpretation: Fragment of an Analysis* (1986)   162
   c. *The Maturational Processes and the Facilitating Environment* (1965)   163
   d. *Playing and Reality* (1971)   166

PART 2 Winnicott's Correspondence

1. Chronological Bibliography of Letters by D. W. Winnicott   173
2. Alphabetical Bibliography of Letters by D. W. Winnicott   185
3. Short Biographies of Winnicott's Correspondents   193

PART 3 Winnicott's Lectures, Broadcasts, and Audio Recordings

1. Winnicott's Lectures   213
2. Winnicott's Broadcasts   233
3. Index of Available Audio Recordings   239
   Introduction to Winnicott's Broadcasts   239
      ANNE KARPF
   The Ordinary Devoted Mother and Her Baby   239
   The Ordinary Devoted Mother and Her Children   239
   Further Audio Material   240

4. **Original Broadcast Scripts**   241
    a. *The New Baby:* Looking Forward to Baby's Arrival (1945)   241
    b. *The New Baby:* Getting to Know Your Baby (1945)   245
    c. Problems of Management: Training Babies (1949)   249
    d. The Ordinary Devoted Mother and Her Baby: My Fan Mail (1952)   253

PART 4 Guide to New Material in the *Collected Works*

1. **Works Published for the First Time**   259

2. **Letters Published for the First Time**   263

3. **Works First Published in a Winnicott Edition**   267

4. **Remarks on Some Chapter Revised for the *Collected Works***   273

PART 5 Selected Drawings and Signatures

1. **Selected Drawings**   279

2. **Selected Signatures**   289

    D. W. W.: A Reflection   295
        CLARE WINNICOTT

Reference List of the *Collected Works*   311
Chronology   343
Contributors   349
Credits   351
Complete Index of the *Collected Works*   353

EDITORS' NOTE

The *Collected Works* comprises eleven volumes of previously published and new texts and a selection of letters, presented in chronological order following either the date of delivery, writing, or first publication, and an accompanying volume of end material. Some undateable items have been grouped together as the final part of Volume 9. For more information on the structure and organisation of the *Collected Works*, see the Note in Volume 12.

This entire collection is also available online, together with many of Winnicott's original audio recordings and an introduction to his collection of broadcasts to parents by journalist and author Anne Karpf, at www.oxfordclinicalpsych.com/winnicott/.

In compiling these collected works, the editors made all reasonable efforts to preserve Winnicott's original writings and publications with minimal editorial intervention. For this reason, some points of style, such as citation format, figure numbering, and spelling vary from piece to piece. For the convenience of the reader, figure numbers have been added in instances where the original figures were unnumbered. All editorial notes are marked with lowercase roman numerals and, in the print edition, appear as footnotes. Winnicott's own notes are marked with Arabic numerals and appear as endnotes. Editorial interpolations in the original text and notes appear in square brackets. Cross-references to works appearing elsewhere in the *Collected Works* have been added to aid the reader. These references are indicated by an abbreviation that includes volume, part, and chapter numbers (e.g., '[CW 2:7:8]' for Volume 2, Part 7, Chapter 8). Although the *Collected Works* is as complete as possible a collection of Winnicott's work, it does not include works which remain inaccessible or which are protected by confidentiality restrictions.

The Collected Works
of D. W. Winnicott

Volume 12, Appendices and Bibliographies

CONTENTS

Note on the Compilation, Structure, and Contents of
the *Collected Works*   liii
ROBERT ADÈS

Introduction to Volume 12: Appendices and Bibliographies   3
ROBERT ADÈS

PART 1 Winnicott's Publications

1. Chronological Bibliography of Works by D. W. Winnicott   25
2. Alphabetical Bibliography of Works by D. W. Winnicott   81
3. Complete Back Catalogue of the Published Books
   of D. W. Winnicott   123
4. Winnicott's Plans for Books   151
5. Reference Lists from Books in Winnicott's Back Catalogue   159
   a. *Collected Papers: Through Paediatrics to Psychoanalysis* (1958)   159
   b. *Holding and Interpretation* (1986)   162
   c. *The Maturational Processes and the Facilitating Environment* (1965)   163
   d. *Playing and Reality* (1971)   166

PART 2 Winnicott's Correspondence

1. Chronological Bibliography of Letters by D. W. Winnicott   173
2. Alphabetical Bibliography of Letters by D. W. Winnicott   185
3. Winnicott's Correspondents   193

PART 3 Winnicott's Lectures, Broadcasts, and Audio Recordings

1. Winnicott's Lectures   213
2. Winnicott's Broadcasts   233
3. Index of Available Audio Recordings   239
   Introduction to Winnicott's Broadcasts
   ANNE KARPF   239

The Ordinary Devoted Mother and Her Baby	239
The Ordinary Devoted Mother and Her Children	239
Further Audio Material	240

4. Original Broadcast Scripts — 241

a. *The New Baby*: Looking Forward to Baby's Arrival (1945)	241
b. *The New Baby*: Getting to Know Your Baby (1945)	245
c. Problems of Management: Training Babies (1949)	249
e. *The Ordinary Devoted Mother and Her Baby*: My Fan Mail (1952)	253

PART 4 Guide to New Material in the *Collected Works*

1. Works Published for the First Time	259
2. Letters Published for the First Time	263
3. Works First Published in a Winnicott Edition	267
4. Remarks on Some Chapters Revised for the *Collected Works*	273

PART 5 Selected Drawings and Signatures

1. Selected Drawings	279
2. Selected Signatures	289

D.W.W.: A Reflection CLARE WINNICOTT	295
Reference List of the *Collected Works*	311
Chronology	343
Contributors	349
Credits	351
Complete Index of the *Collected Works*	353

NOTE ON THE COMPILATION, STRUCTURE, AND CONTENTS OF THE *COLLECTED WORKS*

Robert Adès

Compiling the Edited Works

These collected writings constitute nearly all the texts that Donald W. Winnicott composed during his lifetime. The majority have already been published in collections compiled by Winnicott or by editors appointed by Clare Winnicott and, after her death, by the Winnicott Trust. The Trust's vision for a complete collection was to present an authoritative reference text with new editorial input to be made available in print and online in order to best disseminate Winnicott's work and to meet the requirements of a modern global audience of practitioners, scholars and general readers.

While the project for a complete works of Winnicott has been in gestation for some three decades,[1] the origin of the current editorial team dates from 2009, when a management board, headed by Amal Treacher Kabesh, was established to manage its progress. A detailed framework for ordering the volumes following a largely thematic arrangement within a chronological outline was begun by editor Elisabeth Young-Bruehl. She selected for inclusion a significant number of new letters, some of which were uncovered by Megan Wolff at the Winnicott archive of the Institute for the History of Psychiatry's Oskar Diethlem Library at Weill Cornell Medical College in New York. After Young-Bruehl's untimely death in 2011, her assistant Clay Pearn, who had already catalogued the new and existing texts and bibliographies and converted them into documents, and her plans, were received by the new editors in London appointed by the Winnicott Trust: Lesley Caldwell and Helen Taylor Robinson. I was engaged by the editors at this time to assess the contents of the Winnicott archive in the Wellcome Library in London and to provide general assistance in research and planning.

In the long process of managing, cataloguing and incorporating the unpublished with the existing work, it became clear that a new approach would be needed in order to marshal the array of materials. The contract for publication with Oxford University Press and its unbounded Oxford Clinical Psychology online platform on which the *Collected Works* was to be released provided the opportunity to develop an alternative system. The General Editors, together with the editorial team, decided that the *Collected Works* would best be served by following a principle of inclusion and by adhering to a strictly chronological structure.

Arrangement of the *Collected Works*

CHRONOLOGY

An important feature of Winnicott's writing is its diversity. His work demonstrates an intellectual breadth that ranges across multiple disciplines and forms of expression, providing a rich literary experience for the reader but actively resisting configuration into categories 'which give a tidy look to the textbooks' ('Autism' [CW 7:3:8]). An unabridged chronology, in the spirit of a *catalogue raisonné*, presents the diversity of his work and the range of his professional involvement without post-facto classification. Laying out his life's productivity in a continuous scroll aspires to provide the reader with a 'formlessness which is what the material is like before it is patterned and cut and shaped and put together' ('Dreaming, Fantasying, Living' [CW 9:3:6]).

Chronological succession must be reckoned by certain selected criteria, and as much of Winnicott's work was written or presented to an audience many years before being published, the first known date of presentation or authorship—rather than the date of first publication—reflects Winnicott's life and his thought with the greatest veracity. Thus the *Collected Works* is more than the sum of his theoretical writings, it is also 'about the analyst, about the analyst's work' ('Primitive Emotional Development' [CW 2:7:8]).

COLLECTIONS CURRENTLY IN PRINT

Much of Winnicott's work remains in circulation in the form of anthologies gathered together at different stages of his career, some in his own chosen arrangement, some posthumously collated by editors. The format of these books itself points to the ways in which he and his editors conceived of his writings at that time—a process that was ongoing and incomplete at his death.[2] Readers looking to experience his writings as they were first produced are encouraged to continue to consult these works, and users of the *Collected Works* online platform can access the structure of the original books via the back catalogue in this volume [CW 12:1:3], along with the reference lists from four books prepared by Winnicott [CW 12:1:4].

His first mature specialist book, *Collected Papers*, was subtitled *Through Paediatrics to Psychoanalysis*, and the linkage of fields expressed in the title could be applied to the *Collected Works* in toto: it, too, is a collected papers ranging not just from paediatrics to psychoanalysis, but through war evacuation to social work, through rheumatic fever to delinquency research, through nursery education to leucotomy, through paediatrics to probation work and through psychoanalysis to parenting.

THE *COLLECTED WORKS*: 'ABOUT THE ANALYST, ABOUT THE ANALYST'S WORK'

Winnicott engaged deeply with all the fields with which he came into contact, living by his remark that one might 'shed this useless layer of knowledge that is intertwined with words and settle down to involvement' ('Environmental Health in Infancy' [CW 8:1:6]). This thread of participation runs throughout his working life, from the young house officer racing one of his child outpatients onto the roof,[3] to the departmental head and Society President. His work across fields and through multiple forms of communication, as presented in the *Collected Works*, demonstrates his commitment to empirical observation and scientific research, a fearless and straight-talking dissent (with sufficient capacity for diplomatic compromise to enable him to spend much of his life leading one clinical department or another), a pragmatic dedication to public service and public debate, and a certain hands-on eccentricity which can perhaps best be summed up—just as he described his own training analyst, James Strachey—as that of a distinctly 'English analyst' ('Obituary of James Strachey' [CW 8:1:14]).

In the discussion of his paper 'Changing Patterns' [CW 12:3:3] (audio file), Winnicott stated 'I am not a bit religious myself . . . as far as I know'. Brought up in a free-thinking household and having attended a Methodist school, Winnicott's personality—well-married with Methodism—tended towards pragmatic dissent from the canon. In 1969, Winnicott underlined this propensity when he wrote to Ian Roger that he saw himself as 'a natural Lollard',[4] an apposite term which captures the coherence between his life and his work. The Lollards, heretics of the late medieval period, were supporters of John Wycliffe, a proponent of translating the Bible into English vernacular for the benefit of the uneducated population who could otherwise not participate in the revelations of the church. The range of audiences to whom Winnicott lectured, and the sheer volume of his clinical experience as demonstrated in the *Collected Works* (he is believed to have seen 60,000 mother-and-baby couples in his career as a paediatrician[5]), is a testament to his own commitment to work in the field and to engage directly with the population at large.

As a theoretician, Winnicott rethought many of the concepts and clinical techniques adhered to by the established training groups of British analytical society. He was the leading figure of the 'Independent' group, an internationally influential thinker and yet, being possessed, like the Lollards, of 'a militant incapacity to accept dogma',[6] did not found a school in his name or indeed accept the commonplace depiction that he was an 'Independent'.

Perhaps he also knew that the word 'lollard' meant *mumbler*—an insult signifying the indistinct or uneducated sound of plain-speaking English. As his producer at the BBC, Isa Benzie, wrote in an internal BBC memo on Winnicott's very particular voice: 'He has on the one hand a desperately bad heart and uses very little voice, and on the other has a life-long professional habit of talking to mentally sick small children in a very, very quiet way'.[7]

The chronological *Collected Works* enables the reader to meet this natural lollard, reflecting the unity of Winnicott the plain-speaking public broadcaster, Winnicott the anti-dogmatic theoretician whose output of technical papers grew to be of lasting global influence,[8] Winnicott the pillar of the child and psychiatric health community and public-minded protestor of health policy, and Winnicott the bustling local practitioner—the difficult but devoted doctor 'who comes down every week and doesn't like social workers and leaves things in a muddle'.[9]

Contents of the *Collected Works*

SELECTION

The *Collected Works* includes journal articles, professional lectures, transcriptions of talks and public broadcasts, reviews and obituaries, as well as personal items, fiction, short notes, poetry and personal correspondence. Amongst the works that are already cornerstones of Winnicott's contributions to professional fields, these *Collected Works* incorporate items which cast him in a more personal light: from his childhood letters from boarding school, doodles or flashes of inspiration jotted down on scraps of paper, unconsolidated fictions and reminiscences, to the letters and notes written in the days before his death. Sculpted and polished works are presented alongside everyday letters, notes and items included in the spirit of his doodle 'Frustrated sculpture (wanted to be an ordinary thing)' [CW 12:5:1]. They provide a human dimension to his work, and are presented here as much for the historian, biographer, enthusiast or casual reader as for the training or practising analyst, therapist or paediatrician.

COMPLEMENTARY MATERIAL

The *Collected Works* provides new indices for each volume, extensive cross-references and editorial annotations, and this final volume comprises a variety of appendices and a complete index for the edition as a whole. Each article is accompanied by a headnote composed of its bibliographical entry, its original provenance and any additional comments relating to its formulation.

Some accompanying material is included where it is pertinent to the context. Correspondence from Thomas Stapleton [CW 4:3:23], Michael Fordham [CW 9:2:2] and the magistrate Roger North [CW 2:6:1], and Robert Graves's letter to *The Times* [CW 7:3:1] are provided in footnotes to Winnicott's own letters. His complete letter on autism [CW 7:1:10] is provided alongside the shortened version as printed in the *Observer* which proved so controversial. On several occasions, the reported discussions of Winnicott's papers are included to help to frame the reception of his work (see the upcoming section 'Winnicott in the Third Person').

BOOKS REPUBLISHED

One consequence of the chronological arrangement of the *Collected Works* is the redistribution of existing volumes of Winnicott's collected papers, with the exception of three complete books prepared by Winnicott and two books published posthumously, all five of which are retained in their original form.

Clinical Notes on Disorders of Childhood, Winnicott's first book, written in 1931, may be found in its entirety in Volume 1, Part 3 [CW 1:3].

Holding and Interpretation, the account of the final six months of an analysis undertaken between 1953 and 1955 and first published in a heavily annotated form in 1972, and in the current edition edited by Masud Khan in 1986, has been placed in Volume 4, Part 4 [CW 4:4:1]. 'Withdrawal and Regression', an account of the same patient and included by Khan as the appendix to that book in 1986, is located chronologically as it was first composed, in 1954 [CW 4:3:29].

Winnicott's working life did not end with his death which, in the *Collected Works,* arrives at the end of Volume 9, Part 3. Volumes 10 and 11 contain three books prepared by Winnicott, and published posthumously.

Therapeutic Consultations in Child Psychiatry [CW 10] is a collection of case studies, sessions, interviews and consultations with children (and one mother) over a ten-year period, compiled by Winnicott and published just after his death in 1971. While some ten of the case studies were published earlier than 1971, this complete work is reproduced whole, retaining the total cumulative meaning he intended it to convey (see Armellini [CW 10:Introduction]).

The Piggle [CW 11:2] and *Human Nature* [CW 11:1], a pair of unfinished works completed and published as whole books after his death, are presented unchanged in Volume 11. Winnicott's analysis of Gabrielle—the 'piggle'—lasted from 1964 to 1966 (occurring alongside the material of Volume 7), and was completed several years before he showed it to the eventual editor, Ishak Ramzy, a young analyst from the Menninger Clinic in Topeka, Kansas. Ramzy used his correspondence with Winnicott from 1969 to guide him in producing the final book, published in 1977, while leaving undone what he considered could have been completed only by Winnicott (Ramzy, Editor's Foreword [CW 11:2]).

Human Nature was largely written in the summer of 1954, originally with the purpose of supplying Winnicott's social work and mental health students at the University of London with the notes on human nature that they were unable to take during his lectures (see Clare Winnicott's 'Preface to *Human Nature*' [CW 11:1]). Winnicott continued to revise and review this collection of notes up until his death; it was eventually published in 1988 together with two synopses giving clues as to its construction—one from 1954 and a second from 1967.

While the essays in *Playing and Reality*, like all of Winnicott's other collections, have been redistributed according to chronology, five of the eleven chapters nevertheless remain grouped together in Part 3 of Volume 9—the end of Winnicott's living work—demonstrating the incredible productivity of his final weeks and months.

TRANSCRIPTIONS

Included here are transcriptions of recordings, some new and some previously published, which are also available in audio format at www.oxfordclinicalpsych.com/winnicott [CW 12:3:3]. Previously published transcribed items which would normally have received some editorial intervention have not been altered, while new transcriptions have been published verbatim. An historically important document—the evidence given by Donald Winnicott and Clare Britton to the Curtis Committee [CW 2:7:9]—*has* been edited, leaving only Winnicott's contributions. The complete transcript is kept in the UK National Archives.

MEMORANDA

As the head of several hospital and clinical departments, Winnicott composed memoranda as evidence for government or institutional committees (see [CW 2:5:3], [CW 2:7:6], [CW 5:1:4], [CW 5:5:4] and [CW 6:2:3]). In the case of the 'Memorandum on Homosexuality and the Law' [CW 5:1:4], the input from his colleague Thomas Stapleton is also published [CW 4:3:23], illustrating the balance which Winnicott struck between writing as himself and writing on behalf of his department.

JUVENILIA

Volume 1, Part 1, essentially included for the biographer, historian and enthusiast, is composed exclusively of Winnicott's childhood letters, school essays and notes and articles he wrote while a medical student.

These early writings shed a light across his life as much as they cast the shadow of his survival of World War I, which broke out when he was seventeen. In 'An Allotted Spanner in the Works' [CW 7:3:37], written in 1967 when he had, according to the psalmist, reached his 'allotted span' of threescore years and ten,[10] Winnicott wrote:

> If I have got anywhere, or contributed anything to the world, then the word *I* includes friends and contemporaries who were killed in the two great wars, who died of cancer or by accident, or who got into trouble and never caught up again.

He returned to this sentiment in 'Not Less than Everything' [CW 9:3:11], 'Individuation' [CW 9:2:10] and, bluntly and without pathos, in a letter to his close friend and colleague John Davis in the final weeks before his death, writing 'I ought to have been killed in World War I, like my friends' [CW 9:3:1]. The early works of Volume 1 open a window for us onto these friends and onto this boy who was not killed with them: of those schoolmates shown in the portrait taken in 1914 [CW 1:Gallery:4]—the first readers of Winnicott's earliest surviving writings, published in Volume 1: ('Smith' [CW 1:1:3], 'The Night Attack' [CW 1:1:6] and 'The Best Remedy' [CW 1:1:8])—F. D. Adam (seated far right) and A. M. Rees (sitting at Winnicott's left shoulder), would be killed in 1918, as would his other classmates, not pictured: William Strang Maclay (d. 1915), Edward Barcroft George (d. 1916) and Leslie Gordon Atkins (d. 1918).[11] While the school friends of Winnicott's youth, along with a generation of young men, gave up their lives in World War I, Winnicott would go on to give his life to changing society in a different way.

Challenges to Compiling the *Collected Works*

UNDATED WORKS

Works about which there is only speculation regarding the date of their authorship have been placed at the end of Volume 9, in Part 4.

INTRODUCTIONS FOR BOOKS NOT REPRODUCED IN THEIR ORIGINAL FORM

The Preface and Acknowledgements to *Through Paediatrics to Psychoanalysis* [CW 5:3:32], the Introduction to *The Maturational Processes and the Facilitating Environment* [CW 7:2:24] and the Preface and Acknowledgements of the *The Family and Individual Development* [CW 7:2:25] (and of this book's Italian translation [CW 7:3:27]) are presented in the years in which they were written. The Introduction to *Playing and Reality* is printed immediately before the group of chapters from that book which remain clustered together in 1971 [CW 9:3:4]. The Introduction to *The Child, the Family and the Outside World* [CW 7:1:17] includes, as a footnote, the Preface to one of the two early incarnations of this book, *The Child and the Family* (1957); its companion *The Child and the Outside World* (1957) did not include a preface or introduction by Winnicott.

While the books for which these various forewords were prepared have been dismantled in the *Collected Works,* they remain accessible in situ online—along with any dedications and reference lists—through the appendix of Winnicott's back catalogue [CW 12:1:3].

REPETITION

Winnicott and his publishers often reused his material and, within a chronological arrangement, it becomes possible to appreciate why and how Winnicott reassessed his own work.

'Winnicott's Wisdom', the name given to a series of four papers printed in a popular parenting magazine in 1967[12] [CW 8:1:13, CW 8:1:16, CW 8:1:17, CW 8:1:22], are reproductions of versions of probably Winnicott's first works for the general public: his essays in *Getting to Know Your Baby*, written more than twenty years previously. Their re-emergence sheds new light on Winnicott's position in the ongoing social debate surrounding child care in the 1960s—not least, perhaps, by demonstrating that, in 1944, he was twenty years ahead of his time.

'Transitional Objects and Transitional Phenomena' is presented in all four versions [CW 3:6:6, CW 4:2:21, CW 5:4:24, CW 9:3:5], each with an extensive headnote discussing its repetition.

'Adolescence: Struggling Through the Doldrums' [CW 6:2:4] was revised for two audiences. Originally given as a lecture to London County Council's children's department, it was first printed in the education journal *New Era in Home and School*. Although Winnicott revised the article for publication in the popular magazine *New Society* as 'Struggling Through the Doldrums' [CW 6:4:7], he returned to the more specialised version when he included it two years later in his 1965 book *The Family and Individual Development*. Rather than provide a series of annotations and analysis of the differences within the texts, the editors have elected to print both versions in full.

'On the Split-off Male and Female Elements' (1966) [CW 7:3:2], originally a lecture to the British Psychoanalytical Society (BPAS) given in 1966, was not published until it was included as part of 'Creativity and Its Origins' [CW 9:3:7] in *Playing and Reality* in 1971. The 1966 lecture alone was published in *Psychoanalytic Explorations* (1989), together with two examples of clinical material from the same patient taken in 1959 [CW 5:5:26] and 1963

[CW 6:4:20], and Winnicott's answers to comments on the lecture [CW 9:1:30], written in 1968–69 and first published in *Psychoanalytic Forum* in 1972. In the *Collected Works*, these five items are presented chronologically rather than grouped together thematically: the two clinical notes from 1959 and 1963, the original lecture from 1966, Winnicott's answers to comments to the paper (including new material printed in the *Collected Works* for the first time) in the late 1960s and the culminating paper 'Creativity and Its Origins' in 1971 [CW 9:3:7]. Accordingly, the original lecture appears, *in media res*, twice. Each of the five chapters includes the relevant cross-references, and the thematic arrangement as published in *Psychoanalytic Explorations* (1989) can be found in the back catalogue [CW 12:1:3].

'Envy: A Male Patient at the End of his Analysis' [CW 6:2:21] is the name given by Winnicott to a short extract of case material from 1961 included by the editors of *Psychoanalytic Explorations* as part of the chapter 'The Beginnings of a Formulation of an Appreciation and Criticism of Klein's Envy Statement' [CW 6:3:7], where the following paragraph was omitted:

> In making this statement I have lost nearly all my objection to Mrs Klein's concept. I am left, however, with the main thing that annoyed me in her presentation of her ideas at Geneva, and also in her book. This is that without mentioning the effect of the mother's failure which brings the infant's intolerance of the assault on his omnipotence to the fore, Mrs Klein jumps over into a statement about inherited aggression. I believe that in practice what she was meeting and calling inherited aggression may well have been the urge to break free from the mother who is reluctant to give up her role. My objection, therefore, has dwindled to something scientific, relatively unimportant, but nevertheless something which I do now after a long period of re-consideration continue to think is a fault in Mrs Klein's presentation.

This important statement has been reinstated in the original case note and presented here as a free-standing chapter [CW 6:2:21]. However, the case material without this paragraph remains a part of 'The Beginnings of a Formulation of an Appreciation and Criticism of Klein's Envy Statement' [CW 6:3:7] as it was originally published in 1989. The same material is therefore printed twice, once as a free-standing case note and again as the extract of a case study used in a paper on Kleinian theory.

CASES IN *THERAPEUTIC CONSULTATIONS* IN CHILD PSYCHIATRY

The repetition and reworking of material occurred extensively in the case of Winnicott's many lectures and articles on therapeutic consultations given during the 1960s. In five of the original publications of these consultations,

Winnicott wrote fresh *précis* of the principle of his therapeutic consultation technique. When twenty-one of these cases were collected together to form the volume *Therapeutic Consultations* these sections were removed from the individual papers and assimilated into the three introductory sections in the book. This alternative expository material has been presented in Volume 10 in the form of appendices.

Furthermore, the two case studies from *Therapeutic Consultations* that were also published in another Winnicott collection appear in the *Collected Works* in both forms:

> 'Dissociation Revealed in a Therapeutic Consultation' [CW 7:2:21], first published in 1965 and reprinted in 1984 in *Deprivation and Delinquency*, is the original version of the case study of 'Ada' [CW 10:3:13].
>
> 'The Value of the Therapeutic Consultation' was written in 1965 without any accompanying case material, but was first published in 1968 along with the full text of the case study 'Ashton'. The case of 'Ashton' alone was then published in *Therapeutic Consultations* in 1971. The original 1965 paper—without 'Ashton'—was posthumously published in *Psychoanalytic Explorations* in 1989, rounding off a palindromic publishing history. The *Collected Works* presents the original essay from 1965 (as published in 1989) [CW 7:2:22] and the case study 'Ashton' (as part of *Therapeutic Consultations*) [CW 10:2:9].

WINNICOTT IN THE THIRD PERSON

The editors chose on the whole to include items which refer to Winnicott in the third person: reports of his lectures, discussions of his papers, and abstracts of his articles. While the extent to which Winnicott himself contributed some of these as synopses or abstracts cannot be known, they form first-hand accounts of papers and lectures which might otherwise have been lost and give an invaluable insight into the reception and handling of his work in its own time.

Several abstracts of Winnicott's articles or lectures are presented for the first time in the *Collected Works*.[13] Two lecture abstracts have been presented as free-standing chapters: 'Enuresis', given to the Royal Society of Medicine [CW 1:2:17], and 'The Wearing of Masks in the Nursing of Premature and Older Infants', given to the British Paediatric Association [CW 2:5:9], which includes Winnicott's first use of the word 'unintegration'. Two further abstracts are published in Volume 2 as footnotes to a relevant surviving paper on the same subject from the same era: 'The Value of Breastfeeding' (psychological)—a lecture given to the British Paediatric Association—is printed in 'Breast Feeding' [CW 2:7:12], and 'Observations of Infant Behaviour During

Routine Clinical Examination' (in support of his memorandum) (1943) is published in the footnotes to 'Observation of Infants in a Set Situation' [CW 2:3:6] as an example of his attempts to disseminate the material of this important paper. Winnicott's contribution to the discussion of Auden's *The Difficult Child* was published as a third-person report [CW 1:4:4], and an additional announcement of Winnicott's contribution to the discussion has been given as a footnote. The report of his paper 'Neurosis in the Child' appears as a footnote in the Introduction to Volume 1 (Ken Robinson) [CW 1:Introduction], where it is quoted at length.

Several early medical papers in Volume 1 Part 2 ([CW 1:2:2], [CW 1:2:3], [CW 1:2:4], [CW 1:2:7], [CW 1:2:9], [CW 1:2:15], [CW 1:2:17], [CW 1:2:19], [CW 1:2:20] and [CW 1:4:18]), include peer discussion of Winnicott's paper along with his replies (or a report of them), and these papers and their discussions have been reproduced in full. There are also a few examples of parenthetical asides relating an unprinted component of Winnicott's presentation (such as [CW 3:3:8]), which have also been retained.

A report of a talk which Winnicott gave on the 'Psychological Aspects of Birching' [CW 2:6:3] has been included as one of very few comments he made on this topic.[14] The minutes of the BPAS (16 February 1944) state that this lecture, given to the Reform League, was reported inaccurately in the *News Chronicle* and that, in response, Winnicott distributed a corrected version to the members of the Society.[15] The manuscript printed here is held in the archive of Roger Money-Kyrle in the Wellcome Library, London. It is not possible to determine whether they are the notes distributed by Winnicott to members (most likely) or Money-Kyrle's own notes on Winnicott's lecture. In either case, the document serves as the only known account of an otherwise lost statement on corporal punishment.

The typed notes for the discussion of Winnicott's paper 'The Birth Trauma' [CW 3:4:11] included within the same document both Winnicott's responses in the first person and a third-person report of the discussion. It is reproduced here in full.

'First Interview with Child May Start Resumption of Maturation' [CW 8:2:27], an anonymously-written report in an American psychiatry magazine of a lecture given a few days prior to 'The Use of an Object' [CW 8:2:28], reproduces largely in his own words one of the many lectures and seminars Winnicott gave during the 1960s on his therapeutic consultation method—in this case, that of the patient described in 'Hesta' [CW 10:2:11]. The reception of Winnicott's work during this trip is a point of continuing debate, and this article and the subsequent discussion by Dr J. C. Hirschberg of the Menninger Clinic of Topeka, Kansas, represent two of the few first-hand examples of the response to a presentation of his therapeutic consultation technique. The account, and its discussion, have therefore been included to add to the context of the surrounding works and to this period.

The *Collected Works* in Print and Online

Oxford Clinical Psychology online brings Winnicott into contact with the professions his work was originally intended for: doctors, psychiatrists and paediatricians, as well as parents, teachers, social workers and psychoanalysts. Online, all works are fully cross-referenced and searchable, providing a powerful tool for tracing Winnicott's work thematically. It is hoped that the user can encounter Winnicott's work in its chronological form, charting his development in a linear progress, while also being provided with the means to view his writing in its original formation and to search by theme or keyword or navigate by means of the extensive cross-references and annotations.

AUDIO

Perhaps most excitingly, the audio resource which Winnicott made his own within the psychoanalytic community—the radio broadcast—has been made free to all without subscription at www.oxfordclinicalpsych.com/winnicott [CW 12:3:3]. In addition to his broadcasts, a few fascinating private recordings of Winnicott lecturing or talking are now available, bringing his words urgently to life for the first time in half a century (see [CW 12:Introduction]). The audio section is introduced with a podcast by Anne Karpf on Winnicott's relationship to broadcasting and his first BBC producers.

IMAGES

Images can be downloaded as PowerPoint slides. Although the print edition is produced in black and white, colour images—when available—are reproduced online.

ANNOTATIONS

As a technical necessity, footnotes in the online edition are presented slightly differently from those in print. In both the printed and the online editions, all editorial annotations are given as footnotes marked with italicised Roman numerals (*i, ii, iii, iv, v*), whereas Winnicott's annotations are presented as endnotes marked with Arabic numerals (1, 2, 3, 4, 5). With no pagination online, all annotations are presented as endnotes, but the Roman/Arabic numeric distinction is retained.

In its original publication, *The Piggle* included Winnicott's commentary in the form of marginalia. Unfortunately, due to the constraints of online layout, such a presentation proved impossible to reproduce and, in this edition, both online and in print, the commentary has been given as footnotes using capitalised Roman numerals (I, II, III, IV, V).

Notes

1. See Christopher Bollas's Foreword to the *Collected Works,* Vol. 1 [CW 1:FM].
2. Winnicott planned numerous different arrangements of his essays for books which were never ultimately realized [CW 12:1:5].
3. 'I feel the heart thumping away, but as the boy is a healthy boy I run with him to the hospital roof'. *Clinical Notes on Disorders of Childhood,* 'Active Heart Disease' [CW 1:3:8].
4. Reported in *Winnicott,* A. Phillips (1988) p. 38. Also in Kahr, B. (2016), p. 31.
5. Quoted from Ishak Ramzy's foreword to *The Piggle* [CW 11:2] and Clare Winnicott's interview with Michael Neve, 1983, in *Free Associations,* 3:167–184, 1992.
6. Masud Khan, 'Introduction to *Through Paediatrics to Psychoanalysis*', Second Ed. 1975.
7. Isa Benzie, Memorandum to Janet Quigley et al., 3 May 1960.
8. In 2016, the two most viewed journal articles (and three of the top five, and six of the top fifteen) on the internationally used Psychoanalytic Electronic Publishing platform are by Winnicott: 'Transitional Objects and Transitional Phenomena' [CW 4:2:21] and 'Hate in the Countertransference' [CW 3:2:1]. Among the most viewed books on the site—a list dominated by the volumes of Freud's *Standard Edition—*three of the nine most viewed are by Winnicott.
9. C. Winnicott (1982), p. 264.
10. That is, 70 years of age. Psalms 90:10.
11. In Kahr, B. (1996), Appendix A.
12. The magazine describes Winnicott as 'one of the world's great acknowledged experts on the mother–baby relationship . . .', '. . . reading D. W. Winnicott is a supreme experience for a mother-to-be. . .'.
13. These should not be confused with the three abstracts which Winnicott wrote of the works of other authors, all of which appear in Volume 1, Part 4.
14. See also his evidence given for the *Curtis Report* [CW 2:7:9].
15. King and Steiner, *The Freud-Klein Controversies* (1991), p. 730.

References

Anon. (1968). First interview with child may start resumption of maturation. [CW 8:2:27]

Armellini, M. (2017). Introduction to Volume 10, *The collected works of D. W. Winnicott.* New York: Oxford University Press. [CW 10:Introduction]

Benzie, I. (3 May 1960). Memorandum to Janet Quigley et al. (BBC R CONT1, D. W. Winnicott, File 1b, 1960–1962). BBC Written Archives, Caversham, UK.

Bollas, C. (2017). Foreword to Volume 1, *The collected works of D. W. Winnicott.* New York: Oxford University Press. [CW 1:FM]

Graves, R. (1966). Letter to the *Times,* Thursday January 13, 1966, p. 11. Issue 56528. [also CW 7:3:1]

Kahr, B. (1996). *D. W. Winnicott: A biographical portrait.* London: Karnac.

Kahr, B. (2016). *Tea with Winnicott.* London: Karnac.

Kantner, J. (2004). *Face to face with children: The life and work of Clare Winnicott* (pp. 97–111). London: Karnac.

Khan, M. (1975). Introduction, in *Collected papers: Through paediatrics to psychoanalysis,* 2nd ed. London: Hogarth.

King, P., & Steiner, R. (1991). *The Freud-Klein controversies 1941–45*. The New Library of Psychoanalysis. London/New York: Tavistock/Routledge.
Neve, M. (1992). Clare Winnicott talks to Michael Neve. *Free Associations*, 3:167–184.
Phillips, A. (1988). *Winnicott*. London: Fontana Paperbacks.
Ramzy, I. (1977). Editor's Foreword, *The Piggle*. [CW 11:2]
Robinson, K. (2017). Introduction to Volume 1, *The collected works of D. W. Winnicott*. New York: Oxford University Press. [CW 1:Introduction]
Winnicott C. (1982). D. W. Winnicott: His life and work. In J. Kanter (Ed.), *Face to face with children: The life and work of Clare Winnicott* (p. 264). London: Karnac.
Winnicott, C. (1988). Preface, *Human Nature*. [CW 11:1]
Winnicott, C. (1992). Interview with Michael Neve, 1983. *Free Associations*, 3, 167–184.
Winnicott, D. W. (1913). Smith. [CW 1:1:3]
Winnicott, D. W. (1914). The best remedy. [CW 1:1:8]
Winnicott, D. W. (1914). The night attack. [CW 1:1:6]
Winnicott, D. W. (1926). Case for diagnosis (? infantile hemiplegia) [CW 1:2:3]
Winnicott, D. W. (1926). Case for diagnosis (? poliomyelitis with some spasticity) [CW 1:2:2]
Winnicott, D. W. (1926). Two cases of post-encephalitic hypernœa. [CW 1:2:4]
Winnicott, D. W. (1928). Encephalitis after measles and chicken-pox. [CW 1:2:9]
Winnicott, D. W. (1928). Facial nerve paralysis. [CW 1:2:7]
Winnicott, D. W. (1929). Symptoms suggesting post-encephalitis. [CW 1:2:15]
Winnicott, D. W. (1930). Enuresis (abstract) [1929]. [CW 1:2:17]
Winnicott, D. W. (1930). Pathological sleeping. [CW 1:2:19]
Winnicott, D. W. (1931). Active heart disease. [CW 1:3:8]
Winnicott, D. W. (1931). Hæmoptysis: Case for diagnosis. [CW 1:2:20]
Winnicott, D. W. (1934). Discussion: Auden *The difficult child*. [CW 1:4:4]
Winnicott, D. W. (1938). Skin changes in relation to emotional disorder. [CW 1:4:18]
Winnicott, D. W. (1941). The observation of infants in a set situation. [CW 2:3:6]
Winnicott, D. W. (1944). The wearing of masks in the nursing of premature and older infants (abstract) [1943]. [CW 2:5:9]
Winnicott, D. W. (1945). Primitive emotional development. [CW 2:7:8]
Winnicott, D. W. (1948). Disorders of childhood. [CW 3:3:8]
Winnicott, D. W. (1949). Hate in the countertransference [1947]. [CW 3:2:1]
Winnicott, D. W. (1953). Transitional objects and transitional phenomena. [CW 4:2:21]
Winnicott, D. W. (1955). Withdrawal and regression [1954]. [CW 4:3:29]
Winnicott, D. W. (1957). Breast feeding [1945]. [CW 2:7:12]
Winnicott, D. W. (1958). *Collected papers: Through paediatrics to psycho-analysis*. London: Tavistock.
Winnicott, D. W. (1958). Preface and acknowledgements to *Through Paediatrics to Psychoanalysis*. [CW 5:3:32]
Winnicott, D. W. (1958). Transitional objects and transitional phenomena. [CW 5:4:24]
Winnicott, D. W. (1962). Adolescence: Struggling through the doldrums [1961]. [CW 6:2:4]
Winnicott, D. W. (1963). Struggling through the doldrums. [CW 6:4:7]
Winnicott, D. W. (1964). Introduction to *The child, the family and the outside world*. [CW 7:1:17]
Winnicott, D. W. (1964, 25 October). Letter to the Observer, *All of mother*. [CW 7:1:10]

Winnicott, D. W. (1965). *The family and individual development.* London: Tavistock.
Winnicott, D. W. (1965). Introduction to *The maturational processes facilitating environment.* [CW 7:2:24]
Winnicott, D. W. (1965). Preface and acknowledgements to the *The family and individual development* [CW 7:2:25]
Winnicott, D. W. (1966). Dissociation revealed in a therapeutic consultation. [CW 7:2:21]
Winnicott, D. W. (1967). Winnicott's wisdom. [CW 8:1:13, CW 8:1:16, CW 8:1:17, CW 8:1:22]
Winnicott, D. W. (1968). The value of the therapeutic consultation [1965]. [CW 7:2:22]
Winnicott, D. W. (1969). Changing patterns in young people (audio). [CW 12:3:3]
Winnicott, D. W. (1969). Obituary: James Strachey. [CW 8:1:14]
Winnicott, D. W. (1969). The use of an object [1968]. [CW 8:2:28]
Winnicott, D. W. (1971). 'Ada aet 8 years'. [CW 10:3:13]
Winnicott, D. W. (1971). 'Ashton aet 12 years'. [CW 10:2:9]
Winnicott, D. W. (1971). Creativity and its origins. [CW 9:3:7]
Winnicott, D. W. (1971). Dreaming, fantasying, living. [CW 9:3:6]
Winnicott, D. W. (1971). 'Hesta aet 16 years'. [CW 10:2:11]
Winnicott, D. W. (1971). Introduction to *Playing and reality.* [CW 9:3:4]
Winnicott, D. W. (1971). *Therapeutic consultations in child psychiatry.* [CW 10]
Winnicott, D. W. (1971). Transitional objects and transitional phenomena. [CW 9:3:5]
Winnicott, D. W. (1972). Holding and interpretation: Fragment of an analysis [1955]. [CW 4:4:1]
Winnicott, D. W. (1977). *The piggle* [1964–1966]. [CW 11:2]
Winnicott, D. W. (1984). *Deprivation and delinquency.* C. Winnicott, R. Shepherd & M. Davis (Eds.). London: Tavistock.
Winnicott, D. W. (1987). Environmental health in infancy [1967]. [CW 8:1:6]
Winnicott, D. W. (1988). *Human nature.* [CW 11:1]
Winnicott, D. W. (1989). The beginnings of a formulation of an appreciation and criticism of Klein's envy statement [1962]. [CW 6:3:7]
Winnicott, D. W. (1989). Clinical material on the theme of a male patient's exploitation of his female self [1959]. [CW 5:5:26]
Winnicott, D. W. (1989). Envy: A male patient at the end of his analysis [1961]. [CW 6:2:21]
Winnicott, D. W. (1989). Further clinical material on the theme of a male patient's exploitation of his female self [1963]. [CW 6:4:20]
Winnicott, D. W. (1989). Individuation [1970]. [CW 9:2:10]
Winnicott, D. W. (1989). Not less than everything [ca. 1968–71]. [CW 9:3:11]
Winnicott, D. W. (1989). On the split-off male and female elements [1966]. [CW 7:3:2]
Winnicott, D. W. (1989). *Psychoanalytic explorations.* C. Winnicott, R. Shepherd & M. Davis (Eds.). Cambridge, MA: Harvard University Press.
Winnicott, D. W. (1996). Autism [1966]. [CW 7:3:8]
Winnicott, D. W. (2003). Preface to the Italian translation of *The family and individual development* [1966]. [CW 7:3:27]
Winnicott, D. W. (2017). An allotted spanner in the works [ca. 1966–67]. [CW 7:3:37]
Winnicott, D. W. (2017). Answers to comments on 'The split-off male and female elements' [1968–69]. [CW 9:1:30]
Winnicott, D. W. (2017). Evidence given to the home office committee on children's homes (the *Curtis Report*) [1945]. [CW 2:7:9]

Winnicott, D. W. (2017). Frustrated sculpture (wanted to be an ordinary thing). [CW 12:5:1]
Winnicott, D. W. (2017). Memorandum on corporal punishment [1945]. [CW 2:7:6]
Winnicott, D. W. (2017). Memorandum on Gisburne House [1955]. [CW 5:5:4]
Winnicott, D. W. (2017). Memorandum on organisational aspects of child care at Paddington Green Children's Hospital [1961]. [CW 6:2:3]
Winnicott, D. W. (2017). Memorandum from Paddington Green Children's Hospital Psychology Department on homosexuality and the law [1955]. [CW 5:1:4]
Winnicott, D. W. (2017). Memorandum on 'The relationship between clinical paediatrics and child psychology' [1943]. [CW 2:5:3]
Winnicott, D. W. (2017). Notes on the discussion held on Dr Winnicott's paper 'The birth trauma' [1949]. [CW 3:4:11]
Winnicott, D. W. (2017). Psychological aspects of birching [1944]. [CW. 2:6:3]
Winnicott, D. W. (2017). Transitional objects and transitional phenomena [1951]. [CW 3:6:6]

Volume 12

Appendices and Bibliographies

Introduction to Volume 12
APPENDICES AND BIBLIOGRAPHIES
Robert Adès

Gallery Figure 1 (p. 19): Oscar Nemon's Statue of Sigmund Freud

Oscar Nemon's statue of Freud was originally intended to be unveiled in bronze in 1936, on Freud's eightieth birthday, at the Psychoanalytic Society in Vienna.[1] But, in 1964, the twice-life-size plaster remained in Nemon's London studio, increasingly vulnerable to decay. Having been taken aback by the work on visits to the studio, Lady Penelope Balogh, a psychotherapist and a biographer of Freud, undertook to have the statue cast in bronze. While Balogh found that a Freud in bronze appealed to many of the wealthy philanthropists and politicians she approached for funds, it also frightened them all. Barbara Docker-Drysdale gave Balogh a crucial piece of advice: to lay her troubles at Winnicott's feet.[2]

Docker-Drysdale proved correct. Lady Balogh wrote that Winnicott 'was emphatic that the psychoanalysts of the world should get it cast. From then on he never spared himself the huge task of arranging the appeal', and in 1968 he established the Freud Statue Committee, with Joyce Coles as Honorary Secretary. Nemon recognised the integrity in Winnicott's determination: 'what mattered most for him was that a debt of honour should be paid from him and his colleagues to Freud, from whom they had received so much encouragement to enable them to persevere in their endeavours'. Nemon was also personally touched by Winnicott's dedication, describing him as having 'a passion for rescuing which was fully applied to me'.[3] Winnicott sometimes spent Saturday mornings in Nemon's studio, playing with clay.[4]

This letter to psychiatrists (Winnicott, 1970) is an example of the culmination of several years of fund-raising efforts:

> Dear Sir,
>
> This is an appeal for a personal contribution from all your readers who may feel that Freud's importance merits that he should be commemorated by a statue.

The Freud Statute Committee has been formed to buy the statue based on a study of Freud and made by Oscar Nemon in 1929 with Freud's co-operation, and to present it to the Borough of Camden so that it may be erected in Hampstead near where Freud lived at the end of his life and where he died. The Borough Council has agreed to accept it and to erect it on a site at the junction of Fitzjohn's Avenue and College Crescent. It is now being cast in bronze.

I personally have taken it upon myself to collect the necessary money. It seemed appropriate first to ask the psychoanalysts of the world to contribute towards this project, and by making personal contact with my colleagues I have been able to raise about £6,500 on behalf of the Committee. There may, however, be many other psychiatrists who would like to contribute. We aim to raise the total to about £10,000.

It is suggested that an appropriate amount would be the equivalent of a consultation fee, but smaller amounts are welcome. To subscribers of £10 the sculptor is giving away a desk-sized bust of Freud about 5 inches high; there is a full-length figurine for subscribers of £15 or more. Cheques should be made payable to the Freud Statue Committee and sent to me at 87 Chester Square, London, SW1.[5]

D. W. Winnicott

A total of £11,000 was raised.[6] The British Psycho-Analytical Society (BPAS) donated £1,000 and the New York Psychoanalytical Society more than £400.[7] The statue was erected in October 1970 and stands a few streets from Freud's home in Maresfield Gardens, London.

The undertaking had consumed Winnicott in his final years. Renata Gaddini wrote that 'Clare Winnicott feared that having now achieved his goal there would be a fall in tension and a decreased attachment to life. All that "had been meaningful in his battle for life" in the last five years was no longer there'.[8] The ceremony itself, of dignitaries and speeches on a brutally cold October day, took its toll on Winnicott: Anne Clancier later told Serge Lebovici that 'his cheeks and lips were blue. I knew he had a bad heart and I was afraid throughout that he might die at any moment. He survived however'.[9]

Placed as if it were the masthead of the Tavistock Clinic, the glare of Nemon's Freud mingles a look of contempt with the 'knowledge and penetration of mankind'[10] that Nemon so admired. Freud's housekeeper, Paula Fichtl, told Freud that Nemon had made him look too angry.

'But I am angry,' replied Freud, 'I am angry with humanity'.[11]

Characteristically, Winnicott envisaged an altogether different mood, delighted with the idea that generations of children (reminiscent of his own work with the Piggle: 'Third Consultation' [CW 11:2:4]) would enjoy clambering over the statue and playing on Freud's head.[12]

Part 1: Winnicott's Publications

The bibliographies of works and letters were compiled in American Psychological Association (APA) style by Clay Pearn and Robert Adès, based on the earlier bibliographies by Masud Khan (1965), Harry Karnac (1996) and Knud Hjulmand (2007).

The chronological bibliography allows the reader to search for a work by its first publication date and by its publication in a previous Winnicott edition. The alphabetical bibliography allows the reader to search for work by all previous titles—including those not used in the *Collected Works*—and including titles of works first published in languages other than English, although excluding later translations of Winnicott's works. Later republications of his articles in other journals or in mixed-author anthologies have not been included. Each item is followed by its CW citation code in the form [CW Volume:Part:Chapter].

As the *Collected Works* as a whole is ordered chronologically, the known date of composition or first presentation takes priority over the date of first publication. However, the chronological bibliography, following APA style, is ordered exclusively by the year of first publication. Accordingly, a work's position in the bibliography does not always correspond to the location of the item in the *Collected Works*. In cases where this differs, the date of composition—and hence the publication's location in the *Collected Works*—is given in square brackets after the title. Date codes given for citations of Winnicott throughout the *Collected Works* follow APA style and therefore correlate to the chronological bibliography.

Uncertain or estimated dates have been indicated with *ca.*—when some estimation is possible—and otherwise marked not dated [n.d.]. Any further information on the history of a work's composition and publication, along with other pertinent information, can be found in its headnote.

Articles that have previously been published under more than one title are labelled with either 'Published here as…' or 'Not published in this form'. A link is given to the title under which the article is published in the *Collected Works*. In order to streamline the bibliography, full publication details are only given at the entry of the title used in the *Collected Works*, while all former titles are linked to this main heading. In the case of articles otherwise related to each other by part-publication, republication or revision, 'See also…' is used to refer the reader to the other relevant entries.

'[Abstract]', given in square brackets after a title, denotes that the chapter is the abstract of a work by Winnicott. This is not to be confused with the three chapters in Volume 1 Part 4 entitled 'Abstract:'—these are examples of Winnicott writing the abstract to another author's work.

Many of Winnicott's works were first written and presented as broadcasts on BBC radio, and broadcasting information is included in these bibliographies. As with lectures, these radio talks appear in the *Collected Works* with the date of their original broadcast which, if different from the date of first publication, is given in square brackets. All broadcasts, without exception, were produced and transmitted by the British Broadcasting Corporation (BBC). An index of Winnicott's broadcasts can be found in CW 12:3:2.

Volume 10, the complete text of *Therapeutic Consultations in Child Psychiatry*, is idiosyncratically numbered; the *Collected Works* has retained Winnicott's numbering of the case studies and his division of the work into three parts, each with its own unnumbered Introduction. Part 1, Chapter 7 is therefore followed by Part 2, Chapter 8 rather than Part 2, Chapter 1. The three Introductions were not given chapter numbers and are listed as [CW 10:1:Introduction], [CW 10:2:Introduction] and [CW 10:3:Introduction]. The same system of coding is used for the general introductions to each volume.

CW 12:1:1. The *Chronological Bibliography* is ordered by the year of first publication, showing each first publication and each republication in a Winnicott volume. Within each year, the works are ordered alphabetically.

Previously published complete books of Winnicott's works are given in bold italics. Each chapter of each book is then listed in the order in which they appeared. The part headings under which certain essays were grouped in some of the original books, most notably in the three *The Child, the Family and the Outside World* books (1957, 1957, 1964) can be seen in the appendix of the back catalogue of Winnicott's publications [CW 12:1:3]. The original reference lists for those books can also be found in this volume [CW 12:1:4].

Items published for the first time in the *Collected Works* are given in alphabetical order at the end of the bibliography, signifying their first publication in 2017.

CW 12:1:2. The *Alphabetical Bibliography* is arranged with the definite and indefinite articles excluded. The alphabetical bibliography includes all titles under which Winnicott's work was published in English, and the non-English language title in the case of first publications in a language other than English. Unlike the chronological bibliography, each title appears in this list only once. All other conventions follow the chronological bibliography. Chapters published in the *Collected Works* for the first time naturally contain no previous publication information.

CW 12:1:3. The *Back Catalogue of Winnicott's Books* shows the complete contents of all published anthologies of his work in chronological order. This list allows the online user, through hyperlinks, to access these books in their original arrangements. This list includes publication details, dedications, original section headings and page numbers for each of the works.

CW 12:1:5. *Reference Lists from Winnicott's Back Catalogue*. Four books produced in Winnicott's lifetime included their own reference lists. These have been reproduced here, allowing the reader to explore the influences credited by

Winnicott in his own work and completing the contents of the Back Catalogue [CW 12:1:3].

   a. *Collected Papers: Through Paediatrics to Psychoanalysis*
   b. *Holding and Interpretation*
   c. *The Maturational Processes and the Facilitating Environment*
   d. *Playing and Reality*

CW 12:1:4. The appendix of *Winnicott's Plans for Books* contains his own unedited plans for projected but unrealised rearrangements of his own work into alternative volumes of collected papers. When the chapter can be identified, the CW code has been given; where there is uncertainty, no guess has been offered.

Part 2: Winnicott's Correspondence

Unlike previous Winnicott bibliographies, lists of correspondence and lists of works have been separated. Letters to journals and newspapers have been included in this list alongside personal correspondence. When the date of dispatch of the letter is known as well as the date of publication, the former is given in brackets preceding the date of publication.

Several of Winnicott's letters from hospital in New York in 1968 were not dated but were marked with a day of the week. The likely order of these letters has been reconstructed, but dates which are uncertain (while the day of the week is known) have been marked with a question mark, rather than 'circa'.

The letters published here represent perhaps a quarter of Winnicott's total correspondence. Many letters are inaccessible, and many more remain restricted for reasons of confidentiality.

Brief *Short Biographies of Winnicott's Correspondents* [CW 12:2:3] have been provided here to aid the reader. Edited versions of these short biographies also appear as part of the headnotes for each letter.

Part 3: Lectures, Broadcasts, Audio

CW 12:3:1. *Winnicott's Lectures.* The primary source for this appendix is a series of lists of Winnicott's engagements compiled by his long-time secretary Joyce Coles. Further sources are available scattered throughout Winnicott's books, from other papers in Winnicott's archive and elsewhere in the public domain. Research on his lectures was also published in Kahr (1996) and Rodman (2003) in their respective biographies of Winnicott.

Lectures published in the *Collected Works* under the same title are cross-referenced. When the lecture is believed to have been given under a different name, the *Collected Works* title is given in square brackets. Presumably due to ill health in 1969 and 1970, some dates, lectures and lecture series had been struck through by Coles, and this is replicated here.

The scale of his involvement with such a wide range of audiences is striking. Winnicott told a group of analysts that 'The most valuable thing has been having to lecture to people who aren't analysts' ('D. W. W. on D. W. W.' [CW 8:1:2]) but it was, nevertheless, a disappointment to him to be so infrequently invited to teach at the BPAS; as he wrote to Sylvia Payne, the society's president in 1953, 'I realised a long time ago that I would not be asked to teach in the Society and therefore I concentrated on teaching teachers' [CW 4:2:13].[13]

CW 12:3:2. *Winnicott's Broadcasts* covers Winnicott's complete radio and television output. This index is to be distinguished from the index of surviving audio material [CW 12:3:3].

Although around sixty recordings and broadcasts can be identified with some certainty, there are likely to be gaps in the record, marking an opportunity for further research. The information available is inconsistent, and the compilation of this list was not without its challenges.

The BBC Written Archive in Caversham, UK, houses microfilms of the scripts of many radio broadcasts whose audio record has been deleted. Not all broadcasts were microfilmed; moreover, the contributors' indexes were compiled to log the catalogue of scripts rather than the actual transmissions. The identity of contributors was not necessarily recorded, and, to further obscure the issue, Winnicott always broadcast anonymously. However, correspondence exists from 1943 between Winnicott and a succession of his producers, and this appendix has been reconstructed from the correspondence in combination with the surviving microfilms and catalogue and contributor indexes.

Several discrepancies exist between the possible sources. 'The Deprived Mother' [CW 2:1:4] and 'Children in the War' [CW 2:2:4] are both listed in Masud Khan's 1965 bibliography as wartime radio broadcasts of 1939. However, in their first publication in 1957, of these two chapters only 'The Deprived Mother' is listed as a broadcast. Neither are to be found in the BBC archives, and the earliest surviving correspondence between Winnicott and his BBC producers dates from four years later. We cannot, however, categorically rule out the possibility that they were broadcast. Joyce Coles noted in the late 1960s that four long-playing gramophone records existed, dating from around 1940, which would indicate the earlier start-date of Winnicott's broadcast career. Nevertheless, the tone of these two early papers is distinctly less approachable than that of the 1940s talks, whose accessibility—as worked on extensively with his producers at this time—is such a *shibboleth* of Winnicott's broadcasting style. If these broadcasts were indeed aired in 1939 they would demonstrate the extent to which Winnicott's radio technique developed under the guiding tutelage of his first known producer, Janet Quigley.[14]

All six chapters of Winnicott's 1945 pamphlet *Getting to Know Your Baby* were described as 'broadcast in 1944' when they were republished in 1957. However, Winnicott noted in his personal copy of this pamphlet that only the first, second, fourth and fifth chapters were broadcast. Winnicott wrote to Quigley in late 1944 that he had just published these original broadcasts with 'a bit added'[15] and, although BBC archives show that Winnicott did give six broadcasts in 1943-44, it seems most likely that the third and sixth chapters of the published pamphlet: 'Infant Feeding' [CW 2:6:13] and 'Support for Normal Parents' [CW 2:6:11], were the 'bits added' and were not, in fact, radio talks.

Conversely, 'What Do We Mean By a Normal Child?' [CW 2:6:10] was certainly broadcast in 1944, despite not being listed as a BBC talk on its publication in 1957.

'The Innate Morality of the Baby' was published in 1957 in the form of its 1949 broadcast, but was extensively revised for republication in 1964 [CW 3:4:30]; the original broadcast script can be found reproduced in this volume [CW 12:3:4c].

CW 12:3:3. *Further Audio Material.* Almost all of Winnicott's BBC recordings, along with most recorded material from this period, were erased and the tapes reused. Fortunately, some audio material—around thirty items—has survived and is available, free of charge, on the web page of the *Collected Works* online, and without subscription at www.oxfordclinicalpsych.com/winnicott [CW audio online 12:3:3].

The audio material presented in the *Collected Works* is introduced with a specially recorded podcast by Anne Karpf, including a deeper discussion of the origins and development of Winnicott's work on the BBC and the social and cultural context of the broadcasts than is provided in these introductory paragraphs. Print readers of the *Collected Works* are urged to listen or download at www.oxfordclinicalpsych.com/winnicott.

The first series of recordings presented here consists of the fourteen chapters of *The Ordinary Devoted Mother and Her Baby*, as published in Part 1 of *The Child and the Family* (1957). These recordings were made some time after this by Winnicott and represent an audio record of this publication, rather than being the original BBC broadcasts. The written chapters were, however, based on the seventeen radio talks which Winnicott gave between 1943 and 1950: his first six broadcasts on *Happy Children* in 1943-44 (published in Volume 2) and the eleven he made for *How's the Baby?* in 1949-50 (published in Volume 3), nine of which were released in print in 1949 as 'The Ordinary Devoted Mother and Her Baby'. All the original talks appeared on the BBC Home Service, with the first series produced by Janet Quigley and the second by Isa Benzie. The written chapters were published in 1957 and sometimes vary from the original 1940s BBC transmissions, some of which exist in the form of microfilm (see also the Index of Broadcasts [CW 12:3:2] and the four original BBC scripts [CW 12:3:4]).

The second section of surviving audio material consists of eleven of the sixteen programmes which Winnicott contributed to the BBC programme *Parents and Children*, including the first nine of Winnicott's 1960 series 'The Ordinary Devoted Mother and Her Children'. The ninth talk seems not to be the original BBC transmission, but a re-recording, again made by Winnicott himself, from a later date. Winnicott also gave the eleventh and thirteenth talks in the series 'The First Five Years', of which the audio transmission of the former, 'Right and Wrong' [CW 6:3:4], is not available.

The collection of audio material concludes with a small number of private recordings of Winnicott talking live, including an electric performance to the Progressive League crowd on 'The Pill' [CW 9:1:23]; three late conference lectures, including his contributions to the discussions; and Winnicott recording his own private notes on Virginia Axline's book, *Play Therapy* [CW 9:1:32].

All Winnicott's recordings are held in the Wellcome Library Moving Image and Sound Collection, London. Private and institutional recordings of his broadcasts are extant and periodically emerge, and we can only hope that this edition will spur on the discovery of further recordings.

Finally, some recordings exist of the presentation and discussion of Winnicott's papers given at Scientific Meetings at the BPAS in the 1960s. They remain confidential and restricted but may be accessed by permission on application through the archivist at the Institute of Psychoanalysis:

> 'A Child Psychiatry Case: Description of a Psychotherapeutic Interview', 7 July 1965.
> 'The Split-off Male and Female Elements to Be Found Clinically in Men and Women: Theoretical Inferences', 2 February 1966 [CW 7:3:2] (see also the later version of this in the published paper [CW 9:3:7], and Winnicott's 'Answers to Comments' on the paper [CW 9:1:30]).
> 'The Location of Cultural Experience', 7 December 1966 (see the published version [CW 7:3:31] and its Addendum [CW 8:1:37]).
> 'Discussion Around Clinical Detail', 15 March 1967.
> 'Towards a Theory of Psychotherapy: The Link with Playing', 18 October 1967 (related to the paper 'Playing: A Theoretical Statement' [CW 8:2:15]).

CW 12:3:4. *Original Broadcast Scripts.*

CW 12:3:4a. The New Baby: *Looking Forward to Baby's Arrival.*

CW 12:3:4b. The New Baby: *Getting to Know Your Baby.* By mid-1945, Winnicott had given two series of talks on the BBC Home Service with Janet Quigley as his producer: *Happy Children*—on new babies—and *Difficult Children*—on issues relating to the war, the evacuation and the return home. The first of these series was published that year in the popular education journal *New Era in Home and School* and immediately reissued as a short pamphlet called 'Getting to Know

Your Baby', which sold for one shilling.[16] Donald's first wife, Alice, provided the cover design, a touchingly naïve woodcut of a mother cradling her sleeping infant (p. 20). In October, Quigley (who was just 'leaving' the BBC to be married), and Isa Benzie, were preparing *The New Baby*, a series of twelve talks on the Home Service, to which Winnicott would contribute these two.

Isa Benzie's vision for *The New Baby*, to be broadcast in the months following the end of the war, demonstrates her and Quigley's desire to sympathetically expand their programming towards a franker, less superficial discourse on mothering:

> I am inclined to think that we should spend most of our time on managing children in respects other than feeding them; I believe that all the agencies concerned, including the Corporation [the BBC], have had a great deal of success with their propaganda for the right food, but I still hear privately of the saddest things going on in other directions even in educated and prosperous families.[17]

In keeping with Quigley's personal input on Winnicott's earlier 1943–44 broadcasts, the correspondence shows that Benzie recommended several pages of edits to 'Looking Forward to Baby's Arrival' [CW 12:4:4a], mostly relating to his section on 'the grim side' of pregnancy. Benzie asked Winnicott to consider the fears of those mothers who were not so easily able to breastfeed, noting that medical propaganda at this time of postwar rationing was putting mothers under tremendous pressure, and reminding him that

> As our audience will be made up very largely not of intellectual women but women exposed to the full force of the prejudice and old wives' tales of their friends, in a series like this we always wish to make people grasp that in very many cases they put up with a lot of discomfort for which there is no need at all.[18]

Benzie supported and encouraged Winnicott's use of the pronoun 'you' to talk directly to the listening expectant mother and, no doubt thinking of their listeners' real experiences, asked that he 'Please don't take away anything about the women and the soldiers'. Winnicott's final script, as was almost always the case, shows that he was malleable and attentive to his producers' advice. While he had worked for two decades with mothers in clinical settings, he needed and made use of Benzie and Quigley to help him to translate his theoretical and therapeutic insights into something identifiable and comprehensible to the general listener.[19]

It was perhaps the emphasis on military analogies and wartime experiences in 'Looking Forward to Baby's Arrival' that contributed to it being overlooked for publication during peacetime, and it seems to have been completely forgotten until now. The eighth talk, 'Getting to Know Your Baby', of autumn 1945

[CW 12:4:4b], was also never published or repeated in its own right, presumably due to its similarity to the more extensive series of the same name that been broadcast and published earlier that year.

CW 12:3:4c. *How's the Baby? Problems of Management: Training Babies.* In early 1949, Winnicott and Isa Benzie resumed a correspondence on the possibility of a broadcast on the use of electric-shock treatment for mental disorders. Benzie remarked that she had been considering asking Winnicott for more programmes on children, to which Winnicott responded with relief, 'Broadcasts about children really interest me four thousand times more than broadcasts about the frontal lobes'.[20]

Winnicott later recalled the meeting with Benzie to discuss the proposed new series:

> I had no interest whatever in telling people what to do.... I didn't know. But I would like to talk to mothers about what they do well ... because each mother is simply devoted to the task in hand, namely the care of an infant. I said that ordinarily this just happens...

Benzie, apparently listening for a good title for the new programme, exclaimed 'Splendid! The Ordinary Devoted Mother'. 'And that', said Winnicott, 'was that'. [21]

The ensuing nine weekly talks were broadcast in autumn 1949, with two further talks commissioned a few months later, all appearing on the BBC Home Service programme *How's the Baby?* The first nine of these broadcasts, many renamed, were published before the year was out by C. Brock & Co. as *The Ordinary Devoted Mother and Her Baby* (1949), a pamphlet that again sold for one shilling. The contents of these two series are reproduced below. The whole set, along with talks from his two BBC series of the mid-1940s, were republished with original work by Tavistock in 1957 in two books: *The Child and the Family* and *The Child and the Outside World*. The title of this—the eighth talk on 'training babies'—there became 'The Innate Morality of the Child', shifting its emphasis from external management to the baby's own internal resources. This chapter was then largely rewritten for its republication in the Penguin paperback *The Child, the Family and the Outside World* in 1964 [CW 3:4:30]. The original broadcast script from 1949, showing the very minor alterations for its publication in 1957, is reproduced here [CW 12:4:4c].

The Ordinary Devoted Mother (1949) in broadcast and in print:
HOW'S THE BABY? BBC HOME SERVICE (1949–50),
BENZIE, I. (PRODUCER):

> Caring for Children and How Babies Develop Their Personalities, 5 October 1949.
> The Mind of a Child, 12 October 1949.
> The Baby and Its Food, 19 October 1949.

> The Passing of Excretions, 26 October 1949.
> No Baby Can Grow Properly Without Love, 2 November 1949.
> The Baby at Feeding Time, 9 November 1949.
> Presenting the World to a Baby, 16 November 1949.
> Problems of Management: Training Babies, 23 November 1949 [CW 12:3:4c].
> Weaning, 30 November 1949.
> Management: Knowing and Learning How to Be a Mother, 22 March 1950.
> Symptoms of Illness, 29 March 1950.

THE ORDINARY DEVOTED MOTHER AND HER BABY (1949), C. BROCK & CO.:

> Introduction
> The Baby as a Going Concern
> Where the Food Goes
> The End of the Digestive Process
> The Baby as a Person
> Close-up of Mother Feeding Baby
> The World in Small Doses
> The Innate Morality of the Baby
> Weaning

CW 12:3:4d. *The Ordinary Devoted Mother and Her Baby: My Fan Mail*. In late 1951, Isa Benzie (now the producer of *Woman's Hour*) asked Winnicott, at the request of Janet Quigley (now the programme's editor), to rebroadcast the 1949 Home Service series *The Ordinary Devoted Mother and Her Baby* for *Woman's Hour*, and to follow it up with a discussion of listeners' responses:

> We are agreed here that there is no point in trying to do a thing differently when once it has been done superbly, and so we are asking for the simple repetition of your earlier series.[22]

Woman's Hour was a daily, morning series broadcast on the Light Programme (now BBC Radio 2), a channel tending—as the name suggests—towards light entertainment. The Home Service (now BBC Radio 4, with the current slogan 'Intelligent Speech') tended to broadcast informative and discursive programmes, typically covering wartime news, discussions and dramas. The transition of Winnicott's work from one channel to the other was not smooth, and, in a long letter to Winnicott on the day before the fifth talk was scheduled, Benzie subtly expressed the difficulties of presenting his ideas to listeners on the new channel:

> Now I am learning that the environment is far more than a question of the number and length of the pieces of time available. We were really *alone* on

the Home Service—you were alone with the listener, and now no one is alone! I find I imagine the listener as interrupted while feeding her baby by the man who has come to read the gas meter. I think the fact is . . . it makes women have a slight feeling of immodesty.[23]

Whatever alterations Benzie had considered making to the series became irrelevant: the next day saw the death of King George VI, and all BBC programming was suspended. After two weeks of postponed broadcasts and 'a long conversation with Dr Winnicott',[24] they decided not to go ahead with the final two programmes, ending 'what has turned out to be a rather short series of talks' [CW 12:3:4d] with the short segment on readers' letters, a broadcast Benzie described as 'harmless'.[25]

The mothers who had taken the time to write in with their thoughts, 'lyrical', 'lurid' and 'fiercely critical', presented a much more valuable resource to Winnicott than the tongue-in-cheek epithet 'fan mail' would imply. Benzie later wrote to Janet Quigley:

> You will perhaps recall his delighted amazement at the quantity and quality of the correspondence, which he recognised as ore from a gold mine, to which a professional worker like himself or his wife . . . normally never can have access.[26]

THE ORDINARY DEVOTED MOTHER AND HER BABY (1952). WOMAN'S HOUR. LIGHT PROGRAMME. BENZIE, I. (PRODUCER):

The Baby as a Going Concern, 9 January 1952
The First Week, 16 January 1952
Breast Feeding, 23 January 1952
Baby Bites, 30 January 1952
6 February 1952 [cancelled]
13 February 1952 [cancelled]
My Fan Mail, 20 February 1952 [CW 12:4:4d]

Part 4: Guide to New Material in the *Collected Works*

CW 12:4:1. *Works Published for the First Time.*

CW 12:4:2. *Letters Published for the First Time.* These are lists of the new works and new letters printed here for the first time, mostly selected from the Winnicott archive in the Institute for the History of Psychiatry's Oskar Diethlem Library at Weill Cornell Medical College in New York, or the Winnicott archive in the library of the Wellcome Trust, London.

CW 12:4:3. *Works First Published in a Winnicott Edition.* This is a list of articles, reviews and letters to journals which have been printed, though not in a collection of Winnicott's works, and which have therefore remained until now unconnected to the rest of Winnicott's œuvre. Nearly the entirety of Volume 1—works from Winnicott's early professional career as a paediatrician—are republished for the first time, along with around twenty-five letters to newspapers and journals, around forty-five reviews, and a handful of other articles or broadcasts.

CW 12:4:4. *Remarks on Some Chapters Revised for the* Collected Works. A brief list and discussion of the few works which have been revised or slightly edited for the *Collected Works*. This typically has taken the form of reinstating Winnicott's original work or separating papers that had been conflated or edited together posthumously.

Reference Lists

The reference lists for each of the eleven volumes collated together in this one volume [CW 12:7:2] were newly researched and compiled by Clay Pearn.

To co-ordinate the references, a new system had to be developed to manage citations. We decided not to follow the APA system ('1968az') due to the unwieldy quantity of items within some years. At the request of Oxford University Press, a single citation code was developed based on the volume, part and chapter numbers of each item to facilitate hyperlinking articles online. If unclear the article name and its publication date are also given.

Notes

1. According to a cutting from the Belgian newspaper *La Dernière Heure*, 1936, courtesy of Lady Aurelia Young. There remains no statue commemorating Freud in Vienna.
2. From 'My Part in the Freud Statue' by Lady Penelope Balogh (n.d., unpublished).
3. Both quotations are from Rodman (2003), p. 372.
4. Clare Winnicott, reported in Rodman (2003), p. 360. See Figure 2 on p. 19 of Volume 9 of the *Collected Works* for Winnicott and Nemon with the Freud statue in Nemon's studio.
5. Winnicott's home and consulting address.
6. Gitelson, F. (1972), p. 119.
7. Kahr, B. (2003), p. 11.
8. Gaddini, R. (2003), p. 40.
9. Clancier, A. and Kalmanovitch, J. (1984), p. 137.
10. Oscar Nemon, Letter to Simone Hotlett, 24 January 1936 (unpublished, courtesy of Lady Aurelia Young).
11. *The Diary of Sigmund Freud 1929–1939*, 24 July 1931.
12. As told by Joyce Coles to Jeannine Kalmanovitch, in Clancier, A. and Kalmanovitch, J. (1984), p. 65.

13. See also 'A 70th Birthday Present' [CW 7:2:20].
14. For an in-depth discussion of the dating of the early broadcasts and Winnicott's relationship to his first BBC producers, see Karpf (2014).
15. Winnicott, D. W., letter to Janet Quigley (28 December 1944).
16. The fact that Winnicott's broadcast series were immediately published in book form—including acknowledgements to his radio colleagues and to the BBC (except, through printer error, in this first instance)—signaled to future producers that Winnicott was an 'expert' on this subject, considerably lending to his appeal.
17. Isa Benzie, letter to Winnicott (2 October 1945).
18. Isa Benzie, letter to Winnicott (4 October 1945).
19. For a detailed analysis of Winnicott's relationship with his producers, see Karpf, A. (2014), and the Introduction to the Audio Material [CW 12:3:3].
20. Winnicott, D. W., letter to Isa Benzie (26 January 1949).
21. Winnicott, D. W., 'The Ordinary Devoted Mother' (1966) [CW 7:3:3], quoted in Karpf, A. (2014), p. 88.
22. Isa Benzie, letter to Winnicott (12 December 1951).
23. Isa Benzie, letter to Winnicott (5 February 1952); see also Karpf, A. (2014), p. 96.
24. Isa Benzie, memorandum to Janet Quigley (21 February 1952).
25. Isa Benzie, memorandum to Janet Quigley (21 February 1952).
26. Isa Benzie, memorandum to Janet Quigley (29 August 1956); see also Karpf, A. (2014), p. 91.

References

Anon. (1936). *La Dernière Heure* (Belgian newspaper). (Courtesy of Lady Aurelia Young).

Axline, V. (1966). *Play therapy*. London: Victor Gollancz.

Balogh, Penelope. (n.d., unpublished). My part in the Freud statue. (Courtesy of Lady Aurelia Young).

Benzie, I. (2 October 1945). Letter to D. W. Winnicott (R51/221 Health, New Baby). BBC Written Archives, Caversham, UK.

Benzie, I. (4 October 1945). Letter to D. W. Winnicott (BBC R CONT1, D.W. Winnicott, File 1a, 1943–59). BBC Written Archives, Caversham, UK.

Benzie, I. (12 December 1951). Letter to D. W. Winnicott (BBC R CONT1, D.W. Winnicott, File 1a, 1943–59). BBC Written Archives, Caversham, UK.

Benzie, I. (5 February 1952). Letter to D. W. Winnicott (BBC R CONT1, D.W. Winnicott, File 1a, 1943–59). BBC Written Archives, Caversham, UK.

Benzie, I. (21 February 1952). Memorandum to Janet Quigley (BBC R CONT1, D.W. Winnicott, File 1a, 1943–59). BBC Written Archives, Caversham, UK.

Benzie, I. (29 August 1956). Memorandum to Janet Quigley (BBC R CONT1, D.W. Winnicott, File 1a, 1943–59). BBC Written Archives, Caversham, UK.

Clancier, A., & Kalmanovitch, J. (Eds.). (1984). *Winnicott and paradox: From birth to creation*. London: Tavistock.

Freud, S. (1992). *The diary of Sigmund Freud, 1929–1939*. Molnar, M. (Ed.). London: Hogarth.

Gaddini, R. (2003). Annotation for Letter to Donald Winnicott, 1 September 1970. In 'Correspondence between Donald W. Winnicott and Renata Gaddini, 1964–1970', *Psychoanalysis and History*, 5, 13–47.

Gitelson, F. H. (1972). Report of the 27th International Psycho-Analytical Congress. *Bulletin of the International Psycho-Analytic Association*, 53, 83–140.

Hjulmand, K. (2007). D. W. Winnicott bibliography. In J. Abram (Ed.), *The language of Winnicott* (pp. 361–435). London: Karnac.

Kahr, B. (1996). *D. W. Winnicott: A biographical portrait*. London: Karnac.

Kahr, B. (2003). Foreword. In J. McDougall (Ed.), *Donald Winnicott the man: reflections and recollections*. London: Karnac.

Karnac, Harry (1996). Bibliography. In R. Shepherd, J. Johns, & H. Taylor Robinson (Eds.), *Thinking about children*. London: Karnac.

Karpf, A. (2014). Constructing and addressing the 'Ordinary Devoted Mother': Donald Winnicott's BBC broadcasts, 1943–1962. *History Workshop Journal*, 78, Autumn 2014.

Karpf, A. (2016) (audio). Introduction to the audio material, *The Collected Works of Winnicott*, Vol. 12. www.oxfordclinicalpsych.com/winnicott. [CW 12:3:3]

Khan, M. (1965). Publications by D. W. Winnicott 1926–1964. In M. Khan (Ed.), *The Maturational processes and the facilitating environment* (pp. 264–276). London: Hogarth.

Nemon, O. (1936, unpublished). Letter to Simone Hotlett, 24 January 1936. (Courtesy of Lady Aurelia Young.)

Rodman, F. R. (2003). *Winnicott: Life and work*. Cambridge, MA: Da Capo Press.

Winnicott, D. W. (1940). Children in the war. [CW 2:2:4]

Winnicott, D. W. (1940). The deprived mother [1939]. [CW 2:1:4]

Winnicott, D. W. (1945). Infant feeding [1944]. [CW 2:6:13]

Winnicott, D. W. (1945). Support for normal parents [1944]. [CW 2:6:11]

Winnicott, D. W. (1946). What do we mean by a normal child? [1944]. [CW 2:6:10]

Winnicott, D. W. (1949). The innate morality of the baby. [CW 12:3:4c (1949 broadcast); CW 3:4:30 (1964)]

Winnicott, D. W. (1949). *The ordinary devoted mother and her baby*. London: C. Brock & Co.

Winnicott, D. W. (1957). *The child and the family*. London: Tavistock.

Winnicott, D. W. (1957). *The child and the outside world*. London: Tavistock.

Winnicott, D. W. (1958). *Collected papers: Through paediatrics to psychoanalysis*. London: Tavistock.

Winnicott, D. W. (1964). *The child, the family and the outside world*. Harmondsworth: Penguin.

Winnicott, D. W. (1965). *The Maturational processes and the facilitating environment*. London: Hogarth.

Winnicott, D. W. (1967). The location of cultural experience [1966]. [CW 7:3:31]

Winnicott, D. W. (1968). Playing: A theoretical statement [1967]. [CW 8:2:15]

Winnicott, D. W. (1970). Letter. *British Journal of Psychiatry*, 116(531), 240.

Winnicott, D. W. (1971). Creativity and its origins. (Includes 'The split-off male and female elements to be found in men and women'.) [CW 9:3:7]

Winnicott, D. W. (1971). *Playing and reality*. London: Tavistock.

Winnicott, D. W. (1971). *The Piggle*. [CW 11:2]

Winnicott, D. W. (1971). The split-off male and female elements to be found clinically in men and women [1966]. [CW 7:3:2]

Winnicott, D. W. (1986). *Holding and interpretation: Fragment of an analysis*. The Institute of Psychoanalysis. London: Karnac.

Winnicott, D. W. (1987). The ordinary devoted mother [1966]. [CW 7:3:3]

Winnicott, D. W. (1989). Addendum to 'The location of cultural experience' [1967]. [CW 8:1:37]

Winnicott, D. W. (1989). Commentary. V. Axline, *Play therapy* (Boston: Houghton Mifflin, 1947) [1965]. [CW 9:1:32]

Winnicott, D. W. (1989). D. W. W. on D. W. W. [1967]. [CW 8:1:2]

Winnicott, D. W. (2016). A 70th birthday present [1965]. [CW 7:2:20]

Winnicott, D. W. (2017). Answers to comments on 'The split-off male and female elements to be found clinically in men and women' [1968–69]. [CW 9:1:30]

Winnicott, D. W. (2017). Getting to know your baby [1945]. [CW 12:4:4b]

Winnicott, D. W. (2017). How's the baby? [1949]. [CW 12:3:4c]

Winnicott, D. W. (2017). Looking forward to baby's arrival [1945]. [CW 12:4:4a]

Winnicott, D. W. (2017). The ordinary devoted mother and her baby: My fan mail [1952]. [CW 12:3:4d]

Winnicott, D. W. (2016). The pill [1969]. [CW 9:1:23]

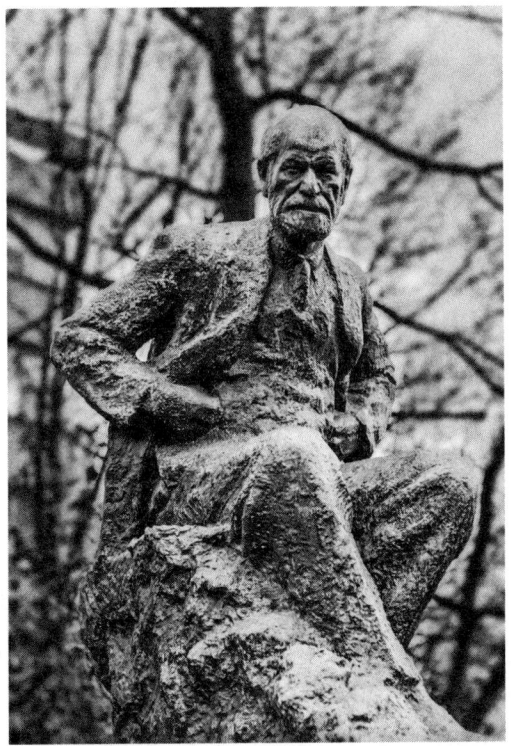

FIGURE 1 Oscar Nemon's Statue of Sigmund Freud, outside the Tavistock Clinic, London. Winnicott devoted much of his final years to raising this memorial to Freud. See the 'Introduction to Volume 12' for Winnicott's contribution [CW 12:Introduction].

PHOTO CREDIT: NEMO ROBERTS, 2016.

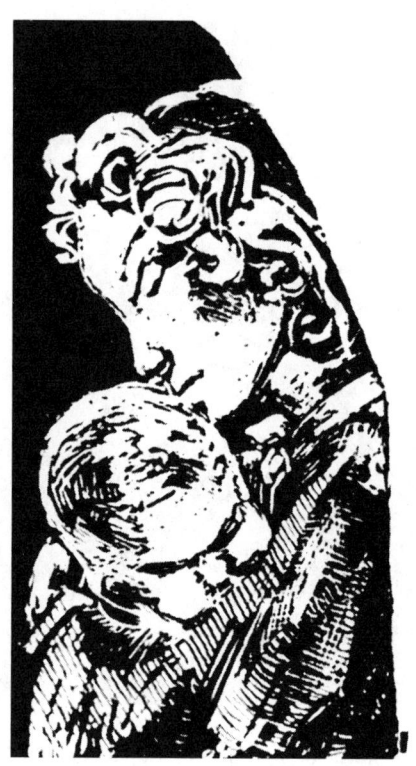

FIGURE 2 Alice Winnicott's woodcut for the cover of Winnicott's pamphlet of BBC broadcasts, *Getting to Know Your Baby* (1945).

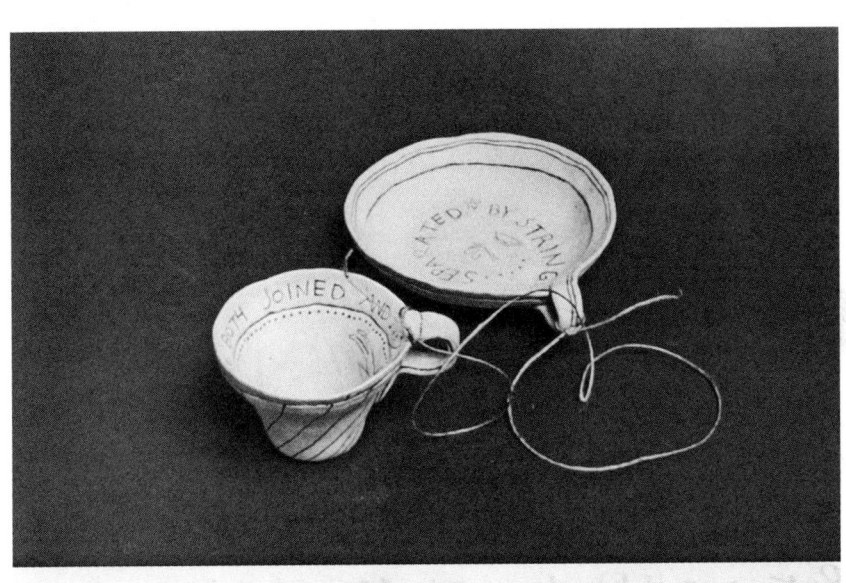

FIGURE 3 A cup and saucer both joined and separated by string (see 'Transitional Objects and Transitional Phenomena' [CW 9:3:5]).
ALISON BRITTON OBE RA.

PART 1

Winnicott's Publications

Chronological Bibliography of Works by D. W. Winnicott

1913

Smith. *The Fortnightly* (The Leys School, Cambridge), 3 October 1913. [CW 1:1:3]

1914

The best remedy. *The Fortnightly* (The Leys School, Cambridge), 12 June 1914. [CW 1:1:8]
The night attack. *The Fortnightly* (The Leys School, Cambridge), 13 February 1914. [CW 1:1:6]

1920

A Shropshire surgeon (Poem). *St Bartholomew's Hospital Journal*, 1920, 27. [CW 1:1:12]
St Bartholomew's Hospital amateur dramatic club. *St Bartholomew's Hospital Journal*, 1920, 27, 152–154. [CW 1:1:13]

1921

A reminder to the binder. *St Bartholomew's Hospital Journal*, 1921, 28, 107. [CW 1:1:14]
The snag. *St Bartholomew's Hospital Journal*, 1921, 28, 188. [CW 1:1:15]

1926

Case for diagnosis (? infantile hemiplegia). *Section for the Study of Disease in Children, Proceedings of the Royal Society of Medicine*, 1926, 19, 47–48. [CW 1:2:3]
Case for diagnosis (? poliomyelitis with some spasticity). *Section for the Study of Disease in Children, Proceedings of the Royal Society of Medicine*, 1926, 19, 46–47. [CW 1:2:2]
Two cases of post-encephalitic hyperpnœa. *Section for the Study of Disease in Children, Proceedings of the Royal Society of Medicine*, 1926, 19, 52–53. [CW 1:2:4]
Varicella encephalitis and vaccinia encephalitis (with N. Gibbs). *British Journal of Children's Diseases*, 1926, 23, 107–127. [CW 1:2:1]

1927

Case of stunted growth. *Proceedings of the Royal Society of Medicine*, 1927, 20(10), 1586. [CW 1:2:5]

The only child. *Maternity and Child Welfare: A Monthly Journal for Workers Among Mothers and Children*, No. 124, April 1927, XI(4). Also published in Viscountess Erleigh (Ed.), *The mind of the growing child* (pp. 47–64). London: Faber/New York: Oxford University Press, 1928. [CW 1:2:6]

1928

Abscess in frontal lobe: Post-mortem findings in a case shown at a previous meeting of the section (with E. O'Flynn). *Proceedings of the Royal Society of Medicine*, 1928, 21(7), 1256–1257. [CW 1:2:11]

Encephalitis after measles and chicken-pox. *Proceedings of the Royal Society of Medicine*, 1928, 21(4), 567. [CW 1:2:9]

Facial nerve paralysis. *Proceedings of the Royal Society of Medicine*, 1928, 21(4), 565–566. [CW 1:2:7]

Facial nerve paralysis, associated with fits. *Proceedings of the Royal Society of Medicine*, 1928, 21(4), 566. [CW 1:2:8]

Muscle weakness, altered gait and absent deep reflexes after measles. *Proceedings of the Royal Society of Medicine*, 1928, 21(7), 1259. [CW 1:2:10]

1929

Hemiplegia noticed after diptheria. *Proceedings of the Royal Society of Medicine*, 1929, 22(4), 392. [CW 1:2:13]

Measles encephalitis. *Proceedings of the Royal Society of Medicine*, 1929, 22(9), 1247–1248. [CW 1:2:14]

Rheumatism in children [1928]. In *Annual report of the London County council: Vol. 3. Report of the school medical officer for the year 1928*. London: P. S. King and Son, 1929. [CW 1:2:12]

Symptoms suggesting post-encephalitis. *Proceedings of the Royal Society of Medicine*, 1929, 22(9), 1248–1249. [CW 1:2:15]

The diagnosis of chorea. *Postgraduate Medical Journal*, 1929, 4(45), 147–153. [CW 1:2:16]

1930

Enuresis [abstract] [1929]. *Proceedings of the Royal Society of Medicine*, 1930, 23(3), 255–256. [CW 1:2:17]

Pathological sleeping. *Proceedings of the Royal Society of Medicine*, 1930, 23(8), 1109–1110. [CW 1:2:19]

Short communication on enuresis. *St Bartholomew's Hospital Journal*, April 1930, 125–127. Also published in R. Shepherd, J. Johns & H. Taylor Robinson (Eds.), *Thinking about children* (pp. 170–175). London: Karnac, 1996. [CW 1:2:18]

1931

Clinical notes on disorders of childhood. London: Heinemann, 1931. [CW 1:3]

Preface. v. [CW 1:3:Preface]

Introduction. 1–6. [CW 1:3:Introduction]

History-taking. 7–21. [CW 1:3:1]

Physical examination. 22–31. [CW 1:3:2]
A note on temperature and the importance of charts. 32–37. [CW 1:3:3]
The nose and throat. 38–41. [CW 1:3:4]
The heart, with special reference to rheumatic carditis. 42–57. [CW 1:3:5]
Rheumatic fever. 58–63. [CW 1:3:6]
The rheumatic clinic. 64–68. [CW 1:3:7]
Active heart disease. 69–75. [CW 1:3:8]
Growing pains. 76–80. [CW 1:3:9]
Arthritis associated with emotional disturbance. 81–86. [CW 1:3:10]
Fidgetiness. 87–97. Also published in *Collected papers: Through paediatrics to psycho-analysis* (pp. 22–30). London: Tavistock, 1958. [CW 1:3:11]
A note on normality and anxiety. 98–121. Also published in *Collected papers: Through paediatrics to psycho-analysis* (pp. 3–21). London: Tavistock, 1958. [CW 1:3:12]
Anxiety (continued). 122–128. [CW 1:3:13]
Disease of the nervous system. 129–142. [CW 1:3:14]
Walking. 143–151. [CW 1:3:15]
Mental defect. 152–156. [CW 1:3:16]
Convulsions, fits. 157–171. [CW 1:3:17]
Micturition disturbances. 172–182. [CW 1:3:18]
Masturbation. 183–190. [CW 1:3:19]
Speech disorders. 191–200. [CW 1:3:20]

Hæmoptysis: Case for diagnosis. *Proceedings of the Royal Society of Medicine*, 1931, 24(7), 855–856. [CW 1:2:20]

Pre-systolic murmur, possibly not due to mitral stenosis. *Proceedings of the Royal Society of Medicine*, 1931, 24(10), 1354. [CW 1:2:21]

1933

Abstract: Alexander, F., 'Psychoanalysis and medicine' (*Mental Hygiene*, 1932, *16*, 63). *International Journal of Psychoanalysis*, 1933, *14*, 108. [CW 1:4:1]

1934

Abstract: Lundholm, H., 'Repression and rationalization' (*British Journal of Medical Psychology*, 1933, *13*(1), 23). *International Journal of Psychoanalysis*, 1934, *15*, 308. [CW 1:4:2]

Discussion: Auden, G. A., 'The difficult child' (*The Journal of the Royal Society for the Promotion of Health*, March 1929, *50*, 157–164). *Journal of State Medicine*, 1934, *42*, 628–630. [CW 1:4:4]

Papular urticaria and the dynamics of skin sensation. *British Journal of Children's Diseases*, 1934, *31*. Also published in R. Shepherd, J. Johns & H. Taylor Robinson (Eds.), *Thinking about children* (pp. 157–169). London: Karnac, 1996. [CW 1:4:3]

1935

Abstract: Barinbaum, M., 'A contribution to the problem of psycho-physical relations with special reference to dermatology'. (*Internationale Zeitschrift für Psychoanalyse*, 1934, *20*, 241–251). *International Journal of Psychoanalysis*, 1935, *16*, 369. [CW 1:4:5]

1936

Contribution to a discussion on enuresis. In *Proceedings of the Royal Society of Medicine*, 1936, 29, 1522–1524. Also published in R. Shepherd, J. Johns & H. Taylor Robinson (Eds.), *Thinking about children* (pp. 151–156). London: Karnac, 1996. [CW 1:4:9]

Review: Aichhorn, A., *Wayward youth* ['Verwahrloste Jugend'] (Leipzig, Vienna and Zurich: Internationaler Psychoanalytischer Verlag, 1925; London: Putnam, 1936). *British Journal of Medical Psychology*, 1936, 16(2), 154–156. [CW 1:4:12]

Review: Rickman, J. (Ed.), *On the bringing up of children* (London: Kegan Paul, 1936). *British Journal of Medical Psychology*, 1936, 16(2), 151–152. [CW 1:4:13]

1938

Notes on a little boy. *New Era in Home and School*, 1938, 19. Also published in R. Shepherd, J. Johns & H. Taylor Robinson (Eds.), *Thinking about children* (pp. 102–103). London: Karnac, 1996. [CW 1:4:16]

Review: Kanner, L., *Child psychiatry* (Springfield, IL: Charles C. Thomas, 1935. London: Ballière, Tindall & Cox, 1937). *International Journal of Psychoanalysis*, 1938, 19, 362–363. Also published in R. Shepherd, J. Johns & H. Taylor Robinson (Eds.), *Thinking about children* (pp. 191–193). London: Karnac, 1996, part of 'Three reviews of books on autism'. [CW 1:4:14]

Shyness and nervous disorders in children. *New Era in Home and School*, 1938, 19. Also published in *The child and the outside world: Studies in developing relationships* (pp. 35–39). London: Tavistock, 1957; and *The child, the family, and the outside world* (pp. 211–215). Harmondsworth: Penguin, 1964. [CW 1:4:17]

Skin changes in relation to emotional disorder. *St John's Hospital Dermatological Society Report*, 1938, 27, 62–73. [CW 1:4:18]

1939

The psychology of juvenile rheumatism. In R. G. Gordon (Ed.), *A survey of child psychiatry* (pp. 28–34). London: Oxford University Press, 1939. [CW 2:1:7]

1940

Children and their mothers. *New Era in Home and School*, 1940, 21. Also published in C. Winnicott, R. Shepherd & M. Davis (Eds.), *Deprivation and delinquency* (pp. 14–21, part of 'Evacuation of small children'). London: Tavistock, 1984. [CW 2:2:2]

Children in the war. *New Era in Home and School*, 1940, 21. Also published in *The child and the outside world: Studies in developing relationships* (pp. 69–74). London: Tavistock, 1957; and C. Winnicott, R. Shepherd & M. Davis (Eds.), *Deprivation and delinquency* (pp. 25–30). London: Tavistock, 1984. [CW 2:2:4]

The deprived mother [1939]. *New Era in Home and School*, 1940, 21(3). Also published in *The child and the outside world: Studies in developing relationships* (pp. 75–82). London: Tavistock, 1957); and C. Winnicott, R. Shepherd & M. Davis (Eds.),

Deprivation and delinquency (pp. 31–38). London: Tavistock, 1984. Broadcast 1939. London: British Broadcasting Corporation. [CW 2:1:4]

1941

On influencing and being influenced. *New Era in Home and School*, 1941, 22. Also published in *The child and the outside world: Studies in developing relationships* (pp. 35–39). London: Tavistock, 1957; and *The child, the family, and the outside world* (pp. 199–204). Harmondsworth: Penguin, 1964. [CW 2:3:3]

The observation of infants in a set situation. *International Journal of Psychoanalysis*, 1941, 22, 229–249. Also published in *Collected papers: Through paediatrics to psycho-analysis* (pp. 52–69). London: Tavistock, 1958. [CW 2:3:6]

Review: Flügel, J. C., *The moral paradox of peace and war* (London: Watts, 1941). *New Era in Home and School*, 1941, 22. [CW 2:3:4]

Review: Isaacs, S., (Ed), *The Cambridge Evacuation Survey: A war time study in social welfare and education* (London: Methuen, 1941). *New Era in Home and School*, 1941, 22. Also published in C. Winnicott, R. Shepherd & M. Davis (Eds.), *Deprivation and delinquency* (pp. 22–24). London: Tavistock, 1984. [CW 2:3:5]

1942

Child department consultations. *International Journal of Psychoanalysis*, 1942, 23, 139–146. Also published in *Collected papers: Through paediatrics to psycho-analysis* (pp. 70–84). London: Tavistock, 1958. [CW 2:4:2]

Review: Middlemore, M. P., *The nursing couple* (London: Hamish Hamilton, 1941). *International Journal of Psychoanalysis*, 1942, 23, 179–180. [CW 2:4:5]

Why children play. *New Era in Home and School*, 1942, 23. Also published in *The child and the outside world: Studies in developing relationships* (pp. 149–152). London: Tavistock, 1957; and *The child, the family, and the outside world* (pp. 143–146). Harmondsworth: Penguin, 1964, revised 1968. [CW 2:4:4]

1943

Delinquency research. *New Era in Home and School*, 1943, 24. [CW 2:5:2]

Observations of infant behaviour during routine clinical examination [abstract]. *Archives of Disease in Childhood*, 1943, 18, 156. Published here as a footnote to 'The observation of infants in a set situation' [CW 2:3:6 (footnote i)]

1944

The magistrate, the psychiatrist and the clinic. *New Era in Home and School*, 1944, 25, 7–8. Also published in C. Winnicott, R. Shepherd & M. Davis (Eds.), *Deprivation and delinquency* (pp. 166–170, as 'Correspondence with a magistrate'). London: Tavistock, 1984. Published here as 'Letter to Roger North'. [CW 2:6:1]

Ocular psychoneuroses of childhood. *Transactions of the Ophthalmological Society of the United Kingdom*, 1944, 64, 46–52, as 'Discussion on ocular psychoneuroses'. Also published in *Collected papers: Through paediatrics to psycho-analysis* (pp. 85–90). London: Tavistock, 1958. [CW 2:6:15]

The problem of homeless children (with C. Britton). *New Education Fellowship Monograph*, No. 1, 1944. Also published in *New Era in Home and School*, 1944, 25(7), 155–161; and J. Kanter (Ed.), *Face to face with children: The life and work of Clare Winnicott* (pp. 97–111). London: Karnac, 2004. [CW 2:6:14]

A tendency in therapeutics. *St Bartholomew's Hospital Journal*, February 1944, 7–9. [CW 2:6:5]

The wearing of masks in the nursing of premature and older infants [abstract] [1943]. *Archives of Disease in Childhood*, 1944, 19(97), 38. [CW 2:5:9]

1945

Getting to know your baby. London: Heinemann, 1945. [Not reprinted in this form in the *Collected Works*]

Preface. v. First published in *Clinical notes on disorders of childhood* (p. v.). London: Heinemann, 1931. [CW 1:3:Preface]

Getting to know your baby [1943]. 1–5. First published in *New Era in Home and School*, 1945, 26. Also published in *The child and the family: First relationships* (pp. 7–12). London: Tavistock, 1957; and *The child, the family, and the outside world* (pp. 19–24). Harmondsworth: Penguin, 1964. Broadcast 10 December 1943, J. Quigley (Producer), *Happy children*. Home Service. London: British Broadcasting Corporation. [CW 2:5:8]

Why do babies cry? [1944]. 5–12. First published in *New Era in Home and School*, 1945, 26. Also published in *The child and the family: First relationships* (pp. 43–52). London: Tavistock, 1957; and *The child, the family, and the outside world* (pp. 58–68). Harmondsworth: Penguin, 1964. Broadcast in two parts, 4 and 11 February 1944, as 'Why does your baby cry?' J. Quigley (Producer), *Happy children*. Home Service. London: British Broadcasting Corporation. [CW 2:6:2]

Infant feeding [1944]. 12–16. First published in *New Era in Home and School*, 1945, 26. Also published in *The child and the family: First relationships* (pp. 18–22). London: Tavistock, 1957; and *The child, the family, and the outside world* (pp. 30–34). Harmondsworth: Penguin, 1964. [CW 2:6:13]

What about father? [1944]. 16–21. First published in *New Era in Home and School*, 1945, 26. Also published in *The child and the family: First relationships* (pp. 81–86). London: Tavistock, 1957; and *The child, the family, and the outside world* (pp. 113–118). Harmondsworth: Penguin, 1964. Broadcast 17 March 1944, as 'Where does Dad come in?' J. Quigley (Producer), *Happy children*. Home Service. London: British Broadcasting Corporation. [CW 2:6:8]

Their standards and yours [1944]. 21–24. First published in *New Era in Home and School*, 1945, 26, 21–24. Also published in *The child and the family: First relationships* (pp. 87–91). London: Tavistock, 1957; and *The child, the family, and the outside world* (pp. 119–123). Harmondsworth: Penguin, 1964. Broadcast 12 May 1944, J. Quigley (Producer), *Happy children*. Home Service. London: British Broadcasting Corporation. [CW 2:6:9]

Postscript [1944]. 25–27. First published in *New Era in Home and School*, 1945, 26, as 'Support for normal parents'. Also published in *The child and the family: First* relationships (pp. 137–140). London: Tavistock, 1957; and *The child, the family, and the outside world* (pp. 173–176). Harmondsworth: Penguin, 1964. Published here as 'Support for normal parents'. [CW 2:6:11]

Getting to know your baby [1943]. *New Era in Home and School*, 1945, 26. Also published in *Getting to know your baby* (pp. 1–5). London: Heinemann, 1945; and *The child and the family: First relationships* (pp. 7–12). London: Tavistock, 1957; and *The child, the family, and the outside world* (pp. 19–24). Harmondsworth: Penguin, 1964. Broadcast 10 December 1943, J. Quigley (Producer), *Happy children*. Home Service. London: British Broadcasting Corporation. [CW 2:5:8]

Infant feeding [1944]. *New Era in Home and School*, 1945, 26. Also published in *Getting to know your baby* (pp. 12–16). London: Heinemann, 1945; and *The child and the family: First relationships* (pp. 18–22). London: Tavistock, 1957; and *The child, the family, and the outside world* (pp. 30–34). Harmondsworth: Penguin, 1964. [CW 2:6:13]

Primitive emotional development. *International Journal of Psychoanalysis*, 1945, 26, 137–143. Also published in *Collected papers: Through paediatrics to psycho-analysis* (pp. 145–156). London: Tavistock, 1958. [CW 2:7:8]

Support for normal parents [1944]. *New Era in Home and School*, 1945, 26. In *Getting to know your baby* (pp. 25–27). London: Heinemann, 1945, as 'Postscript'. Also published in *The child and the family: First relationships* (pp. 137–140). London: Tavistock, 1957; and *The child, the family, and the outside world* (pp. 173–176). Harmondsworth: Penguin, 1964. [CW 2:6:11]

Their standards and yours [1944]. *New Era in Home and School*, 1945, 26. Also published in *Getting to know your baby* (pp. 21–24). London: Heinemann, 1945; and *The child and the family: First relationships* (pp. 87–91). London: Tavistock, 1957; and in *The child, the family, and the outside world* (pp. 119–123). Harmondsworth: Penguin, 1964. Broadcast 12 May 1944, J. Quigley (Producer), *Happy children*. Home Service. London: British Broadcasting Corporation. [CW 2:6:9]

Thinking and the unconscious. *The Liberal Magazine*, March 1945, 125–126. Also published in C. Winnicott, R. Shepherd & M. Davis (Eds.), *Home is where we start from: Essays by a psychoanalyst* (pp. 169–171). Harmondsworth: Penguin, 1986. [CW 2:7:4]

Towards an objective study of human nature. *New Era in Home and School*, 1945, 26, as 'Talking about psychology'; reissued in 1952, 33(3), as 'What is psychoanalysis?' Also published in *The child and the outside world: Studies in developing relationships* (pp. 125–133). London: Tavistock, 1957; and R. Shepherd, J. Johns & H. Taylor Robinson (Eds.), *Thinking about children* (pp. 3–12). London: Karnac, 1996. [CW 2:7:11]

The value of breastfeeding (psychological) [abstract]. *Archives of Disease in Childhood*, 1945, 20(104), 186. Published here as a footnote in 'Breast feeding' [CW 2:7:12 (footnote *i*)]

What about father? [1944]. *New Era in Home and School*, 1945, 26. Also published in *Getting to know your baby* (pp. 16–21). London: Heinemann, 1945; and *The child and the family: First relationships* (pp. 81–86). London: Tavistock, 1957; and *The child, the family, and the outside world* (pp. 113–118). Harmondsworth: Penguin, 1964. Broadcast 17 March 1944, as 'Where does Dad come in?' J. Quigley (Producer), *Happy children*. Home Service. London: British Broadcasting Corporation. [CW 2:6:8]

Why do babies cry? [1944]. *New Era in Home and School*, 1945, 26. Also published in *Getting to know your baby* (pp. 5–12). London: Heinemann, 1945; and *The child and the family: First relationships* (pp. 43–52). London: Tavistock, 1957; and *The child, the family, and the outside world* (pp. 58–68). Harmondsworth: Penguin, 1964; and *Parents*, 1967, 22(8), as 'Winnicott's wisdom: Why babies cry'. Broadcast in two parts, 4 and 11 February 1944, as 'Why does your baby cry?' J. Quigley (Producer), *Happy children*. Home Service. London: British Broadcasting Corporation. [CW 2:6:2]

1946

Educational diagnosis. *National Froebel Foundation Bulletin*, 1946, 41, 3. Also published in *The child and the outside world: Studies in developing relationships* (pp. 29–34). London: Tavistock, 1957; and *The child, the family, and the outside world* (pp. 205–210). Harmondsworth: Penguin, 1964. [CW 3:1:2]

Some psychological aspects of juvenile delinquency [1944]. *New Era in Home and School*, 1946, 27(10), 295. Also published in *Delinquency Research*, 1946, 24(5); and *The child and the outside world: Studies in developing relationships* (pp. 181–187). London: Tavistock, 1957; and C. Winnicott, R. Shepherd & M. Davis (Eds.), *Deprivation and delinquency* (pp. 113–119). London: Tavistock, 1984. [CW 3:1:7] See also 'Aspects of juvenile delinquency'.

What do we mean by a normal child? [1944]. *New Era in Home and School*, 1946, 27. Also published in *The child and the family: First relationships* (pp. 100–106). London: Tavistock, 1957; and *The child, the family, and the outside world* (pp. 124–130). Harmondsworth: Penguin, 1964. Broadcast 23 June 1944, J. Quigley (Producer), *Happy children*. Home Service. London: British Broadcasting Corporation. [CW 2:6:10]

1947

The child and sex. *The Practitioner*, 1947, 158. Also published in *The child and the outside world: Studies in developing relationships* (pp. 153–166). London: Tavistock, 1957; and *The child, the family, and the outside world* (pp. 147–160). Harmondsworth: Penguin, 1964. [CW 3:2:5]

Further thoughts on babies as persons. *New Era in Home and School*, 1947, 28(10), 179, as 'Babies are persons'. Also published in *The child and the outside world: Studies in developing relationships* (pp. 134–140). London: Tavistock, 1957; and *The child, the family, and the outside world* (pp. 85–92). Harmondsworth: Penguin, 1964. [CW 3:2:4]

Physical therapy of mental disorder. *British Medical Journal*, 1947, 1(4506), 688–689. Also published in C. Winnicott, R. Shepherd & M. Davis (Eds.), *Psycho-analytic explorations* (pp. 534–541, part of 'Physical therapy of mental disorder: Convulsion therapy'). Cambridge, MA: Harvard University Press, 1989. [CW 3:2:2]

Residential management as treatment for difficult children: The evolution of a wartime hostels scheme (with C. Britton). *Human Relations*, 1(1), 87–97. Also published in *The child and the outside world: Studies in developing relationships* (pp. 98–116, as part of 'Residential management as treatment for difficult children'). London: Tavistock, 1957; and C. Winnicott, R. Shepherd & M. Davis (Eds.), *Deprivation and delinquency* (pp. 54–72, as part of 'Residential management as treatment for difficult children'). London: Tavistock, 1984. [CW 3:2:3]

1948

Children's hostels in war and peace [1946]. *British Journal of Medical Psychology*, 1948, *21*(3), 175. Also published in *The child and the outside world: Studies in developing relationships* (pp. 117–121). London: Tavistock, 1957; and C. Winnicott, R. Shepherd & M. Davis (Eds.), *Deprivation and delinquency* (pp. 73–77). London: Tavistock, 1984. [CW 3:1:1]

Disorders of childhood. *The Journal of the Royal Institute of Public Health and Hygiene*, 1948, *11*(7), 244. [CW 3:3:8]

Obituary: Isaacs, Susan. *Nature*, 1948, *162*(4127), 881. Also published in C. Winnicott, R. Shepherd & M. Davis (Eds.), *Psycho-analytic explorations* (pp. 385–387). Cambridge, MA: Harvard University Press, 1989. [CW 3:3:11]

Paediatrics and psychiatry. *British Journal of Medical Psychology*, 1948, *21*(4), 229–240. Also published in *Collected papers: Through paediatrics to psycho-analysis* (pp. 157–173). London: Tavistock, 1958. [CW 3:3:2]

Review: Bowley, A., *The psychology of the unwanted child* (Edinburgh: E. & S. Livingstone, 1947). *British Medical Journal*, 1948, *2*(4566), 78. [CW 3:3:6]

Review: Child Study Association of America. *Parents' questions* (New York, London: Harper & Bros., 1947). *British Medical Journal*, 1948, *2*(4569), 257. [CW 3:3:7]

Review: Freud, A., Hoffer, W. (Eds.), *The psychoanalytic study of the child* (Vol. 2). (London: Imago, 1946). *British Medical Journal*, 21 August 1948, *2*(4572), 389. [CW 3:3:9]

Review: Wolff, W., *The personality of the preschool child* (New York: Grune & Stratton, 1946). *British Medical Journal*, 1948, *2*(4581), 747. [CW 3:3:10]

1949

Hate in the countertransference [1947]. *International Journal of Psychoanalysis*, 1949, *30*, 68–74. Also published in *Collected papers: Through paediatrics to psycho-analysis* (pp. 194–203). London: Tavistock, 1958. [CW 3:2:1]

Leucotomy. *British Medical Student's Journal*, 1949, *3*. Also published in C. Winnicott, R. Shepherd & M. Davis (Eds.), *Psycho-analytic explorations* (pp. 543–547, part of 'Physical therapy of mental disorder: Leucotomy'). Cambridge, MA: Harvard University Press, 1989. [CW 3:4:21]

The ordinary devoted mother and her baby. (1949). London: C. A. Brock. [Not reprinted in this form in the *Collected Works*]

> Introduction. 3–6. Also published in *The child and the family: First relationships* (pp. 3–6, as 'A man looks at motherhood'). London: Tavistock, 1957; and *The child, the family, and the outside world* (pp. 15–18, as 'A man looks at motherhood'). Harmondsworth: Penguin, 1964. [CW 3:4:23]
>
> The baby as a going concern. 7–11. Also published in *The child and the family: First relationships* (pp. 13–17). London: Tavistock, 1957; and *The child, the family, and the outside world* (pp. 25–29). Harmondsworth: Penguin, 1964. Broadcast 12 October 1949, as

'The mind of a child'. I. Benzie (Producer), *How's the baby?* Home Service. London: British Broadcasting Corporation. [CW 3:4:24]

Where the food goes. 12–16. Also published in *The child and the family: First relationships* (pp. 23–27). London: Tavistock, 1957; and *The child, the family, and the outside world* (pp. 35–39). Harmondsworth: Penguin, 1964. Broadcast 19 October 1949, as 'The baby and its food'. I. Benzie (Producer), *How's the baby?* Home Service. London: British Broadcasting Corporation. [CW 3:4:25]

The end of the digestive process. 17–21. Also published in *The child and the family: First relationships* (pp. 28–32). London: Tavistock, 1957; and *The child, the family, and the outside world* (pp. 40–44). Harmondsworth: Penguin, 1964. Broadcast 26 October 1949, as 'The passing of excretions'. I. Benzie (Producer), *How's the baby?* Home Service. London: British Broadcasting Corporation. [CW 3:4:26]

The baby as a person. 22–26. Also published in *The child and the family: First relationships* (pp. 33–37). London: Tavistock, 1957; and *The child, the family, and the outside world* (pp. 75–79). Harmondsworth: Penguin, 1964. Broadcast 2 November 1949, as 'No baby can grow properly without love'. I. Benzie (Producer), *How's the baby?* Home Service. London: British Broadcasting Corporation. [CW 3:4:27]

Close-up of mother feeding baby. 27–31. Also published in *The child and the family: First relationships* (pp. 38–42). London: Tavistock, 1957; and *The child, the family, and the outside world* (pp. 45–49). Harmondsworth: Penguin, 1964. Broadcast 9 November 1949, as 'The baby at feeding time'. I. Benzie (Producer), *How's the baby?* Home Service. London: British Broadcasting Corporation. [CW 3:4:28]

The world in small doses. 32–37. Also published in *The child and the family: First relationships* (pp. 53–58). London: Tavistock, 1957; and *The child, the family, and the outside world* (pp. 69–74). Harmondsworth: Penguin, 1964. Broadcast 16 November 1949, as 'Presenting the world to a baby'. I. Benzie (Producer), *How's the baby?* London: British Broadcasting Corporation. [CW 3:4:29]

The innate morality of the baby. 38–42. Also published in *The child and the family: First relationships* (pp. 59–63). London: Tavistock, 1957; and *The child, the family, and the outside world* (pp. 93–97). Harmondsworth: Penguin, 1964. Broadcast 23 November 1949, as 'Problems of management: Training babies' [CW 12:3:4c]. I. Benzie (Producer), *How's the baby?* London: British Broadcasting Corporation. [CW 3:4:30]

Weaning. 43–47. Also published in *The child and the family: First relationships* (pp. 64–68). London: Tavistock, 1957; and *The child, the family, and the outside world* (pp. 80–84). Harmondsworth: Penguin, 1964. Broadcast 30 November 1949. I. Benzie (Producer), *How's the baby?* London: British Broadcasting Corporation. [CW 3:4:31]

Review: Harms, E. (Ed.), *Handbook of child guidance* (New York: Child Care Publications, 1947). *British Medical Journal*, 1949, 2(4622), 321. [CW 3:4:15]

Review: Hill, A., *Art versus illness* (London: George Allen and Unwin, 1948). *British Journal of Medical Psychology*, 1949, 22. Also published in C. Winnicott, R. Shepherd & M. Davis (Eds.), *Psycho-analytic explorations* (pp. 555–557, as part of the chapter 'Occupational therapy'). Cambridge, MA: Harvard University Press, 1989. [CW 3:4:22]

Sex education in schools. *Medical Press*, 1949, 222. Also published in *The child and the outside world: Studies in developing relationships* (pp. 40–44). London: Tavistock, 1957; and *The child, the family, and the outside world* (pp. 216–220). Harmondsworth: Penguin, 1964. [CW 3:4:35]

Young children and other people. *Young Children*, 1949, 1. Also published in *The child and the family: First relationships* (pp. 92–99). London: Tavistock, 1957; and *The child, the family, and the outside world* (pp. 103–110). Harmondsworth: Penguin, 1964. [CW 3:4:32]

1950

Childhood psychosis. *British Medical Journal*, 1950, 1(4659), 944–945. [CW 3:5:5]

Review: Stein, L., *The infancy of speech and the speech of infancy* (London: Methuen, 1949). *British Journal of Medical Psychology*, 1950, 23, 120–121. [CW 3:5:8]

Some thoughts on the meaning of the word democracy. *Human Relations*, 1950, 3. Also published in *The family and individual development* (pp. 155–169). London: Tavistock, 1965; and C. Winnicott, R. Shepherd & M. Davis (Eds.), *Home is where we start from: Essays by a psychoanalyst* (pp. 239–259). Harmondsworth: Penguin, 1986. [CW 3:5:17]

1951

The foundation of mental health. *British Medical Journal*, 1951, 1(4719), 1373–1374. Also published in C. Winnicott, R. Shepherd & M. Davis (Eds.), *Deprivation and delinquency* (pp. 168–171). London: Tavistock, 1984. [CW 3:6:4]

Review: Evans, P. R. & MacKeith, R., *Infant feeding and feeding difficulties* (London: Churchill). *British Journal of Medical Psychology*, 1951, 24(4), 304–305. [CW 3:6:18]

Review: Freud, A., Hoffer, W., Glover, E. (Eds.), *The psychoanalytic study of the child* (Vol. 3–4, Vol. 5) (London: Imago, 1949). *British Medical Journal*, 13 October 1951, 2(4736), 894. [CW 3:6:12]

Review: Jones, E., *Papers on psycho-analysis* (5th ed., London: Ballière, 1948). *British Journal of Medical Psychology*, 1951, 24(2). [CW 3:6:17]

Review: Milner, M., *On not being able to paint* (London: Heinemann, 1950). *British Journal of Medical Psychology*, 1951, 24(1), 75–76, as 'Critical notice'. Also published in C. Winnicott, R. Shepherd & M. Davis (Eds.), *Psycho-analytic explorations* (pp. 390–392). Cambridge, MA: Harvard University Press, 1989. [CW 3:6:15]

Review: *Problems of infancy and childhood. Transactions of the Third Conference* (New York: Josiah Macy, Jr. Foundation, 1949). *British Journal of Medical Psychology*, 1951, 24(2). [CW 3:6:16]

Review: Watson, J. A. F., *The child and the magistrate* (London: Jonathan Cape. 1950). *British Medical Journal*, 1951, 1(4696), 22. [CW 3:6:1]

Review: Wickes, F., *The inner world of man: With psychological drawings and paintings* (London: Methuen, 1950). *Lancet*, 14 July 1951, 258(6672), 66. [CW 3:6:7]

Review: Ziman, E., *Jealousy in children* (London: Victor Gollancz, 1951). *British Medical Journal*, 1951, 2(4730), 532. [CW 3:6:10]

1952

Visiting children in hospital [1951]. *Child-Family Digest*, October 1952; and *New Era in Home and School*, 1952, 33. Also published in *The child and the family: First relationships* (pp. 121–126). London: Tavistock, 1957; and *The child, the family, and the outside world* (pp. 221–226). Harmondsworth: Penguin, 1964. Broadcast in two parts, 16 and 23 May 1951. I. Benzie (Producer), *Woman's hour*. London: British Broadcasting Corporation. [CW 3:6:5]

1953

Mother, teacher and the child's needs (with other members of the joint WHO-UNESCO expert group). First published in *Problems in education* (Vol. 9). New York: UNESCO, 1953. Also published in *The child and the outside world: Studies in developing relationships* (pp. 14–23, as 'The child's needs and the role of the mother in the early stages'). London: Tavistock, 1957; and in *The child, the family, and the outside world* (pp. 189–198). Harmondsworth: Penguin, 1964. [CW 4:2:20]

Psychoses and child care [1952]. *British Journal of Medical Psychology*, 1953, 26(1), 68–74. Also published in *Collected papers: Through paediatrics to psycho-analysis* (pp. 219–228). London: Tavistock, 1958. [CW 4:1:5]

Review: Bowlby, J., *Maternal care and mental health* (Geneva: WHO, 1951). *British Journal of Medical Psychology*, 1953, 26. Also published in C. Winnicott, R. Shepherd & M. Davis (Eds.), *Psycho-analytic explorations* (pp. 423–426). Cambridge, MA: Harvard University Press, 1989. [CW 4:2:10]

Review: Burlingham, D., *Twins: A study of three pairs of identical twins* (London: Imago, 1952). *British Medical Journal*, 1953, 1(4812), 714. [CW 4:2:6]

Review: Burlingham, D., *Twins: A study of three pairs of identical twins* (London: Imago, 1952). *New Era in Home and School*, 1953, 34. Also published in C. Winnicott, R. Shepherd & M. Davis (Eds.), *Psycho-analytic explorations* (pp. 408–412), Cambridge, MA: Harvard University Press, 1989. [CW 4:2:7]

Review: Erikson, E., *Childhood and society* (London: Imago, 1951). *British Medical Journal*, 1953, 2(4847), 1205. [CW 4:2:16]

Review: Glover, E., *Psychoanalysis and child psychiatry* (London: Imago, 1953). *British Medical Journal*, 1953, 2(4836), 609. [CW 4:2:11]

Review: Rosen, J. N., *Direct analysis*: Selected Papers (New York: Grune & Stratton, 1953). *British Journal of Psychology*, 1953, 44, 384. [CW 4:2:17]

Review: Senn, M. (Ed.), *Problems of infancy and childhood: Transactions of the sixth conference* (New York: Josiah Macy, Jr. Foundation, 1953). *British Medical Journal*, 1953, 2(4837), 664. [CW 4:2:12]

Review (with M. M. R. Khan): Fairbairn, W. R. D., *Psychoanalytic studies of the personality* (London: Tavistock, 1952). *International Journal of Psycho-Analysis*, 1953, 34. Also published in C. Winnicott, R. Shepherd & M. Davis (Eds.), *Psycho-analytic explorations* (pp. 413–422). Cambridge, MA: Harvard University Press, 1989. [CW 4:2:18]

Symptom tolerance in paediatrics: A case history. *Proceedings of the Royal Society of Medicine*, 1953, 46. Also published in *Collected papers: Through paediatrics to psychoanalysis* (pp. 101–117). London: Tavistock, 1958. [CW 4:2:4]

Transitional objects and transitional phenomena: A study of the first Not-Me possession [1951]. *International Journal of Psychoanalysis*, 1953, 34, 89–97. [CW: 4:2:21] Also published in *Collected papers: Through paediatrics to psycho-analysis* (pp. 229–242). London: Tavistock, 1958. [CW 5:4:24]; and *Playing and reality* (pp. 1–25) London:

Tavistock, 1971. [CW 9:3:5]; and *The collected works of D. W. Winnicott*. New York: Oxford University Press, 2017 [1951 version] [CW 3:6:6]

1954

Mind and its relation to the psyche-soma [1949]. *British Journal of Medical Psychology*, 1954, 27(4), 201–209. Also published in *Collected papers: Through paediatrics to psycho-analysis* (pp. 243–254). London: Tavistock, 1958. [CW 3:4:20]

Needs of the under-fives. *Nursery Journal*, 1954, 44, as 'The needs of the under-fives in a changing society'. Also published in *The child and the outside world: Studies in developing relationships* (pp. 3–13). London: Tavistock, 1957, as 'Needs of the under-fives in a changing society'; and *The child, the family, and the outside world* (pp. 179–188). Harmondsworth: Penguin, 1964. [CW 4:3:18]

Pitfalls in adoption. *Medical Press*, 1954, 232(6031). Also published in *The child and the outside world: Studies in developing relationships* (pp. 45–51). London: Tavistock, 1957; and R. Shepherd, J. Johns & H. Taylor Robinson (Eds.), *Thinking about children* (pp. 128–135). London: Karnac, 1996. [CW 4:3:30]

Preface. Stevenson, O., 'The first treasured possession. A study of the part played by specially loved objects and toys in the lives of certain children'. *The Psychoanalytic Study of the Child*, 1954, 9, 199–201 (International Universities Press, 1954). [CW 4:3:31]

Review: Bakwin, H. & Bakwin, R. M., *Clinical management of behavior disorders in children* (Philadelphia: Saunders, 1953). *British Medical Journal*, 1954, 2(4885), 453. [CW 4:3:22]

Review: Jackson, J., *Aggression and its interpretation* (London: Methuen, 1952). *British Medical Journal*, 1954, 1(4875), 1363. [CW 4:3:17]

Review: Slavson, S. R., *Child psychotherapy* (New York: Columbia University Press, 1952). *British Medical Journal*, 1954, 1(4871), 1135. [CW 4:3:12]

Two adopted children [1953]. *Case Conference*, 1954, 1. Also published in *The child and the outside world: Studies in developing relationships* (pp. 52–65). London: Tavistock, 1957; and R. Shepherd, J. Johns & H. Taylor Robinson (Eds.), *Thinking about children* (pp. 113–127). London: Karnac, 1996. [CW 4:2:19]

1955

Adopted children in adolescence. First published in *Report of Residential Conference, Standing Conference of Societies Registered for Adoption*, July 1955. Also published in R. Shepherd, J. Johns & H. Taylor Robinson (Eds.), *Thinking about children* (pp. 136–148). London: Karnac, 1996. [CW 5:1:12]

A case managed at home. *Case Conference*, 1955, 2, as 'Childhood psychosis: A case managed at home'. Also published in *Collected papers: Through paediatrics to psycho-analysis* (pp. 118–126). London: Tavistock, 1958. [CW 5:1:18]

The depressive position in normal emotional development [1954]. *British Journal of Medical Psychology*, 1955, 28(2–3), 89–100. Also published in *Collected papers: Through paediatrics to psycho-analysis* (pp. 262–277). London: Tavistock, 1958. [CW 4:3:5]

Foreword. Graham Malleson, J., *Any wife or any husband* (2nd ed.) London: Heinemann, 1955. [CW 5:1:19]

Metapsychological and clinical aspects of regression within the psychoanalytical set-up [1954]. *International Journal of Psychoanalysis*, 1955, 36, 16-26. Also published in *Collected papers: Through paediatrics to psycho-analysis* (pp. 278-294). London: Tavistock, 1958. [CW 4:3:6]

Withdrawal and regression [1954]. *Revue Française de Psychanalyse*, 1955, 19, 1-2, as 'Repli et régression'. Also published in *Psyche*, 1956, 10, 1956-1957; and in *Collected papers: Through paediatrics to psycho-analysis* (pp. 255-261). London: Tavistock, 1958; and *Holding and interpretation: Fragment of an analysis* [1955] (pp. 187-192, as 'Appendix: Withdrawal and regression'). London: Karnac, 1986. [CW 4:3:29]

1956

Clinical varieties of transference [1955]. *International Journal of Psychoanalysis*, 1956, 37, 386-388, as 'On transference'. Also published in *Collected papers: Through paediatrics to psycho-analysis* (pp. 295-299). London: Tavistock, 1958. [CW 5:1:11]

1957

The child and the family: First relationships. London: Tavistock, 1957. [Not reprinted in this form in the *Collected Works*]

Preface. ix. [Part of CW 7:1:17]

A man looks at motherhood [1949]. 3-6. In *The ordinary devoted mother and her baby* (pp. 3-6, 'Introduction'). London: C. A. Brock, 1949. Also published in *The child, the family, and the outside world* (pp. 15-18). Harmondsworth: Penguin, 1964. [CW 3:4:23]

Getting to know your baby [1943]. 7-12. First published in *New Era in Home and School*, 1945, 26. Also published in *Getting to know your baby* (pp. 1-5). London: Heinemann, 1945; and *The child, the family, and the outside world* (pp. 19-24). Harmondsworth: Penguin, 1964. Broadcast 10 December 1943. J. Quigley (Producer), *Happy children*. Home Service. London: British Broadcasting Corporation. [CW 2:5:9]

The baby as a going concern. 13-17. First published in *The ordinary devoted mother and her baby* (pp. 7-11). London: C. A. Brock, 1949. Also published in *The child, the family, and the outside world* (pp. 25-29). Harmondsworth: Penguin, 1964. Broadcast 12 October 1949, as 'The mind of a child'. I. Benzie (Producer), *How's the baby?* Home Service. London: British Broadcasting Corporation. [CW 3:4:24]

Infant feeding [1944]. 18-22. First published in *New Era in Home and School*, 1945, 26. Also published in *Getting to know your baby* (pp. 12-16). London: Heinemann, 1945; and *The child, the family, and the outside world* (pp. 30-34). Harmondsworth: Penguin, 1964. [CW 2:6:13]

Where the food goes. 23-27. First published in *The ordinary devoted mother and her baby* (pp. 12-16). London: C. A. Brock, 1949. Also published in *The child, the family, and the outside world* (pp. 35-39). Harmondsworth: Penguin, 1964. Broadcast 19 October 1949, as 'The baby and its food'. I. Benzie (Producer), *How's the baby?* Home Service. London: British Broadcasting Corporation. [CW 3:4:25]

The end of the digestive process. 28–32. First published in *The ordinary devoted mother and her baby* (pp. 17–21). London: C. A. Brock, 1949. Also published in *The child, the family, and the outside world* (pp. 40–44). Harmondsworth: Penguin, 1964. Broadcast 26 October 1949, as 'The passing of excretions'. I. Benzie (Producer), *How's the baby?* Home Service. London: British Broadcasting Corporation. [3:4:26]

The baby as a person. 33–37. First published in *The ordinary devoted mother and her baby* (pp. 22–26). London: C. A. Brock, 1949. Also published in *The child, the family, and the outside world* (pp. 75–79). Harmondsworth: Penguin, 1964. Broadcast 2 November 1949, as 'No baby can grow properly without love'. I. Benzie (Producer), *How's the baby?* Home Service. London: British Broadcasting Corporation. [CW 3:4:27]

Close-up of mother feeding baby. 38–42. First published in *The ordinary devoted mother and her baby* (pp. 27–31). London: C. A. Brock, 1949. Also published in *The child, the family, and the outside world* (pp. 45–49). Harmondsworth: Penguin, 1964. Broadcast 9 November 1949, as 'The baby at feeding time'. I. Benzie (Producer), *How's the baby?* Home Service. London: British Broadcasting Corporation. [CW 3:4:28]

Why do babies cry? [1944]. 43–52. First published in *New Era in Home and School*, 1945, 26. Also published in *Getting to know your baby* (pp. 5–12). London: Heinemann, 1945; and *The child, the family, and the outside world* (pp. 58–68). Harmondsworth: Penguin, 1964; and *Parents*, 1967, 22(8), as 'Winnicott's wisdom: Why babies cry'. Broadcast in two parts, 4 and 11 February 1944, as 'Why does your baby cry?' J. Quigley (Producer), *Happy children*. Home Service. London: British Broadcasting Corporation. [CW 2:6:2]

The world in small doses. 53–58. First published in *The ordinary devoted mother and her baby* (pp. 32–37). London: C. A. Brock, 1949. Also published in *The child, the family, and the outside world* (pp. 69–74). Harmondsworth: Penguin, 1964. Broadcast 16 November 1949, as 'Presenting the world to a baby'. I. Benzie (Producer), *How's the baby?* Home Service. London: British Broadcasting Corporation. [CW 3:4:29]

The innate morality of the baby. 59–63. In *The ordinary devoted mother and her baby* (pp. 38–42). London: C. A. Brock, 1949. Also published in *The child, the family, and the outside world* (pp. 93–97). Harmondsworth: Penguin, 1964. Broadcast 23 November 1949, as 'Problems of management: Training babies' [CW 12:3:4c]. I. Benzie (Producer), *How's the baby?* Home Service. London: British Broadcasting Corporation. [CW 3:4:30]

Weaning. 64–68. First published in *The ordinary devoted mother and her baby* (pp. 43–47). London: C. A. Brock, 1949. Also published in *The child, the family, and the outside world* (pp. 80–84). Harmondsworth: Penguin, 1964. Broadcast 30 November 1949. I. Benzie (Producer), *How's the baby?* Home Service. London: British Broadcasting Corporation. [CW 3:4:31]

Knowing and learning [1950]. 69–73. Also published in C. Winnicott, R. Shepherd & M. Davis (Eds.), *Babies and their mothers* (pp. 15–21). Reading, MA: Addison-Wesley, 1987; and *Winnicott on the child* (pp. 19–23). Cambridge, MA: Perseus, 2002. Broadcast 22 March 1950, as 'Knowing and learning how to be a mother'. I. Benzie (Producer), *How's the baby?* Home Service. London: British Broadcasting Corporation. [CW 3:5:14]

Instincts and normal difficulties [1950]. 74–78. Also published in *The child, the family, and the outside world* (pp. 98–102). Harmondsworth: Penguin, 1964. Broadcast 29 March 1950, as 'Symptoms of illness'. I. Benzie (Producer), *How's the baby?* Home Service. London: British Broadcasting Corporation. [CW 3:5:15]

What about father? [1944]. 81–86. First published in *New Era in Home and School*, 1945, 26; and *Getting to know your baby* (pp. 16–21). London: Heinemann, 1945. Also published in *The child, the family, and the outside world* (pp. 113–118). Harmondsworth: Penguin, 1964. Broadcast 17 March 1944, as 'Where does Dad come in?' J. Quigley (Producer), *Happy children*. Home Service. London: British Broadcasting Corporation. [CW 2:6:8]

Their standards and yours [1944]. 87–91. First published in *New Era in Home and School*, 1945, 26; and *Getting to know your baby* (pp. 21–24). London: Heinemann, 1945. Also published in *The child, the family, and the outside world* (pp. 119–123). Harmondsworth: Penguin, 1964. Broadcast 12 May 1944. J. Quigley (Producer), *Happy children*. Home Service. London: British Broadcasting Corporation. [CW 2:6:9]

Young children and other people. 92–99. First published in *Young Children*, 1949, 1. Also published in *The child, the family, and the outside world* (pp. 103–110). Harmondsworth: Penguin, 1964. [CW 3:4:32]

What do we mean by a normal child? [1944]. 100–106. First published in *New Era in Home and School*, 1946, 27. Also published in *The child, the family, and the outside world* (pp. 124–130). Harmondsworth: Penguin, 1964. Broadcast 23 June 1944. J. Quigley (Producer), *Happy children*. Home Service. London: British Broadcasting Corporation. [CW 2:6:10]

The only child [1945]. 107–111. Also published in *The child, the family, and the outside world* (pp. 131–136). Harmondsworth: Penguin, 1964. Broadcast 2 February 1945. J. Quigley (Producer), *Difficult children*. Home Service. London: British Broadcasting Corporation. [CW 2:7:1]

Twins [1945]. 112–116. Also published in *The child, the family, and the outside world* (pp. 137–142). Harmondsworth: Penguin, 1964. Broadcast 27 April 1945. J. Quigley & D. Bridgman (Producers), *Difficult children*. Home Service. London: British Broadcasting Corporation. [CW 2:7:5]

Stealing and telling lies [1949]. 117–120. Also published in *The child, the family, and the outside world* (pp. 161–166). Harmondsworth: Penguin, 1964. [CW 3:4:33]

Visiting children in hospital [1951]. 121–126. First published in *Child-Family Digest*, 1952; and *New Era in Home and School*, 1952, 33. Also published in *The child, the family, and the outside world* (pp. 221–226). Harmondsworth: Penguin, 1964. Broadcast in two parts, 16 and 23 May 1951. I. Benzie (Producer), *Woman's hour*. Light Programme. London: British Broadcasting Corporation. [CW 3:6:5]

On adoption [1955]. 127–130. Broadcast 23 February 1955, as 'Homeless children and childless homes'. I. Benzie (Producer), *Woman's hour*. Light Programme. London: British Broadcasting Corporation. [CW 5:1:2]

First experiments in independence [1955]. 131–136. Also published in *The child, the family, and the outside world* (pp. 167–172). Harmondsworth: Penguin, 1964. [CW 5:1:20]

Support for normal parents [1944]. 137–140. First published in *New Era in Home and School*, 1945, 26. Also published in *Getting to know your baby* (pp. 25–27, as 'Postscript'). London: Heinemann, 1945; and *The child, the family, and the outside world* (pp. 173–176). Harmondsworth: Penguin, 1964. [CW 2:6:11]

Postscript: The mother's contribution to society. 141–144. Also published in C. Winnicott, R. Shepherd & M. Davis (Eds.), *Home is where we start from: Essays by a psychoanalyst* (pp. 123–127, as 'The mother's contribution to society'). Harmondsworth: Penguin, 1986; and *Winnicott on the child* (pp. 202–206, as 'The mother's contribution to society'). Cambridge, MA: Perseus, 2002. [CW 5:3:30]

The child and the outside world: Studies in developing relationships. London: Tavistock, 1957. [Not reprinted in this form in the *Collected Works*]

    Needs of the under-fives in a changing society [1954]. 3–13. *Nursery Journal*, 1954, 44. Also published in *The child, the family, and the outside world* (pp. 179–188, as 'Needs of the under-fives'). Harmondsworth: Penguin, 1964. [CW 4:3:18]

    The child's needs and the role of the mother in the early stages. 14–23. Published here as 'Mother, teacher, and the child's needs'. [CW 4:2:20]

    On influencing and being influenced. 35–39. First published in *New Era in Home and School*, 1941, 22. Also published in *The child, the family, and the outside world* (pp. 199–204). Harmondsworth: Penguin, 1964. [CW 2:3:3]

    Educational diagnosis. 29–34. First published in *National Froebel Foundation Bulletin*, 1946 41, 3. Also published in *The child, the family, and the outside world* (pp. 205–210). Harmondsworth: Penguin, 1964. [CW 3:1:2]

    Shyness and nervous disorders in children. 35–39. First published in *New Era in Home and School*, 1938, 19. Also published in *The child, the family, and the outside world* (pp. 211–215).Harmondsworth: Penguin, 1964. [CW 1:4:17]

    Sex education in schools. 40–44. First published in *Medical Press*, 1949, 222. Also published in *The child, the family, and the outside world* (pp. 216–220). Harmondsworth: Penguin, 1964. [CW 3:4:35]

    Pitfalls in adoption. 45–51. First published in *Medical Press*, 1954, 232(6031). Also published in R. Shepherd, J. Johns & H. Taylor Robinson (Eds.), *Thinking about children* (pp. 128–135). London: Karnac, 1996. [CW 4:3:30]

    Two adopted children [1953]. 52–65. First published in *Case Conference*, 1954, 1. Also published in R. Shepherd, J. Johns & H. Taylor Robinson (Eds.), *Thinking about children* (pp. 113–127). London: Karnac, 1996. [CW 4:2:19]

    Children in the war. 69–74. First published in *New Era in Home and School*, 1940, 21. Also published in C. Winnicott, R. Shepherd & M. Davis (Eds.), *Deprivation and delinquency* (pp. 25–30). London: Tavistock, 1984. [CW 2:2:4]

    The deprived mother [1939]. 75–82. First published in *New Era in Home and School*, 1940, 21(3). Also published in C. Winnicott, R. Shepherd & M. Davis (Eds.), *Deprivation and delinquency* (pp. 31–38). London: Tavistock, 1984. Broadcast 1939. London: British Broadcasting Corporation. [CW 2:1:4]

    The evacuated child [1945]. 83–87. Also published in C. Winnicott, R. Shepherd & M. Davis (Eds.), *Deprivation and delinquency* (pp. 39–43). London: Tavistock, 1984. Broadcast 16 February 1945. J. Quigley & D. Bridgman (Producers), *Difficult children*. Home Service. London: British Broadcasting Corporation. [CW 2:7:2]

    The return of the evacuated child [1945]. 88–92. Also published in C. Winnicott, R. Shepherd & M. Davis (Eds.), *Deprivation and delinquency* (pp. 44–48). London: Tavistock, 1984. Broadcast 23 February 1945. J. Quigley & D. Bridgman (Producers), *Difficult children*. Home Service. London: British Broadcasting Corporation. [CW 2:7:3]

    Home again [1945]. 93–97. Also published in C. Winnicott, R. Shepherd & M. Davis (Eds.), *Deprivation and delinquency* (pp. 49–53). London: Tavistock, 1984. Broadcast 22 June 1945. J. Quigley & D. Bridgman (Producers), *Health magazine*. Home Service. London: British Broadcasting Corporation. [CW 2:7:7]

    Residential management as treatment for difficult children (with C. Britton). 98–116. First published in part, as 'Residential management as treatment for difficult children: The evolution of a wartime hostels scheme'. *Human Relations*, *1*(1), 87–97; and, in part, in 'The problem of homeless children'. *New Education Fellowship Monograph*, No. 1, 1944. Also published in C. Winnicott, R. Shepherd & M. Davis (Eds.), *Deprivation and delinquency* (pp. 54–72). London: Tavistock, 1984. [CW 3:2:3]

Children's hostels in war and peace [1946]. 117–121. First published in *British Journal of Medical Psychology*, 1948, *21*(3), 175. Also published in C. Winnicott, R. Shepherd & M. Davis (Eds.), *Deprivation and delinquency* (pp. 73–77). London: Tavistock, 1984. [CW 3:1:1]

Towards an objective study of human nature. 125–133. First published in *New Era in Home and School*, 1945, *26*, as 'Talking about psychology'; reissued in *33*(3), 1952, as 'What is psychoanalysis?' Also published in R. Shepherd, J. Johns & H. Taylor Robinson (Eds.), *Thinking about children* (pp. 3–12). London: Karnac, 1996. [CW 2:7:11]

Further thoughts on babies as persons. 134–140. *New Era in Home and School*, 1947, *28*(10), 179, as 'Babies are persons'. Also published in *The child, the family, and the outside world* (pp. 85–92). Harmondsworth: Penguin, 1964. [CW 3:2:4]

Breast feeding [1945, revised 1954]. 141–148. Also published in *The child, the family, and the outside world* (pp. 50–57). Harmondsworth: Penguin, 1964. [CW 2:7:12]

Why children play. 149–152. First published in *New Era in Home and School*, 1942, *23*. Also published in *The child, the family, and the outside world* (pp. 143–146). Harmondsworth: Penguin, 1964, revised 1968. [CW 2:4:4]

The child and sex. 153–166. First published in *The Practitioner*, 1947, *158*. Also published in *The child, the family, and the outside world* (pp. 147–160). Harmondsworth: Penguin, 1964. [CW 3:2:5]

Aggression. [ca. 1939]. 167–175. Also published in C. Winnicott, R. Shepherd & M. Davis (Eds.), *Deprivation and delinquency* (pp. 84–92). London: Tavistock, 1984, part of 'Aggression and its roots'. [CW 2:1:8]

The impulse to steal [1949]. 176–180. [CW 3:4:34]

Some psychological aspects of juvenile delinquency. 181–187. First published in *New Era in Home and School*, 1946, *27*. Also published in *Delinquency Research*, 1946, *24*; and C. Winnicott, R. Shepherd & M. Davis (Eds.), *Deprivation and delinquency* (pp. 113–119). London: Tavistock, 1984. [CW 3:1:7] See also 'Aspects of juvenile delinquency'.

The contribution of psycho-analysis to midwifery. *Nursing Mirror*, May 1957. Also published in *The family and individual development* (pp. 106–113). London: Tavistock, 1965; and C. Winnicott, R. Shepherd & M. Davis (Eds.), *Babies and their mothers* (pp. 69–81). Reading, MA: Addison-Wesley, 1987; and *Winnicott on the child* (pp. 56–64). Cambridge, MA: Perseus, 2002. [CW 5:3:15]

Health education through broadcasting. *Mother and Child*, 1957, *28*. Also published in C. Winnicott, C. Bollas, M. Davis & R. Shepherd (Eds.), *Talking to parents* (pp. 1–6). Reading, MA: Addison-Wesley, 1993; and *Winnicott on the child* (pp. 95–98). Cambridge, MA: Perseus, 2002. [CW 5:3:31]

Review: Foote, E. J., *Six children* (London: Thomas, 1956). *British Medical Journal*, 1957, *1*(5027), 1105. [CW 5:3:14]

1958

The capacity to be alone [1957]. *International Journal of Psychoanalysis*, 1958, *39*, 416–420. Also published in *Psyche*, 1958, *12*, as 'Über die Fähigkeit, allein zu sein'; and *The maturational processes and the facilitating environment: Studies in the theory of emotional development* (pp. 29–36). London: Hogarth, 1965. [CW 5:3:20]

Child analysis in the latency period. *A Criança Portuguesa*, 1958, *17*. Also published in *The maturational processes and the facilitating environment: Studies in the theory of emotional development* (pp. 115–123). London: Hogarth, 1965. [CW 5:4:13]

Collected papers: Through paediatrics to psycho-analysis. London: Tavistock, 1958. Second edition with an introduction by M. M. R. Khan. London: Hogarth and the Institute of Psycho-Analysis, 1975. [Not reprinted in this form in the *Collected Works*]

Preface and acknowledgements. ix–x. [CW 5:3:32]

A note on normality and anxiety. 3–21. First published in *Clinical notes on disorders of childhood* (pp. 98–121). London: Heinemann, 1931. [CW 1:3:12]

Fidgetiness. 22–30. First published in *Clinical notes on disorders of childhood* (pp. 87–97). London: Heinemann, 1931. [CW 1:3:11]

Appetite and emotional disorder [1936]. 33–51. [CW 1:4:11]

The observation of infants in a set situation. 52–69. First published in *International Journal of Psychoanalysis*, 1941, *22*, 229–249. [CW 2:3:6]

Child department consultations. 70–84. First published in *International Journal of Psychoanalysis*, 1942, *23*, 139–146. [CW 2:4:2]

Ocular psychoneuroses of childhood. 85–90. First published in *Transactions of the Ophthalmological Society of the United Kingdom*, 1944, *64*, 46–52, as 'Discussion on ocular psychoneuroses'. [CW 2:6:15]

Reparation in respect of mother's organised defence against depression [1948]. 91–96. [CW 3:3:1]

Anxiety associated with insecurity [1952]. 97–100. [CW 4:1:11]

Symptom tolerance in paediatrics: A case history. 101–117. First published in *Proceedings of the Royal Society of Medicine*, 1953, *46*. [CW 4:2:4]

A case managed at home. 118–126. First published in *Case Conference*, 1955, *2*, as 'Childhood psychosis: A case managed at home'. [CW 5:1:18]

The manic defence. [1935]. 129–144. [CW 1:4:6]

Primitive emotional development. 145–156. First published in *International Journal of Psychoanalysis*, 1945, *26*, 137–143. [CW 2:7:8]

Paediatrics and psychiatry. 157–173. First published in *British Journal of Medical Psychology*, 1948, *21*(4), 229–240. [CW 3:3:2]

Birth memories, birth trauma, and anxiety [1949]. 174–193. [CW 3:4:8]

Hate in the countertransference [1947]. 194–203. First published in *International Journal of Psychoanalysis*, 1949, *30*, 69–74. [CW 3:2:1]

Aggression in relation to emotional development [1950]. 204–218. [CW 3:5:2]

Psychoses and child care [1952]. 219–228. First published in *British Journal of Medical Psychology*, 1953, *26*(1), 68–74. [CW 4:1:5]

Transitional objects and transitional phenomena. 229–242. [CW 5:4:24] First published in *International Journal of Psychoanalysis*, 1953, *34*, 89–97, as 'Transitional objects and transitional phenomena: A study of the first Not-Me possession'. [CW 4:2:21]. Also published in *Playing and reality* (pp. 1–25). London: Tavistock, 1971. [CW 9:3:5]; and *The collected works of D. W. Winnicott*. New York: Oxford University Press, 2017 [1951 version] [CW 3:6:6]

Mind and its relation to the psyche-soma [1949]. 243–254. First published in *British Journal of Medical Psychology*, 1954, *27*(4), 201–209. [CW 3:4:20]

Withdrawal and regression [1954]. 255–261. First published in *Revue Française de Psychanalyse*, 1955, *19*, 1–2, as 'Repli et régression'. Also published in *Psyche, 10*, 1956–1957; and *Holding and interpretation: Fragment of an analysis* [1955], The Institute of Psychoanalysis (pp. 187–192 'Appendix'). London: Karnac, 1986. [CW 4:3:29]

The depressive position in normal emotional development [1954]. 262–277. First published in *British Journal of Medical Psychology*, 1955, *28*(2–3), 89–100. [CW 4:3:5]

Metapsychological and clinical aspects of regression within the psychoanalytical set-up [1954]. 278–294. First published in *International Journal of Psychoanalysis*, 1955, *36*, 16–26. [CW 4:3:6]

Clinical varieties of transference [1955]. 295–299. *International Journal of Psychoanalysis*, 1956, *37*, 386–388, as 'On transference'. [CW 5:1:11]

Primary maternal preoccupation [1956]. 300–305. [CW 5:2:16]

The antisocial tendency [1956]. 306–315. Also published in C. Winnicott, R. Shepherd & M. Davis (Eds.), *Deprivation and delinquency* (pp. 120–131). London: Tavistock, 1984. [CW 5:2:8]

Paediatrics and childhood neurosis [1956]. 316–321. [CW 5:2:11]

On the contribution of direct child observation to psychoanalysis [1957]. *Revue Française de Psychanalyse*, 1958, 22, as 'Discussion sur la contribution de l'observation directe de l'enfant à la psychanalyse'. Also published in *The maturational processes and the facilitating environment: Studies in the theory of emotional development* (pp. 109–114). London: Hogarth, 1965. [CW 5:3:21]

The first year of life. *Medical Press*, March 1958, as 'Modern views on the emotional development in the first year of life'. Also published in *The family and individual development* (pp. 3–14). London: Tavistock, 1965. [CW 5:4:6]

Foreword. *The case as the patient sees it: Psycho-analysis* [1957]. London: National Association of Mental Health, 1958. [CW 5:3:17]

Funeral address for Ernest Jones. *International Journal of Psychoanalysis*, 1958, *39*, 305–306. Also published in C. Winnicott, R. Shepherd & M. Davis (Eds.), *Psycho-analytic explorations* (pp. 405–407). Cambridge, MA: Harvard University Press, 1989. [CW 5:4:3]

Obituary: Jones, Ernest. *International Journal of Psychoanalysis*, 1958, *39*, 298–303. Also published in C. Winnicott, R. Shepherd & M. Davis (Eds.), *Psycho-analytic explorations* (pp. 393–404). Cambridge, MA: Harvard University Press, 1989. [CW 5:4:21]

Obituary: Wilson, Dr Ambrose Cyril. *International Journal of Psychoanalysis*, 1958, *39*, 617. [CW 5:4:22]

Psycho-analysis and the sense of guilt [1956]. In J. D. Sutherland (Ed.), *Psychoanalysis and contemporary thought* (pp. 15–32). London: Hogarth, 1958. Also published in *The maturational processes and the facilitating environment: Studies in the theory of emotional development* (pp. 15–28). London: Hogarth, 1965. [CW 5:2:7]

Review: Balint, M., *The doctor, his patients and the illness* (London: Pitman, 1957). *International Journal of Psychoanalysis*, 1958, *39*, 425–427. Also published in C. Winnicott, R. Shepherd & M. Davis (Eds.), *Psycho-analytic explorations* (pp. 438–442). Cambridge, MA: Harvard University Press, 1989. [CW 5:4:23]

Review: Eissler, R. S., Freud, A., Hartmann, H., Kris, E. (Eds.), *The psychoanalytic study of the child* (Vol. 11) (London: Imago, 1956). *British Medical Journal*, 22 March 1958, *1*(5072), 692. [CW 5:4:5]

Review: Eissler, R. S., Freud, A., Hartmann, H., Kris, E. (Eds.), *The psychoanalytic study of the child* (Vol. 12) (London: Imago, 1957). *British Medical Journal*, 4 October 1958, *2*(5100), 838. [CW 5:4:15]

Theoretical statement of the field of child psychiatry. In A. Holzel & J. P. M. Tizard (Eds.), *Modern trends in paediatrics* (pp. 250–262, part of the chapter 'Child psychiatry'). London: Butterworth, 1958. Also published in *The family and individual development* (pp. 97–105). London: Tavistock, 1965. [CW 5:4:25]

1959

Obituary: Friedmann, Oscar. *International Journal of Psychoanalysis*, 1959, *40*, 247–248. [CW 5:5:25]

Review: Klein, M., *Envy and gratitude* (London: Tavistock, 1957). *Case Conference*, 1959, *5*, as 'On envy'. Also published in C. Winnicott, R. Shepherd & M. Davis (Eds.), *Psycho-analytic explorations* (pp. 443–446). Cambridge, MA: Harvard University Press, 1989. [CW 5:5:1]

Review: Robertson, J., *Going to hospital with mother* (film) (London: Tavistock Institute of Human Relations, 1958). *International Journal of Psychoanalysis*, 1959, *40*, 62–63. [CW 5:5:23]

1960

Countertransference [1959]. *British Journal of Medical Psychology*, 1960, *33*(1), 17–21. Also published in *The maturational processes and the facilitating environment: Studies in the theory of emotional development* (pp. 158–168). London: Hogarth, 1965. [CW 5:5:20]

Obituary: Klein, Melanie. *British Medical Journal*, 1 October, 1960, *2*(5204), 1026. [CW 6:1:15]

String: A technique of communication. *Journal of Child Psychology and Psychiatry*, 1960, *1*(1), 49–52, as 'String'. Also published in *The maturational processes and the facilitating environment: Studies in the theory of emotional development* (pp. 153–157). London: Hogarth, 1965; and *Playing and reality* (pp. 15–20, part of 'Transitional objects and transitional phenomena'). London: Tavistock, 1971. [CW 6:1:20]

The theory of the parent-infant relationship. *International Journal of Psychoanalysis*, 1960, *41*, 585–595. Also published in *The maturational processes and the facilitating environment: Studies in the theory of emotional development* (pp. 37–55). London: Hogarth, 1965. [CW 6:1:21]

1961

The effect of psychotic parents on the emotional development of the child [1959]. *British Journal of Psychiatric Social Work*, 1961, *6*(1), 13–20. Also published in *The family and individual development* (pp. 69–78). London: Tavistock, 1965. [CW 5:5:21]

Integrative and disruptive factors in family life [1957]. *Canadian Medical Association Journal*, 1961, *84*(15), 814–815, as 'Integrating and disruptive factors in family life'. Also published in *The family and individual development* (pp. 40–49). London: Tavistock, 1965). [CW 5:3:26]

The paediatric department of psychology. *St Mary's Hospital Gazette*, 1961, 67. Also published in R. Shepherd, J. Johns & H. Taylor Robinson (Eds.), *Thinking about children* (pp. 227–230). London: Karnac, 1996, as 'Training for child psychiatry: the paediatric department of psychology'. [CW 6:2:19]

Review: Simey, T. S., *The concept of love in child care* (Oxford University Press, 1961). *New Statesman*, 5 May 1961. [CW 6:2:8]

Review: Soddy, K., *Clinical child psychiatry* (London: Baillière, Tindall and Cox, 1960). *British Medical Journal*, 1961, 1, 1443. [CW 6:2:10]

1962

Adolescence: Struggling through the doldrums [1961]. *New Era in Home and School*, 1962, October, 43(8), as 'Adolescence'. Also published in *The family and individual development* (pp. 79–87). London: Tavistock, 1965. [CW 6:2:4] See also 'Struggling through the doldrums'.

A child psychiatry interview. *St Mary's Hospital Gazette*, 1962, 68. Also published in *Therapeutic consultations in child psychiatry* (pp. 105–109, as '"Rosemary" aet 10 years'). London: Hogarth, 1971. Published here as '"Rosemary" aet 10 years'. [CW 10:1:6]

Review: Bergeron, M., *Psychologie du premier âge* (Paris: Presses universitaires de France, 1961). *Archive of Diseases in Childhood*, 1962, 37. [CW 6:3:16]

Review: Eissler, R. S., Freud, A., Hartmann, H., Kris, M. (Eds.), *The psychoanalytic study of the child* (Vol. 15) (London: Imago, 1960). *British Medical Journal*, 3 February 1962, 1(5274), 305–306. [CW 6:3:1]

Review: Jones, E. (Ed.), *Letters of Sigmund Freud 1873–1939* (London: Hogarth, 1961). *British Journal of Psychology*, 1962, 53. Also published in C. Winnicott, R. Shepherd & M. Davis (Eds.), *Psycho-analytic explorations* (pp. 474–477). Cambridge, MA: Harvard University Press, 1989. [CW 6:3:15]

Review: Lebovici, S. & McDougall, J., *Un cas de psychose infantile* (Paris: Presses universitaires de France, 1960). *Journal of Child Psychology and Psychiatry*, 1962, 3(1), 63–64. [CW 6:3:17]

The theory of the parent-infant relationship: Contributions to discussion. *International Journal of Psychoanalysis*, 1962, 43, 256–257. [CW 6:3:14]

The theory of the parent-infant relationship. Further remarks. *International Journal of Psychoanalysis*, 1962, 43, 238–239. Also published in C. Winnicott, R. Shepherd & M. Davis (Eds.), *Psycho-analytic explorations* (pp. 73–75). Cambridge, MA: Harvard University Press, 1989. [CW 6:3:13]

1963

Dependence in infant-care, in child-care, and in the psycho-analytic setting [1962]. *International Journal of Psychoanalysis*, 1963, 44, 339–344. Also published in *The maturational processes and the facilitating environment: Studies in the theory of emotional development* (pp. 249–259). London: Hogarth, 1965. [CW 6:3:9]

The development of the capacity for concern [1962]. *Bulletin of the Menninger Clinic*, 1963, 27. Also published in *The maturational processes and the facilitating environment: Studies in the theory of emotional development* (pp. 73–82). London: Hogarth,

1965; and C. Winnicott, R. Shepherd & M. Davis (Eds.), *Deprivation and delinquency* (pp. 100-105). London: Tavistock, 1984; and *Winnicott on the child* (pp. 215-220). Cambridge, MA: Perseus, 2002. [CW 6:3:11]

The mentally ill in your caseload. In J. F. S. King (Ed.), *New thinking for changing needs* (pp. 50-66). London: The Association of Social Workers, 1963. Also published in *The maturational processes and the facilitating environment: Studies in the theory of emotional development* (pp. 217-229). London: Hogarth, 1965. [CW 6:4:5]

Morals and education [1962]. In W. R. Niblett (Ed.), *Moral education in a changing society* (pp. 96-111, as 'The young child at home and at school'). London: Faber, 1963. Also published in *The maturational processes and the facilitating environment: Studies in the theory of emotional development* (pp. 93-105). London: Hogarth, 1965. [CW 6:3:18]

A psychotherapeutic consultation: A case of stammering. *A Criança Portuguesa*, 1963, 21. Introduction published in [CW 10: Appendix 3]. Also published in *Therapeutic consultations in child psychiatry* (pp. 110-126, as '"Alfred" aet 10 years'). London: Hogarth, 1971. Published here as '"Alfred" aet 10 years'. [CW 10:1:7]

Regression as therapy illustrated by the case of a boy whose pathological dependence was adequately met by the parents. *British Journal of Medical Psychology*, 1963, 36. Also published in *Therapeutic consultations in child psychiatry* (pp. 239-269, as '"Cecil" aet 21 months at first consultation'). London: Hogarth, 1971. Published here as '"Cecil" aet 21 months at first consultation'. [CW 10:3:14]

Review: Eissler, R. S., Freud, A., Hartmann, H. & Kris, M. (Eds.) *The psychoanalytic study of the child* (Vol. 16) (London: Imago, 1961). *British Medical Journal*, 26 January 1963, 1(5325), 253. [CW 6:4:1]

Review: Goldfarb, W., *Childhood schizophrenia* (Cambridge, MA: Harvard University Press, 1961). *British Journal of Psychiatric Social Work*, 1963, 7(1), 50-51. Also published in R. Shepherd, J. Johns & H. Taylor Robinson (Eds.), *Thinking about children* (pp. 193-194). London: Karnac, 1996. [CW 6:4:17]

Review: Searles, H. F., *The non-human environment* (New York: International Universities Press, 1960). *International Journal of Psychoanalysis*, 1963, 44, 237-238. Also published in C. Winnicott, R. Shepherd & M. Davis (Eds.), *Psychoanalytic explorations* (pp. 478-481). Cambridge, MA: Harvard University Press, 1989. [CW 6:4:16]

Struggling through the doldrums. *New Society*, 25 April 1963 1(30), 8-11. Also published in C. Winnicott, R. Shepherd & M. Davis (Eds.), *Deprivation and delinquency* (pp. 145-155). London: Tavistock, 1984. [CW 6:4:7]

Training for child psychiatry [1962]. *Journal of Child Psychology and Psychiatry*, 1963, 4(2), 85-91. Also published in *The maturational processes and the facilitating environment: Studies in the theory of emotional development* (pp. 193-202). London: Hogarth, 1965. [CW 6:3:5]

1964

The child, the family, and the outside world. Harmondsworth: Penguin, 1964. [Not reprinted in this form in the *Collected Works*]

Introduction. 9-11. [CW 7:1:17]

A man looks at motherhood [1949]. 15-18. First published in *The ordinary devoted mother and her baby* (pp. 3-6, 'Introduction'). London: Tavistock, 1957. Also published in *The child and the family: First relationships* (pp. 3–6, 'Introduction'). London: Tavistock, 1957. [CW 3:4:23]

Getting to know your baby [1943]. 19–24. First published in *New Era in Home and School*, 1945, 26. Also published in *Getting to know your baby* (pp. 1–5). London: Heinemann, 1945; and *The child and the family: First relationships* (pp. 7–12). London: Tavistock, 1957. Broadcast 10 December 1943. J. Quigley (Producer), *Happy children*. Home Service. London: British Broadcasting Corporation. [CW 2:5:8]

The baby as a going concern. 25–29. First published in *The ordinary devoted mother and her baby* (pp. 7–11). London: C. A. Brock, 1949. Also published in *The child and the family: First relationships* (pp. 13–17). London: Tavistock, 1957. Broadcast 12 October 1949, as 'The mind of a child'. I. Benzie (Producer). *How's the baby?* Home Service. London: British Broadcasting Corporation. [CW 3:4:24]

Infant feeding [1944]. 30–34. First published in *New Era in Home and School*, 1945, 26. Also published in *Getting to know your baby* (pp. 12–16). London: Heinemann, 1945; and *The child and the family: First relationships* (pp. 18–22). London: Tavistock, 1957. [CW 2:6:13]

Where the food goes. 35–39. First published in *The ordinary devoted mother and her baby* (pp. 12–16). London: C. A. Brock, 1949. Also published in *The child and the family: First relationships* (pp. 23–27). London: Tavistock, 1957. Broadcast 19 October 1949, as 'The baby and its food'. I. Benzie (Producer), *How's the baby?* Home Service. London: British Broadcasting Corporation. [CW 3:4:25]

The end of the digestive process. 40–44. First published in *The ordinary devoted mother and her baby* (pp. 17–21). London: C. A. Brock, 1949. Also published in *The child and the family: First relationships* (pp. 28–32). London: Tavistock, 1957. Broadcast 26 October 1949, as 'The passing of excretions'. I. Benzie (Producer), *How's the baby?* Home Service. London: British Broadcasting Corporation. [CW 3:4:26]

Close-up of mother feeding baby. 45–49. First published in *The ordinary devoted mother and her baby* (pp. 27–31). London: C. A. Brock, 1949. Also published in *The child and the family: First relationships* (pp. 38–42). London: Tavistock, 1957. Broadcast 9 November 1949, as 'The baby at feeding time'. I. Benzie (Producer), *How's the baby?* Home Service. London: British Broadcasting Corporation. [CW 3:4:28]

Breast feeding [1945, revised 1954]. 50–57. First published in *The child and the outside world* (pp. 141–148). London: Tavistock, 1957. [CW 2:7:12]

Why do babies cry? [1944]. 58–68. First published in *New Era in Home and School*, 1945, 26. Also published in *Getting to know your baby* (pp. 5–12). London: Heinemann, 1945; and *The child and the family: First relationships* (pp. 43–52). London: Tavistock, 1957; and *Parents*, 1967, 22(8), as 'Winnicott's wisdom: Why babies cry'. Broadcast in two parts, 4 and 11 February 1944, as 'Why does your baby cry?' J. Quigley (Producer), *Happy children*. Home Service. London: British Broadcasting Corporation. [CW 2:6:2]

The world in small doses. 69–74. First published in *The ordinary devoted mother and her baby* (pp. 32–37). London: C. A. Brock, 1949. Also published in *The child and the family: First relationships* (pp. 53–58). London: Tavistock, 1957. Broadcast 16

November 1949, as 'Presenting the world to a baby'. I. Benzie (Producer), *How's the baby?* Home Service. London: British Broadcasting Corporation. [CW 3:4:29]

The baby as a person. 75–79. First published in *The ordinary devoted mother and her baby* (pp. 22–26). London: C. A. Brock, 1949. Also published in *The child and the family: First relationships* (pp. 33–37). London: Tavistock, 1957. Broadcast 2 November 1949, as 'No baby can grow properly without love'. I. Benzie (Producer), *How's the baby?* Home Service. London: British Broadcasting Corporation. [3:4:27]

Weaning. 80–84. First published in *The ordinary devoted mother and her baby* (pp. 43–47). London: C. A. Brock, 1949. Also published in *The child and the family: First relationships* (pp. 64–68). London: Tavistock, 1957. Broadcast 30 November 1949. I. Benzie (Producer), *How's the baby?* Home Service. London: British Broadcasting Corporation. [CW 3:4:31]

Further thoughts on babies as persons. 85–92. First published in *New Era in Home and School*, 1947, 28(10), p. 179, as 'Babies are persons'. Also published in *The child and the outside world: Studies in developing relationships* (pp. 134–140). London: Tavistock, 1957. [CW 3:2:4]

The innate morality of the baby. 93–97. First published in *The ordinary devoted mother and her baby* (pp. 38–42). London: C. A. Brock, 1949. Also published in *The child and the family: First relationships* (pp. 59–63). London: Tavistock, 1957. Broadcast 23 November 1949, as 'Problems of management: Training babies' [CW 12:3:4c]. I. Benzie (Producer), *How's the baby?* Home Service. London: British Broadcasting Corporation. [CW 3:4:30]

Instincts and normal difficulties [1950]. 98–102. First published in *The child and the family: First relationships* (pp. 74–78). London: Tavistock, 1957. Broadcast 29 March 1950, as 'Symptoms of illness'. I. Benzie (Producer), *How's the baby?* Home Service. London: British Broadcasting Corporation. [CW 3:5:15]

Young children and other people. 103–110. First published in *Young Children*, 1949, 1. Also published in *The child and the family: First relationships* (pp. 92–99). London: Tavistock, 1957. [CW 3:4:32]

What about father? [1944]. 113–118. First published in *New Era in Home and School*, 1945, 26. Also published in *Getting to know your baby* (pp. 16–21). London: Heinemann, 1945; and *The child and the family: First relationships* (pp. 81–86). London: Tavistock, 1957. Broadcast 17 March 1944, as 'Where does Dad come in?' J. Quigley (Producer), *Happy children*. Home Service. London: British Broadcasting Corporation. [CW 2:6:8]

Their standards and yours [1944]. 119–123. First published in *New Era in Home and School*, 1945, 26. Also published in *Getting to know your baby* (pp. 21–24). London: Heinemann, 1945; and *The child and the family: First relationships* (pp. 87–91). London: Tavistock, 1957. Broadcast 12 May 1944. J. Quigley (Producer), *Happy children*. Home Service. London: British Broadcasting Corporation. [CW 2:6:9]

What do we mean by a normal child? [1944]. 124–130. First published in *New Era in Home and School*, 1946, 27. Also published in *The child and the family: First relationships* (pp. 100–106). Home Service. London: Tavistock, 1957. Broadcast 23 June 1944. J. Quigley (Producer), *Happy children*. Home Service. London: British Broadcasting Corporation. [CW 2:6:10]

The only child [1945]. 131–136. First published in *The child and the family: First relationships* (pp. 107–111). London: Tavistock, 1957. Broadcast 2 February 1945. J.

Quigley (Producer), *Difficult children*. London: British Broadcasting Corporation. [CW 2:7:1]

Twins [1945]. 137–142. First published in *The child and the family: First relationships* (pp. 112–116). London: Tavistock, 1957. Broadcast 27 April 1945. J. Quigley & D. Bridgman (Producers), *Difficult children*. Home Service. London: British Broadcasting Corporation. [CW 2:7:5]

Why children play [revised 1968]. 143–146. First published in *New Era in Home and School*, 1942, 23. Also published in *The child and the outside world: Studies in developing relationships* (pp. 149–152). London: Tavistock, 1957. [CW 2:4:4]

The child and sex. 147–160. First published in *The Practitioner*, 1947, 158. Also published in *The child and the outside world: Studies in developing relationships* (pp. 153–166). London: Tavistock, 1957. [CW 3:2:5]

Stealing and telling lies [1949]. 161–166. First published in *The child and the family: First relationships* (pp. 117–120). London: Tavistock, 1957. [CW 3:4:33]

First experiments in independence [1955]. 167–172. First published in *The child and the family: First relationships* (pp. 131–136). London: Tavistock, 1957. [CW 5:1:20]

Support for normal parents [1944]. 173–176. First published in *New Era in Home and School*, 1945, 26. Also published in *Getting to know your baby* (pp. 25–27). London: Heinemann, 1945, as 'Postscript'; and *The child and the family: First relationships* (pp. 137–140). London: Tavistock, 1957. Broadcast 1944 as part of J. Quigley (Producer), *Happy children*. Home Service. London: British Broadcasting Corporation. [CW 2:6:11]

Needs of the under-fives [1954]. 179–188. First published in *Nursery Journal*, 1954, 44, as 'The needs of the under-fives in a changing society'. Also published in *The child and the outside world: Studies in developing relationships* (pp. 3–13, as 'Needs of the under-fives in a changing society'). London: Tavistock, 1957. [CW 4:3:18]

Mother, teacher, and the child's needs (with other members of the joint WHO-UNESCO expert group). 189–198. First published in *Problems in education* (Vol. 9, as 'The child's needs and the role of the mother in the early stages'). New York: Unesco 1953. Also published in *The child and the outside world: Studies in developing relationships* (pp. 14–23). London: Tavistock, 1957. [CW 4:2:20]

On influencing and being influenced. 199–204. First published in *New Era in Home and School*, 1941, 22. Also published in *The child and the outside world: Studies in developing relationships* (pp. 35–39). London: Tavistock, 1957. [CW 2:3:3]

Educational diagnosis. 205–210. First published in *National Froebel Foundation Bulletin*, 1946, 41, 3. Also published in *The child and the outside world: Studies in developing relationships* (pp. 29–34). London: Tavistock, 1957. [CW 3:1:2]

Shyness and nervous disorders in children. 211–215. First published in *New Era in Home and School*, 1938, 19. Also published in *The child and the outside world: Studies in developing relationships* (pp. 35–39). London: Tavistock, 1957. [CW 1:4:17]

Sex education in schools. 216–220. First published in *Medical Press*, 1949, 222. Also published in *The child and the outside world: Studies in developing relationships* (pp. 40–44). London: Tavistock, 1957. [CW 3:4:35]

Visiting children in hospital [1951]. 221–226. First published in *Child-Family Digest*, October, 1952. Also published in *New Era in Home and School*, 1952, 33; and *The child and the family: First relationships* (pp. 121–126). London: Tavistock, 1957. Broadcast in two parts, 16 and 23 May 1951. I. Benzie (Producer), *Woman's hour*. Light Programme. London: British Broadcasting Corporation. [CW 3:6:5]

Aspects of juvenile delinquency. 227–231. Published here as 'Some psychological aspects of juvenile delinquency'. [CW 3:1:7]

Roots of aggression. 232–239. Also published in C. Winnicott, R. Shepherd & M. Davis (Eds.), *Deprivation and delinquency* (pp. 92–99, part of 'Aggression and its roots'). London: Tavistock, 1984. [CW 7:1:18]

Deductions drawn from a psychotherapeutic interview with an adolescent. In *Report of the 20th Child Guidance Inter-Clinic Conference*. London: The National Association for Mental Health, 1964. Also published in C. Winnicott, R. Shepherd & M. Davis (Eds.), *Psycho-analytic explorations* (pp. 325–340). Cambridge, MA: Harvard University Press, 1989. [CW 7:1:5]

Foreword. Torrie, M., *The widow's child*. Richmond, Surrey: Cruse Club, 1964. [CW 7:1:12]

The neonate and his mother. *Acta Paediatrica Latina*, 1964, 17. Also published in C. Winnicott, R. Shepherd & M. Davis (Eds.), *Babies and their mothers* (pp. 35–49, as 'The newborn and his mother'). Reading, MA: Addison-Wesley, 1987; and *Winnicott on the child* (pp. 32–42, as 'The newborn and his mother'). Cambridge, MA: Perseus, 2002. [CW 7:1:4]

Review: Jung, C. G., *Memories, dreams, reflections* (London: Collins and Routledge, 1963). *International Journal of Psychoanalysis*, 1964, 45, 450–454. Also published in C. Winnicott, R. Shepherd & M. Davis (Eds.), *Psycho-analytic explorations* (pp. 482–492). Cambridge, MA: Harvard University Press, 1989. [CW 7:1:16]

Review: Riese, H., *Heal the hurt child* (Chicago: Chicago University Press, 1963). *New Society*, 30 January 1964, 3(70), 27. [CW 7:1:2]

The value of depression [1963]. *British Journal of Psychiatric Social Work*, 1964, 7; and *The Observer*, 31 May 1964, as 'Strength out of misery'. Also published in C. Winnicott, R. Shepherd & M. Davis (Eds.), *Home is where we start from: Essays by a psychoanalyst* (pp. 71–79). Harmondsworth: Penguin, 1986. [CW 6:4:10]

Youth will not sleep. *New Society*, 28 May 1964, 3(87), 5. Also published in C. Winnicott, R. Shepherd & M. Davis (Eds.), *Deprivation and delinquency* (pp. 156–158). London: Tavistock, 1984. [CW 7:1:7]

1965

A child psychiatry case illustrating delayed reaction to loss. In M. Schur (Ed.), *Drives, affects, behavior: Essays in memory of Marie Bonaparte* (Vol. 2, pp. 212–242). New York: International Universities Press, 1965. Also published in C. Winnicott, R. Shepherd & M. Davis (Eds.), *Psycho-analytic explorations* (pp. 341–368). Cambridge, MA: Harvard University Press, 1989. [CW 7:2:23]

Child therapy: A case of anti-social behaviour. In J. G. Howells (Ed.), *Modern perspectives in child psychiatry* (pp. 523–533). London: Oliver & Boyd, 1965. Introduction published in [CW 10: Appendix 5]. Also published in *Therapeutic consultations in child psychiatry* (pp. 270–295, as '"Mark" aet 12 years'). London: Hogarth, 1971. Published here as '"Mark" aet 12 years'. [CW 10:3:15]

A clinical study of the effect of a failure of the average expectable environment on a child's mental functioning. *International Journal of Psychoanalysis*, 1965, 46, 81–87. Introduction published in [CW 10: Appendix 2]. Also published in *Therapeutic consultations in child psychiatry* (pp. 64–88, in part, as '"Bob" aet 6 years'). London: Hogarth, 1971. Published here as '"Bob" aet 6 years'. [CW 10:1:4]

The family and individual development. London: Tavistock, 1965. (Second edition, with an introduction by Martha Nussbaum, London and New York: Routledge Classics, 2006.) [Not reprinted in this form in the *Collected Works*]

Preface. vii. [CW 7:2:25]

The first year of life: Modern views on the emotional development. 3–14. First published in *Medical Press*, March 1958, as 'Modern views on the emotional development in the first year of life'. [CW 5:4:6]

The relationship of a mother to her baby at the beginning [1960]. 15–20. [CW 6:1:8]

Growth and development in immaturity [1950]. 21–29. [CW 3:5:16]

On security [1960]. 30–33. Also published in C. Winnicott, C. Bollas, M. Davis & R. Shepherd (Eds.), *Talking to parents* (pp. 87–93, as 'Security'). Reading, MA: Addison-Wesley, 1993; and *Winnicott on the child* (pp. 155–159, as 'Security'). Cambridge, MA: Perseus, 2002. Broadcast 18 April 1960, as 'Too much security?' I. Benzie (Producer), *Parents and children*. Network Three. London: British Broadcasting Corporation. [CW 6:1:9]

The five-year-old [1962]. 34–39. Also published in C. Winnicott, C. Bollas, M. Davis & R. Shepherd (Eds.), *Talking to parents* (pp. 111–120, as 'Now they are five'). Reading, MA: Addison-Wesley, 1993; and *Winnicott on the child* (pp. 171–177, as 'Now they are five'). Cambridge, MA: Perseus, 2002. Broadcast 25 June 1962, as 'The first five years 13: Now they are five'. S. Waterhouse (Producer), *Parents and children*. Network Three. London: British Broadcasting Corporation. [CW 6:3:6]

Integrative and disruptive factors in family life [1957]. 40–49. First published in *Canadian Medical Association Journal*, 1961 84(15), 814–815, as 'Integrating and disruptive factors in family life'. [CW 5:3:26]

The family affected by depressive illness in one or both parents [1958]. 50–60. [CW 5:4:17]

The effect of psychosis on family life [1960]. 61–68. [CW 6:1:6]

The effect of psychotic parents on the emotional development of the child [1959]. 69–78. First published in *British Journal of Psychiatric Social Work*, 1961, 6(1), 13–20. [CW 5:5:21]

Adolescence: Struggling through the doldrums [1961]. 79–87. First published in *New Era in Home and School*, October 1962, 43(8), as 'Adolescence'. [CW 6:2:4] See also 'Struggling through the doldrums'.

The family and emotional maturity [1960]. 88–94. Also published in *Winnicott on the child* (pp. 207–214). Cambridge, MA: Perseus, 2002. [CW 6:1:17]

Theoretical statement of the field of child psychiatry. 97–105. First published in A. Holzel & J. P. M. Tizard (Eds.), *Modern trends in paediatrics* (pp. 250–262, part of the chapter 'Child psychiatry'). London: Butterworth, 1958. [CW 5:4:25]

Advising parents [1957]. 114–120. Also published in *Winnicott on the child* (pp. 193–201). Cambridge, MA: Perseus, 2002. [CW 5:3:27]

Casework with mentally ill children [1959]. 121–131. [CW 5:5:15]

The contribution of psycho-analysis to midwifery. 106–113. First published in *Nursing Mirror*, 1957 (two parts, 17 and 24 May). Also published in C. Winnicott, R. Shepherd & M. Davis (Eds.), *Babies and their mothers* (pp. 69–81). Reading, MA: Addison-Wesley, 1987; and *Winnicott on the child* (pp. 56–64). Cambridge, MA: Perseus, 2002. [CW 5:3:15]

The deprived child and how he can be compensated for loss of family life [1950]. In *The family and individual development* (pp. 132–145). London: Tavistock, 1965. [CW 3:5:9]

Group influences and the maladjusted child: The school aspect [1955]. 146–154. Also published in C. Winnicott, R. Shepherd & M. Davis (Eds.), *Deprivation and delinquency* (pp. 189–199). London: Tavistock, 1984. [CW 5:1:9]

Some thoughts on the meaning of the word democracy. 155–169. First published in *Human Relations*, 1950, 3. Also published in C. Winnicott, R. Shepherd & M. Davis (Eds.), *Home is where we start from: Essays by a psychoanalyst* (pp. 239–259). Harmondsworth: Penguin, 1986. [CW 3:5:17]

The maturational processes and the facilitating environment: Studies in the theory of emotional development. London: Hogarth, 1965. [Not reprinted in this form in the *Collected Works*]

Introduction. 9–11. [CW 7:2:24]

Acknowledgement. 11. [CW 7:2:24 (footnote)]

Psycho-analysis and the sense of guilt [1956]. 15–28. First published in J. D. Sutherland (Ed.), *Psychoanalysis and contemporary thought* (pp. 15–32). London: Hogarth, 1958. [CW 5:2:7]

The capacity to be alone [1957]. 29–36. First published in *International Journal of Psychoanalysis*, 1958, *39*, 416–420. Also published in *Psyche*, 1958, *12*, as 'Über die Fähigkeit, allein zu sein'. [CW 5:3:20]

The theory of the parent-infant relationship. 37–55. First published in *International Journal of Psychoanalysis*, 1960, *41*, 585–595. [CW 6:1:21]

Ego integration in child development [1962]. 56–63. [CW 6:3:19]

Providing for the child in health and crisis [1962]. 64–72. [CW 6:3:10]

The development of the capacity for concern [1962]. 73–82. First published in *Bulletin of the Menninger Clinic*, 1963, *27*. Also published in C. Winnicott, R. Shepherd & M. Davis (Eds.), *Deprivation and delinquency* (pp. 100–105). London: Tavistock, 1984; and *Winnicott on the child* (pp. 215–220). Cambridge, MA: Perseus, 2002. [6:3:11]

From dependence towards independence in the development of the individual [1963]. 83–92. [CW 6:4:11]

Morals and education [1962]. 93–105. First published in W. R. Niblett (Ed.), *Moral education in a changing society* (pp. 96–111, as 'The young child at home and at school'). London: Faber, 1963. [CW 6:3:18]

On the contribution of direct child observation to psycho-analysis [1957]. 109–114. First published in *Revue Française de Psychanalyse*, 1958, *22*, as 'Discussion sur la contribution de l'observation directe de l'enfant à la psychanalyse'. [CW 5:3:21]

Child analysis in the latency period. 115–123. First published in *A Criança Portuguesa*, 1958, *17*. [CW 5:4:13]

Classification: Is there a psycho-analytic contribution to psychiatric classification? [1959, 1964]. 124–139. [CW 5:5:5]

Ego distortion in terms of true and false self [1960]. 140–152. [CW 6:1:22]

String: A technique of communication. 153–157. First published in *Journal of Child Psychology and Psychiatry*, 1960, *1*(1), 49–52, as 'String'. Also published in *Playing and reality* (pp. 15–20, part of 'Transitional objects and transitional phenomena'). London: Tavistock, 1971. [CW 6:1:20]

Countertransference [1959]. 158–165. First published in *British Journal of Medical Psychology*, 1960, *33*(1), 17–21. [CW 5:5:20]

The aims of psycho-analytical treatment [1962]. 166–170. [CW 6:3:2]

A personal view of the Kleinian contribution [1962]. 171–178. [CW 6:3:8]

Communicating and not communicating leading to a study of certain opposites [1963]. 179–192. [CW 6:4:8]

Training for child psychiatry [1962]. 193–202. First published in *Journal of Child Psychology and Psychiatry*, 1963, *4*(2), 75–136. [CW 6:3:5]

Psychotherapy of character disorders [1963]. 203–216. Also published in C. Winnicott, R. Shepherd & M. Davis (Eds.), *Deprivation and delinquency* (pp. 241–255). London: Tavistock, 1984. [CW 6:4:9]

The mentally ill in your caseload. 217–229. First published in J. F. S. King (Ed.), *New thinking for changing needs* (pp. 50–66). London: The Association of Social Workers, 1963. [CW 6:4:5]

Psychiatric disorder in terms of infantile maturational processes [1963]. 230–241. [CW 6:4:12]

Hospital care supplementing intensive psychotherapy in adolescence [1963]. 242–248. [CW 6:4:13]

Dependence in infant-care, in child-care, and in the psycho-analytic setting [1962]. 249–259. First published in *International Journal of Psychoanalysis*, 1963, *44*, 339–344. [CW 6:3:9]

The price of disregarding psychoanalytic research. In *The price of mental health. Report of the National Association for Mental Health Annual Conference* (London, 1965), as 'The price of disregarding research findings'. Also published in C. Winnicott, R. Shepherd & M. Davis (Eds.), *Home is where we start from: Essays by a psychoanalyst* (pp. 172–182). Harmondsworth: Penguin, 1986. [CW 7:2:4]

Review: Erikson, E. H., *Childhood and society* (London: Hogarth, 1965). *New Society*, 30 September 1965, *6*(156), 35. Also published in C. Winnicott, R. Shepherd & M. Davis (Eds.), *Psycho-analytic explorations* (pp. 493–494). Cambridge, MA: Harvard University Press, 1989. [CW 7:2:14]

Review: Kirk, H. D., *Shared fate: A theory of adoption and mental health* (New York: The Free Press of Glencoe/London: Collier-Macmillan, 1964). *New Society*, 9 September 1965, *6*(154), 29. [CW 7:2:26]

1966

Becoming deprived as a fact: A psychotherapeutic consultation. *Journal of Child Psychotherapy*, 1966, *1*(4), 5–12. [CW 10:Appendix 6]. Also published in *Therapeutic consultations in child psychiatry* (pp. 315–330, as ' "Ruth" aet 8 years'). London: Hogarth, 1971. Published here as ' "Ruth" aet 8 years'. [CW 10:3:17]

Comment on obsessional neurosis and 'Frankie' [1965]. *International Journal of Psychoanalysis*, 1966, *47*, 143–144. Also published in C. Winnicott, R. Shepherd & M. Davis (Eds.), *Psycho-analytic explorations* (pp. 158–160). Cambridge, MA: Harvard University Press, 1989. [CW 7:2:10]

Discussion. Alger, I., 'The clinical handling of the analyst's response'. *Psychoanalytic Forum*, 1966, *1*. [CW 7:3:36]

A psychoanalytic view of the antisocial tendency. In R. Slovenko (Ed.), *Crime, law and corrections* (pp. 102–130). Springfield, IL: Charles C. Thomas, 1966. Published here as 'Dissociation revealed in a therapeutic consultation'. [CW 10:3:13] Includes ' "Ada" aet 8 years'.

Psycho-somatic illness in its positive and negative aspects [1964]. *International Journal of Psychoanalysis*, 1966, 47, 510–516. Also published in C. Winnicott, R. Shepherd & M. Davis (Eds.), *Psycho-analytic explorations* (pp. 103–114, in the chapter 'Psycho-somatic disorder'). Cambridge, MA: Harvard University Press, 1989. [CW 7:1:6]

Review: Axline, V., *Dibs in search of self* (Harmondsworth: Penguin, 1964). *New Society*, 28 April 1966, 7(187), 25. [CW 7:3:10]

Review: Chess, S., Thomas, A. & Birch, H., *Your child is a person* (London: Peter Davies, 1966). *Medical News*, October 1966. [CW 7:3:25]

Review: Clyne, M. B., *Absent: School refusal as an expression of disturbed family relationships* (London: Tavistock, 1966). *New Society*, 29 September 1966, 8(209), 507–508. [CW 7:3:22]

Review: Eissler, R. S., Freud, A., Hartmann, H., Kris, M. (Eds.), *The psychoanalytic study of the child* (Vol. 20) (London: Hogarth, 1966). *British Medical Journal*, 17 December 1966, 2(5528), 1510–1511. [CW 7:3:14]

Review: Eppel, E. M. & Eppel, M., *Adolescents and morality* (London: Routledge & Kegan Paul, 1966). *New Society*, 15 September 1966, 8(207), 417–418. Also published in R. Shepherd, J. Johns & H. Taylor Robinson (Eds.), *Thinking about children* (pp. 48–50, as 'Out of the mouths of adolescents'). London: Karnac, 1996. [CW 7:3:20]

Review: Goodacre, I., *Adoption policy & practice* (London: George Allen & Unwin, 1966). *New Society*, 24 November 1966, 8(217), 806–807. [CW 7:3:30]

Review: Lask, A., *Asthma: Attitude & milieu* (London: Tavistock, 1966). *New Society*, 17 November 1966, 8(216), 771. [CW 7:3:26]

Review: Rimland, B., *Infantile autism* (New York: Appleton-Century-Crofts, 1964). *British Medical Journal*, 10 September 1966, 2(5514), 634. Also published in R. Shepherd, J. Johns & H. Taylor Robinson (Eds.), *Thinking about children* (pp. 195–196, part of 'Three reviews of books on autism'). London: Karnac, 1996. [CW 7:3:18]

1967

Eine kinderbeobachtung. *Psyche*, 1967, 21. Also published in C. Winnicott, R. Shepherd & M. Davis (Eds.), *Psycho-analytic explorations* (pp. 499–505). Cambridge, MA: Harvard University Press, 1989. Published here as 'A tribute on the occasion of Willi Hoffer's seventieth birthday'. [CW 8:1:11]

The location of cultural experience. [1966] *International Journal of Psychoanalysis*, 1967, 48, 368–372. Also published in *Playing and reality* (pp. 95–103). London: Tavistock, 1971. [CW 7:3:31]

Mirror-role of mother and family in child development. In P. Lomas (Ed.), *The predicament of the family: A psychoanalytical symposium* (pp. 26–33). London: Hogarth, 1967. Also published in *Playing and reality* (pp. 111–118). London: Tavistock, 1971. [CW 8:1:38]

Review: Clyne, M. B., *Absent: School refusal as an expression of disturbed family relationships* (London: Tavistock, 1966). *British Medical Journal*, 1967, 3(5557), 99, as 'Dynamic psychiatry and the G.P.' [CW 8:1:15]

Review: A collection of children's books. *New Society*, 7 December 1967, *10*(271), 835, as 'Small things for small people'. [CW 8:1:35]
Review: LeShan, E. J., *How to survive parenthood* (Harmondsworth: Penguin, 1965). *New Society*, 26 October 1967, *10*(265), 601. [CW 8:1:28]
Review: Stewart, S., *A home from home* (London: Longmans, Green & Co., 1967). *New Society*, 25 May 1967, *9*(243), 772–773. Also published in C. Winnicott, R. Shepherd & M. Davis (Eds.), *Deprivation and delinquency* (pp. 200–201, as 'The persecution that wasn't'). London: Tavistock, 1984. [CW 8:1:10]
Review: Thomson, H., *The successful stepparent* (London: W. H. Allen, 1966). *New Society*, 13 April 1967, *9*(237), 545–546. [CW 8:1:7]
Winnicott's wisdom: Hobgoblins and good habits. *Parents*, 1967, *22*(9), 63–65. [CW 8:1:22]
Winnicott's wisdom: How a baby begins to feel sorry and to make amends. *Parents*, 1967, *22*(7), 32–35. [CW 8:1:16]
Winnicott's wisdom: The meaning of mother love. *Parents*, 1967, *22*(6), 22–23. [CW 8:1:13]
Winnicott's wisdom: Why do babies cry? *Parents*, 1967, *22*(8), 22–23. [CW 8:1:17]

1968

The aetiology of infantile schizophrenia in terms of adaptive failure [1967]. *Recherches*, 1968 (special issue 'Enfance aliénée', 2), as 'La schizophrénie infantile en termes d'échec d'adaption'. Also published in R. Shepherd, J. Johns & H. Taylor Robinson (Eds.), *Thinking about children* (pp. 218–233). London: Karnac, 1996. [CW 8:1:25]
Children learning. In *The human family and God*. London: Christian Teamwork Institute of Education, 1968. Also published in C. Winnicott, R. Shepherd & M. Davis (Eds.), *Home is where we start from: Essays by a psychoanalyst* (pp. 142–149). Harmondsworth: Penguin, 1986; and *Winnicott on the child* (pp. 232–238). Cambridge, MA: Perseus, 2002. [CW 8:2:16]
Communication between infant and mother, and mother and infant, compared and contrasted. In W. G. Joffe (Ed.), *What is psychoanalysis* (pp. 15–25). London: The Institute of Psycho-Analysis/Bailliere, Tindall & Cassell, 1968. Also published in C. Winnicott, R. Shepherd & M. Davis (Eds.), *Babies and their mothers* (pp. 89–103). Reading, MA: Addison-Wesley, 1987; and *Winnicott on the child* (pp. 70–81). Cambridge, MA: Perseus, 2002. [CW 8:2:2]
The concept of clinical regression compared with that of defence organization [1967]. In S. H. Eldred & M. Vanderpol (Eds.), *Psychotherapy in the designed therapeutic milieu*. (International Psychiatry Clinics. Vol. 5, pp. 193–199). Boston: Little, Brown and Co., 1968, as 'Clinical regression compared with defense organization'. Also published in C. Winnicott, R. Shepherd & M. Davis (Eds.), *Psycho-analytic explorations* (pp. 193–199). Cambridge, MA: Harvard University Press, 1989. [CW 8:1:29]
Delinquency as a sign of hope [1967]. *Prison Service Journal*, 1968, 7. Also published in C. Winnicott, R. Shepherd & M. Davis (Eds.), *Home is where we start from: Essays by a psychoanalyst* (pp. 90–100). Harmondsworth: Penguin, 1986. [CW 8:1:8]
Environmental health in infancy [1967]. *Maternal and Child Care*, 1968, 4, in part, as 'Infant feeding and emotional development'. Also published in R. Shepherd, J. Johns & H. Taylor Robinson (Eds.), *Thinking about children* (pp. 39–41, in part, as 'The bearing of emotional development on feeding problems' [1967]).

London: Karnac, 1996. First published in this form in C. Winnicott, R. Shepherd & M. Davis (Eds.), *Babies and their mothers* (pp. 59-68). Reading, MA: Addison-Wesley, 1987; and then in *Winnicott on the child* (pp. 49-55). Cambridge, MA: Perseus, 2002. [CW 8:1:6]

Foreword. Dockar-Drysdale, B., *Collected papers: Vol. 3. Therapy in child care* (pp. ix-x). London: Longman, 1968. [CW 8:2:45]

Foreword. Tod, R. J. N. (Ed.), *Disturbed children* (pp. vii-viii). London: Longman, 1968. [CW 8:2:8]

La interrelación en términos de identificaciones cruzadas. *Revista de Psicoanálisis*, 1968, 25. Published in *Playing and reality* (pp. 129-137, as part of the chapter 'Interrelating apart from instinctual drive and in terms of cross-identifications'). London: Tavistock, 1971. Published here as 'Interrelating in terms of cross-identifications'. [CW 9:3:8]

The non-pharmacological treatment of psychosis in childhood [1967]. In H. Stutte & H. Harbauer (Eds.), *Concilium paedopsychiatricum*. Proceedings of the 3rd European Congress of Paedopsychiatry, Wiesbaden, 4-9 May 1967. Basel/New York: S. Karger, 1968. [CW 8:1:9]

Note of contribution. (25th International Psycho-Analytical Congress Symposium on Child Analysis and Paediatrics, Copenhagen, 1967) [1967]. *International Journal of Psychoanalysis*, 1968, 49, 279. Published here as part of the headnote to ' "Iiro" aet 9 years 9 months' [CW 10:Appendix 1]

Playing: A theoretical statement [1967]. *International Journal of Psychoanalysis*, 1968, 49, 591-599, as 'Playing: Its theoretical status in the clinical situation'. Also published in *Playing and reality* (pp. 38-52). London: Tavistock, 1971. [CW 8:2:15]

Review: Burton, L., *Vulnerable children. Three studies of children in conflict: Accident involved children, sexually assaulted children, and children with asthma* (London: Routledge & Kegan Paul, 1968). *New Society*, 25 April 1968, 11(291), 613. [CW 8:2:11]

Review: Clegg, A. & Megson, B., *Children in distress* (Harmondsworth: Penguin, 1968). *New Society*, 7 November 1968, 12(319), 688. [CW 8:2:25]

Review: Eissler, R. S., Freud, A., Hartmann, H., Kris, M. (Eds.), *The psychoanalytic study of the child* (Vol. 22) (London: Hogarth, 1967). *New Society*, 16 May 1968, 11(294), 726-727. [CW 8:2:13]

Review: Sandström, C. I., *The psychology of childhood and adolescence* (Harmondsworth: Penguin, 1968 [originally published as 'Barn- och ungdomspsykologi'. Almqvist & Wiksell, 1961]). *National Marriage Guidance Council Journal*, 1968, 11. [CW 8:2:46]

Review: Storr, C. A., *Human aggression* (Harmondsworth: Penguin, 1968). *New Statesman*, 5 July 1968, 76, 15-18. [CW 8:2:18]

Sleep refusal in children. *Medical News Magazine* (Suppl. Paediatrics, pp. 8-9), July 1968. Also published in R. Shepherd, J. Johns & H. Taylor Robinson (Eds.), *Thinking about children* (pp. 42-45). London: Karnac, 1996. [CW 8:2:19]

The squiggle game [1964, 1968]. In C. Winnicott, R. Shepherd & M. Davis (Eds.), *Psychoanalytic explorations* (pp. 299-317). Cambridge, MA: Harvard University Press, 1989. Published, in part, in *Voices: The Art and Science of Psycho-therapy*, 1968, 4, 98-112. Also published, in part, in G. Biermann (Ed.), *Handbuch der Kinderpsychotherapie* (pp. 269-277, as 'Die volle Nutzung der ersten Behandlungsstunde. Beitrag zu Problemen der Kinderanalyse' or 'Meeting the challenge of the case'). Munchen/Basel: Ernst Reinhardt Verlag, 1968. Includes 'Case of L'. Also published in *Therapeutic consultations in child psychiatry* (pp. 42–63, as ' "Eliza" aet 7½ years'). London: Hogarth, 1971. [CW 8:2:47]

The value of the therapeutic consultation [1965]. In E. Miller (Ed.), *Foundations of child psychiatry* (pp. 593–608, together with ' "Ashton" aet 12 years'). Oxford, UK: Pergamon, 1968. Also published in C. Winnicott, R. Shepherd & M. Davis (Eds.), *Psycho-analytic explorations* (pp. 318–324). Cambridge, MA: Harvard University Press, 1989. [CW 7:2:22]

1969

Adolescent process and the need for personal confrontation. *Pediatrics*, 1969, 44. Published here as 'Death and murder in the adolescent process', as part of 'Contemporary concepts of adolescent development and their implications for higher education'. [CW 9:3:9] See also 'Adolescent immaturity'.

Breast-feeding as communication [1968]. *Maternal and Child Care*, 1969, 5. Also published in C. Winnicott, R. Shepherd & M. Davis (Eds.), *Babies and their mothers* (pp. 23–33). Reading, MA: Addison-Wesley, 1987; and *Winnicott on the child* (pp. 24–31). Cambridge, MA: Perseus, 2002. [CW 8:2:26]

Changing patterns: The young person, the family and society [1968]. In *Proceedings of the British Student Health Association Twentieth Conference* (Newcastle, UK, 1968), 1969. Published here as part of 'Contemporary concepts of adolescent development and their implications for higher education'. [CW 9:3:9] See also 'Adolescent immaturity'.

Do progressive schools give too much freedom to the child? [1965] In M. Ash (Ed.), *Who are the progressives now?* (pp. 165–170, as 'Contribution to conference at Dartington Hall'). London: Routledge & Kegan Paul, 1969. Also published in C. Winnicott, R. Shepherd & M. Davis (Eds.), *Deprivation and delinquency* (pp. 209–213, together with 'Notes made in the train' [1956] [CW 7:2:6], part of the chapter 'Do progressive school give too much freedom to the child?'). London: Tavistock, 1984. [CW 7:2:5]

Foreword. Gardner, D. E. M., *Susan Isaacs* (pp. 5–6). London: Methuen, 1969. Also published in C. Winnicott, R. Shepherd & M. Davis (Eds.), *Psycho-analytic explorations* (pp. 387–389). Cambridge, MA: Harvard University Press, 1989. [CW 8:2:22]

Foreword. Milner, M., *The hands of the living God* [1967]. London: Hogarth, 1969. [CW 8:1:12]

A link between paediatrics and child psychology: Clinical observations [1968]. *Dynamische Psychiatrie*, 1969, 2, as 'Eine Verbindung zwischen Kinderheilkunde und Kinderpsychologie, klinische Betrachtungen'. Also published in R. Shepherd, J. Johns & H. Taylor Robinson (Eds.), *Thinking about children* (pp. 255–276). London: Karnac, 1996. [CW 8:2:14]

Obituary: Strachey, James. *International Journal of Psychoanalysis*, 1969, 50, 129–131. Also published in C. Winnicott, R. Shepherd & M. Davis (Eds.), *Psycho-analytic explorations* (pp. 506–510). Cambridge, MA: Harvard University Press, 1989. [CW 8:1:14]

Physiotherapy and human relations. *Physiotherapy*, 1969, 55, as 'Human relations'. Also published in C. Winnicott, R. Shepherd & M. Davis (Eds.), *Psycho-analytic explorations* (pp. 561–568). Cambridge, MA: Harvard University Press, 1989. [CW 9:1:14]

Preface. Lebovici, S. & McDougall, J., *Dialogue with Sammy: A psycho-analytical contribution to the understanding of child psychosis*. London: Hogarth, 1969 (Originally published as *Un cas de psychose infantile*, Paris: Presses universitaires de France, 1960). [CW 9:1:27]

Review: Freud, A., *Indications for child analysis and other papers* (New York: International Universities Press, 1968; London: Hogarth, 1969). *New Society*, 21 August 1969, 14(360), 297. Also published in C. Winnicott, R. Shepherd & M. Davis (Eds.), *Psycho-analytic explorations* (pp. 511–512). Cambridge, MA: Harvard University Press, 1989. [CW 9:1:20]

The use of an object and relating through identifications [1968]. *International Journal of Psychoanalysis*, 1969, 50, 711–716, as 'The use of an object'. Also published in *Playing and reality* (pp. 86–94). London: Tavistock, 1971; and C. Winnicott, R. Shepherd & M. Davis (Eds.), *Psycho-analytic explorations* (pp. 218–227, as part of the chapter 'On "The use of an object"'). Cambridge, MA: Harvard University Press, 1989. [CW 8:2:28]

1970

Contribution to 'The final number'. *Case Conference*, 1970, 16(12). [CW 9:2:5]

Day dreaming. *Your Child*, 1970, 2. [CW 9:2:14]

The mother-infant experience of mutuality [1969]. In E. J. Anthony & T. Benedek (Eds.), *Parenthood: Its psychology and psychopathology* (pp. 245–256). Boston: Little, Brown & Co., 1970. Also published in C. Winnicott, R. Shepherd & M. Davis (Eds.), *Psycho-analytic explorations* (pp. 251–260). Cambridge, MA: Harvard University Press, 1989. [CW 9:1:28]

1971

Basis for self in body [1970]. *Nouvelle Revue de Psychanalyse*, 1971, 3, as 'Le corps et le self'. Also published in C. Winnicott, R. Shepherd & M. Davis (Eds.), *Psycho-analytic explorations* (pp. 261–271). Cambridge, MA: Harvard University Press, 1989. [CW 9:2:12]

The concept of a healthy individual [1967]. In J. D. Sutherland (Ed.), *Towards community mental health* (pp. 1–16). London: Tavistock, 1971. Also published in C. Winnicott, R. Shepherd & M. Davis (Eds.), *Home is where we start from: Essays by a psychoanalyst* (pp. 21–38). Harmondsworth: Penguin, 1986. [CW 8:1:4]

Playing and reality. London: Tavistock, 1971. [Not reprinted in this form in the Collected Works]

Acknowledgements. ix.

Introduction. xi–xiii. [CW 9:3:4]

Transitional objects and transitional phenomena. 1–25. [CW 9:3:5]. First published in *International Journal of Psychoanalysis*, 1953, 34, 89–97, as 'Transitional objects and transitional phenomena: A study of the first Not-Me possession' [CW: 4:2:21]. Also published in *Collected papers: Through paediatrics to psycho-analysis* (pp. 229–242). London: Tavistock, 1958. [CW 5:4:24]; and *The collected works of D. W. Winnicott*. New York: Oxford University Press, 2017 [1951 version] [CW 3:6:6]

Dreaming, fantasying and living: A case-history describing a primary dissociation. 26–37. [CW 9:3:6]

Playing: A theoretical statement [1967]. 38–52. First published in *International Journal of Psychoanalysis*, 1968, *49*, as 'Playing: Its theoretical status in the clinical situation'. [CW 8:2:15]

Playing: Creative activity and the search for the self. 53–64. [CW 8:1:27]

Creativity and its origins. 65–85. [CW 9:3:7] Includes 'The split-off male and female elements to be found in men and women'.

The use of an object and relating through identifications [1968]. 86–94. First published in *International Journal of Psychoanalysis*, 1969, *50*, 711–716, as 'The use of an object'. Also published in C. Winnicott, R. Shepherd & M. Davis (Eds.), *Psycho-analytic explorations* (pp. 218–227, as part of the chapter 'On "The use of an object"'). Cambridge, MA: Harvard University Press, 1989. [CW 8:2:28]

The location of cultural experience [1966]. 95–103. First published in *International Journal of Psychoanalysis*, 1967, *48*, 368–372. [CW 7:3:31]

The place where we live. 104–110. [CW 8:2:1]

Mirror-role of mother and family in child development. 111–118. First published in P. Lomas (Ed.), *The predicament of the family: A psychoanalytical symposium* (pp. 26–33). London: Hogarth, 1967. [CW 8:1:38]

Interrelating apart from instinctual drive and in terms of cross-identifications. 119–137. [CW 9:3:8] See also 'La interrelación en términos de identificaciones cruzadas'.

Contemporary concepts of adolescent development and their implications for higher education [1968]. 138–150. *Proceedings of the British Student Health Association*, 1969, in part, as 'Changing patterns: The young person, the family and society'. Also published in *Pediatrics*, 1969, *44* (as 'Adolescent process and the need for personal confrontation', part of the section 'Death and murder in the adolescent process'); and C. Winnicott, R. Shepherd & M. Davis (Eds.), *Home is where we start from: Essays by a psychoanalyst* (pp. 150–166, as 'Adolescent immaturity'). Harmondsworth: Penguin, 1986. [CW 9:3:9]

Tailpiece. 151. [CW 9:3:10]

A psychotherapeutic consultation in child psychiatry: A comparative study of the dynamic processes. In S. Arieti (Ed.), *The world biennial of psychiatry and psychotherapy* (Vol. 1, pp. 377–399). New York: Basic, 1971. Introduction published in [CW 10: Appendix 4]. Also published in *Therapeutic consultations in child psychiatry* (pp. 194–214, as '"Milton" aet 8 years'). London: Hogarth, 1971. [CW 10:2:12]

Therapeutic consultations in child psychiatry. London: Hogarth, 1971.

Introduction (Part One). 1–11. [CW 10:1:Introduction]

'Iiro' aet 9 years 9 months, Case 1. 12–27. [CW 10:1:1]

'Robin' aet 5 years. 28–41. [CW 10:1:2]

'Eliza' aet 7½ years. 42–63. Also published in G. Biermann (Ed.), *Handbuch der Kinderpsychotherapie* (pp. 269–277, as part of 'Die volle Nutzung der ersten Behandlungsstunde. Beitrag zu Problemen der Kinderanalyse'). München/Basel: Ernst Reinhardt Verlag, 1968; and in *Voices: The Art and Science of Psycho-therapy*, 1968, *4*, 98–112 (as part of the chapter 'The squiggle game'); and in C. Winnicott, R. Shepherd & M. Davis (Eds.), *Psycho-analytic explorations* (pp. 299–317, as 'Case of L', part of the chapter 'The squiggle game'). Cambridge, MA: Harvard University Press, 1989. [CW 10:1:3]

'Bob' aet 6 years. 64–88. [CW 10:1:4] See also 'A clinical study of the effect of a failure of the average expectable environment on a child's mental functioning'.
'Robert' aet 9 years. 89–104. [CW 10:1:5]
'Rosemary', aet 10 years. 105–109. [CW 10:1:6] See also 'A child psychiatry interview'.
'Alfred' aet 10 years 110–126. [CW 10:1:7] See also 'A psychotherapeutic consultation: A case of stammering'. [CW 10:1:7]
Introduction (Part Two). 127–128. [CW 10:2:Introduction]
'Charles' aet 9 years. 129–146. [CW 10:2:8]
'Ashton' aet 12 years. 147–160. Published in E. Miller (Ed.), *Foundations of child psychiatry* (pp. 593–608, as part of 'The value of the therapeutic consultation'). Oxford, UK: Pergamon, 1968. [CW 10:2:9]
'Albert' aet 7 years 9 months. 161–175. [CW 10:2:10]
'Hesta' aet 16 years. 176–193. [CW 10:2:11]
'Milton', aet 8 years. 194–214. [CW 10:2:12] See also 'A psychotherapeutic consultation in child psychiatry: A comparative study of the dynamic processes'.
Introduction (Part Three). 215–219. [CW 10:3:Introduction]
'Ada' aet 8 years. 220–238. [CW 10:3:13] First published in R. Slovenko (Ed.), *Crime, law and corrections* (pp. 102–130, as 'Psychotherapeutic interview', part of the chapter 'A psychoanalytic view of the antisocial tendency'). Springfield, IL: Charles C. Thomas, 1966; and in C. Winnicott, R. Shepherd & M. Davis (Eds.), *Deprivation and delinquency* (pp. 256–282, as Dissociation revealed in a therapeutic consultation'). London: Tavistock, 1984. [CW 7:2:21]
'Cecil' aet 21 months at first consultation. 239–269. [CW 10:3:14] See also 'Regression as therapy illustrated by the case of a boy whose pathological dependence was adequately met by the parents'.
'Mark', aet 12 years. 270–295. [CW 10:3:15] See also 'Child therapy: A case of anti-social behaviour'. [CW 10:3:15]
'Peter' aet 13 years. 296–314. [CW 10:3:16]
'Ruth', aet 8 years. 315–330. [CW 10:3:17] See also 'Becoming deprived as a fact: A psychotherapeutic consultation'.
'Mrs X' aet 30 years. 332–341. [CW 10:3:18]
'Lily' aet 5 years. 342–343. [CW 10:3:19]
'Jason' aet 8 years 9 months. 344–379. [CW 10:3:20]
'George' aet 13 years. 380–396. [CW 10:3:21]

1972

Answers to comments on 'The split-off male and female elements' [1968–1969]. Published, in part, in *Psychoanalytic Forum*, 1972, 4; and, in part, in C. Winnicott, R. Shepherd & M. Davis (Eds.), *Psycho-analytic explorations* (pp. 189–192). Cambridge, MA: Harvard University Press, 1989. [CW 9:1:30]
Holding and interpretation: Fragment of an analysis [1955]. First published in P. L. Giovacchini (Ed.), *Tactics and techniques in psychoanalytic therapy* (pp. 455–693, as 'Fragment of an analysis'). London: Hogarth, 1972. Also published in *Holding and interpretation: Fragment of an analysis* (pp. 19–186). The Institute of Psychoanalysis. London: Karnac, 1986. [CW 4:4:1]

Mother's madness appearing in the clinical material as an ego-alien factor [1969]. In P. L. Giovacchini (Ed.), *Tactics and techniques in psychoanalytic therapy* (pp. 405–413). London: Hogarth, 1972. Also published in C. Winnicott, R. Shepherd & M. Davis (Eds.), *Psycho-analytic explorations* (pp. 375–382). Cambridge, MA: Harvard University Press, 1989. [CW 9:1:29]

1974

Fear of breakdown [ca. 1963–1964]. *International Review of Psycho-Analysis*, 1974, *1*, 103–108. Also published in C. Winnicott, R. Shepherd & M. Davis (Eds.), *Psycho-analytic explorations* (pp. 87–95). Cambridge, MA: Harvard University Press, 1989. [CW 6:4:21]

1977

The Piggle [1964–1966]. *An account of the psycho-analytic treatment of a little girl* (I. Ramzy, Ed.). London: Hogarth, 1977. [CW 11:2]

1982

Foreword. Briance, P., *Childbirth with confidence* [n.d., ca. 1959–1971] (London: Dick-Read School for Natural Birth, 1982). [CW 5:5:24]

1984

Deprivation and delinquency (C. Winnicott, R. Shepherd & M. Davis, Eds.). London: Tavistock, 1984. [Not reprinted in this form in the *Collected Works*]

Introduction by Clare Winnicott. 1–4.
Evacuation of small children. 14–21. Published, in part, in a letter to the *British Medical Journal* (with J. Bowlby & E. Miller), on 16 December 1939, titled, 'Evacuation of small children' [CW 2:1:6]. Published here as 'Children and their mothers'. [CW 2:2:2]
Review: Isaacs, S. (Ed.), *The Cambridge evacuation survey: A war time study in social welfare and education* (London: Methuen, 1941). 22–24. First published in *New Era in Home and School*, 1941, 22. [CW 2:3:5]
Children in the war. 25–30. First published in *New Era in Home and School*, 1940, *21*. Also published in *The child and the outside world: Studies in developing relationships* (pp. 69–74). London: Tavistock, 1957. [CW 2:2:4]
The deprived mother [1939]. 31–38. First published in *New Era in Home and School*, 1940, *21*(3). Also published in *The child and the outside world: Studies in developing relationships* (pp. 75–82). London: Tavistock, 1957. Broadcast 1939. London: British Broadcasting Corporation. [CW 2:1:4]
The evacuated child [1945]. 39–43. First published in *The child and the outside world: Studies in developing relationships* (pp. 83–87). London: Tavistock, 1957.

Broadcast 16 February 1945. J. Quigley & D. Bridgman (Producers), *Difficult children*. Home Service. London: British Broadcasting Corporation. [CW 2:7:2]

The return of the evacuated child [1945]. 44–48. First published in *The child and the outside world: Studies in developing relationships* (pp. 88–92). London: Tavistock, 1957. Broadcast 23 February 1945. J. Quigley & D. Bridgman (Producers), *Difficult children*. Home Service. London: British Broadcasting Corporation. [CW 2:7:3]

Home again [1945]. 49–53. First published in *The child and the outside world: Studies in developing relationships* (pp. 93–97). London: Tavistock, 1957. Broadcast 22 June 1945. J. Quigley & D. Bridgman (Producers), *Health magazine*. Home Service. London: British Broadcasting Corporation. [CW 2:7:7]

Residential management as treatment for difficult children (with C. Britton). 54–72. First published, in part, in 'Residential management as treatment for difficult children: The evolution of a wartime hostels scheme'. *Human Relations*, 1(1), 87–97. Also published, in part, as 'The problem of homeless children'. *New Education Monograph*, No. 1, 1944. [CW 2:6:14]; and in *The child and the outside world: Studies in developing relationships* (pp. 98–116). London: Tavistock, 1957. [CW 3:2:3]

Children's hostels in war and peace [1946]. 73–77. First published in *British Journal of Medical Psychology*, 1948, 21(3), 175–180. Also published in *The child and the outside world: Studies in developing relationships* (pp. 117–121). London: Tavistock, 1957. [CW 3:1:1]

Aggression and its roots. 84–92 [Not reprinted in this form in the *Collected Works*]. Published, in part, in *The child and the outside world: Studies in developing relationships* (pp. 167–175, as 'Aggression'). London: Tavistock, 1957. [CW 2:1:8] Also published, in part, in *The child, the family, and the outside world* (pp. 232–239, as 'Roots of Aggression' [1964]). Harmondsworth: Penguin, 1964. [CW 7:1:18]

The development of the capacity for concern [1962]. 100–105. First published in *Bulletin of the Menninger Clinic*, 1963, 27. Also published in *The maturational processes and the facilitating environment: Studies in the theory of emotional development* (pp. 73–82). London: Hogarth, 1965; and *Winnicott on the child* (pp. 215–220). Cambridge, MA: Perseus, 2002. [CW 6:3:11]

The absence of a sense of guilt [1966]. 106–112. [CW 7:3:32]

Some psychological aspects of juvenile delinquency. 113–119. First published in *New Era in Home and School*, 1946, 27(10), 295. Also published in *Delinquency Research*, 1946, 24(5); and *The child and the outside world: Studies in developing relationships* (pp. 181–187). London: Tavistock, 1957. [CW 3:1:7] See also 'Aspects of juvenile delinquency'.

The antisocial tendency [1956]. 120–131. First published in *Collected papers: Through paediatrics to psycho-analysis* (pp. 306–315). London: Tavistock, 1958. [CW 5:2:8]

The psychology of separation [1958]. 132–135. [CW 5:4:7]

Aggression, guilt and reparation [1960]. 136–144. Also published in C. Winnicott, R. Shepherd & M. Davis (Eds.), *Home is where we start from: Essays by a psychoanalyst* (pp. 80–89). Harmondsworth: Penguin, 1986. [CW 6:1:10]

Struggling through the doldrums. 145–155. First published in *New Society*, 25 April 1963, 1(30), 8–11. [CW 6:4:7] See also 'Adolescence: Struggling through the doldrums'

Youth will not sleep. 156–158. First published in *New Society*, 28 May 1964, 3(87), 5. [CW 7:1:7]

Correspondence with a magistrate. 166–170. First published in *New Era in Home and School*, 1944, 25, as 'The magistrate, the psychiatrist and the clinic. Published here as 'Letter to Roger North'. [CW 2:6:1]

The foundation of mental health. 168–171. First published in *British Medical Journal*, 1951, 1(4719), 1373–1374. [CW 3:6:4]

The deprived child and how he can be compensated for loss of family life [1950]. 172–188. First published in *The family and individual development* (pp. 132–145). London: Tavistock, 1965. [CW 3:5:10]

Group influences and the maladjusted child: The school aspect [1955]. 189–199. First published in *The family and individual development* (pp. 146–154). London: Tavistock, 1965. [CW 5:1:9]

The persecution that wasn't. 200–201. First published in *New Society*, 25 May 1967, 9(243), 772–773. (London: Longmans, Green & Co., 1967). Published here as 'Review: Stewart, S., *A home from home*'. [CW 8:1:10]

Comments on the Report of the Committee on Punishment in Prisons and Borstals [1961]. 202–208. [CW 6:2:22]

Do progressive schools give too much freedom to the child? [1965]. 209–213. (Including 'Notes made in the train' [1956] [CW 7:2:6]). First published in M. Ash (Ed.), *Who are the progressives now?* (pp. 165–170, as 'Contribution to conference at Dartington Hall'). London: Routledge & Kegan Paul, 1969. [CW 7:2:5]

Residential care as therapy [1970]. 220–228. [CW 9:2:9]

Varieties of psychotherapy [1961]. 232–240. Also published in C. Winnicott, R. Shepherd & M. Davis (Eds.), *Home is where we start from: Essays by a psychoanalyst* (pp. 101–111). Harmondsworth: Penguin, 1986. [CW 6:2:5]

Psychotherapy of character disorders [1963]. 241–255. First published in *The maturational processes and the facilitating environment: Studies in the theory of emotional development* (pp. 203–216). London: Hogarth, 1965. [CW 6:4:9]

Dissociation revealed in a therapeutic consultation. 256–282. Also published in R. Slovenko (Ed.), *Crime, law and corrections* (pp. 102–130, as 'A psychoanalytic view of the antisocial tendency'). Springfield, IL: Charles C. Thomas, 1966.as. [CW 7:2:21] Includes '"Ada" aet 8 years'.

Freedom [ca. 1969]. *Nouvelle Revue de Psychanalyse*, 1984, 30, as 'Liberté'. Also published in C. Winnicott, R. Shepherd & M. Davis (Eds.), *Home is where we start from: Essays by a psychoanalyst* (pp. 228–232). Harmondsworth: Penguin, 1986. [CW 9:1:16]

Sum, I am [1968]. *Mathematics Teaching*, March 1984. Also published in C. Winnicott, R. Shepherd & M. Davis (Eds.), *Home is where we start from: Essays by a psychoanalyst* (pp. 55–64). Harmondsworth: Penguin, 1986. [CW 8:2:10]

1986

***Holding and interpretation: Fragment of an analysis*. The Institute of Psychoanalysis. London: Karnac, 1986.** [Not reprinted in this form in the *Collected Works*]

Holding and interpretation: Fragment of an analysis [1955]. 19–186. First published in P. L. Giovacchini (Ed.), *Tactics and techniques in psychoanalytic therapy* (pp.

455–693, as 'Fragment of an analysis' [A. Flarsheim, Ed.]). London: Hogarth, 1972. [CW: 4:4:1]

Appendix: Withdrawal and regression [1954]. 187–192. First published in *Revue Française de Psychanalyse*, 1955, *19*, 1–2, as 'Repli et régression'. Also published in *Psyche, 10*, 1956–1957; and *Collected papers: Through paediatrics to psycho-analysis* (pp. 255–261). London: Tavistock, 1958, as 'Withdrawal and regression'. [CW 4:3:29]

Home is where we start from: Essays by a psychoanalyst (C. Winnicott, R. Shepherd & M. Davis, Eds.). Harmondsworth: Penguin, 1986. [Not reprinted in this form in the *Collected Works*]

Psychoanalysis and science: Friends or relations? [1961]. 13–18. [CW 6:2:9]

The concept of a healthy individual [1967]. 21–38. First published in John D. Sutherland (Ed.), *Towards community mental health* (pp. 1–16). London: Tavistock, 1971. [CW 8:1:4]

Living creatively [1970]. 39–54. [CW 9:2:11]

Sum, I am [1968]. 55–64. First published in *Mathematics Teaching*, March 1984. [CW 8:2:10]

The concept of the false self [1964]. 65–70. [CW 7:1:1]

The value of depression [1963]. 71–79. First published in *British Journal of Psychiatric Social Work*, 1964, *7*(3), 123–127; and *The Observer*, 31 May 1964, p. 33, as 'Strength out of misery'. [CW 6:4:10]

Aggression, guilt and reparation [1960]. 80–89. First published in C. Winnicott, R. Shepherd & M. Davis (Eds.), *Deprivation and delinquency* (pp. 136–144). London: Tavistock, 1984. [CW 6:1:10]

Delinquency as a sign of hope [1967]. 90–100. First published in *Prison Service Journal*, 1968, *7*. [CW 8:1:8]

Varieties of psychotherapy [1961]. 101–111. First published in C. Winnicott, R. Shepherd & M. Davis (Eds.), *Deprivation and delinquency* (pp. 232–240). London: Tavistock, 1984. [CW 6:2:5]

Cure [1970]. 112–120. [CW 9:2:8]

The mother's contribution to society. 123–127. First published in *The child and the family: First relationships* (pp. 141–144, as 'Postscript: The mother's contribution to society'). London: Tavistock, 1957. Also published in *Winnicott on the child* (pp. 202–206). Cambridge, MA: Perseus, 2002. [CW 5:3:30]

The child in the family group [1966]. 128–141. Also published in *Winnicott on the child* (pp. 221–231). Cambridge, MA: Perseus, 2002. [CW 7:3:17]

Children learning. 142–149. First published in *The human family and God*. London: Christian Teamwork Institute of Education, 1968. Also published in *Winnicott on the child* (pp. 232–238). Cambridge, MA: Perseus, 2002. [CW 8:2:16]

Adolescent immaturity. 150–166. Published here as 'Contemporary concepts of adolescent development and their implications for higher education'. [CW 9:3:9]

Thinking and the unconscious. 169–171. First published in *The Liberal Magazine*, March 1945, 125–126. [CW 2:7:4]

The price of disregarding psychoanalytic research. 172–182. First published in *The Price of Mental Health. Report of the National Association for Mental Health Annual Conference* (London, 1965), as 'The price of disregarding research findings'. [CW 7:2:4]

This feminism [1964]. 183–194. [CW 7:1:14]

The pill and the moon [1969]. 195–208. [Not printed in this form in the *Collected Works*]. Published here as 'The pill'. [CW 9:1:23]; and as 'Moon landing'. [CW 9:1:18]

Discussion of war aims. [1940]. 210–220. [CW 2:2:3]

Berlin walls [1969]. 221–227. [CW 9:1:25]

Freedom [ca. 1969]. 228–232. First published in *Nouvelle Revue de Psychanalyse*, 1984, 30, as 'Liberté'. [CW 9:1:16]. Including 'The threat to freedom' [1969]. 232–238 [CW 9:1:17]

Some thoughts on the meaning of the word democracy. 239–259. First published in *Human Relations*, 1950, 3. Also published in *The family and individual development* (pp. 155–169). London: Tavistock, 1965. [CW 3:5:17]

The place of the monarchy [1970]. 260–268. [CW 9:2:6]

1987

Babies and their mothers (C. Winnicott, R. Shepherd & M. Davis, Eds.). Reading, MA: Addison-Wesley, 1987. [Not reprinted in this form in the *Collected Works*] Also published as Part 1 of *Winnicott on the child*. Cambridge, MA: Perseus, 2002.

The ordinary devoted mother [1966]. 3–14. Also published in *Winnicott on the child* (pp. 11–18). Cambridge, MA: Perseus, 2002.[CW 7:3:3]

Knowing and learning [1950]. 15–21. First published in *The child and the family: First relationships* (pp. 69–73). London: Tavistock, 1957. Also published in *Winnicott on the child* (pp. 19–23). Cambridge, MA: Perseus, 2002. Broadcast 22 March 1950, as 'Knowing and learning how to be a mother'. I. Benzie (Producer), *How's the baby?* Home Service. London: British Broadcasting Corporation. [CW 3:5:14]

Breast-feeding as communication [1968]. 23–33. First published in *Maternal and Child Care*, 1969, 5. Also published in *Winnicott on the child* (pp. 24–31). Cambridge, MA: Perseus, 2002. [CW 8:2:26]

The newborn and his mother. 35–49. First published in *Acta Paediatrica Latina*, 1964, 17, as 'The neonate and his mother'. Also published in *Winnicott on the child* (pp. 32–42). Cambridge, MA: Perseus, 2002. [CW 7:1:4]

The beginning of the individual [1966]. 51–58. Also published in *Winnicott on the child* (pp. 43–48). Cambridge, MA: Perseus, 2002. [CW 7:3:34]

Environmental health in infancy [1967]. 59–68. Published, in part, in *Maternal and Child Care*, 1968, 4, as 'Infant feeding and emotional development'. Also published in R. Shepherd, J. Johns & H. Taylor Robinson (Eds.), *Thinking about children* (pp. 39–41, in part, as 'The bearing of emotional development on feeding problems' [1967]). London: Karnac, 1996; and in *Winnicott on the child* (pp. 49–55). Cambridge, MA: Perseus, 2002. [CW 8:1:6]

The contribution of psycho-analysis to midwifery. 69–81. First published in *Nursing Mirror*, May 1957. Also published in *The family and individual development* (pp. 106–113). London: Tavistock, 1965; and *Winnicott on the child* (pp. 56–64). Cambridge, MA: Perseus, 2002. [CW 5:3:15]

Dependence in child care. 83–88. First published in *Your Child*, 1970, 2, as 'Dependence'. Also published in *Winnicott on the child* (pp. 65–69). Cambridge, MA: Perseus, 2002. [CW 9:2:15]

Communication between infant and mother, and mother and infant, compared and contrasted. 89–103. First published in W. G. Joffe (Ed.), *What is psychoanalysis?* (pp. 15–25). London: The Institute of Psycho-Analysis/Bailliere, Tindall & Cassell, 1968. Also published in *Winnicott on the child* (pp. 70–81). Cambridge, MA: Perseus, 2002. [CW 8:2:2]

The spontaneous gesture: Selected letters (F. R. Rodman, Ed.). **Cambridge, MA: Harvard University Press, 1987.** [Not reprinted in this form in the *Collected Works*]

1988

Human nature (C. Bollas, M. Davis & R. Shepherd, Eds.). **London: Free Association Books, 1988.** [CW 11:1]

1989

Psycho-analytic explorations (C. Winnicott, R. Shepherd & M. Davis, Eds.). **Cambridge, MA: Harvard University Press, 1989.** [Not reprinted in this form in the *Collected Works*]

D. W. W.: A reflection. Introduction by Clare Winnicott. 1–18. [CW 12:1:5] Includes 'Sleep (Poem)'.
Early disillusion [1939]. 21–23. [CW 2:1:5]
Knowing and not knowing: A clinical example [n.d.]. 24–25. [CW 9:4:4]
A point in technique [n.d.]. 26–27. [CW 9:4:5]
Play in the analytic situation [1954]. 28–29. [CW 4:3:28]
Fragments concerning varieties of clinical confusion [1956]. 30–33. [CW 5:2:4]
Excitement in the aetiology of coronary thrombosis [1957]. 34–38. [CW 5:3:29]
Hallucination and dehallucination [1957]. 39–42. [CW 5:3:23]
Ideas and definitions [n.d., ca. early 1950s]. 43–44. [CW 9:4:1]
Psychogenesis of a beating fantasy [1958]. 45–48. [CW 5:4:4]
Nothing at the centre [1959]. 49–52. [CW 5:5:10]
The fate of the transitional object [1959]. 53–58. [CW 5:5:22]
Notes on play [n.d.]. 59–63. [CW 9:4:8]
Psycho-neurosis in childhood [1961]. 64–72. [CW 6:2:17]
The theory of the parent-infant relationship. Further remarks. 73–75. First published in *International Journal of Psycho-Analysis*, 1962, 43, 238–239. [CW 6:3:13]
A note on a case involving envy [1963]. 76–78. [CW 6:4:3]
Perversions and pregenital fantasy [1963]. 79–80. [CW 6:4:18]
Two notes on the use of silence [1963]. 81–86. [CW 6:4:19]
Fear of breakdown [ca. 1963–1964]. 87–95. First published in *International Review of Psycho-Analysis*, 1974, 1, 103–108. [CW 6:4:21]
The importance of the setting in meeting regression in psycho-analysis [1964]. 96–102. [CW 7:1:9]
Psycho-somatic disorder. 103–118. [Not reprinted in this form in the *Collected Works*].
  I. Psycho-somatic illness in its positive and negative aspects [1964]. 103–114. First published in *International Journal of Psycho-Analysis*, 1966, 47, 510–516 [CW 7:1:6];
  II. Additional note on psycho-somatic disorder [1969]. 115–118 [CW 9:1:21]
The psychology of madness: A contribution from psycho-analysis [1965]. 119–129. [CW 7:2:18]

The concept of trauma in relation to the development of the individual within the family [1965]. 130–148. [CW 7:2:7]

Notes on withdrawal and regression [1965]. 149–151. Published here as part of 'Case notes for a psychoanalytic seminar: Withdrawal, regression, male identification'. [CW 7:2:19]

New light on children's thinking [1965]. 152–157. [CW 7:2:1]

Comment on obsessional neurosis and 'Frankie' [1965]. 158–160. First published in *International Journal of Psycho-Analysis*, 1966, *47*, 143–144. [CW 7:2:10]

A note on the mother-foetus relationship [n.d., ca. 1960s]. 161–162. [CW 9:4:11]

Absence and presence of a sense of guilt illustrated in two patients [1966]. 163–167. Published here as part 2 of 'The absence of a sense of guilt'. [CW 7:3:32]

On the split-off male and female elements. 169–192. [Not published in this form in the *Collected Works*]. I. The split-off male and female elements to be found in men and women [1966]. 169–183. First published in *Playing and reality* (pp. 72–85, as part of the chapter 'Creativity and its origins'). London: Tavistock, 1971. Also published in J. Lindon (Ed.), *Psychoanalytic forum* (Vol. 4). New York: International Universities Press, 1972. [CW 7:3:2] II. Clinical Material [1959–1963] 183–188. [Not published in this form in the *Collected Works*] Published, in part, as 'Clinical material on the theme of a male patient's exploitation of his female self [1959] [CW 5:5:26]; also published, in part, as 'Further clinical material on the theme of a male patient's exploitation of his female self' [1963]. [CW 6:4:20] III. Answer to comments. 189–192. First published in *Psychoanalytic forum* (Vol. 4, as part of 'Answers to comments on "The split-off male and female elements"' [1968–1969]). [CW 9:1:30] See also 'Creativity and its origins'.

The concept of clinical regression compared with that of defence organization [1967]. 193–199. First published in S. H. Eldred & M. Vanderpol (Eds.), *Psychotherapy in the designed therapeutic milieu. International Psychiatry Clinics* (Vol. 5, as 'Clinical regression compared with defense organization') Boston: Little, Brown and Co., 1968. [CW 8:1:29]

Addendum to 'The location of cultural experience' [1967]. 200–202. [CW 8:1:37]

Playing and culture [1968]. 203–206. [CW 8:2:9]

Interpretation in psycho-analysis [1968]. 207–212. [CW 8:2:6]

Thinking and symbol-formation [1968]. 213–216. [CW 8:2:48]

On 'The use of an object'. 217–246. [Not published in this form in the *Collected Works*]. I. The use of an object and relating through identifications [1968]. 218–227. First published in *International Journal of Psychoanalysis*, 1969, *50*, 711–716, as 'The use of an object'. Also published in *Playing and reality* (pp. 86–94). London: Tavistock, 1971. [CW 8:2:28] II. D. W. W's dream related to reviewing Jung [1963]. 228–230 [CW 6:4:15] III. Notes made on the train: Part 2 [1965]. 231–233. First published as part of the chapter 'Do progressive schools give too much freedom to the child?' in C. Winnicott, R. Shepherd & M. Davis (Eds.), *Deprivation and delinquency* (pp. 214–219). London: Tavistock, 1984. Published here as Part 2 of 'Notes made in the train' [CW 7:2:6] IV. The use of the word 'use' [1968]. 233–235 [CW 8:2:5] V. Clinical illustration of 'The use of an object' [1968]. 235–238 [CW 8:2:29] VI. Comments on my paper 'The use of an object'

[1968]. 238–240 [CW 8:2:38] VII. The use of an object in the context of *Moses and Monotheism* [1969]. 240–246. [CW 9:1:4]

Development of the theme of the mother's unconscious as discovered in psycho-analytic practice [1969]. 247–250. [CW 9:1:15]

The mother-infant experience of mutuality [1969]. 251–260. First published in E. J. Anthony & T. Benedek (Eds.), *Parenthood: Its psychology and psychopathology* (pp. 245–256). Boston: Little, Brown & Co., 1970. [CW 9:1:28]

On the basis for self in body. 261–283. [Not published in this form in the *Collected Works*]. I. Basis for self in body [1970]. 261–271. First published in *Nouvelle Revue de Psychanalyse*, 1971, 3, as 'Le corps et le self'. [CW 9:2:12] II. Two further clinical examples [1970]. 272–283. [CW 9:2:13]

Individuation [1970]. 284–288. [CW 9:2:10]

Private practice [1955]. 291–298. [CW 5:1:7]

The squiggle game [1964, 1968]. 299–317 Published, in part, in *Voices: The Art and Science of Psycho-therapy*, 1968, 4, 98–112. Also published, in part, as 'Die volle Nutzung der ersten Behandlungsstunde'. In G. Biermann (Ed.), *Handbuch der Kinderpsychotherapie* (pp. 269–277). Munchen/Basel: Ernst Reinhardt Verlag, 1968. Includes 'Case of L', also published in *Therapeutic consultations in child psychiatry* (pp. 42–63, as '"Eliza" aet 7½ years'). London: Hogarth, 1971. [CW 8:2:47]

The value of the therapeutic consultation [1965]. 318–324. First published, together with '"Ashton" aet 12 years', in E. Miller (Ed.), *Foundations of child psychiatry* (pp. 593–608, as 'The value of the therapeutic consultation'). Oxford, UK: Pergamon, 1968. [CW 7:2:22]

Deductions drawn from a psychotherapeutic interview with an adolescent. 325–340. First published in *Report of the 20th Child Guidance Inter-Clinic Conference, 1964*. London: The National Association for Mental Health, 1964. [CW 7:1:5]

A child psychiatry case illustrating delayed reaction to loss. 341–368. First published in M. Schur (Ed.), *Drives, affects, behavior: Essays in memory of Marie Bonaparte* (Vol. 2, pp. 212–242). New York: International Universities Press, 1965. [CW 7:2:23]

Physical and emotional disturbances in an adolescent girl [1968]. 369–374. [CW 8:2:3]

Mother's madness appearing in the clinical material as an ego-alien factor [1969]. 375–382. First published in P. L. Giovacchini (Ed.), *Tactics and techniques in psychoanalytic therapy* (pp. 405–413). London: Hogarth, 1972. [CW 9:1:29]

Susan Issacs. 385–390. [Not published in this form in the *Collected Works*] I. Obituary, Susan Isaacs. 385–387. First published in *Nature*, 1948, 162(4127), 881. [CW 3:3:11] II. Foreword. D. E. M. Gardner, *Susan Isaacs* (pp. 387–389). London: Methuen, 1969. [CW 8:2:22]

Review: Milner, M., *On not being able to paint*. (London: Heinemann, 1950). 390–392. First published in *British Journal of Medical Psychology*, 1951, 24, as 'Critical notice'. [CW 3:6:15]

Ernest Jones. 393–404. I. Obituary. First published in *International Journal of Psycho-Analysis*, 1958, 39, 298–303. [CW 5:4:21] II. Funeral address. 405–407. First published in *International Journal of Psycho-Analysis*, 1958, 39, 305–306. [CW 5:4:3]

Review: Burlingham, D., *Twins: A study of three pairs of identical twins* (London: Imago, 1952). 408–412. First published in *New Era in Home and School*, 1953, 34 [CW 4:2:7]

Review (with M. M. R. Khan): Fairbairn, W. R. D., *Psychoanalytic studies of the personality* (London: Tavistock, 1952). 413–422. First published in *International Journal of Psycho-Analysis*, 1953, *34*, 329–332. [CW 4:2:18]

John Bowlby. 423–432. I. Review: J. Bowlby, *Maternal care and mental health* (Geneva: WHO, 1951). 423–426. First published in *British Journal of Medical Psychology*, 1953, 26. [CW 4:2:10] II. Discussion of 'Grief and mourning in infancy' by John Bowlby [1959]. 426–432. [CW 5:5:17]

Michael Balint. 433–442. I. Character types: The foolhardy and the cautious. On '*Funfairs, thrills and regressions*' by M. Balint [1954]. 433–438. [CW 4:3:26] II. Review: M. Balint, *The doctor, his patients and the illness* (London: Pitman, 1957). 438–442. First published in *International Journal of Psycho-Analysis*, 1958, 39, 425–427. [CW 6:4:23]

Melanie Klein: On her concept of envy. 443–464. [Not reprinted in this form in the *Collected Works*] I. Review: M. Klein, *Envy and gratitude* (London: Tavistock, 1957). 443–446. First published in *Case Conference*, 1959, 5, as 'On envy' [CW 5:5:1] II. The beginnings of a formulation of an appreciation and criticism of Klein's envy statement [1962]. 447–457. [CW 6:3:7] Also published, in part and expanded, in 'Envy: A male patient near the end of his analysis' [1961]. [CW 6:2:21] III. Roots of aggression [1968]. 458–461 [CW 8:2:21] IV. Contribution to a symposium on envy and jealousy [1969]. 462–464. [CW 9:1:8]

Comments on J. Sandler's 'On the concept of the superego' (*The psychoanalytic study of the child* (Vol. 15) 1960). 465–473. [CW 6:1:19]

Review: E. Jones (Ed.), *Letters of Sigmund Freud 1873–1939* (London: Hogarth, 1961). 474–477. First published in *British Journal of Psychology*, 1962, 53. [CW 6:3:15]

Review: H. F. Searles, *The non-human environment* (New York: International Universities Press, 1960). 478–481. First published in *International Journal of Psycho-Analysis*, 1963, 44, 237–238. [CW 6:4:16]

Review: C. G. Jung, *Memories, dreams, reflections* (London: Collins and Routledge, 1963). 482–492. First published in *International Journal of Psycho-Analysis*, 1964, 45, 450–454. [CW 7:1:16]

Review: E. H. Erikson, *Childhood and society* (London: Hogarth, 1965). 493–494. First published in *New Society*, 30 September 1965, 6(156), 35. [CW 7:2:14]

Commentary. V. Axline, *Play therapy* (Boston: Houghton Mifflin, 1947) [1965]. 495–498. [CW 9:1:32]

A tribute on the occasion of Willi Hoffer's seventieth birthday. 499–505. First published in *Psyche*, 1967, *21*, as 'Eine Kinderbeobachtung'. [CW 8:1:11]

Obituary, James Strachey. 506–510. First published in *International Journal of Psycho-Analysis*, 1969, 50, 129–131. [CW 8:1:14]

Review: A. Freud, *Indications for child analysis and other papers* (New York: International Universities Press, 1968; London: Hogarth, 1969). 511–512. First published in *New Society*, 21 August 1969, 14(360), 297. [CW 9:1:20]

Physical therapy of mental disorder: Convulsion therapy. 515–541. [Not printed in this form in the *Collected Works*] I. Treatment of mental disease by induction of fits. [CW 2:5:6] II. Shock treatment of mental disorder, letter to the *British Medical Journal*, 1943, 2(4329), 829–830. [CW 2:5:10] III. Shock therapy, letter to the *British Medical Journal*, 1944, 1(4336), 234–235. [CW: 2:6:4] IV. Introduction to a symposium on the psycho-analytic contribution to the theory of shock therapy. [CW 2:6:6] V. Kinds of psychological effect of shock therapy. [CW 2:6:7] VI. Physical therapy of mental disorder. *British Medical Journal*, 1947, 1(4506), 688–689. [CW 3:2:2]

Physical therapy of mental disorder: Leucotomy. 543–554. [Not published in this for in the *Collected Works*]. I. Prefrontal leucotomy, letter to *Lancet*, 10 April 1943, *241*(6241), 475. [CW 2:5:4] II. Leucotomy. *British Medical Student's Journal*, 1949, 3. [CW 3:4:21] III. Notes on the general implications of leucotomy. [CW 3:6:14] IV. Prefrontal leucotomy, letter to the *British Medical Journal*, 1956, 1(4960), 229–230. [CW 5:2:2]

Occupational therapy. 555–557. First published in *British Journal of Medical Psychology*, 1949, 22, as 'Review: Hill, A., *Art versus illness*' (London: George Allen and Unwin, 1948). [CW 3:4:22]

Physiotherapy and human relations. 561–568. First published in *Physiotherapy*, 1969, 55, as 'Human relations'. [CW 9:1:14]

Postscript: D. W. W. on D. W. W. [1967]. 569–582. Published here as 'D. W. W. on D. W. W.'. [CW 8:1:2]

1991

Resolution K: On scientific aims in psychoanalysis [1942]. Published in P. King & R. Steiner (Eds.), *The Freud-Klein controversies 1941–45. New Library of Psychoanalysis*, *11*, 87–89. London and New York: Tavistock/Routledge, 1991. [CW 2:4:1]

1993

Talking to parents **(C. Winnicott, C. Bollas, M. Davis & R. Shepherd, Eds.). [Introduction by T. Berry Brazelton] Reading, MA: Addison-Wesley, 1993.** Also published as Part Two of in *Winnicott on the child*. Cambridge, MA: Perseus, 2002. [Not reprinted in this form in the *Collected Works*]

Health education through broadcasting. 1–6. First published in *Mother and Child*, 1957, 28. Also published in *Winnicott on the child* (pp. 95–98). Cambridge, MA: Perseus, 2002. [CW 5:3:31]

For stepparents [1955]. 7–13. Also published in *Winnicott on the child* (pp. 99–103). Cambridge, MA: Perseus, 2002. Broadcast in three parts, 7–9 June 1955. I. Benzie (Producer), *Woman's hour*. Light Programme. London: British Broadcasting Corporation. [CW 5:1:10]

What do we know about babies as cloth suckers? [1956]. 15–20. Also published in *Winnicott on the child* (pp. 104–107). Cambridge, MA: Perseus, 2002. Broadcast 31 January 1956. I. Benzie (Producer), *Woman's hour*. Light Programme. London: British Broadcasting Corporation. [CW 5:2:1]

Saying 'No' [1960]. 21–39. Also published in *Winnicott on the child* (pp. 108–121). Cambridge, MA: Perseus, 2002. Broadcast as parts 1–3 of 'The ordinary devoted mother and her children', 25 January, 1 and 8 February 1960. I. Benzie & E. Brewer

(Producers), *Parents and children*. Network Three. London: British Broadcasting Corporation. [CW 6:1:1]

Jealousy [1960]. 41–64. Also published in *Winnicott on the child* (pp. 122–138). Cambridge, MA: Perseus, 2002. Broadcast as parts 4–7 of 'The ordinary devoted mother and her children', 15, 22, 29 February and 7 March 1960. I. Benzie & E. Brewer (Producers), *Parents and children*. Network Three. London: British Broadcasting Corporation. [CW 6:1:4]

What irks? [1960]. 65–86. Also published in *Winnicott on the child* (pp. 139–154). Cambridge, MA: Perseus, 2002. Broadcast as parts 8–9 of 'The ordinary devoted mother and her children', 14 and 21 March 1960. I. Benzie & E. Brewer (Producers), *Parents and children*. Network Three. London: British Broadcasting Corporation. [CW 6:1:7]

Security [1960]. 87–93. First published in *The family and individual development* (pp. 30–33, as 'On security'). London: Tavistock, 1965. Also published in *Winnicott on the child* (pp. 155–159). Cambridge, MA: Perseus, 2002. Broadcast 18 April 1960, as 'Too much security?' I. Benzie (Producer), *Parents and children*. Network Three. London: British Broadcasting Corporation. Published here as 'On security'. [CW 6:1:9]

Feeling guilty [1961]. 95–103. Also published in *Winnicott on the child* (pp. 160–166). Cambridge, MA: Perseus, 2002. Broadcast 13 March 1961, as 'Guilt feelings in young mothers. A discussion with Clare Rayner'. E. Crowther (Producer), *Parents and children*. Network Three. London: British Broadcasting Corporation. [CW 6:2:6]

The development of a child's sense of right and wrong [1962]. 105–110. Also published in *Winnicott on the child* (pp. 167–170). Cambridge, MA: Perseus, 2002. Broadcast 11 June 1962 as 'The first five years: 11. The development of a child's sense of right and wrong'. S. Waterhouse (Producer), *Parents and children*. Network Three. London: British Broadcasting Corporation. [CW 6:3:4]

Now they are five. 111–120. First published in *The family and individual development* (pp. 34–39, as 'The five-year-old'). London: Tavistock, 1965. Also published in *Winnicott on the child* (pp. 171–177). Cambridge, MA: Perseus, 2002. Broadcast 25 June 1962, as 'The first five years: 13. Now they are five'. S. Waterhouse (Producer), *Parents and children*. Network Three. London: British Broadcasting Corporation. Published here as 'The five-year-old' [CW 6:3:6]

The building up of trust [1969]. 121–134. Also published in *Winnicott on the child* (pp. 178–187). Cambridge, MA: Perseus, 2002. [CW 9:1:26]

1996

Thinking about children (R. Shepherd, J. Johns & H. Taylor Robinson, Eds.). London: Karnac, 1996. [Not reprinted in this form in the *Collected Works*]

Towards an objective study of human nature. 3–12. First published in *New Era in Home and School*, 1945, 26, as 'Talking about psychology'; reissued in 1952, 33(3), as 'What is psychoanalysis?' Also published in *The child and the outside world: Studies in developing relationships* (pp. 125–133). London: Tavistock, 1957. [CW 2:7:11]

'Yes, but how do we know it's true?' [1950]. 13–18. [CW 3:5:18]

Primary introduction to external reality: The early stages [1948]. 21–28. [CW 3:3:12]

Environmental needs; the early stages; total dependence and essential independence [1948]. 29–36. [CW 3:3:13]

The bearing of emotional health on feeding problems. 39–41. [Not reprinted in this form in the *Collected Works*] Published as part of 'Environmental health in infancy' [CW 8:1:6], in C. Winnicott, R. Shepherd & M. Davis (Eds.), *Babies and their mothers* (pp. 59–68). Reading, MA: Addison-Wesley, 1987; and *Winnicott on the child* (pp. 49–55). Cambridge, MA: Perseus, 2002.

Sleep refusal in children. (42–45). First published in *Medical News Magazine*. (Suppl. Paediatrics, pp. 8–9), July 1968. [CW 8:2:19]

The effect of loss on the young [1968]. 46–47. [CW 8:2:12]

Out of the mouths of adolescents. 48–50. First published in *New Society*, 15 September 1966, 8(207), 417–418. Published here as 'Review: E. M. Eppel & M. Eppel, *Adolescents and morality*'. [CW 7:3:20]

The delinquent and habitual offender [ca. 1939]. 51–53. [CW 2:1:3]

A clinical approach to family problems: The family [1959]. 54–56. [CW 5:5:27]

Mental hygiene of the pre-school child [1936]. 59–76. [CW 1:4:9]

The teacher, the parent and the doctor [1936]. 77–93. [CW 1:4:10]

A clinical example of symptomatology following the birth of a sibling [1931]. 97–101. [CW 1:2:22]

Notes on a little boy. 102–103. First published in *New Era in Home and School*, 1938, *19*. [CW 1:4:16]

The niffle [n.d.]. 104–109. [CW 9:4:10]

Two adopted children [1953]. 113–127. First published in *Case Conference*, 1954, *1*. Also published in *The child and the outside world: Studies in developing relationships* (pp. 52–65). London: Tavistock, 1957. [CW 4:2:19]

Pitfalls in adoption. 128–135. First published in *Medical Press*, 1954, 232(6031). Also published in *The child and the outside world: Studies in developing relationships* (pp. 45–51). London: Tavistock, 1957. [CW 4:3:30]

Adopted children in adolescence. 136–148. First published in *Report of Residential Conference, Standing Conference of Societies Registered for Adoption*, July 1955. [CW 5:1:12]

Contribution to a discussion on enuresis. 151–156. First published in *Proceedings of the Royal Society of Medicine*, 1936, *29*, 1522–1524. [CW 1:4:9]

Papular urticaria and the dynamics of skin sensation. 157–169. First published in the *British Journal of Children's Diseases*, 1934, *31*. [CW 1:4:3]

Short communication on enuresis. 170–175. First published in *St Bartholomew's Hospital Journal*, April 1930. [CW 1:2:18]

Child psychiatry: The body as affected by psychological factors [1931]. 176–178. [CW 1:2:23]

On cardiac neurosis in children [1966]. 179–188. [CW 7:3:16]

Three reviews of books on autism. 191–196. [Not reprinted in this form in the *Collected Works*] I. 'Review: L. Kanner, *Child psychiatry* (Springfield, IL: Charles C. Thomas, 1935. London: Ballière, Tindall & Cox, 1937). *International Journal of Psycho-Analysis*, 1938, *19*, 362–363. [CW 1:4:15] II. Review: B. Rimland, *Infantile autism*

(New York: Appleton-Century-Crofts, 1964). *British Medical Journal*, 2(5514), 634, 1966. [CW 7:3:18] III. Review: W. Goldfarb, *Childhood schizophrenia* (Cambridge, MA: Harvard University Press, 1961). First published in *British Journal of Psychiatric Social Work*, 1963, 7(1), 50–51. [CW 6:4:16]

Autism [1966]. 197–217. [CW 7:3:8]

The aetiology of infantile schizophrenia in terms of adaptive failure [1967]. 218–223. First published in *Recherches*, 1968 (special issue 'Enfance aliénée', 2), as 'La schizophrénie infantile en termes d'échec d'adaption'. [CW 8:1:25]

Training for child psychiatry: The paediatric department of psychology [1960]. 227–230. First published in *St Mary's Hospital Gazette*, 1961, 67, as 'The paediatric department of psychology'. Published here as 'The paediatric department of psychology'. [CW 6:2:19]

Notes on the time factor in treatment [1961]. 231–234. [CW 6:2:11]

The Association for Child Psychology and Psychiatry observed as a group phenomenon [1967]. 235–254. [CW 8:1:3]

A link between paediatrics and child psychology: Clinical observations [1968]. 255–276. First published in *Dynamische Psychiatrie*, 1969, 2, as 'Eine Verbindung zwischen Kinderheilkunde und Kinderpsychologie, klinische Betrachtungen'. [CW 8:2:14]

Child psychiatry, social work and alternative care [1970]. 277–281. [CW 9:2:3]

2002

Winnicott on the child [with introductions by T. Berry Brazelton, Stanley I. Greenspan, and Benjamin Spock]. Cambridge, MA: Perseus, 2002. Part 1 first published as *Babies and their mothers* (C. Winnicott, R. Shepherd & M. Davis, Eds.). Reading, MA: Addison-Wesley, 1987; Part 2 first published as *Talking to parents* (C. Winnicott, C. Bollas, M. Davis & R. Shepherd, Eds.). Reading, MA: Addison-Wesley, 1993. [Not reprinted in this form in the *Collected Works*]

The ordinary devoted mother [1966]. 11–18. First published in C. Winnicott, R. Shepherd & M. Davis (Eds.), *Babies and their mothers* (pp. 3–14). Reading, MA: Addison-Wesley, 1987. [CW 7:3:3]

Knowing and learning [1950]. 19–23. First published in *The child and the family: First relationships* (pp. 69–73). London: Tavistock, 1957. Also published in C. Winnicott, R. Shepherd & M. Davis (Eds.), *Babies and their mothers* (pp. 15–21). Reading, MA: Addison-Wesley, 1987. Broadcast 22 March 1950, as 'Knowing and learning, how to be a mother'. I. Benzie (Producer), *How's the baby?* Home Service. London: British Broadcasting Corporation. [CW 3:5:14]

Breast-feeding as communication [1968]. 24–31. First published in *Maternal and Child Care*, 1969, 5. Also published in C. Winnicott, R. Shepherd & M. Davis (Eds.), *Babies and their mothers* (pp. 23–33). Reading, MA: Addison-Wesley, 1987. [CW 8:2:26]

The newborn and his mother. 32–42. First published in *Acta Paediatrica Latina*, 1964, 17, as 'The neonate and his mother'. Also published in C. Winnicott, R. Shepherd & M. Davis (Eds.), *Babies and their mothers* (pp. 35–49). Reading, MA: Addison-Wesley, 1987. [CW 7:1:4]

The beginning of the individual [1966]. 43–48. First published in C. Winnicott, R. Shepherd & M. Davis (Eds.), *Babies and their mothers* (pp. 51–58). Reading, MA: Addison-Wesley, 1987. [CW 7:3:34]

Environmental health in infancy [1967]. 49–55. Published in *Maternal and Child Care*, 1968, 4, in part, as 'Infant feeding and emotional development'; also published, in part, in R. Shepherd, J. Johns & H. Taylor Robinson (Eds.), *Thinking about children* (pp. 39–41, in part, as 'The bearing of emotional development on feeding problems' [1967]). London: Karnac, 1996. First published in this form in C. Winnicott, R. Shepherd & M. Davis (Eds.), *Babies and their mothers* (pp. 59–68). Reading, MA: Addison-Wesley, 1987; and in *Winnicott on the child* (pp. 49–55). Cambridge, MA: Perseus, 2002. [CW 8:1:6]

The contribution of psycho-analysis to midwifery. 56–64. First published in *Nursing Mirror*, May 1957. Also published in *The family and individual development* (pp. 106–113). London: Tavistock, 1965; and C. Winnicott, R. Shepherd & M. Davis (Eds.), *Babies and their mothers* (pp. 69–81). Reading, MA: Addison-Wesley, 1987. [CW 5:3:15]

Dependence in child care. 65–69. First published in *Your Child*, 1970, 2, as 'Dependence'. Also published in C. Winnicott, R. Shepherd & M. Davis (Eds.), *Babies and their mothers* (pp. 83–88). Reading, MA: Addison-Wesley, 1987. [CW 9:2:15]

Communication between infant and mother, and mother and infant, compared and contrasted. 70–81. First published in W. G. Joffe (Ed.), *What is psychoanalysis?* (pp. 15–25). London: The Institute of Psycho-Analysis/Bailliere, Tindall & Cassell, 1968. Also published in C. Winnicott, R. Shepherd & M. Davis (Eds.), *Babies and their mothers* (pp. 89–103). Reading, MA: Addison-Wesley, 1987. [CW 8:2:2]

Health education through broadcasting. 95–98. First published in *Mother and Child*, 1957, 28. Also published in C. Winnicott, C. Bollas, M. Davis & R. Shepherd (Eds.), *Talking to parents* (pp. 1–6). Reading, MA: Addison-Wesley, 1993. [CW 5:3:31]

For stepparents [1955]. 99–103. First published in C. Winnicott, C. Bollas, M. Davis & R. Shepherd (Eds.), *Talking to parents* (pp. 7–13). Reading, MA: Addison-Wesley, 1993. Broadcast in three parts, 7–9 June 1955, I. Benzie (Producer), *Woman's hour*. Light Programme. London: British Broadcasting Corporation. [CW 5:1:10]

What do we know about babies as cloth suckers? [1956]. 104–107. First published in C. Winnicott, C. Bollas, M. Davis & R. Shepherd (Eds.), *Talking to parents* (pp. 15–20). Reading, MA: Addison-Wesley, 1993. Broadcast 31 January 1956. I. Benzie (Producer), *Woman's hour*. Light Programme. London: British Broadcasting Corporation. [CW 5:2:1]

Saying 'No' [1960]. 108–121. First published in C. Winnicott, C. Bollas, M. Davis & R. Shepherd (Eds.), *Talking to parents* (pp. 21–39). Reading, MA: Addison-Wesley, 1993. Broadcast as parts 1–3 of 'The ordinary devoted mother and her children', 25 January, 1 and 8 February 1960. I. Benzie & E. Brewer (Producers), *Parents and children*. Network Three. London: British Broadcasting Corporation. [CW 6:1:1]

Jealousy [1960]. 122–138. First published in C. Winnicott, C. Bollas, M. Davis & R. Shepherd (Eds.), *Talking to parents* (pp. 41–64). Reading, MA: Addison-Wesley, 1993. Broadcast as parts 4–7 of 'The ordinary devoted mother and her children',

15, 22, 29 February and 7 March 1960. I. Benzie & E. Brewer (Producers), *Parents and children*. Network Three. London: British Broadcasting Corporation. [CW 6:1:4]

What irks? [1960]. 139–154. First published in C. Winnicott, C. Bollas, M. Davis & R. Shepherd (Eds.), *Talking to parents* (pp. 68–86). Reading, MA: Addison-Wesley, 1993. Broadcast as parts 8–9 of 'The ordinary devoted mother and her children', 14 and 21 March 1960. I. Benzie & E. Brewer (Producers), *Parents and children*. Network Three. London: British Broadcasting Corporation. [CW 6:1:7]

Security [1960]. 155–159. First published in *The family and individual development* (pp. 30–33). London: Tavistock, 1965, as 'On security'. Also published in C. Winnicott, C. Bollas, M. Davis & R. Shepherd (Eds.), *Talking to parents* (pp. 87–93). Reading, MA: Addison-Wesley, 1993. Broadcast 18 April 1960, as 'Too much security?' I. Benzie (Producer), *Parents and children*. Network Three. London: British Broadcasting Corporation. Published here as 'On security' [CW 6:1:9]

Feeling guilty [1961]. 160–166. First published in C. Winnicott, C. Bollas, M. Davis & R. Shepherd (Eds.), *Talking to parents* (pp. 95–103). Reading, MA: Addison-Wesley, 1993. Broadcast 13 March 1961, as 'Guilt feelings in young mothers. A discussion with Clare Rayner'. E. Crowther (Producer), *Parents and children*. Network Three. London: British Broadcasting Corporation. [CW 6:2:6]

The development of a child's sense of right and wrong [1962]. 167–170. First published in C. Winnicott, C. Bollas, M. Davis & R. Shepherd (Eds.), *Talking to parents* (pp. 105–110). Reading, MA: Addison-Wesley, 1993. Broadcast 11 June 1962 as 'The first five years: 11. The development of a child's sense of right and wrong'. S. Waterhouse (Producer), *Parents and Children*. Network Three. London: British Broadcasting Corporation. [CW 6:3:4]

Now they are five. 171–177. First published in *The family and individual development* (pp. 34–39, as 'The five-year-old' [1962]). London: Tavistock, 1965. Also published in C. Winnicott, C. Bollas, M. Davis & R. Shepherd (Eds.), *Talking to parents* (pp. 111–120, as 'Now they are five'). Reading, MA: Addison-Wesley, 1993. Broadcast 25 June 1962, as 'The first five years: 13. Now they are five'. S. Waterhouse (Producer), *Parents and children*. Network Three. London: British Broadcasting Corporation. Published here as 'The five-year-old'. [CW 6:3:6]

The building up of trust [1969]. 178–187. First published in C. Winnicott, C. Bollas, M. Davis & R. Shepherd (Eds.), *Talking to parents* (pp. 121–134). Reading, MA: Addison-Wesley, 1993. [CW 9:1:26]

Advising parents [1957]. 193–201. First published in *The family and individual development* (pp. 114–120). London: Tavistock, 1965. [CW 5:3:27]

The mother's contribution to society. 202–206. First published in *The child and the family: First relationships* (pp. 141–144, as 'Postscript: The mother's contribution to society'). London: Tavistock, 1957. Also published in C. Winnicott, R. Shepherd & M. Davis (Eds.), *Home is where we start from: Essays by a psychoanalyst* (pp. 123–127). Harmondsworth: Penguin, 1986. [CW 5:3:30]

The family and emotional maturity [1960]. 207–214. First published in *The family and individual development* (pp. 88–94). London: Tavistock, 1965. [CW 6:1:17]

The development of the capacity for concern [1962]. 215–220. First published in *Bulletin of the Menninger Clinic*, 1963, 27. Also published in *The maturational processes and the facilitating environment: Studies in the theory of emotional development* (pp.

73–82). London: Hogarth, 1965; and C. Winnicott, R. Shepherd & M. Davis (Eds.), *Deprivation and delinquency* (pp. 100–105). London: Tavistock, 1984. [CW 6:3:11]

The child in the family group [1966]. 221–231. First published in C. Winnicott, R. Shepherd & M. Davis (Eds.), *Home is where we start from: Essays by a psychoanalyst* (pp. 128–141). Harmondsworth: Penguin, 1986. [CW 7:3:17]

Children learning. 232–238. First published in *The human family and God*. London: Christian Teamwork Institute of Education, 1968. Also published in C. Winnicott, R. Shepherd & M. Davis (Eds.), *Home is where we start from: Essays by a psychoanalyst* (pp. 142–149). Harmondsworth: Penguin, 1986. [CW 8:2:16]

2003

Ditty on Enoch Powell, in a letter to Peter Tizard [ca. 1968]. In F. R. Rodman (Ed.), *Winnicott: Life and work* (p. 393). Cambridge, MA: Perseus, 2003. [CW 9:4:13]

Moon landing (Poem) [1969]. In C. Winnicott, R. Shepherd & M. Davis (Eds.), *Home is where we start from: Essays by a psychoanalyst* (pp. 208–209, part of 'The pill and the moon'). Harmondsworth: Penguin, 1986. Also published, in part, in F. R. Rodman (Ed.), *Winnicott: Life and work* (pp. 416–417). Cambridge, MA: Perseus, 2003. [CW 9:1:18]

Preface. R. Gaddini's Italian translation of *The family and individual development* [1966]. *Psychoanalysis and History*, 2003, 5. [CW 7:3:27]

The tree (poem) [1963]. In F. R. Rodman (Ed.), *Winnicott: Life and work* (pp. 289–291). Cambridge, MA: Perseus, 2003. [CW 6:4:14]

2013

Notes for the Vienna Congress [1971]. Published, in part, in J. Abram (Ed.), *Donald Winnicott today* (pp. 302–330, as 'D. W. W.'s notes on the Vienna Congress 1971: A consideration of Winnicott's theory of aggression and an interpretation of the clinical implications'). London: Routledge, 2013. [CW 9:3:12]

Previously Unpublished

A 70th birthday present [1965]. [CW 7:2:20]

Address introducing Margaret Mead, VIIIth Ernest Jones Lecture (British Psychoanalytical Society) [1957]. [CW 5:3:4]

An allotted spanner in the works [n.d., ca. 1966–1967]. [CW 7:3:37]

Answers to comments on 'The split-off male and female elements' [1968–1969]. Published, in part, in *Psychoanalytic Forum*, 1972, 4; and, in part, in C. Winnicott, R. Shepherd & M. Davis Eds.), *Psycho-analytic explorations* (pp. 189–192). Cambridge, MA: Harvard University Press, 1989. [CW 9:1:30]

Chards pil... [1968]. [CW 8:2:4]

The child, the family and the offender: Response to a Home Office White Paper [1965]. [CW 7:2:12]

Cleopatra anamnesis [n.d.]. [CW 9:4:9]

Clinical material: Theme of 'Two', also theme of 'Black' [1965]. [CW 7:2:13]

Comment: Sandler, J., 'Problems of research in psycho-analysis' [1961]. [CW 6:2:12]
Considerations in the study of homosexuality [1963]. [CW 6:4:4]
The day-dreamer [n.d.]. [CW 9:4:2]
Delinquency: Continued [ca. 1930s]. [CW 2:1:9]
A doctor looks at the psychiatric social worker [1943]. [CW 2:5:1]
Enuresis: Notes for a lecture to the Tavistock Children's Department [n.d., ca. 1949]. [CW 3:4:36]
Evidence given to the Home Office Committee on Children's Homes [1945]. [CW 2:7:9]
Found objects and waifs [n.d.]. [CW 9:4:7]
Further clinical illustration of 'The use of an object' [1968]. [CW 8:2:30]
Getting to know your baby (1945). Broadcast 14 November 1945. I. Benzie (Producer), *The New Baby*. Home Service. London: British Broadcasting Corporation. [CW 12:3:4b]
The Gwrw Tree [1948]. [CW 3:3:4]
The infancy of Juliet [1949]. [CW 3:4:4]
Looking forward to your baby's arrival. Broadcast 10 October 1945. I. Benzie (Producer), *The New Baby*. Home Service. London: British Broadcasting Corporation. [CW 12:3:4a]
'Matti', aet 12 years: A therapeutic consultation [1961]. [CW 6:2:15]
Meet to be stolen from. [n.d., ca. 1939–1945] [CW 2:3:7]
Memorandum from Paddington Green Children's Hospital Psychology Department on homosexuality and the law [1955]. [CW 5:1:4]
Memorandum on corporal punishment [1945]. [CW 2:7:6]
Memorandum on Gisburne House [1959]. [CW 5:5:4]
Memorandum on organizational aspects of child care at Paddington Green Children's Hospital (Psychology Department) [1961]. [CW 6:2:3]
Memorandum on 'The relationship between clinical paediatrics and child psychology' [1943]. [CW 2:5:3]
Note on infant observation [n.d., after 1957]. [CW 9:4:6]
A note on regression and reassurance [1955]. [CW 5:1:21]
Notes for a discussion on technique in analysis of psychotics [n.d.]. [CW 9:4:3]
Notes on adolescence [ca. 1956]. [CW 5:2:17]
Notes on the discussion held on Dr Winnicott's paper 'The birth trauma' [1949]. [CW 3:4:11]
Not less than everything [extracts] [ca. 1968–1971]. Reprinted from C. Winnicott 'D. W. W.: A reflection', in C. Winnicott, R. Shepherd & M. Davis (Eds.), *Psycho-analytic explorations* (pp. 423–426). Cambridge, MA: Harvard University Press, 1989. [CW 9:3:11]
On in-patient treatment for rheumatic fever and chorea. [n.d., c. 1923–1931]. [CW 1:2:24]
On 'Separation anxiety' by J. Bowlby [1958]. [CW 5:4:18]
On the occasion of the publication of the *Standard Edition* of Freud [1966]. [CW 7:3:23]
The ordinary devoted mother and her baby: The first week. Broadcast 16 January 1952. I. Benzie (Producer), *Woman's hour*. Light Programme. London: British Broadcasting Corporation. [CW 4:1:1]
The ordinary devoted mother and her baby: Baby bites. Broadcast 30 January 1952. I. Benzie (Producer), *Woman's hour*. Light Programme. London: British Broadcasting Corporation. [CW 4:1:2]
The ordinary devoted mother and her baby: My fan mail. Broadcast 20 February 1952. I. Benzie (Producer), *Woman's hour*. Light Programme. London: British Broadcasting Corporation. [CW 12:3:4d]

Outline for a study in the sociology of knowledge [n.d.]. [CW 9:4:12]
A personal statement on child psychiatry [1970]. [CW 9:2:4]
Problems of management: Training babies. Broadcast 23 November 1949. I. Benzie (Producer), *How's the baby?* Home Service. London: British Broadcasting Corporation. [CW 12:3:4c]. See also 'The innate morality of the baby'.
The psychoanalyst and child psychiatry, a matter of economics [1962]. [CW 6:3:12]
Psychological aspects of birching [1944]. [CW 2:6:3]
Psychological aspects of juvenile delinquency (a talk to probation officers) [n.d., ca. 1940s]. [CW 3:1:8]
Psychologists as a group [1969]. [CW 9:1:31]
Remarks on a discussion of Balint's paper on technique [1957]. [CW 5:3:8]
Report on Q Camps [1941]. [CW 2:3:1]
Review: Freud, A., *Normality and pathology in childhood* (New York: International Universities Press, 1965) [1965]. [CW 7:2:16]
Sakari: A therapeutic consultation [1961]. [CW 6:2:16]
Social aspects of autism [1966]. [CW 7:3:7]
Some principles of child analysis [1969]. [CW 9:1:9]
Spoken comments on obsessional neurosis and 'Frankie' [1965]. [CW 7:2:11]
A study of envy and gratitude [1956]. [CW 5:2:5]
The toddler, the second adoption, telling children about adoption [n.d., ca. mid 1950s]. [CW 5:1:23]
Trips into partisanship [1967]. [CW 8:1:30]
The unconscious [1953]. [CW 4:2:8]
The unconscious [1966]. [CW 7:3:29]
What is worthwhile in medicine [ca. 1917–1923]. [CW 1:1:16]
Where angels fear to tread, or, a comment on generic teaching [1958]. [CW 5:4:9]

Unpublished

Last Will and Testament [1965]. Published in Brett Kahr, *D. W. Winnicott: A biographical portrait* (pp. 147–148). London: Karnac, 1996.
Plea for a kind of Christianity [ca. 1917–1923]. Winnicott Archive, held in the Wellcome Library, London.
Poem [written after C. O. Conference at Southport, with Clare Britton (Winnicott)]. In F. R. Rodman (Ed.), *Winnicott: Life and work* (p. 393). Cambridge, MA: Perseus, 2003.

Alphabetical Bibliography of Works by D. W. Winnicott

A 70th birthday present [1965]. [CW 7:2:20]

Abscess in frontal lobe: Post-mortem findings in a case shown at a previous meeting of the section (with E. O'Flynn). *Proceedings of the Royal Society of Medicine*, 1928, 21(7), 1256–1257. [CW 1:2:11]

Absence and presence of a sense of guilt illustrated in two patients [1966]. In C. Winnicott, R. Shepherd & M. Davis (Eds.), *Psycho-analytic explorations* (pp. 163–167). Cambridge, MA: Harvard University Press, 1989. [Part 2 of 'The absence of a sense of guilt', CW 7:3:32]

The absence of a sense of guilt [1966]. In C. Winnicott, R. Shepherd & M. Davis (Eds.), *Deprivation and delinquency* (pp. 106–112). London: Tavistock, 1984. [CW 7:3:32]

Abstract: Alexander, F., 'Psychoanalysis and medicine' (*Mental Hygiene*, 1932, *16*, 63). *International Journal of Psychoanalysis*, 1933, *14*, 108. [CW 1:4:1]

Abstract: Barinbaum, M., 'A contribution to the problem of psycho-physical relations with special reference to dermatology' (*Internationale Zeitschrift für Psychoanalyse*, 1934, *20*, 241–251). *International Journal of Psychoanalysis*, 1935, *16*, 369. [CW 1:4:5]

Abstract: Lundholm, H., 'Repression and rationalization' (*British Journal of Medical Psychology*, 1933, *13*(1), 23). *International Journal of Psychoanalysis*, 1934, *15*, 308. [CW 1:4:2]

Active heart disease. In *Clinical notes on disorders of childhood* (pp. 69–75). London: Heinemann, 1931. [CW 1:3:8]

'Ada' aet 8 years. In *Therapeutic consultations in child psychiatry* (pp. 220–238). London: Hogarth, 1971. [CW 10:3:13] Also published in R. Slovenko (Ed.), *Crime, law and corrections* (pp. 102–130, as 'Psychotherapeutic interview', part of the chapter 'A psychoanalytic view of the antisocial tendency'). Springfield, IL: Charles C. Thomas, 1966; and C. Winnicott, R. Shepherd & M. Davis (Eds.), Deprivation and delinquency (pp. 256–282, as 'Psychotherapeutic interview', part of the chapter 'Dissociation revealed in a therapeutic consultation'). London: Tavistock, 1984. [CW 7:2:21]

Addendum to 'The location of cultural experience' [1967]. In C. Winnicott, R. Shepherd & M. Davis (Eds.), *Psycho-analytic explorations* (pp. 200–202). Cambridge, MA: Harvard University Press, 1989. [CW 8:1:37]

Additional note on psycho-somatic disorder [1969]. In C. Winnicott, R. Shepherd & M. Davis (Eds.), *Psycho-analytic explorations* (pp. 115–118, in the chapter 'Psycho-somatic disorder'). Cambridge, MA: Harvard University Press, 1989. [CW 9:1:21]

Address introducing Margaret Mead, 8th Ernest Jones Lecture, British Psychoanalytical Society [1957]. [CW 5:3:4]

Adolescence: Struggling through the doldrums [1961]. *New Era in Home and School*, 43(8), 1962 October, as 'Adolescence'. Also published in *The family and individual development* (pp. 79–87). London: Tavistock, 1965. [CW 6:2:4] See also 'Struggling through the doldrums'. [CW 6:4:7]

Adolescent immaturity. In C. Winnicott, R. Shepherd & M. Davis (Eds.), *Home is where we start from: Essays by a psychoanalyst* (pp. 150–166). Published here as 'Contemporary concepts of adolescent development and their implications for higher education'. [CW 9:3:9]

Adolescent process and the need for personal confrontation. *Pediatrics*, 1969, 44. Published here as 'Death and murder in the adolescent process', as part of 'Contemporary concepts of adolescent development and their implications for higher education'. [CW 9:3:9] See also 'Adolescent immaturity'.

Adopted children in adolescence. First published in *Report of Residential Conference, Standing Conference of Societies Registered for Adoption*, July 1955. Also published in R. Shepherd, J. Johns & H. Taylor Robinson (Eds.), *Thinking about children* (pp. 136–148). London: Karnac, 1996. [CW 5:1:12]

Advising parents [1957]. First published in *The family and individual development* (pp. 114–120). London: Tavistock, 1965. Also published in *Winnicott on the child* (pp. 193–201). Cambridge, MA: Perseus, 2002. [CW 5:3:27]

The aetiology of infantile schizophrenia in terms of adaptive failure [1967]. *Recherches*, 1968 (special issue 'Enfance aliénée', 2), as 'La schizophrénie infantile en termes d'échec d'adaption'. Also published in R. Shepherd, J. Johns & H. Taylor Robinson (Eds.), *Thinking about children* (pp. 218–233). London: Karnac, 1996. [CW 8:1:25]

Aggression [ca. 1939]. In *The child and the outside world* (pp. 167–175). London: Tavistock, 1957. Also published in C. Winnicott, R. Shepherd & M. Davis (Eds.), *Deprivation and delinquency* (pp. 84–92, part of 'Aggression and its roots'). London: Tavistock, 1984. [CW 2:1:8]

Aggression, guilt and reparation [1960]. In C. Winnicott, R. Shepherd & M. Davis (Eds.), *Deprivation and delinquency* (pp. 136–144). London: Tavistock, 1984. Also published in C. Winnicott, R. Shepherd & M. Davis (Eds.), *Home is where we start from: Essays by a psychoanalyst* (pp. 80–89). Harmondsworth: Penguin, 1986. [CW 6:1:10]

Aggression in relation to emotional development [1950]. In *Collected papers: Through paediatrics to psycho-analysis* (pp. 204–218). London: Tavistock, 1958. [CW 3:5:2]

The aims of psycho-analytical treatment [1962]. In *The maturational processes and the facilitating environment: Studies in the theory of emotional development* (pp. 166–170). London: Hogarth, 1965. [CW 6:3:2]

'Albert' aet 7 years 9 months. In *Therapeutic consultations in child psychiatry* (pp. 161–175). London: Hogarth, 1971. [CW 10:2:10]

'Alfred' aet 10 years. In *Therapeutic consultations in child psychiatry* (pp. 110–126). London: Hogarth, 1971. [CW 10:1:7] See also 'A psychotherapeutic consultation: A case of stammering'.

An allotted spanner in the works [n.d., ca. 1966–1967]. [CW 7:3:38]

Answers to comments on 'The split-off male and female elements' [1968–1969]. Published, in part, in *Psychoanalytic Forum*, 1972, 4; and, in part, in C. Winnicott, R. Shepherd & M. Davis (Eds.), *Psycho-analytic explorations* (pp. 189–192). Cambridge, MA: Harvard University Press, 1989. [CW 9:1:30]

The antisocial tendency [1956]. In *Collected papers: Through paediatrics to psycho-analysis* (pp. 306–315). London: Tavistock, 1958. Also published in C. Winnicott, R. Shepherd & M. Davis (Eds.), *Deprivation and delinquency* (pp. 120–131). London: Tavistock, 1984. [CW 5:2:8]

Anxiety associated with insecurity [1952]. In *Collected papers: Through paediatrics to psycho-analysis* (pp. 97–100). London: Tavistock, 1958. [CW 4:1:11]

Anxiety (continued). In *Clinical notes on disorders of childhood* (pp. 122–128). London: Heinemann, 1931. [CW 1:3:13]

Appendix: Withdrawal and regression [1954]. In *Holding and interpretation: Fragment of an analysis* (pp. 187–192). London: Karnac, 1986. Published here as 'Withdrawal and regression'. [CW 4:3:29]

Appetite and emotional disorder [1936]. In *Collected papers: Through paediatrics to psycho-analysis* (pp. 33–51). London: Tavistock, 1958. [CW 1:4:11]

Arthritis associated with emotional disturbance. In *Clinical notes on disorders of childhood* (pp. 81–86). London: Heinemann, 1931. [CW 1:3:10]

'Ashton' *aet* 12 years. In *Therapeutic consultations in child psychiatry* (pp. 147–160). London: Hogarth, 1971. Also published in E. Miller (Ed.), *Foundations of child psychiatry* (pp. 593–608, as part of 'The value of the therapeutic consultation'). Oxford, UK: Pergamon, 1968. [CW 10:2:9]

Aspects of juvenile delinquency. In *The child, the family, and the outside world* (pp. 227–231). Harmondsworth: Penguin, 1964. Published here as 'Some psychological aspects of juvenile delinquency'. [CW 3:1:7]

The Association for Child Psychology and Psychiatry observed as a group phenomenon [1967]. In R. Shepherd, J. Johns & H. Taylor Robinson (Eds.), *Thinking about children* (pp. 235–254). London: Karnac, 1996. [CW 8:1:3]

Autism [1966]. In R. Shepherd, J. Johns & H. Taylor Robinson (Eds.), *Thinking about children* (pp. 197–217). London: Karnac, 1996. [CW 7:3:8]

Babies and their mothers (C. Winnicott, R. Shepherd & M. Davis, Eds.). Reading, MA: Addison-Wesley, 1987. Also published as Part 1 of **Winnicott on the child**. Cambridge, MA: Perseus, 2002. [Not reprinted in this form in the *Collected Works*]

Babies are persons. *New Era in Home and School*, 1947, 28(10), 179. Also published in *The child and the outside world: Studies in developing relationships* (pp. 134–140, as 'Further thoughts on babies as persons'). London: Tavistock, 1957; and *The child, the family, and the outside world* (pp. 85–92, as 'Further thoughts on babies as persons'). Harmondsworth: Penguin, 1964. Published here as 'Further thoughts on babies as persons'. [CW 3:2:4]

The baby as a going concern. In *The ordinary devoted mother and her baby* (pp. 7–11). London: C. A. Brock, 1949. Also published in *The child and the family: First relationships* (pp. 13–17). London: Tavistock, 1957; and *The child, the family, and the outside world* (pp. 25–29). Harmondsworth: Penguin, 1964. Broadcast 12 October 1949, as 'The mind of a child'. I. Benzie (Producer), *How's the baby?* Home Service. London: British Broadcasting Corporation. [CW 3:4:24]

The baby as a person. In *The ordinary devoted mother and her baby* (pp. 22–26). London: C. A. Brock, 1949. Also published in *The child and the family: First relationships* (pp. 33–37). London: Tavistock, 1957; and *The child, the family, and the outside world* (pp. 75–79). Harmondsworth: Penguin, 1964. Broadcast 2 November 1949, as 'No baby can grow properly without love'. I. Benzie (Producer), *How's the baby?* Home Service. London: British Broadcasting Corporation. [CW 3:4:27]

Basis for self in body [1970]. *Nouvelle Revue de Psychanalyse*, 1971, 3, as 'Le corps et le self'. Also published in C. Winnicott, R. Shepherd & M. Davis (Eds.), *Psycho-analytic explorations* (pp. 261–271). Cambridge, MA: Harvard University Press, 1989. [CW 9:2:12]

The bearing of emotional development on feeding problems. In R. Shepherd, J. Johns & H. Taylor Robinson (Eds.), *Thinking about children* (pp. 39–41). London: Karnac, 1996. Published here, together with 'Infant feeding and emotional development', as 'Environmental health in infancy'. [CW 8:1:6]

Becoming deprived as a fact: A psychotherapeutic consultation. *Journal of Child Psychotherapy*, 1966, 1(4), 5–12. [CW 10: Appendix 6] Also published in *Therapeutic consultations in child psychiatry* (pp. 315–330, as '"Ruth" aet 8 years'). London: Hogarth, 1971. Published here as '"Ruth" aet 8 years'. [CW 10:3:17]

The beginning of the individual [1966]. In C. Winnicott, R. Shepherd & M. Davis (Eds.) *Babies and their mothers* (pp. 51–58). Reading, MA: Addison-Wesley, 1987. Also published in *Winnicott on the child* (pp. 43–48). Cambridge, MA: Perseus, 2002. [CW 7:3:34]

The beginnings of a formulation of an appreciation and criticism of Klein's envy statement [1962]. In C. Winnicott, R. Shepherd & M. Davis (Eds.), *Psycho-analytic explorations* (pp. 447–457, in the chapter 'Melanie Klein: On her concept of envy'). Cambridge, MA: Harvard University Press, 1989. [CW 6:3:7]

Berlin walls [1969]. In C. Winnicott, R. Shepherd, & M. Davis (Eds.), *Home is where we start from: Essays by a psychoanalyst* (pp. 221–227). Harmondsworth: Penguin 1986. [CW 9:1:25]

The best remedy. *The Fortnightly* (The Leys School, Cambridge), 12 June 1914. [CW 1:1:8]

Birth memories, birth trauma and anxiety [1949]. In *Collected papers: Through paediatrics to psycho-analysis* (pp. 174–193). London: Tavistock, 1958. [CW 3:4:8]

'Bob' aet 6 years. In *Therapeutic consultations in child psychiatry* (pp. 64–88). London: Hogarth, 1971. [CW 10:1:4]. See also 'A clinical study of the effect of a failure of the average expectable environment on a child's mental functioning'.

Breast feeding [1945, revised 1954]. In *The child and the outside world* (pp. 141–148). London: Tavistock, 1957. Also published in *The child, the family, and the outside world* (pp. 50–57). Harmondsworth: Penguin, 1964. [CW 2:7:12]

Breast-feeding as communication [1968]. *Maternal and Child Care*, 1969, 5. Also published in C. Winnicott, R. Shepherd & M. Davis (Eds.), *Babies and their mothers* (pp. 23–33). Reading, MA: Addison-Wesley, 1987; and *Winnicott on the child* (pp. 24–31). Cambridge, MA: Perseus, 2002. [CW 8:2:26]

The building up of trust [1969]. In C. Winnicott, C. Bollas, M. Davis & R. Shepherd (Eds.), *Talking to parents* (pp. 121–134). Reading, MA: Addison-Wesley, 1993. Also published in *Winnicott on the child* (pp. 178–187). Cambridge, MA: Perseus, 2002. [CW 9:1:26]

The capacity to be alone [1957]. *International Journal of Psychoanalysis*, 1958, 39, 416–420. Also published in *Psyche*, 1958, 12, as 'Über die Fähigkeit, Allein zu Sein'; and *The maturational processes and the facilitating environment: Studies in the theory of emotional development* (pp. 29–36). London: Hogarth, 1965. [CW 5:3:20]

Case for diagnosis (? infantile hemiplegia). *Section for the Study of Disease in Children, Proceedings of the Royal Society of Medicine*, 1926, 19, 47–48. [CW 1:2:3]

Case for diagnosis (? poliomyelitis with some spasticity). *Section for the Study of Disease in Children, Proceedings of the Royal Society of Medicine*, 1926, *19*, 46–47. [CW 1:2:2]

A case managed at home. *Case Conference*, 1955, 2, as 'Childhood psychosis: A case managed at home'. Also published in *Collected papers: Through peadiatrics to psycho-analysis* (pp. 118–126). London: Tavistock, 1958. [CW 5:1:18]

Case notes for a psychoanalytic seminar: Withdrawal, regression, male identification [1965]. In C. Winnicott, R. Shepherd & M. Davis (Eds.), *Psycho-analytic explorations* (pp. 149–151, in part, as 'Notes on withdrawal and regression'). Cambridge, MA: Harvard University Press, 1989. [CW 7:2:19]

Case of stunted growth. *Proceedings of the Royal Society of Medicine*, 1927, *20*(10), 1586. [CW 1:2:5]

Casework with mentally ill children [1959]. In *The family and individual development* (pp. 121–131). London: Tavistock, 1965. [CW 5:5:15]

'Cecil' aet 21 months at first consultation. In *Therapeutic consultations in child psychiatry* (pp. 239–269). London: Hogarth, 1971. [CW 10:3:14] See also 'Regression as therapy illustrated by the case of a boy whose pathological dependence was adequately met by the parents'.

Changing patterns: The young person, the family and society. In *Proceedings of the British Student Health Association Twentieth Conference* (Newcastle, UK, 1968), 1969. Published here as part of 'Contemporary concepts of adolescent development and their implications for higher education'. [CW 9:3:9] See also 'Adolescent immaturity'.

Character types: The foolhardy and the cautious. On M. Balint '*Funfairs, thrills and regressions*' [1954]. In C. Winnicott, R. Shepherd & M. Davis (Eds.), *Psycho-analytic explorations* (pp. 433–437). Cambridge, MA: Harvard University Press, 1989. [CW 4:3:26]

Chards pil. . . [1968]. [CW 8:2:4]

'Charles' aet 9 years. In *Therapeutic consultation in child psychiatry* (pp. 129–146). London: Hogarth, 1971. [CW 10:2:8]

Child analysis in the latency period. *A Criança Portuguesa*, 1958, *17*. Also published in *The maturational processes and the facilitating environment: Studies in the theory of emotional development* (pp. 115–123). London: Hogarth, 1965. [CW 5:4:13]

The child and sex. *The Practitioner*, 1947, *158*. Also published in *The child and the outside world: Studies in developing relationships* (pp. 153–166). London: Tavistock, 1957; and *The child, the family, and the outside world* (pp. 147–160). Harmondsworth: Penguin, 1964. [CW 3:2:5]

The child and the family: First relationships. London: Tavistock, 1957. [Not reprinted in this form in the *Collected Works*]

The child and the outside world: Studies in developing relationships. London: Tavistock, 1957. [Not reprinted in this form in the *Collected Works*]

Child department consultations. *International Journal of Psychoanalysis*, 1942, *23*, 139–146. Also published in *Collected papers: Through paediatrics to psycho-analysis* (pp. 70–84). London: Tavistock, 1958. [CW 2:4:2]

Childhood psychosis. *British Medical Journal*, 1950, *1*, 944–945. [CW 3:5:5]

The child in the family group [1966]. In C. Winnicott, R. Shepherd & M. Davis (Eds.), *Home is where we start from: Essays by a psychoanalyst* (pp. 128–141). Harmondsworth: Penguin, 1986. Also published in *Winnicott on the child* (pp. 221–231). Cambridge, MA: Perseus, 2002. [CW 7:3:17]

A child psychiatry case illustrating delayed reaction to loss. In M. Schur (Ed.), *Drives, affects, behavior: Essays in memory of Marie Bonaparte* (Vol. 2, pp. 212–242). New York: International Universities Press, 1965. Also published in C. Winnicott, R. Shepherd & M. Davis (Eds.), *Psycho-analytic explorations* (pp. 341–368). Cambridge, MA: Harvard University Press, 1989. [CW 7:2:23]

A child psychiatry interview. *St Mary's Hospital Gazette,* 1962, 68. Also published in *Therapeutic consultations in child psychiatry* (pp. 105–109, as ' "Rosemary" aet 10 years'). London: Hogarth, 1971. Published here as ' "Rosemary" aet 10 years'. [CW 10:1:6]

Child psychiatry, social work and alternative care [1970]. In R. Shepherd, J. Johns & H. Taylor Robinson (Eds.), *Thinking about children* (pp. 277–281). London: Karnac, 1996. [CW 9:2:3]

Child psychiatry: The body as affected by psychological factors [1931]. In R. Shepherd, J. Johns & H. Taylor Robinson (Eds.), *Thinking about children* (pp. 176–178). London: Karnac, 1996. [CW 1:2:23]

The child's needs and the role of the mother in the early stages. In *The child and the outside world: Studies in developing relationships* (pp. 14–23). London: Tavistock, 1957. Published here as 'Mother, teacher, and the child's needs'. [CW 4:2:20]

Children and their mothers. *New Era in Home and School,* 1940, 21. Also published in C. Winnicott, R. Shepherd & M. Davis (Eds.), *Deprivation and delinquency* (pp. 14–21, part of 'Evacuation of small children'). London: Tavistock, 1984. [CW 2:2:2]

Children in the war. *New Era in Home and School,* 1940, 21. Also published in *The child and the outside world: Studies in developing relationships* (pp. 69–74). London: Tavistock, 1957; and C. Winnicott, R. Shepherd & M. Davis (Eds.), *Deprivation and delinquency* (pp. 25–30). London: Tavistock, 1984. [CW 2:2:4]

Children learning. In *The human family and god*. London: Christian Teamwork Institute of Education, 1968. Also published in C. Winnicott, R. Shepherd & M. Davis (Eds.), *Home is where we start from: Essays by a psychoanalyst* (pp. 142–149). Harmondsworth: Penguin, 1986; and *Winnicott on the child* (pp. 232–238). Cambridge, MA: Perseus, 2002. [CW 8:2:16]

Children's hostels in war and peace [1946]. First published in *British Journal of Medical Psychology,* 1948, 21(3), 175–180. Also published in *The child and the outside world: Studies in developing relationships* (pp. 117–121). London: Tavistock, 1957; and C. Winnicott, R. Shepherd & M. Davis (Eds.), *Deprivation and delinquency* (pp. 73–77). London: Tavistock, 1984. [CW 3:1:1]

The child, the family and the offender: Response to a Home Office White Paper [1965]. [CW 7:2:12]

The child, the family, and the outside world. Harmondsworth: Penguin, 1964. [Not reprinted in this form in the *Collected Works*]

Child therapy: A case of anti-social behaviour. In J. G. Howells (Ed.), *Modern perspectives in child psychiatry* (pp. 523–533). London: Oliver & Boyd, 1965. Introduction published in [CW 10: Appendix 5]. Also published in *Therapeutic consultations in child psychiatry* (pp. 270–295, as ' "Mark" aet 12 years'). London: Hogarth, 1971. Published here as ' "Mark" aet 12 years'. [CW 10:3:15]

Classification: Is there a psycho-analytic contribution to psychiatric classification? [1959, 1964]. In *The maturational processes and the facilitating environment: Studies in the theory of emotional development* (pp. 124–139). London: Hogarth, 1965. [CW 5:5:5]

Cleopatra anamnesis [n.d.]. [CW 9:4:9]
A clinical approach to family problems: The family [1959]. In R. Shepherd, J. Johns & H. Taylor Robinson (Eds.), *Thinking about children* (pp. 54–56). London: Karnac, 1996. [CW 5:5:27]
A clinical example of symptomatology following the birth of a sibling [1931]. In R. Shepherd, J. Johns & H. Taylor Robinson (Eds.), *Thinking about children* (pp. 97–101). London: Karnac, 1996. [CW 1:2:22]
Clinical illustration of 'The use of an object' [1968]. In C. Winnicott, R. Shepherd & M. Davis (Eds.), *Psycho-analytic explorations* (pp. 235–238, part of the chapter 'The use of an object'). Cambridge, MA: Harvard University Press, 1989. [CW 8:2:29]
Clinical material on the theme of a male patient's exploitation of his female self [1959]. In C. Winnicott, R. Shepherd & M. Davis (Eds.), *Psycho-analytic explorations* (pp. 183–188, part of 'Clinical Material [1959–1963]' in the chapter 'On the split-off male and female elements'). Cambridge, MA: Harvard University Press, 1989. [CW 5:5:26]
Clinical material: Theme of 'Two', also Theme of 'Black' [1965]. [CW 7:2:13]
Clinical material [1959–1963]. In C. Winnicott, R. Shepherd & M. Davis (Eds.), *Psycho-analytic explorations* (pp. 183–188, in the chapter 'On the split-off male and female elements'). Cambridge, MA: Harvard University Press, 1989. Published, in part, as 'Clinical material on the theme of a male patient's exploitation of his female self' [1959] [CW 5:5:26]; and, in part, as 'Further clinical material on the theme of a male patient's exploitation of his female self' [1963]. [CW 6:4:20]
Clinical notes on disorders of childhood. London: Heinemann, 1931. [CW 1:3]
Clinical regression compared with defense organization. In S. H. Eldred & M. Vanderpol (Eds.), *Psychotherapy in the designed therapeutic milieu. International Psychiatry Clinics* (Vol. 5). Boston: Little, Brown, 1968. Published here as 'The concept of clinical regression compared with that of defence organization'. [CW 8:1:29]
A clinical study of the effect of a failure of the average expectable environment on a child's mental functioning. *International Journal of Psychoanalysis*, 1965, 46, 81–87. Introduction published in [CW 10: Appendix 2] Also published in *Therapeutic consultations in child psychiatry* (pp. 64–88, in part, as '"Bob" aet 6 years'). London: Hogarth, 1971. Published here as '"Bob" aet 6 years'. [CW 10:1:4]
Clinical varieties of transference [1955]. *International Journal of Psychoanalysis*, 1956, 37, 386–388, as 'On transference'. Also published in *Collected papers: Through paediatrics to psycho-analysis* (pp. 295–299). London: Tavistock, 1958. [CW 5:1:11]
Close-up of mother feeding baby. In *The ordinary devoted mother and her baby* (pp. 27–31). London: C. A. Brock, 1949. Also published in *The child and the family: First relationships* (pp. 38–42). London: Tavistock, 1957; and *The child, the family, and the outside world* (pp. 45–49). Harmondsworth: Penguin, 1964. Broadcast 9 November 1949, as 'The baby at feeding time'. I. Benzie (Producer), *How's the baby?* Home Service. London: British Broadcasting Corporation. [CW 3:4:28]
Collected papers: Through paediatrics to psycho-analysis. London: Tavistock, 1958. Second edition with introduction by M. M. R. Khan. London: Hogarth and The Institute of Psycho-Analysis, 1975. [Not reprinted in this form in the *Collected Works*]
Commentary. V. Axline, *Play therapy*. (Boston: Houghton Mifflin, 1947) [1965]. In C. Winnicott, R. Shepherd & M. Davis (Eds.), *Psycho-analytic explorations* (pp. 495–198). Cambridge, MA: Harvard University Press, 1989. [CW 9:1:32]

Comment on obsessional neurosis and 'Frankie' [1965]. *International Journal of Psychoanalysis*, 1966, 47, 143–144. Also published in C. Winnitcott, R. Shepherd & M. Davis (Eds.), *Psycho-analytic explorations* (pp. 158–160). Cambridge, MA: Harvard University Press, 1989. [CW 7:2:10]

Comment: Sandler, J., 'Problems of research in psycho-analysis' [1961]. [CW 6:2:12]

Comments on Joseph Sandler's 'On the concept of the superego' (*The psycho-analytic study of the child* (Vol. 15) 1960). In C. Winnicott, R. Shepherd & M. Davis (Eds.), *Psycho-analytic explorations* (pp. 465–473). Cambridge, MA: Harvard University Press, 1989. [CW 6:1:19]

Comments on my paper 'The use of an object' [1968]. In C. Winnicott, R. Shepherd & M. Davis (Eds.), *Psycho-analytic explorations* (pp. 238–240, part of the chapter 'The use of an object'). Cambridge, MA: Harvard University Press, 1989. [CW 8:2:38]

Comments on the *Report of the Committee on Punishment in Prisons and Borstals* [1961]. In C. Winnicott, R. Shepherd & M. Davis (Eds.), *Deprivation and delinquency* (pp. 202–208). London: Tavistock, 1984. [CW 6:2:22]

Communicating and not communicating leading to a study of certain opposites [1963]. In *The maturational processes and the facilitating environment: Studies in the theory of emotional development* (pp. 179–192). London: Hogarth, 1965. [CW 6:4:8]

Communication between infant and mother, and mother and infant, compared and contrasted. In W. G. Joffe (Ed.), *What is psychoanalysis?* (pp. 15–25). London: The Institute of Psycho-Analysis/Bailliere, Tindall & Cassell, 1968. Also published in C. Winnicott, R. Shepherd & M. Davis (Eds.), *Babies and their mothers* (pp. 89–103). Reading, MA: Addison-Wesley, 1987; and *Winnicott on the child* (pp. 70–81). Cambridge, MA: Perseus, 2002. [CW 8:2:2]

The concept of a healthy individual [1967]. In John D. Sutherland (Ed.), *Towards community mental health* (pp. 1–16). London: Tavistock, 1971. Also published in C. Winnicott, R. Shepherd & M. Davis (Eds.), *Home is where we start from: Essays by a psychoanalyst* (pp. 21–38). Harmondsworth: Penguin, 1986. [CW 8:1:4]

The concept of clinical regression compared with that of defence organization [1967]. In S. H. Eldred & M. Vanderpol (Eds.), *Psychotherapy in the designed therapeutic milieu. International Psychiatry Clinics* (Vol. 5, pp. 193–199, as 'Clinical regression compared with defense organization'). Boston: Little, Brown, 1968. Also published in C. Winnicott, R. Shepherd & M. Davis (Eds.), *Psycho-analytic explorations* (pp. 193–199). Cambridge, MA: Harvard University Press, 1989. [CW 8:1:29]

The concept of the false self [1964]. In C. Winnicott, R. Shepherd, & M. Davis, Eds, *Home is where we start from: Essays by a psychoanalyst* (pp. 65–70). Harmondsworth: Penguin, 1986. [CW 7:1:1]

The concept of trauma in relation to the development of the individual within the family [1965]. In C. Winnicott, R. Shepherd & M. Davis (Eds.), *Psycho-analytic explorations* (pp. 130–148). Cambridge, MA: Harvard University Press, 1989. [CW 7:2:7]

Considerations in the study of homosexuality [1963]. [CW 6:4:4]

Contemporary concepts of adolescent development and their implications for higher education [1968]. *Proceedings of the British Student Health Association*, 1969, in part, as 'Changing patterns: The young person, the family and society'. Also published in *Pediatrics*, 1969, 44 (as 'Adolescent process and the need for personal confrontation', part of the section 'Death and murder in the adolescent process'); and *Playing and reality* (pp. 138–150). London: Tavistock, 1971; and C. Winnicott, R. Shepherd &

M. Davis (Eds.), *Home is where we start from: Essays by a psychoanalyst* (pp. 150–166, as 'Adolescent immaturity'). Harmondsworth: Penguin, 1986. [CW 9:3:9]

The contribution of psycho-analysis to midwifery. *Nursing Mirror*, May 1957. Also published in *The family and individual development* (pp. 106–113). London: Tavistock, 1965; and C. Winnicott, R. Shepherd & M. Davis (Eds.), *Babies and their mothers* (pp. 69–81). Reading, MA: Addison-Wesley, 1987; and *Winnicott on the child* (pp. 56–64). Cambridge, MA: Perseus, 2002. [CW 5:3:15]

Contribution to a discussion on enuresis. In *Proceedings of the Royal Society of Medicine*, 1936, 29, 1522–1524. Also published in R. Shepherd, J. Johns & H. Taylor Robinson (Eds.), *Thinking about children* (pp. 151–156). London: Karnac, 1996. [CW 1:4:9]

Contribution to a symposium on envy and jealousy [1969]. In C. Winnicott, R. Shepherd & M. Davis (Eds.), *Psycho-analytic explorations* (pp. 462–464, in the chapter 'Melanie Klein: On her concept of envy'). Cambridge, MA: Harvard University Press, 1989. [CW 9:1:8]

Contribution to conference at Dartington Hall. In M. Ash (Ed.), *Who are the progressives now?* (pp. 165–170). London: Routledge & Kegan Paul, 1969. Published here as 'Do progressive schools give too much freedom to the child?' [CW 7:2:5]

Contribution to 'The final number'. *Case Conference*, 1970, 16(12). [CW 9:2:5]

Convulsions, fits. In *Clinical notes on disorders of childhood* (pp. 157–171). London: Heinemann, 1931. [CW 1:3:17]

Correspondence with a magistrate. First published in *New Era in Home and School*, 1944, 25, 7–8, as 'The magistrate, the psychiatrist and the clinic'. Also published in C. Winnicott, R. Shepherd & M. Davis (Eds.), *Deprivation and delinquency* (pp. 166–170). Published here as 'Letter to Roger North'. [CW 2:6:1]

Countertransference [1959]. *British Journal of Medical Psychology*, 1960, 33(1), 17–21. Also published in *The maturational processes and the facilitating environment: Studies in the theory of emotional development* (pp. 158–168). London: Hogarth, 1965. [CW 5:5:20]

Creativity and its origins. In *Playing and reality* (pp. 68–85). London: Tavistock, 1971. [CW 9:3:7]. Includes 'The split-off male and female elements to be found in men and women'.

Critical notice. *British Journal of Medical Psychology*, March 1951, 24. Published here as 'Review: Milner, M., *On not being able to paint*'. [CW 3:6:15]

Cure [1970]. In C. Winnicott, R. Shepherd & M. Davis (Eds.), *Home is where we start from: Essays by a psychoanalyst* (pp. 112–120). Harmondsworth: Penguin 1986. [CW 9:2:8]

The day-dreamer (short story) [n.d., ca. 1950s–1960s]. [CW 9:4:2]

Day dreaming. *Your Child*, 1970, 2. [CW 9:2:14]

Deductions drawn from a psychotherapeutic interview with an adolescent. In *Report of the 20th Child Guidance Inter-Clinic Conference, 1964*. London: The National Association for Mental Health, 1964. Also published in C. Winnicott, R. Shepherd & M. Davis (Eds.), *Psycho-analytic explorations* (pp. 325–340). Cambridge, MA: Harvard University Press, 1989. [CW 7:1:5]

Delinquency as a sign of hope [1967]. *Prison Service Journal*, 1968, 7. Also published in C. Winnicott, R. Shepherd & M. Davis (Eds.), *Home is where we start from: Essays by a psychoanalyst* (pp. 90–100). Harmondsworth: Penguin, 1986. [CW 8:1:8]

Delinquency: Continued [ca. 1930s]. [CW 2:1:9]

Delinquency research. *New Era in Home and School*, 1943, 24. [CW 2:5:2]

The delinquent and habitual offender [ca. 1939]. In R. Shepherd, J. Johns & H. Taylor Robinson (Eds.), *Thinking about children* (pp. 51–53). London: Karnac, 1996. [CW 2:1:3]

Dependence in infant-care, in child-care, and in the psycho-analytic setting [1962]. *International Journal of Psychoanalysis*, 1963, 44, 339–344. Also published in *The maturational processes and the facilitating environment: Studies in the theory of emotional development* (pp. 249–259). London: Hogarth, 1965. [CW 6:3:9]

Dependence in child care. *Your Child*, 1970, 2, as 'Dependence'. Also published in C. Winnicott, R. Shepherd & M. Davis (Eds.), *Babies and their mothers* (pp. 83–88). Reading, MA: Addison-Wesley, 1987; and *Winnicott on the child* (pp. 65–69). Cambridge, MA: Perseus, 2002. [CW 9:2:15]

The depressive position in normal emotional development [1954]. *British Journal of Medical Psychology*, 1955, 28(2–3), 89–100. Also published in *Collected papers: Through paediatrics to psycho-analysis* (pp. 262–277). London: Tavistock, 1958. [CW 4:3:5]

Deprivation and delinquency (C. Winnicott, R. Shepherd & M. Davis, Eds.). London: Tavistock, 1984. [Not reprinted in this form in the *Collected Works*]

The deprived child and how he can be compensated for loss of family life [1950]. In *The family and individual development*. London: Tavistock, 1965. [CW 3:5:10]

The deprived mother [1939]. *New Era in Home and School*, 1940, 21(3). Also published in *The child and the outside world: Studies in developing relationships* (pp. 75–82). London: Tavistock, 1957); and C. Winnicott, R. Shepherd & M. Davis (Eds.), *Deprivation and delinquency* (pp. 31–38). London: Tavistock, 1984. Broadcast 1939. London: British Broadcasting Corporation. [CW 2:1:4]

The development of a child's sense of right and wrong [1962]. In C. Winnicott, C. Bollas, M. Davis & R. Shepherd (Eds.), *Talking to parents* (pp. 105–110). Reading, MA: Addison-Wesley, 1993. Also published in *Winnicott on the child* (pp. 167–170). Cambridge, MA: Perseus, 2002. Broadcast 11 June 1962 as 'The first five years: 11. The development of a child's sense of right and wrong'. S. Waterhouse (Producer), *Parents and children*. Network Three. London: British Broadcasting Corporation. [CW 6:3:4]

The development of the capacity for concern [1962]. *Bulletin of the Menninger Clinic*, 1963, 27. Also published in *The maturational processes and the facilitating environment: Studies in the theory of emotional development* (pp. 73–82). London: Hogarth, 1965; and C. Winnicott, R. Shepherd & M. Davis (Eds.), *Deprivation and delinquency* (pp. 100–105). London: Tavistock, 1984; and *Winnicott on the child* (pp. 215–220). Cambridge, MA: Perseus, 2002. [CW 6:3:11]

Development of the theme of the mother's unconscious as discovered in psycho-analytic practice [1969]. In C. Winnicott, R. Shepherd & M. Davis (Eds.), *Psycho-analytic explorations* (pp. 247–250). Cambridge, MA: Harvard University Press, 1989. [CW 9:1:15]

The diagnosis of chorea. *Postgraduate Medical Journal*, 1929, 4(45), 147–153. [CW 1:2:16]

Die volle Nutzung der ersten Behandlungsstunde. In G. Bierman (Ed.), *Handbuch der Kinderpsychotherapie* (pp. 269–277). München/Basel: Ernst Reinhardt Verlag, 1968. Includes '"Eliza" aet 7½ years'. See also 'The squiggle game'.

Discussion: Alger, I., 'The clinical handling of the analyst's response'. *Psychoanalytic Forum*, 1966, *1*. [CW 7:3:36]

Discussion: Auden, G. A., 'The difficult child' (*The Journal of the Royal Society for the Promotion of Health*, March 1929, 50, 157–164). *Journal of State Medicine*, 1934, 42, 628–630. [CW 1:4:4]

Discussion: 'Grief and mourning in infancy' by John Bowlby (*The Psychoanalytic Study of the Child*, 1960, 15) [1959]. In C. Winnicott, R. Shepherd & M. Davis (Eds.), *Psychoanalytic explorations* (pp. 426–432). Cambridge, MA: Harvard University Press, 1989. [CW 5:5:17]

Discussion of war aims [1940]. In C. Winnicott, R. Shepherd & M. Davis, (Eds.), *Home is where we start from: Essays by a psychoanalyst* (pp. 210–220). Harmondsworth: Penguin, 1986. [CW 2:2:3]

Discussion on ocular psychoneuroses. *Transactions of the Ophthalmological Society of the United Kingdom*, 1944 64, 46–52. Published here as 'Ocular psychoneuroses of childhood'. [CW 2:6:15]

Discussion sur la contribution de l'observation directe de l'enfant à la psychanalyse. *Revue Française de Psychanalyse*, 1958, 22. Published here as 'On the contribution of direct child observation to psycho-analysis'. [CW 5:3:21]

Disease of the nervous system. In *Clinical notes on disorders of childhood* (pp. 129–142). London: Heinemann, 1931. [CW 1:3:14]

Disorders of childhood. *The Journal of the Royal Institute of Public Health and Hygiene*, 1948, 11(7), 244. [CW 3:3:8]

Dissociation revealed in a therapeutic consultation. In C. Winnicott, R. Shepherd & M. Davis (Eds.), *Deprivation and delinquency* (pp. 256–282). London: Tavistock, 1984. Also published in R. Slovenko (Ed.), *Crime, law and corrections* (pp. 102–130, as 'A psychoanalytic view of the antisocial tendency'). Springfield, IL: Charles C. Thomas, 1966. Published here as 'Dissociation revealed in a therapeutic consultation'. [CW 7:2:21] Includes '"Ada" aet 8 years'.

Ditty on Enoch Powell, in a letter to Peter Tizard [ca. 1968]. In F. R. Rodman (Ed.), *Winnicott: Life and work* (p. 393). Cambridge, MA: Perseus, 2003. [CW 9:4:13]

A doctor looks at the psychiatric social worker [1943]. [CW 2:5:1]

Do progressive schools give too much freedom to the child? [1965]. In M. Ash (Ed.), *Who are the progressives now?* (pp. 165–170, as 'Contribution to conference at Dartington Hall'). London: Routledge & Kegan Paul, 1969. Also published in C. Winnicott, R. Shepherd & M. Davis (Eds.), *Deprivation and delinquency* (pp. 209–213, together with 'Notes made in the train', as part of the chapter 'Do progressive schools give too much freedom to the child?'). London: Tavistock, 1984. [CW 7:2:5]

Dreaming, fantasying and living: A case-history describing a primary dissociation. In *Playing and reality* (pp. 26–37). London: Tavistock, 1971. [CW 9:3:6]

D. W. W. on D. W. W. [1967]. In C. Winnicott, R. Shepherd & M. Davis (Eds.), *Psychoanalytic explorations* (pp. 569–582, as 'Postscript: D. W. W. on D. W. W.'). Cambridge, MA: Harvard University Press, 1989. [CW 8:1:2]

D. W. W.'s dream related to reviewing Jung [1963]. In C. Winnicott, R. Shepherd & M. Davis (Eds.), *Psycho-analytic explorations* (pp. 228–230, part of the chapter 'The use of an object'). Cambridge, MA: Harvard University Press, 1989. [CW 6:4:15]

Dynamic psychiatry and the G.P. *British Medical Journal*, 1967, 3(5557). Published here as 'Review: Clyne, M. B., *Absent: School refusal as an expression of disturbed family relationships*'. [CW 8:1:15]

Early disillusion [1939]. In C. Winnicott, R. Shepherd & M. Davis (Eds.), *Psycho-analytic explorations* (pp. 21–23). Cambridge, MA: Harvard University Press, 1989. [CW 2:1:5]

Educational diagnosis. *National Froebel Foundation Bulletin*, 1946, *41*, 3. Also published in *The child and the outside world: Studies in developing relationships* (pp. 29–34). London: Tavistock, 1957; and *The child, the family, and the outside world* (pp. 205–210). Harmondsworth: Penguin, 1964. [CW 3:1:2]

The effect of loss on the young [1968]. In R. Shepherd, J. Johns & H. Taylor Robinson (Eds.), *Thinking about children* (pp. 46–47). London: Karnac, 1996. [CW 8:2:12]

The effect of psychosis on family life [1960]. In *The family and individual development* (pp. 61–68). London: Tavistock, 1965. [CW 6:1:6]

The effect of psychotic parents on the emotional development of the child [1959]. *British Journal of Psychiatric Social Work*, 1961, *6*(1), 13–20. Also published in *The family and individual development* (pp. 69–78). London: Tavistock, 1965. [CW 5:5:21]

Ego distortion in terms of true and false self [1960]. In *The maturational processes and the facilitating environment: Studies in the theory of emotional development* (pp. 140–152). London: Hogarth, 1965. [CW 6:1:22]

Ego integration in child development [1962]. In *The maturational processes and the facilitating environment: Studies in the theory of emotional development* (pp. 56–63). London: Hogarth, 1965. [CW 6:3:19]

Eine Kinderbeobachtung. *Psyche*, 1967, *21*. Published here as 'A tribute on the occasion of Willi Hoffer's seventieth birthday'. [CW 8:1:11]

Eine Verbindung zwischen Kinderheilkunde und Kinderpsychologie, klinische Betrachtungen. *Dynamische Psychiatrie*, 1969, *2*. Published here as 'A link between paediatrics and child psychology: Clinical observations'. [CW 8:2:14]

'Eliza' aet 7½ years. In *Therapeutic consultations in child psychiatry* (pp. 42–63). London: Hogarth, 1971. Also published in G. Biermann (Ed.), *Handbuch der Kinderpsychotherapie* (pp. 269–277, as part of 'Die volle Nutzung der ersten Behandlungsstunde. Beitrag zu Problemen der Kinderanalyse' or 'Meeting the challenge of the case'). München/Basel: Ernst Reinhardt Verlag, 1968; and, in part, in *Voices: The Art and Science of Psycho-therapy*, 1968, *4*, 98–112 (as part of the chapter 'The squiggle game'); and in C. Winnicott, R. Shepherd & M. Davis (Eds.), *Psychoanalytic explorations* (pp. 299–317, as 'Case of L', part of the chapter 'The squiggle game'). Cambridge, MA: Harvard University Press, 1989. Published here as ' "Eliza" aet 7½ years'. [CW 10:1:3].

Encephalitis after measles and chicken-pox. In *Proceedings of the Royal Society of Medicine*, 1928, *21*(4), 567. [CW 1:2:9]

The end of the digestive process. In *The ordinary devoted mother and her baby* (pp. 17–21). London: C. A. Brock, 1949. Also published in *The child and the family: First relationships* (pp. 28–32). London: Tavistock, 1957; and *The child, the family, and the outside world* (pp. 40–44). Harmondsworth: Penguin, 1964. Broadcast 26 October 1949, as 'The passing of excretions'. I. Benzie (Producer), *How's the baby?* Home Service. London: British Broadcasting Corporation. [CW 3:4:26]

Enuresis [abstract] [1929]. In *Proceedings of the Royal Society of Medicine*, 1930, *23*(3), 255–256. [CW 1:2:17]

Enuresis: Notes for a lecture to the Tavistock Children's Department [n.d., ca. 1949]. [CW 3:4:36]

Environmental health in infancy [1967]. *Maternal and Child Care*, 1968, 4, in part, as 'Infant feeding and emotional development'. Also published in R. Shepherd, J. Johns & H. Taylor Robinson (Eds.), *Thinking about children* (pp. 39–41, in part, as 'The bearing of emotional development on feeding problems' [1967]). London: Karnac, 1996. First published in this form in C. Winnicott, R. Shepherd & M. Davis (Eds.), *Babies and their mothers* (pp. 59–68). Reading, MA: Addison-Wesley, 1987; and then in *Winnicott on the child* (pp. 49–55). Cambridge, MA: Perseus, 2002. [CW 8:1:6]

Environmental needs; the early stages; total dependence and essential independence [1948]. In R. Shepherd, J. Johns & H. Taylor Robinson (Eds.), *Thinking about children* (pp. 29–36). London: Karnac, 1996. [CW 3:3:13]

Envy: A male patient near the end of his analysis [1961]. Part of 'The beginnings of a formulation of an appreciation and criticism of Klein's envy statement'. In C. Winnicott, R. Shepherd & M. Davis (Eds.), *Psycho-analytic explorations* (pp. 447–457, part of the chapter 'Melanie Klein: On her concept of envy'). Cambridge, MA: Harvard University Press, 1989. [CW 6:2:21]

The evacuated child [1945]. In *The child and the outside world: Studies in developing relationships* (pp. 83–87). London: Tavistock, 1957. Also published in C. Winnicott, R. Shepherd & M. Davis (Eds.), *Deprivation and delinquency* (pp. 39–43). London: Tavistock, 1984. Broadcast 16 February 1945. J. Quigley & D. Bridgman (Producers), *Difficult children*. Home Service. London: British Broadcasting Corporation. [CW 2:7:2]

Evacuation of small children. In C. Winnicott, R. Shepherd & M. Davis (Eds.), *Deprivation and delinquency* (pp. 14–21). Published, in part, in a letter to the *British Medical Journal* (W. J. Bowlby & E. Miller), 16 December 1939, titled, 'Evacuation of small children' [CW 2:1:6]. Published here as 'Children and their mothers'. [CW 2:2:2].

Evidence given to the Home Office Committee on Children's Homes [1945]. [CW 2:7:9]

Excitement in the aetiology of coronary thrombosis [1957]. In C. Winnicott, R. Shepherd & M. Davis (Eds.), *Psycho-analytic explorations* (pp. 34–38). Cambridge, MA: Harvard University Press, 1989. [CW 5:3:29]

Facial nerve paralysis, associated with fits. In *Proceedings of the Royal Society of Medicine*, 1928, 21(4), 566. [CW 1:2:8]

Facial nerve paralysis. *Proceedings of the Royal Society of Medicine*, 1928, 21(4), 565–566. [CW 1:2:7]

The family affected by depressive illness in one or both parents [1958]. In *The family and individual development* (pp. 50–60). London: Tavistock, 1965. [CW 5:4:17]

The family and emotional maturity [1960]. In *The family and individual development* (pp. 88–94). London: Tavistock, 1965. Also published in *Winnicott on the child* (pp. 207–214). Cambridge, MA: Perseus, 2002. [CW 6:1:17]

The family and individual development. London: Tavistock, 1965. (Second edition, with an introduction by Martha Nussbaum). London and New York: Routledge Classics, 2006. [Not reprinted in this form in the *Collected Works*]

The fate of the transitional object [1959]. In C. Winnicott, R. Shepherd & M. Davis (Eds.), *Psycho-analytic explorations* (pp. 53–58). Cambridge, MA: Harvard University Press, 1989. [CW 5:5:22]

Fear of breakdown [ca. 1963–1964]. *International Review of Psychoanalysis*, 1974, 1, 103–108. Also published in C. Winnicott, R. Shepherd & M. Davis (Eds.), *Psycho-analytic explorations* (pp. 87–95). Cambridge, MA: Harvard University Press, 1989. [CW 6:4:21]

Feeling guilty [1960]. In C. Winnicott, C. Bollas, M. Davis & R. Shepherd (Eds.), *Talking to parents* (pp. 95–103). Reading, MA: Addison-Wesley, 1993. Also published in *Winnicott on the child* (pp. 160–166). Cambridge, MA: Perseus, 2002. Broadcast 13 March 1961, as 'Guilt feelings in young mothers. A discussion with Clare Rayner'. E. Crowther (Producer), *Parents and children*. Network Three. London: British Broadcasting Corporation. [CW 6:2:6]

Fidgetiness. In *Clinical notes on disorders of childhood* (pp. 87–97). London: Heinemann, 1931. Also published in *Collected papers: Through paediatrics to psycho-analysis* (pp. 22–30). London: Tavistock, 1958. [CW 1:3:11]

First experiments in independence [1955]. In *The child and the family: First relationships* (pp. 131–136). London: Tavistock, 1957; and *The child, the family, and the outside world* (pp. 167–172). Harmondsworth: Penguin, 1964. [CW 5:1:20]

The first year of life: Modern views on the emotional development. *Medical Press*, March 1958, as 'Modern views on the emotional development in the first year of life'. Also published in *The family and individual development* (pp. 3–14). London: Tavistock, 1965. [CW 5:4:6]

The five-year-old [1962]. In *The family and individual development* (pp. 34–39). London: Tavistock, 1965. Also published in C. Winnicott, C. Bollas, M. Davis & R. Shepherd (Eds.), *Talking to parents* (pp. 111–120, as 'Now they are five'). Reading, MA: Addison-Wesley, 1993; and *Winnicott on the child* (pp. 171–177, as 'Now they are five'). Cambridge, MA: Perseus, 2002. Broadcast 25 June 1962, under the title 'The first five years: 13. Now they are five'. S. Waterhouse (Producer), *Parents and children*. Network Three. London: British Broadcasting Corporation. [CW 6:3:6]

For stepparents [1955]. In C. Winnicott, C. Bollas, M. Davis & R. Shepherd (Eds.), *Talking to parents* (pp. 7–13). Reading, MA: Addison-Wesley, 1993. Also published in *Winnicott on the child* (pp. 99–103). Cambridge, MA: Perseus, 2002. Broadcast in three parts, 7–9 June 1955, I. Benzie (Producer), *Woman's hour*. Light Programme. London: British Broadcasting Corporation. [CW 5:1:10]

Foreword. Briance, P., *Childbirth with confidence* [n.d., ca. 1959–1971]. London: Dick-Read School for Natural Birth, 1982. [CW 5:5:24]

Foreword. *The case as the patient sees it: Psycho-analysis* [1957]. London: National Association of Mental Health, 1958. [CW 5:3:17]

Foreword. Dockar-Drysdale, B., Therapy in child care. In *Collected papers: Vol. 3. Therapy in child care* (pp. ix–x). London: Longman, 1968. [CW 8:2:45]

Foreword. Gardner, D. E. M., *Susan Isaacs* (pp. 5–6). London: Methuen, 1969. Also published in C. Winnicott, R. Shepherd & M. Davis (Eds.), *Psycho-analytic explorations* (pp. 387–389). Cambridge, MA: Harvard University Press, 1989. [CW 8:2:22]

Foreword. Malleson, J. Graham, *Any wife or any husband* (2nd ed.). London: Heinemann, 1955. [CW 5:1:19]

Foreword. Milner, M., *The hands of the living God* [1967]. London: Hogarth, 1969. [CW 8:1:12]

Foreword. Tod, R. J. N. (Ed.), *Disturbed children* (pp. vii–viii). London: Longman, 1968. [CW 8:2:8]

Foreword. Torrie, M., *The widow's child*. Richmond, Surrey, UK: Cruse Club, 1964. [CW 7:1:12]

The foundation of mental health. *British Medical Journal*, 16 June 1951, *1*(4719), 1373–1374. Also published in C. Winnicott, R. Shepherd & M. Davis (Eds.), *Deprivation and delinquency* (pp. 168–171). London: Tavistock, 1984. [CW 3:6:4]

Found objects and waifs [n.d.]. [CW 9:4:7]

Fragment of an analysis [1955]. A. Flarsheim (Ed.). In Peter L. Giovacchini (Ed.), *Tactics and techniques in psychoanalytic therapy* (pp. 455-693) London: Hogarth, 1972. Published here as 'Holding and interpretation: Fragment of an analysis'. [CW 4:4:1]

Fragments concerning varieties of clinical confusion [1956]. In C. Winnicott, R. Shepherd & M. Davis (Eds.), *Psycho-analytic explorations* (pp. 30-33). Cambridge, MA: Harvard University Press, 1989. [CW 5:2:4]

Freedom [ca. 1969]. *Nouvelle Revue de Psychanalyse*, 1984, 30, as 'Liberté'. Also published in C. Winnicott, R. Shepherd & M. Davis (Eds.), *Home is where we start from: Essays by a psychoanalyst* (pp. 228-232). Harmondsworth: Penguin, 1986. [CW 9:1:16]

From dependence towards independence in the development of the individual [1963]. In *The maturational processes and the facilitating environment: Studies in the theory of emotional development* (pp. 83-92). London: Hogarth, 1965. [CW 6:4:11]

Funeral address for Ernest Jones. *International Journal of Psychoanalysis*, 1958, 39, 305-306. Also published in C. Winnicott, R. Shepherd & M. Davis (Eds.), *Psycho-analytic explorations* (pp. 405-407). Cambridge, MA: Harvard University Press, 1989. [CW 5:4:3]

Further clinical illustration of 'The use of an object' [1968]. [CW 8:2:30]

Further clinical material on the theme of a male patient's exploitation of his female self [1963]. In C. Winnicott, R. Shepherd & M. Davis (Eds.), *Psycho-analytic explorations* (pp. 183-188, as part of 'Clinical Material [1959-1963]', in the chapter 'On the split-off male and female elements'). Cambridge, MA: Harvard University Press, 1989. [CW 6:4:20]

Further thoughts on babies as persons. In *The child and the outside world: Studies in developing relationships* (pp. 134-140). London: Tavistock, 1957; and *The child, the family, and the outside world* (pp. 85-92). Harmondsworth: Penguin, 1964. [CW 3:2:4]. See also 'Babies as persons'.

'George' aet 13 years. In *Therapeutic consultations in child psychiatry* (pp. 380-396). London: Hogarth, 1971. [CW 10:3:21]

Getting to know your baby. London: Heinemann, 1945. [Not reprinted in this form in the Collected Works]

Getting to know your baby [1943]. *New Era in Home and School*, 1945, 26. Also published in *Getting to know your baby* (pp. 1-5). London: Heinemann, 1945; and *The child, the family, and the outside world* (pp. 19-24). Harmondsworth: Penguin, 1964. Broadcast 10 December 1943. Quigley, J. (Producer), *Happy Children*. Home Service. London: British Broadcasting Corporation. [CW 2:5:8]

Getting to know your baby. Broadcast 14 November 1945. I. Benzie (Producer), *The new baby*. Home Service. London: British Broadcasting Corporation, 14 November 1945. [CW 12:3:4b]

Group influences and the maladjusted child: The school aspect. [1955]. In *The family and individual development* (pp. 146-154). London: Tavistock, 1965. Also published in C. Winnicott, R. Shepherd & M. Davis (Eds.), *Deprivation and delinquency* (pp. 189-199). London: Tavistock, 1984. [CW 5:1:9]

Growing pains. In *Clinical notes on disorders of childhood* (pp. 76-80). London: Heinemann, 1931. [CW 1:3:9]

Growth and development in immaturity [1950]. In *The family and individual development* (pp. 21-29). London: Tavistock, 1965. [CW 3:5:16]

The Gwrw tree [1948]. [CW 3:3:4]

Hæmoptysis: Case for diagnosis. *Proceedings of the Royal Society of Medicine*, 1931, 24(7), 855–856. [CW 1:2:20]

Hallucination and dehallucination [1957]. In C. Winnicott, R. Shepherd & M. Davis (Eds.), *Psycho-analytic explorations* (pp. 39–42). Cambridge, MA: Harvard University Press, 1989. [CW 5:3:23]

Hate in the countertransference [1947]. *International Journal of Psychoanalysis*, 1949, 30, 69–74. Also published in *Collected papers: Through paediatrics to psycho-analysis* (pp. 194–203). London: Tavistock, 1958. [CW 3:2:1]

Health education through broadcasting. *Mother and Child*, 1957, 28. Also published in C. Winnicott, C. Bollas, M. Davis & R. Shepherd (Eds.), *Talking to parents* (pp. 1–6). Reading, MA: Addison-Wesley, 1993; and *Winnicott on the child* (pp. 95–98). Cambridge, MA: Perseus, 2002. [CW 5:3:31]

The heart, with special reference to rheumatic carditis. In *Clinical notes on disorders of childhood* (pp. 42–57). London: Heinemann, 1931. [CW 1:3:5]

Hemiplegia noticed after diphtheria. *Proceedings of the Royal Society of Medicine*, 1929, 22(4), 392. [CW 1:2:13]

'Hesta' aet 16 years. In *Therapeutic consultations in child psychiatry* (pp. 176–193). London: Hogarth, 1971. [CW 10:2:11]

History-taking. In *Clinical notes on disorders of childhood* (pp. 7–21). London: Heinemann, 1931. [CW 1:3:1]

Holding and interpretation: Fragment of an analysis [1955]. In Peter L. Giovacchini (Ed.), *Tactics and techniques in psychoanalytic therapy* (pp. 455–693, as 'Fragment of an analysis' [A. Flarsheim, Ed.]). London: Hogarth, 1972. Also published in *Holding and interpretation: Fragment of an analysis* (pp. 19–186). The Institute of Psychoanalysis. London: Karnac, 1986. [CW 4:4:1]

Holding and interpretation: Fragment of an analysis. The Institute of Psychoanalysis. London: Karnac, 1986. [Not reprinted in this form in the *Collected Works*]

Home again [1945]. In *The child and the outside world* (pp. 93–97). London: Tavistock, 1957. Also published in C. Winnicott, R. Shepherd & M. Davis (Eds.), *Deprivation and delinquency* (pp. 49–53). London: Tavistock, 1984. Broadcast 22 June 1945. J. Quigley & D. Bridgman (Producers), *Health Magazine*. Home Service. London: British Broadcasting Corporation. [CW 2:7:7]

Home is where we start from: Essays by a psychoanalyst (C. Winnicott, R. Shepherd & M. Davis, Eds.). Harmondsworth: Penguin, 1986. [Not reprinted in this form in the *Collected Works*]

Hospital care supplementing intensive psychotherapy in adolescence [1963]. In *The maturational processes and the facilitating environment: Studies in the theory of emotional development* (pp. 242–248). London: Hogarth, 1965. [CW 6:4:13]

Human nature (C. Bollas, M. Davis & R. Shepherd, Eds.). London: Free Association Books, 1988. [CW 11:1]

Human relations. *Physiotherapy*, 1969, 55. Published here as 'Physiotherapy and human relations'. [CW 9:1:14]

Ideas and definitions [n.d., ca. early 1950s]. In C. Winnicott, R. Shepherd & M. Davis (Eds.), *Psycho-analytic explorations* (pp. 43–44). Cambridge, MA: Harvard University Press, 1989. [CW 9:4:1]

'Iiro' aet 9 years 9 months, Case 1. In *Therapeutic consultations in child psychiatry* (pp. 12–27). London: Hogarth, 1971. [CW 10:1:1]

The importance of the setting in meeting regression in psycho-analysis [1964]. In C. Winnicott, R. Shepherd & M. Davis (Eds.), *Psycho-analytic explorations* (pp. 96–102). Cambridge, MA: Harvard University Press, 1989. [CW 7:1:9]

The impulse to steal [1949]. In *The child and the outside world* (pp. 176–180). London: Tavistock, 1957. [CW 3:4:34]

Individuation [1970]. In C. Winnicott, R. Shepherd & M. Davis (Eds.), *Psycho-analytic explorations* (pp. 284–288). Cambridge, MA: Harvard University Press, 1989. [CW 9:2:10]

The infancy of Juliet [1949]. [CW 3:4:4]

Infant feeding [1944]. *New Era in Home and School*, 1945, 26. Also published in *Getting to know your baby* (pp. 12–16). London: Heinemann, 1945; and *The child and the family: First relationships* (pp. 18–22). London: Tavistock, 1957; and *The child, the family, and the outside world* (pp. 30–34). Harmondsworth: Penguin, 1964. [CW 2:6:13]

Infant feeding and emotional development. *Maternal and Child Care*, 1968, 4. Published here, together with 'The bearing of emotional development on feeding problems', as 'Environmental health in infancy'. [CW 8:1:6]

The innate morality of the baby. In *The ordinary devoted mother and her baby* (pp. 38–42). London: C. A. Brock, 1949. Also published in *The child and the family: First relationships* (pp. 59–63). London: Tavistock, 1957; and *The child, the family, and the outside world* (pp. 93–97). Harmondsworth: Penguin, 1964. Broadcast 23 November 1949, as 'Problems of management: Training babies' [CW 12:3:4c]. I. Benzie (Producer), *How's the baby?* Home Service. London: British Broadcasting Corporation. [CW 3:4:30]

Instincts and normal difficulties [1950]. In *The child and the family: First relationships* (pp. 74–78). London: Tavistock, 1957. Also published in *The child, the family, and the outside world* (pp. 98–102). Harmondsworth: Penguin, 1964. Broadcast 29 March 1950, as 'Symptoms of illness'. I. Benzie (Producer), *How's the baby?* Home Service. London: British Broadcasting Corporation. [CW 3:5:15]

Integrative and disruptive factors in family life [1957]. *Canadian Medical Association Journal*, 84(15), 814–815, 15 April 1961, as 'Integrating and disruptive factors in family life'. Also published in *The family and individual development* (pp. 40–49). London: Tavistock, 1965. [CW 5:3:26]

Interpretation in psycho-analysis [1968]. In C. Winnicott, R. Shepherd & M. Davis (Eds.), *Psycho-analytic explorations* (pp. 207–212). Cambridge, MA: Harvard University Press, 1989. [CW 8:2:6]

Interrelating in terms of cross-identification. *Revista de Psicoanálisis*, 1968, 25 (as 'La interrelación en términos de identificaciones cruzadas'). Published in *Playing and reality* (pp. 129–137, part of the chapter 'Interrelating apart from instinctual drive and in terms of cross-identifications'). London: Tavistock, 1971. [CW 9:3:8]

Interrelating apart from instinctual drive and in terms of cross-identifications. In *Playing and reality* (pp. 119–137). London: Tavistock, 1971. [CW 9:3:8]

Introduction. In *Clinical notes on disorders of childhood* (pp. 1–6). London: Heinemann, 1931. [CW 1:3]

Introduction. In *The ordinary devoted mother and her baby* (pp. 3–6). London: C. A. Brock, 1949. Published here as 'A man looks at motherhood'. [CW 3:4:23]

Introduction. In *Playing and reality* (pp. xi–xiii). London: Tavistock, 1971. [CW 9:3:4]

Introduction. In *The child, the family, and the outside world* (pp. 9–11). Harmondsworth: Penguin Books, 1964. [CW 7:1:17]

Introduction. In *The maturational processes and the facilitating environment: Studies in the theory of emotional development* (pp. 9–10). London: Hogarth, 1965. [CW 7:2:24]

Introduction to a symposium on the psycho-analytic contribution to the theory of shock therapy [1944]. In C. Winnicott, R. Shepherd & M. Davis (Eds.), *Psycho-analytic explorations* (pp. 525–528, part of the chapter 'Physical therapy of mental disorder: Convulsion therapy'). Cambridge, MA: Harvard University Press, 1989. [CW 2:6:6]

'Jason' aet 8 years 9 months. In *Therapeutic consultations in child psychiatry* (pp. 344–379). London: Hogarth, 1971. [CW 10:3:20]

Jealousy [1960]. In C. Winnicott, C. Bollas, M. Davis & R. Shepherd (Eds.), *Talking to parents* (pp. 41–64). Reading, MA: Addison-Wesley, 1993. Also published in *Winnicott on the child* (pp. 122–138). Cambridge, MA: Perseus, 2002. Broadcast as parts 4–7 of 'The ordinary devoted mother and her children', 15, 22, 29 February and 7 March 1960, I. Benzie & E. Brewer (Producers), *Parents and children*. Network Three. London: British Broadcasting Corporation. [CW 6:1:4]

Kinds of psychological effect of shock therapy [1944]. In C. Winnicott, R. Shepherd & M. Davis (Eds.), *Psycho-analytic explorations* (pp. 529–533, part of the chapter 'Physical therapy of mental disorder: Convulsion therapy'). Cambridge, MA: Harvard University Press, 1989. [CW 2:6:7]

Knowing and learning [1950]. In *The child and the family* (pp. 69–73). London: Tavistock, 1957. Also published in C. Winnicott, R. Shepherd & M. Davis (Eds.), *Babies and their mothers* (pp. 15–21). Reading, MA: Addison-Wesley, 1987; and *Winnicott on the child* (pp. 19–23). Cambridge, MA: Perseus, 2002. Broadcast 22 March 1950, as 'Knowing and learning how to be a mother'. I. Benzie (Producer), *How's the baby?* Home Service. London: British Broadcasting Corporation. [CW 3:5:14]

Knowing and not knowing: A clinical example [n.d.]. In C. Winnicott, R. Shepherd & M. Davis (Eds.), *Psycho-analytic explorations* (pp. 24–25). Cambridge, MA: Harvard University Press, 1989. [CW 9:4:4]

La interrelación en términos de identificaciones cruzadas. *Revista de Psicoanálisis*, 1968, 25. Published here as 'Interrelating in terms of cross identifications', part of the chapter 'Interrelating apart from instinctual drive and in terms of cross-identifications'. [CW 9:3:8]

La schizophrénie infantile en termes d'échec d'adaption. *Recherches*, 1968 (special issue 'Enfance aliénée', 2). Published here as 'The aetiology of infantile schzophrenia in terms of adaptive failure'. [CW 8:1:25]

Le corps et le self. *Nouvelle Revue de Psychanalyse*, 1971, 3. Published here as 'Basis for self in body'. [CW 9:2:12]

Leucotomy. *British Medical Student's Journal*, 1949, 3. Also published in C. Winnicott, R. Shepherd & M. Davis (Eds.) *Psycho-analytic explorations* (pp. 543–547, part of the chapter 'Physical therapy of mental disorder: Leucotomy'). Cambridge, MA: Harvard University Press, 1989. [CW 3:4:21]

Liberté. *Nouvelle Revue de Psychanalyse*, 1984, 30. Published here as 'Freedom'. [CW 9:1:16]

'Lily' aet 5 years. In *Therapeutic consultations in child psychiatry* (pp. 342–343). London: Hogarth, 1971. [CW 10:3:19]

A link between paediatrics and child psychology: Clinical observations [1968]. *Dynamische Psychiatrie*, 1969, 2, as 'Eine Verbindung zwischen Kinderheilkunde und Kinderpsychologie, klinische Betrachtungen'. Also published in R. Shepherd, J. Johns & H. Taylor Robinson (Eds.), *Thinking about children* (pp. 255–276). London: Karnac, 1996. [CW 8:2:14]

Living creatively [1970]. In C. Winnicott, R. Shepherd & M. Davis (Eds.), *Home is where we start from: Essays by a psychoanalyst* (pp. 39–54). Harmondsworth: Penguin, 1986. [CW 9:2:11]

The location of cultural experience [1966]. *International Journal of Psychoanalysis*, 1967, 48, 368–372. Also published in *Playing and reality* (pp. 95–103). London: Tavistock, 1971. [CW 7:3:31]

Looking forward to your baby's arrival. Broadcast 10 October 1945. I. Benzie (Producer), *The New Baby*. Home Service. London: British Broadcasting Corporation. [CW 12:3:4a]

The magistrate, the psychiatrist and the clinic. *New Era in Home and School*, 1944, 24, 7–8. Also published in C. Winnicott, R. Shepherd & M. Davis (Eds.), *Deprivation and delinquency* (pp. 166–170, as part of the chapter 'Correspondence with a magistrate'). Published here as 'Letter to Roger North'. [CW 2:6:1]

The manic defence [1935]. In *Collected papers: Through paediatrics to psycho-analysis* (pp. 129–144). London: Tavistock, 1958. [CW 1:4:6]

A man looks at motherhood [1949]. In *The ordinary devoted mother and her baby* (pp. 3–6, 'Introduction'). London: C. A. Brock, 1949. Also published in *The child and the family: First relationships* (pp. 3–6, 'Introduction'). London: Tavistock, 1957; and *The child, the family, and the outside world* (pp. 15–18). Harmondsworth: Penguin Books, 1964. [CW 3:4:23]

'Mark' aet 12 years. In *Therapeutic consultations in child psychiatry* (pp. 270–295). London: Hogarth, 1971. [CW 10:3:15]. See also 'Child therapy: A case of anti-social behaviour'.

Masturbation. In *Clinical notes on disorders of childhood* (pp. 183–190). London: Heinemann, 1931. [CW 1:3:19]

'Matti', aet 12 years: A therapeutic consultation [1961]. [CW 6:2:15]

The maturational processes and the facilitating environment: Studies in the theory of emotional development. London: Hogarth, 1965. [Not reprinted in this form in the Collected Works]

Measles encephalitis. *Proceedings of the Royal Society of Medicine*, 1929, 22(9), 1247–1248. [CW 1:2:14]

Meeting the challenge of the case in child psychiatry. See 'The squiggle game'.

Meet to be stolen from [n.d., ca. 1939–1945]. [CW 2:3:7]

Memorandum from Paddington Green Children's Hospital Department on homosexuality and the law [1955]. [CW 5:1:4]

Memorandum on corporal punishment [1945]. [CW 2:7:6]

Memorandum on Gisburne House [1959]. [CW 5:5:4]

Memorandum on organizational aspects of child care at Paddington Green Hospital [1961]. [CW 6:2:3]

Memorandum on 'The relationship between clinical paediatrics and child psychology' [1943]. [CW 2:5:3]

Mental defect. In *Clinical notes on disorders of childhood* (pp. 152–156). London: Heinemann, 1931. [CW 1:3:16]

Mental hygiene of the pre-school child [1936]. In R. Shepherd, J. Johns & H. Taylor Robinson (Eds.), *Thinking about children* (pp. 59–76). London: Karnac, 1996. [CW 1:4:9]

The mentally ill in your caseload. In J. F. S. King (Ed.), *New thinking for changing needs* (pp. 50–66). London: The Association of Social Workers, 1963. Also published in *The maturational processes and the facilitating environment: Studies in the theory of emotional development* (pp. 217–229). London: Hogarth, 1965. [CW 6:4:5]

Metapsychological and clinical aspects of regression within the psychoanalytical set-up [1954]. *International Journal of Psychoanalysis*, 1955, 36, 16–26. Also published in *Collected papers: Through paediatrics to psycho-analysis* (pp. 278–294). London: Tavistock, 1958. [CW 4:3:6]

Micturition disturbances. In *Clinical notes on disorders of childhood* (pp. 172–182). London: Heinemann, 1931. [CW 1:3:18]

'Milton' aet 8 years. In *Therapeutic consultations in child psychiatry* (pp. 194–214). London: Hogarth, 1971. [CW 10:2:12] See also 'A psychotherapeutic consultation in child psychiatry: A comparative study of the dynamic processes'.

Mind and its relation to the psyche-soma [1949]. *British Journal of Medical Psychology*, 1954, 27(4), 201–209. Also published in *Collected papers: Through paediatrics to psycho-analysis* (pp. 243–254). London: Tavistock, 1958. [CW 3:4:20]

Mirror-role of mother and family in child development. In P. Lomas (Ed.), *The predicament of the family: A psychoanalytical symposium* (pp. 26–33). London: Hogarth, 1967. Also published in *Playing and reality* (pp. 111–118). London: Tavistock, 1971. [CW 8:1:38]

Modern views on the emotional development in the first year of life. *Medical Press*, March 1958. Published here as 'Modern views on the emotional development in the first year of life'. [CW 5:4:6]

Moon landing (Poem) [1969]. In C. Winnicott, R. Shepherd, M. Davis (Eds.), *Home is where we start from: Essays by a psychoanalyst* (pp. 208–209). Harmondsworth: Penguin, 1986, part of 'The pill and the moon'. Also published, in part, in F. Robert Rodman (Ed.), *Winnicott: Life and work* (pp. 416–417). Cambridge, MA: Perseus, 2003. [CW 9:1:18]

Morals and education [1962]. In W. R. Niblett (Ed.), *Moral education in a changing society* (pp. 96–111, as 'The young child at home and at school'). London: Faber, 1963. Also published in *The maturational processes and the facilitating environment: Studies in the theory of emotional development* (pp. 93–105). London: Hogarth, 1965. [CW 6:3:18]

The mother-infant experience of mutuality [1969]. In E. J. Anthony & T. Benedek (Eds.), *Parenthood: Its psychology and psychopathology* (pp. 245–256). Boston: Little, Brown & Co., 1970. Also published in C. Winnicott, R. Shepherd & M. Davis (Eds.), *Psycho-analytic explorations* (pp. 251–260). Cambridge, MA: Harvard University Press, 1989. [CW 9:1:28]

The mother's contribution to society. In *The child and the family* (pp. 141–144, as 'Postscript: The mother's contribution to society'). London: Tavistock, 1957. Also published in C. Winnicott, R. Shepherd & M. Davis (Eds.), *Home is where we start from: Essays by a psychoanalyst* (pp. 123–127). Harmondsworth: Penguin, 1986; and *Winnicott on the child* (pp. 202–206). Cambridge, MA: Perseus, 2002. [CW 5:3:30]

Mother's madness appearing in the clinical material as an ego-alien factor [1969]. In P. L. Giovacchini (Ed.), *Tactics and techniques in psychoanalytic therapy* (pp. 405–413). London: Hogarth, 1972. Also published in C. Winnicott, R. Shepherd & M. Davis (Eds.), *Psycho-analytic explorations* (pp. 375–382). Cambridge, MA: Harvard University Press, 1989. [CW 9:1:29]

Mother, teacher and the child's needs (with other members of the joint WHO-UNESCO expert group). First published in *Problems in education* (Vol. 9). New York: UNESCO, 1953. Also published in *The child and the outside world: Studies in developing relationships* (pp. 14–23, as 'The child's needs and the role of the mother in the early stages'). London: Tavistock, 1957; and *The child, the family, and the outside world* (pp. 189–198). Harmondsworth: Penguin, 1964. [CW 4:2:20]

'Mrs X' aet 30 years. In *Therapeutic consultations in child psychiatry* (pp. 332–341). London: Hogarth, 1971. [CW 10:3:18]

Muscle weakness, altered gait and absent deep reflexes after measles. *Proceedings of the Royal Society of Medicine*, 1928, *21*(7), 1259. [CW 1:2:10]

Needs of the under-fives. *Nursery Journal*, 1954, *44*, as 'The needs of the under-fives in a changing society'. Also published in *The child and the outside world: Studies in developing relationships* (pp. 3–13). London: Tavistock, 1957, as 'Needs of the under-fives in a changing society'; and *The child, the family, and the outside world* (pp. 179–188). Harmondsworth: Penguin, 1964. [CW 4:3:18]

The neonate and his mother. *Acta Paediatrica Latina*, 1964, *17*. Also published in C. Winnicott, R. Shepherd & M. Davis (Eds.), *Babies and their mothers* (pp. 35–49). Reading, MA: Addison-Wesley, 1987; and *Winnicott on the child* (pp. 32–42, as 'The newborn and his mother'). Cambridge, MA: Perseus, 2002. [CW 7:1:4]

The newborn and his mother. In *Winnicott on the child* (pp. 32–42). Cambridge, MA: Perseus, 2002. Published here as 'The neonate and his mother'. [CW 7:1:4]

New light on children's thinking [1965]. In C. Winnicott, R. Shepherd & M. Davis (Eds.), *Psycho-analytic explorations* (pp. 152–157). Cambridge, MA: Harvard University Press, 1989. [CW 7:2:1]

The niffle [n.d.]. In R. Shepherd, J. Johns & H. Taylor Robinson (Eds.), *Thinking about children* (pp. 104–109). London: Karnac, 1996 (pp. 104–109). [CW 9:4:10]

The night attack. *The Fortnightly* (The Leys School, Cambridge), 13 February 1914. [CW 1:1:6]

The non-pharmacological treatment of psychosis in childhood [1967]. In H. Stutte & H. Harbauer (Eds.), *Concilium paedopsychiatricum*. Proceedings of the 3rd European Congress of Paedopsychiatry, Wiesbaden, 4–9 May 1967. Basel/New York: S. Karger, 1968. [CW 8:1:9]

The nose and throat. In *Clinical notes on disorders of childhood* (pp. 38–41). London: Heinemann, 1931. [CW 1:3:4]

Note of contribution (25th International Psycho-Analytical Congress Symposium on Child Analysis and Paediatrics, Copenhagen, 1967) [1967]. *International Journal of Psychoanalysis*, 1968, *49*, 279. Published here as part of the headnote to '"Iiro" aet 9 years 9 months'. [CW 10:Appendix 1]

A note on a case involving envy [1963]. In C. Winnicott, R. Shepherd & M. Davis (Eds.), *Psycho-analytic explorations* (pp. 76–78). Cambridge, MA: Harvard University Press, 1989. [CW 6:4:3]

Note on infant observation [n.d., after 1957]. [CW 9:4:6]

A note on normality and anxiety. In *Clinical notes on disorders of childhood* (pp. 98–121). London: Heinemann, 1931. Also published in *Collected papers: Through paediatrics to psycho-analysis* (pp. 3–21). London: Tavistock, 1958. [CW 1:3:12]

A note on regression and reassurance [1955]. [CW 5:1:21]

A note on temperature and the importance of charts. In *Clinical notes on disorders of childhood* (pp. 32–37). London: Heinemann, 1931. [CW 1:3:3]

A note on the mother-foetus relationship [n.d., ca. 1960s]. In C. Winnicott, R. Shepherd & M. Davis (Eds.), *Psycho-analytic explorations* (pp. 161–162). Cambridge, MA: Harvard University Press, 1989. [CW 9:4:11]

Notes for a discussion on technique in analysis of psychotics [n.d.]. [CW 9:4:3]

Notes for the Vienna Congress [1971]. In J. Abram (Ed.), *Donald Winnicott today* (pp. 302–330), as 'D. W. W.'s notes on the Vienna Congress 1971: A consideration of Winnicott's theory of aggression and an interpretation of the clinical implications'. London: Routledge, 2013. [CW 9:3:12]

Notes made in the train [1965]. In C. Winnicott, R. Shepherd & M. Davis (Eds.), *Deprivation and delinquency* (pp. 214–219, as part of the chapter 'Do progressive schools give too much freedom to the child?'). London: Tavistock, 1984. Part 2 published in C. Winnicott, R. Shepherd & M. Davis (Eds.), *Psycho-analytic explorations* (pp. 231–233, as 'Notes made on the train, Part 2'). Cambridge, MA: Harvard University Press, 1989. [CW 7:2:6]

Notes made on the train [1965]. In C. Winnicott, R. Shepherd & M. Davis (Eds.), *Psycho-analytic explorations* (pp. 231–233). Also published as Part 2 of 'Notes made in the train', in C. Winnicott, R. Shepherd & M. Davis (Eds.), *Deprivation and delinquency* (pp. 214–219, part of the chapter 'Do progressive schools give too much freedom to the child?'). Published here as Part 2 of 'Notes made in the train'. [CW 7:2:6]

Notes on adolescence [ca. 1956]. [CW 5:2:17]

Notes on a little boy. *New Era in Home and School*, 1938, 19. Also published in R. Shepherd, J. Johns & H. Taylor Robinson (Eds.), *Thinking about children* (pp. 102–103). London: Karnac, 1996. [CW 1:4:16]

Notes on play [n.d.]. In C. Winnicott, R. Shepherd & M. Davis (Eds.), *Psycho-analytic explorations* (pp. 59–63). Cambridge, MA: Harvard University Press, 1989. [CW 9:4:8]

Notes on the discussion held on Dr Winnicott's paper 'The birth trauma' [1949]. [CW 3:4:11]

Notes on the general implications of leucotomy [1951]. In C. Winnicott, R. Shepherd & M. Davis (Eds.), *Psycho-analytic explorations* (pp. 548–552, part of the chapter 'Physical therapy of mental disorder: Leucotomy'). Cambridge, MA: Harvard University Press, 1989. [CW 3:6:14]

Notes on the time factor in treatment [1961]. In R. Shepherd, J. Johns & H. Taylor Robinson (Eds.), *Thinking about children* (pp. 231–234). London: Karnac, 1996. [CW 6:2:11]

Notes on withdrawal and regression [1965]. In C. Winnicott, R. Shepherd & M. Davis (Eds.), *Psycho-analytic explorations* (pp. 149–151). Cambridge, MA: Harvard University Press, 1989. Published as part of 'Case notes for a psychoanalytic seminar: Withdrawal, regression, male identification'. [CW 7:2:19]

Nothing at the centre [1959]. In C. Winnicott, R. Shepherd & M. Davis (Eds.), *Psychoanalytic explorations* (pp. 49–52). Cambridge, MA: Harvard University Press, 1989. [CW 5:5:10]

Not less than everything [extracts] [ca. 1968–1971]. In C. Winnicott, R. Shepherd & M. Davis (Eds.), *Psycho-analytic explorations* (pp. 1–18). Cambridge, MA: Harvard University Press, 1989 (Reprinted from C. Winnicott (Ed.), 'D. W. W.: A Reflection'). [CW 9:3:11]

Now they are five. In C. Winnicott, C. Bollas, M. Davis & R. Shepherd (Eds.), *Talking to parents* (pp. 111–120). Reading, MA: Addison-Wesley, 1993; and *Winnicott on the child* (pp. 171–177). Cambridge, MA: Perseus, 2002. Published here as 'The five-year-old'. [CW 6:3:6]

Obituary: Friedmann, Oscar. *International Journal of Psychoanalysis*, 1959, 40, 247–248. [CW 5:5:25]

Obituary: Isaacs, Susan. *Nature*, 1948, 163. Also published in C. Winnicott, R. Shepherd & M. Davis (Eds.), *Psycho-analytic explorations* (pp. 385–387). Cambridge, MA: Harvard University Press, 1989. [CW 3:3:11]

Obituary: Jones, Ernest. *International Journal of Psychoanalysis*, 1958, 39, 298–303. Also published in C. Winnicott, R. Shepherd & M. Davis (Eds.), *Psycho-analytic explorations* (pp. 393–404). Cambridge, MA: Harvard University Press, 1989. [CW 5:4:21]

Obituary: Klein, Melanie. *British Medical Journal*, 1 October, 1960, 2(5204), 1026. [CW 6:1:15]

Obituary: Strachey, James. *International Journal of Psychoanalysis*, 1969, 50, 129–131. Also published in C. Winnicott, R. Shepherd & M. Davis (Eds.), *Psycho-analytic explorations* (pp. 506–510). Cambridge, MA: Harvard University Press, 1989. [CW 8:1:14]

Obituary: Wilson, Ambrose Cyril. *International Journal of Psychoanalysis*, 1958, 39, 617. [CW 5:4:22]

Observations of infant behaviour during routine clinical examination [abstract]. *Archives of Disease in Childhood*, 1943, 18, 156. Published here as a footnote to 'The observation of infants in a set situation'. [CW 2:3:6 (footnote *i*)]

The observation of infants in a set situation. *International Journal of Psychoanalysis*, 1941, 22, 229–249. Also published in *Collected papers: Through paediatrics to psycho-analysis* (pp. 52–69). London: Tavistock, 1958. [CW 2:3:6]

Ocular psychoneuroses of childhood. *Transactions of the Ophthalmological Society of the United Kingdom*, 1944 64, 46–52, as 'Discussion on ocular psychoneuroses'. Also published in *Collected papers: Through paediatrics to psycho-analysis* (pp. 85–90). London: Tavistock, 1958. [CW 2:6:15]

On adoption. In *The child and the family* (pp. 127–130). London: Tavistock, 1957. Broadcast 23 February 1955, as 'Homeless children and childless homes'. I. Benzie (Producer), *Woman's hour*. Light Programme. London: British Broadcasting Corporation. [CW 5:1:2]

On cardiac neurosis in children [1966]. In R. Shepherd, J. Johns & H. Taylor Robinson (Eds.), *Thinking about children*. London: Karnac, 1996 (pp. 179–188). [CW 7:3:16]

On envy. *Case Conference*, 1959, 5. Published here as 'Review: Klein, M., *Envy and gratitude*'. [CW 5:5:1]

On influencing and being influenced. *New Era in Home and School*, 1941, 22. Also published in *The child and the outside world: Studies in developing relationships* (pp. 35–39).

London: Tavistock, 1957; and *The child, the family, and the outside world* (pp. 199–204). Harmondsworth: Penguin, 1964. [CW 2:3:3]

On in-patient treatment for rheumatic fever and chorea [n.d., ca. 1923–1931]. [CW 1:2:24]

The only child [1945]. In *The child and the family* (pp. 107–111). London: Tavistock, 1957. Also published in *The child, the family, and the outside world* (pp. 131–136). Harmondsworth: Penguin, 1964. Broadcast 2 February 1945. J. Quigley (Producer), *Difficult children*. Home Service. London: British Broadcasting Corporation. [CW 2:7:1]

The only child. *Maternity and Child Welfare*, April 1927, 124, 11(4). Also published in Viscountess Erleigh (Ed.), *The mind of the growing child* (pp. 47–64). London: Faber, 1928; New York: Oxford University Press, 1928. [CW 1:2:6]

On security [1960]. In *The family and individual development* (pp. 30–33). London: Tavistock, 1965. Also published in C. Winnicott, C. Bollas, M. Davis & R. Shepherd (Eds.), *Talking to parents* (pp. 87–93, as 'Security'). Reading, MA: Addison-Wesley, 1993; and *Winnicott on the child* (pp. 155–159, as 'Security'). Cambridge, MA: Perseus, 2002. Broadcast 18 April 1960, as 'Too much security?' I. Benzie (Producer), *Parents and children*. Network Three. London: British Broadcasting Corporation. [CW 6:1:9]

On '*Separation Anxiety*' by J. Bowlby [1958]. [CW 5:4:18]

On the contribution of direct child observation to psycho-analysis [1957]. *Revue Française de Psychanalyse*, 1958, 22, as 'Discussion sur la contribution de l'observation directe de l'enfant à la psychanalyse'. Also published in *The maturational processes and the facilitating environment: Studies in the theory of emotional development* (pp. 109–114). London: Hogarth, 1965. [CW 5:3:21]

On the occasion of the publication of the *Standard Edition* of Freud [1966]. [CW 7:3:23]

On transference. *International Journal of Psychoanalysis*, 1956, 37, 386–388. Published here as 'Clinical varieties of transference'. [CW 5:1:11]

The ordinary devoted mother and her baby. **London: C. A. Brock, 1949.** [Not reprinted in this form in the *Collected Works*]

The ordinary devoted mother [1966]. In C. Winnicott, R. Shepherd & M. Davis (Eds.) *Babies and their mothers* (pp. 3–14). Reading, MA: Addison-Wesley, 1987. Also published in *Winnicott on the child* (pp. 11–18). Cambridge, MA: Perseus, 2002. [CW 7:3:3]

The ordinary devoted mother and her baby: Baby bites. Broadcast 30 January 1952, I. Benzie (Producer), *Woman's hour*. Light Programme. London: British Broadcasting Corporation. [CW 4:1:2]

The ordinary devoted mother and her baby: The first week. Broadcast 16 January 1952. I. Benzie (Producer), *Woman's hour*. Light Programme. London: British Broadcasting Corporation. [CW 4:1:1]

The ordinary devoted mother and her baby: My fan mail. Broadcast 20 February 1952. I. Benzie (Producer), *Woman's hour*. Light Programme. London: British Broadcasting Corporation. [CW 12:3:4d]

Outline for a study in the sociology of knowledge [n.d.]. [CW 9:4:12]

Out of the mouths of adolescents. In R. Shepherd, J. Johns & H. Taylor Robinson (Eds.), *Thinking about children* (pp. 48–50). London: Karnac, 1996. Published here as 'Review: Eppel, E. M. & Eppel, M., *Adolescents and morality*'. [CW 7:3:20]

The paediatric department of psychology [1960]. In *St Mary's Hospital Gazette*, 1961, 67. Also published in R. Shepherd, J. Johns & H. Taylor Robinson (Eds.), *Thinking about children* (pp. 227–230, as 'Training for child psychiatry: The paediatric department of psychology'). London: Karnac, 1996. [CW 6:2:19]

Paediatrics and childhood neurosis [1956]. In *Collected papers: Through paediatrics to psycho-analysis* (pp. 316–321). London: Tavistock, 1958. [CW 5:2:11]

Paediatrics and psychiatry. *British Journal of Medical Psychology*, 1948, 21(4), 229–240. Also published in *Collected papers: Through paediatrics to psycho-analysis* (pp. 157–173). London: Tavistock, 1958. [CW 3:3:2]

Papular urticaria and the dynamics of skin sensation. *British Journal of Children's Diseases*, 1934, *31*. Also published in R. Shepherd, J. Johns & H. Taylor Robinson (Eds.), *Thinking about children* (pp. 157–169). London: Karnac, 1996. [CW 1:4:3]

Pathological sleeping. *Proceedings of the Royal Society of Medicine*, 1930, 23(8), 1109–1110. [CW 1:2:19]

The persecution that wasn't. *New Society*, 18 May 1967. Also published in C. Winnicott, R. Shepherd & M. Davis (Eds.), *Deprivation and delinquency* (pp. 200–201). London: Tavistock, 1984. Published here as 'Review: Stewart, S., *A home from home*'. [CW 8:1:10]

A personal statement on child psychiatry [1970]. [CW 9:2:4]

A personal view of the Kleinian contribution [1962]. In *The maturational processes and the facilitating environment: Studies in the theory of emotional development* (pp. 171–178). London: Hogarth, 1965. [CW 6:3:8]

Perversions and pregenital fantasy [1963]. In C. Winnicott, R. Shepherd & M. Davis (Eds.), *Psycho-analytic explorations* (pp. 79–80). Cambridge, MA: Harvard University Press, 1989. [CW 6:4:18]

'Peter' aet 13 years. In *Therapeutic consultations in child psychiatry* (pp. 296–314). London: Hogarth, 1971. [CW 10:3:16]

Physical and emotional disturbances in an adolescent girl [1968]. In C. Winnicott, R. Shepherd & M. Davis (Eds.), *Psycho-analytic explorations* (pp. 369–374). Cambridge, MA: Harvard University Press, 1989. [CW 8:2:3]

Physical examination. In *Clinical notes on disorders of childhood* (pp. 22–31). London: Heinemann, 1931. [CW 1:3:2]

Physical therapy of mental disorder. *British Medical Journal*, 1947, 1(4506), 688–689. Also published in C. Winnicott, R. Shepherd & M. Davis (Eds.), *Psycho-analytic explorations* (pp. 534–541, part of 'Physical therapy of mental disorder: Convulsion therapy'). Cambridge, MA: Harvard University Press, 1989. [CW 3:2:2]

Physiotherapy and human relations. *Physiotherapy*, 1969, *55*, as 'Human relations'. Also published in C. Winnicott, R. Shepherd & M. Davis (Eds.), *Psycho-analytic explorations* (pp. 561–568). Cambridge, MA: Harvard University Press, 1989. [CW 9:1:14]

The Piggle [1964–1966]. *The Piggle: An account of the psycho-analytic treatment of a little girl* (I. Ramzy, Ed.). London: Hogarth, 1977. [CW 11:2:1–17]

The pill [1969]. In C. Winnicott, R. Shepherd & M. Davis (Eds.) *Home is where we start from: Essays by a psychoanalyst* (pp. 195–208). Harmondsworth: Penguin, 1986, part of 'The Pill and the Moon'. [CW 9:1:23]

Pitfalls in adoption. *Medical Press*, 1954, 232(6031). Also published in *The child and the outside world: Studies in developing relationships* (pp. 45–51). London: Tavistock, 1957; and R. Shepherd, J. Johns & H. Taylor Robinson (Eds.), *Thinking about children* (pp. 128–135). London: Karnac, 1996. [CW 4:3:30]

The place of the monarchy [1970]. In C. Winnicott, R. Shepherd & M. Davis (Eds.) *Home is where we start from: Essays by a psychoanalyst* (pp. 260–268). Harmondsworth: Penguin, 1986. [CW 9:2:6]

The place where we live. In *Playing and reality* (pp. 104–110). London: Tavistock, 1971. [CW 8:2:1]

Play in the analytic situation [1954]. In C. Winnicott, R. Shepherd & M. Davis (Eds.), *Psycho-analytic explorations* (pp. 28–29). Cambridge, MA: Harvard University Press, 1989. [CW 4:3:28]

Playing and culture [1968]. In C. Winnicott, R. Shepherd & M. Davis (Eds.), *Psycho-analytic explorations* (pp. 203–206). Cambridge, MA: Harvard University Press, 1989. [CW 8:2:9]

Playing and reality. London: Tavistock, 1971. [Not reprinted in this form in the *Collected Works*]

Playing: A theoretical statement [1967]. *International Journal of Psychoanalysis*, 1968, 49, 591–599, as 'Playing: Its theoretical status in the clinical situation'. Also published in *Playing and reality* (pp. 38–52). London: Tavistock, 1971. [CW 8:2:15]

Playing: Creative activity and the search for the self. In *Playing and reality* (pp. 53–64). London: Tavistock, 1971. [CW 8:1:27]

Playing: Its theoretical status in the clinical situation. *International Journal of Psychoanalysis*, 1968, 49, 591–599. Published here as 'Playing: A theoretical statement'.

Plea for a kind of Christianity (St Barts Christian Union) [ca. 1917–1932]. Not published here.

A point in technique [n.d.]. In C. Winnicott, R. Shepherd & M. Davis (Eds.), *Psycho-analytic explorations* (pp. 26–27). Cambridge, MA: Harvard University Press, 1989. [CW 9:4:5]

Postscript: The mother's contribution to society. In *The child and the family* (pp. 141–144). London: Tavistock, 1957. Published here as 'The mother's contribution to society'. [CW 5:3:30]

Preface. In *Collected papers: Through paediatrics to psychoanalysis* (pp. ix–x). London: Tavistock, 1958. [CW 5:3:32]

Preface. In *The child and the family: First relationships* (p. ix). London: Tavistock, 1957. [CW 7:1:17]

Preface. In *Clinical notes on disorders of childhood* (p. v). London: Heinemann, 1931. [CW 1:3]

Preface. In *The family and individual development* (p. vii). London: Tavistock, 1965. [CW 7:2:25]

Preface. In O. Stevenson, 'The first treasured possession. A study of the part played by specially loved objects and toys in the lives of certain children'. *The psychoanalytic study of the child* (Vol. 9), 1954, 199–201 (International Universities Press, 1954). [CW 4:3:31]

Preface. In R. Gaddini's Italian translation of *The family and individual development* [1965]. *Psychoanalysis and History*, 2003, 5. [CW 7:3:27]

Preface. In S. Lebovici & J. McDougall, *Dialogue with Sammy: A psycho-analytical contribution to the understanding of child psychosis*. London: Hogarth, 1969. Originally published as *Un cas de psychose infantile*. Paris: Presses universitaires de France, 1960. [CW 9:1:27]

Pre-systolic murmur, possibly not due to mitral stenosis (case history). *Proceedings of the Royal Society of Medicine*, 1931, 24(10), 1354. [CW 1:2:21]

The price of disregarding psychoanalytic research. In *The price of mental health. Report of the National Association for Mental Health Annual Conference* (London, 1965), as 'The price of disregarding research findings'. Also published in C. Winnicott, R. Shepherd & M. Davis (Eds.), *Home is where we start from: Essays by a psychoanalyst* (pp. 172–182). Harmondsworth: Penguin, 1986. [CW 7:2:4]

Primary introduction to external reality: The early stages [1948]. In R. Shepherd, J. Johns & H. Taylor Robinson (Eds.), *Thinking about children* (pp. 21–28). London: Karnac, 1996. [CW 3:3:12]

Primary maternal preoccupation [1956]. In *Collected papers: Through paediatrics to psychoanalysis* (pp. 300–305). London: Tavistock, 1958. [CW 5:2:16]

Primitive emotional development. *International Journal of Psychoanalysis*, 1945, 26, 137–143. Also published in *Collected papers: Through paediatrics to psycho-analysis* (pp. 145–156). London: Tavistock, 1958. [CW 2:7:8]

Private practice [1955]. In C. Winnicott, R. Shepherd & M. Davis (Eds.), *Psycho-analytic explorations* (pp. 291–298). Cambridge, MA: Harvard University Press, 1989. [CW 5:1:7]

The problem of homeless children (with C. Britton). *New Education Fellowship Monograph*, No. 1, 1944. Also published in *New Era in Home and School*, 1944, 25(7), 155–161; and J. Kanter (Ed.), *Face to face with children: The life and work of Clare Winnicott* (pp. 97–111). London: Karnac, 2004. [CW 2:6:14]

Problems of management: Training babies. Broadcast 23 November 1949. I. Benzie (Producer), *How's the baby?* Home Service. London: British Broadcasting Corporation. [CW 12:3:4c] See also 'The innate morality of the baby'.

Providing for the child in health and crisis [1962]. In *The maturational processes and the facilitating environment: Studies in the theory of emotional development* (pp. 64–72). London: Hogarth, 1965. [CW 6:3:10]

Psychiatric disorder in terms of infantile maturational processes [1963]. In *The maturational processes and the facilitating environment: Studies in the theory of emotional development* (pp. 230–241). London: Hogarth, 1965. [CW 6:4:12]

Psychoanalysis and science: Friends or relations? [1961]. In C. Winnicott, R. Shepherd & M. Davis (Eds.), *Home is where we start from: Essays by a psychoanalyst* (pp. 13–18). Harmondsworth: Penguin, 1986. [CW 6:2:9]

Psycho-analysis and the sense of guilt [1956]. In John D. Sutherland (Ed.), *Psychoanalysis and contemporary thought* (pp. 1–16). London: Hogarth, 1958. Also published in *The maturational processes and the facilitating environment: Studies in the theory of emotional development* (pp. 15–28). London: Hogarth, 1965. [CW 5:2:7]

The psychoanalyst and child psychiatry, a matter of economics [1962]. [CW 6:3:12]

Psycho-analytic explorations (C. Winnicott, R. Shepherd & M. Davis, Eds.). Cambridge, MA: Harvard University Press, 1989. [Not reprinted in this form in the Collected Works]

A psychoanalytic view of the antisocial tendency. In R. Slovenko (Ed.), *Crime, law and corrections* (pp. 102–130). Springfield, IL: Charles C. Thomas, 1966. Published here as 'Dissociation revealed in a therapeutic consultation' [CW 7:2:21]. Includes '"Ada" aet 8 years'.

Psychogenesis of a beating fantasy [1958]. In C. Winnicott, R. Shepherd & M. Davis (Eds.), *Psycho-analytic explorations* (pp. 45–48). Cambridge, MA: Harvard University Press, 1989. [CW 5:4:4]

Psychological aspects of birching [1944]. [CW 2:6:3]

Psychological aspects of juvenile delinquency (a talk to probation officers) [n.d., ca. 1940s]. [CW 3:1:8]

Psychologists as a group [1969]. [CW 9:1:31]

The psychology of juvenile rheumatism. In R. G. Gordon (Ed.), *A survey of child psychiatry* (pp. 28–34). London: Oxford University Press, 1939. [CW 2:1:7]

The psychology of madness [1965]: A contribution from psycho-analysis. In C. Winnicott, R. Shepherd & M. Davis (Eds.), *Psycho-analytic explorations* (pp. 119–129). Cambridge, MA: Harvard University Press, 1989. [CW 7:2:18]

The psychology of separation [1958]. In C. Winnicott, R. Shepherd & M. Davis (Eds.), *Deprivation and delinquency* (pp. 132–135). London: Tavistock, 1984. [CW 5:4:7]

Psycho-neurosis in childhood [1961]. In C. Winnicott, R. Shepherd & M. Davis (Eds.), *Psycho-analytic explorations* (pp. 64–72). Cambridge, MA: Harvard University Press, 1989. [CW 6:2:17]

Psychoses and child care [1952]. *British Journal of Medical Psychology*, 1953, 26(1), 68–74. Also published in *Collected papers: Through paediatrics to psycho-analysis* (pp. 219–228). London: Tavistock, 1958. [CW 4:1:5]

Psycho-somatic illness in its positive and negative aspects [1964]. *International Journal of Psychoanalysis*, 1966, 47, 510–516. Also published in C. Winnicott, R. Shepherd & M. Davis (Eds.), *Psycho-analytic explorations* (pp. 103–114, part of the chapter 'Psycho-somatic disorder'). Cambridge, MA: Harvard University Press, 1989. [CW 7:1:6]

A psychotherapeutic consultation: A case of stammering. *A Criança Portuguesa*, 1963, 21. Introduction published in [CW 10: Appendix 3] Also published in *Therapeutic consultations in child psychiatry* (pp. 110–126, as '"Alfred" aet 10 years'). London: Hogarth, 1971. Published here as '"Alfred" aet 10 years'. [CW 10:1:7]

A psychotherapeutic consultation in child psychiatry: A comparative study of the dynamic processes. In S. Arieti (Ed.), *The world biennial of psychiatry and psychotherapy* (Vol. 1, pp. 377–399). New York: Basic, 1971. Introduction published in [CW 10: Appendix 4]. Also published in *Therapeutic consultations in child psychiatry* (pp. 194–214, as '"Milton" aet 8 years'). London: Hogarth, 1971. Published here as '"Milton" aet 8 years'. [CW 10:2:12]

Psychotherapy of character disorders [1963]. In *The maturational processes and the facilitating environment: Studies in the theory of emotional development* (pp. 203–216). London: Hogarth, 1965. Also published in C. Winnicott, R. Shepherd & M. Davis (Eds.), *Deprivation and delinquency* (pp. 241–255). London: Tavistock, 1984. [CW 6:4:9]

Regression as therapy illustrated by the case of a boy whose pathological dependence was adequately met by the parents. *British Journal of Medical Psychology*, 1963, 36(1), 1–12. Also published in *Therapeutic consultations in child psychiatry* (pp. 239–269, as '"Cecil" aet 21 months at first consultation'). London: Hogarth, 1971. Published here as '"Cecil" aet 21 months at first consultation'. [CW 10:3:14]

The relationship of a mother to her baby at the beginning [1960]. In *The family and individual development* (pp. 15–20). London: Tavistock, 1965 (pp. 15–20). [CW 6:1:8]

Remarks on a discussion of Balint's paper on technique [1957]. [CW 5:3:8]

A reminder to the binder. *St Bartholomew's Hospital Journal*, 1921, 28, 107. [CW 1:1:14]

Reparation in respect of mother's organised defence against depression [1948]. *Collected papers: Through paediatrics to psycho-analysis* (pp. 91–96). London: Tavistock, 1958. [CW 3:3:1]

Repli et regression. *Revue Française de Psychanalyse*, 1955, *19*, 1–2. Published here as 'Withdrawal and regression'. [CW 4:3:29]

Report on Q camps [1941]. [CW 2:3:1]

Residential management as treatment for difficult children (with C. Britton). In *The child and the outside world: Studies in developing relationships* (pp. 98–116). London: Tavistock, 1957. First published, in part, in 'Residential management as treatment for difficult children: The evolution of a wartime hostels scheme'. *Human Relations*, *1*(1), 87–97; and, in part, in 'The problem of homeless children'. *New Education Fellowship Monograph*, No. 1, 1944. Also published in C. Winnicott, R. Shepherd & M. Davis (Eds.), *Deprivation and delinquency* (pp. 54–72). London: Tavistock, 1984. [CW 3:2:3]

Resolution K: On scientific aims in psychoanalysis [1942]. In P. King & R. Steiner (Eds.), *The Freud-Klein controversies 1941–1945. New Library of Psychoanalysis* (Vol. 11, pp. 87–89). London and New York: Tavistock/Routledge, 1991. [CW 2:4:1]

Residential care as therapy [1970]. In C. Winnicott, R. Shepherd & M. Davis (Eds.), *Deprivation and delinquency* (pp. 220–228). London: Tavistock, 1984. [CW 9:2:9]

The return of the evacuated child [1945]. In *The child and the outside world* (pp. 88–92). London: Tavistock, 1957. Also published in C. Winnicott, R. Shepherd & M. Davis (Eds.), *Deprivation and delinquency* (pp. 44–48). London: Tavistock, 1984. Broadcast 23 February 1945. J. Quigley & D. Bridgman (Producers), *Difficult children*. Home Service. London: British Broadcasting Corporation. [CW 2:7:3]

Review: *A collection of children's books*. *New Society*, 7 December 1967, *10*(271), 835, as 'Small things for small people'. [CW 8:1:35]

Review: Aichhorn, A., *Wayward youth* (Originally published as 'Verwahrloste Jugend', Leipzig, Vienna and Zurich: Internationaler Psychoanalytischer Verlag, 1925; London: Putnam, 1936). *British Journal of Medical Psychology*, 1936, *16*(2), 154–156. [CW 1:4:12]

Review: Axline, V., *Dibs in search of self* (Harmondsworth: Penguin, 1964). *New Society*, 28 April 1966, *7*(187), 25. [CW 7:3:10]

Review: Bakwin, H. & Bakwin, R. M., *Clinical management of behavior disorders in children* (Philadelphia: Saunders, 1953). *British Medical Journal*, 21 August 1954, *2*(4885), 453. [CW 4:3:22]

Review: Balint, M., *The doctor, his patients and the illness* (London: Pitman, 1957). *International Journal of Psychoanalysis*, 1958, *39*, 425–427. Also published in C. Winnicott, R. Shepherd & M. Davis (Eds.), *Psycho-analytic explorations* (pp. 438–442). Cambridge, MA: Harvard University Press, 1989. [CW 5:4:23]

Review: Bergeron, M., *Psychologie du premier âge* (Paris: Presses universitaires de France, 1961). *Archive of Diseases in Childhood*, 1962, *37*. [CW 6:3:16]

Review: Bowlby, J., *Maternal care and mental health* (Geneva: WHO 1951). *British Journal of Medical Psychology*, 1953, *26*. Also published in C. Winnicott, R. Shepherd & M. Davis (Eds.), *Psycho-analytic explorations* (pp. 423–426). Cambridge, MA: Harvard University Press, 1989. [CW 4:2:10]

Review: Bowley, A., *The psychology of the unwanted child* (Edinburgh: E. & S. Livingstone, 1947). *British Medical Journal*, 10 July 1948, *2*(4566), 78. [CW 3:3:6]

Review: Burlingham, D., *Twins: A study of three pairs of identical twins* (London: Imago, 1952). *British Medical Journal*, 28 March 1953, *1*(4812), 714. [CW 4:2:6]

Review: Burlingham, D., *Twins: A study of three pairs of identical twins* (London: Imago, 1952). *New Era in Home and School*, 1953, 34. Also published in C. Winnicott, R. Shepherd & M. Davis (Eds.), *Psycho-analytic explorations* (pp. 408–412), Cambridge, MA: Harvard University Press, 1989. [CW 4:2:7]

Review: Burton, L., *Vulnerable children. Three studies of children in conflict: Accident involved children, sexually assaulted children, and children with asthma* (London: Routledge & Kegan Paul, 1968). *New Society*, 25 April 1968, 11(291), 613. [CW 8:2:11]

Review: Chess, S., Thomas, A. & Birch, H., *Your child is a person* (London: Peter Davies, 1966). *Medical News*, October 1966. [CW 7:3:25]

Review: Child Study Association of America. *Parents' questions* (New York, London: Harper & Bros., 1947). *British Medical Journal*, July 31 1948, 2, 257. [CW 3:3:7]

Review: Clegg, A. & Megson, B., *Children in distress* (Harmondsworth: Penguin Books, 1968). *New Society*, 7 November 1968, 12(319), 688. [CW 8:2:25]

Review: Clyne, M. B., *Absent: School refusal as an expression of disturbed family relationships.* (London: Tavistock, 1966). *New Society*, 8(209), 507–508, 29 September 1966. [CW 7:3:22]

Review: Clyne, M. B., *Absent: School refusal as an expression of disturbed family relationships.* (London: Tavistock, 1966). *British Medical Journal*, 1967, 3(5557), 99, as 'Dynamic psychiatry and the G.P.' [CW 8:1:15]

Review: Eissler, R. S., Freud, A., Hartmann, H. & Kris, E. (Eds.), *The psychoanalytic study of the child* (Vol. 11) (London: Imago, 1956). *British Medical Journal*, 22 March 1958, 1(5072), 692. [CW 5:4:5]

Review: Eissler, R. S., Freud, A., Hartmann, H. & Kris, E. (Eds.), *The psychoanalytic study of the child* (Vol. 12) (London: Imago, 1957). *British Medical Journal*, 4 October 1958, 2(5100), 838. [CW 5:4:15]

Review: Eissler, R. S., Freud, A., Hartmann, H. & Kris, M. (Eds.), *The psychoanalytic study of the child* (Vol. 15) (London: Imago, 1960). *British Medical Journal*, 3 February, 1962, 1(5274), 305–306. [CW 6:3:1]

Review. Eissler, R. S., Freud, A., Hartmann, H. & Kris, M. (Eds.), *The psychoanalytic study of the child* (Vol. 16) (London: Imago, 1961). *British Medical Journal*, 26 January 1963, 1(5325), 253. [CW 6:4:1]

Review: Eissler, R. S., Freud, A., Hartmann, H. & Kris, M. (Eds.), *The psychoanalytic study of the child* (Vol. 20). (London: Hogarth, 1966). *British Medical Journal*, 17 December, 1966, 2(5528), 1510. [CW 7:3:14]

Review: Eissler, R. S., Freud, A., Hartmann, H. & Kris, M. (Eds.) *The psychoanalytic study of the child* (Vol. 22). (London: Hogarth, 1967). *New Society*, 16 May 1968, 11(294), 726-727. [CW 8:2:13]

Review: Eppel, E. M. & Eppel, M., *Adolescents and morality* (London: Routledge & Kegan Paul, 1966). *New Society*, 15 September 1966, 8(207), 417–418. Also published in R. Shepherd, J. Johns & H. Taylor Robinson (Eds.), *Thinking about children* (pp. 48–50, as 'Out of the mouths of adolescents'). London: Karnac, 1996. [CW 7:3:20]

Review: Erikson, E., *Childhood and society* (London: Hogarth, 1965). *British Medical Journal*, November 28 1953, 2(4847), 1205. [CW 4:2:16]

Review: Erikson, E. H., *Childhood and society* (London: Hogarth, 1965). *New Society*, 30 September 1965, 6(156), 35. Also published in C. Winnicott, R. Shepherd &

M. Davis (Eds.), *Psycho-analytic explorations* (pp. 493–494). Cambridge, MA: Harvard University Press, 1989. [CW 7:2:14]

Review: Evans, P. R. & MacKeith, R., *Infant feeding and feeding difficulties* (London: Churchill). *British Journal of Medical Psychology*, December 1951, 24(4), 304–305. [CW 3:6:18]

Review: Flügel, J. C., *The moral paradox of peace and war* (London: Watts, 1941). *New Era in Home and School*, 1941, 22. [CW 2:3:4]

Review: Foote, E. J., *Six children* (London: Thomas, 1956). *British Medical Journal*, 11 May 1957, *1*, 1105. [CW 5:3:14]

Review: Freud, A., *Indications for child analysis and other papers* (New York: International Universities Press, 1968; London: Hogarth, 1969). *New Society*, 21 August 1969, *14*(360), 297. Also published in C. Winnicott, R. Shepherd & M. Davis (Eds.), *Psychoanalytic explorations* (pp. 511–512). Cambridge, MA: Harvard University Press, 1989. [CW 9:1:20]

Review: Freud, A., *Normality and pathology in childhood* (New York: International Universities Press, 1965) [1965]. [CW 7:2:16]

Review: Freud, A. & Hoffer, W. (Eds.), *The psychoanalytic study of the child* (Vol. 2) (London: Imago, 1946). *British Medical Journal*, August 21 1948, 2(4572), 389. [CW 3:3:9]

Review: Freud, A., Hoffer, W. & Glover, E. (Eds.), *The psychoanalytic study of the child* (Vols. 3–4, Vol. 5). (London: Imago, 1949). *British Medical Journal*, 13 October 1951, 2(4736), 894. [CW 3:6:12]

Review: Glover, E., *Psycho-analysis and child psychiatry* (London: Imago, 1953). *British Medical Journal*, 12 September 1953, 2(4836), 609. [CW 4:2:11]

Review: Goldfarb, W., *Childhood schizophrenia* (Cambridge, MA: Harvard University Press, 1961). *British Journal of Psychiatric Social Work*, 1963, 7(1), 50–51. Also published in R. Shepherd, J. Johns & H. Taylor Robinson (Eds.), *Thinking about children* (pp. 193–194). London: Karnac, 1996. [CW 6:4:17]

Review: Goodacre, I., *Adoption policy & practice* (London: George Allen & Unwin, 1966). *New Society*, 24 November 1966, 8(217), 806–807. [CW 7:3:30]

Review: Harms, E. (Ed.), *Handbook of child guidance*. (New York: Child Care Publications, 1947) *British Medical Journal*, 6 August 1949, 2, 321. [CW 3:4:15]

Review: Hill, A., *Art versus illness* (London: George Allen and Unwin, 1948). *British Journal of Medical Psychology*, 1949, 22. Also published in C. Winnicott, R. Shepherd & M. Davis (Eds.), *Psycho-analytic explorations* (pp. 555–557, part of the chapter 'Occupational therapy'). Cambridge, MA: Harvard University Press, 1989. [CW 3:4:22]

Review: Isaacs, S., et al. (Eds.), *The Cambridge Evacuation Survey: A war time study in social welfare and education* (London: Methuen, 1941). *New Era in Home and School*, 1941, 22. Also published in C. Winnicott, R. Shepherd & M. Davis (Eds.), *Deprivation and delinquency* (pp. 22–24). London: Tavistock, 1984. [CW 2:3:5]

Review: Jackson, L., *Aggression and its interpretation* (London: Methuen, 1952). *British Medical Journal*, 12 June 1954, 1(4875), 1363. [CW 4:3:17]

Review: Jones, E. (Ed.), *Letters of Sigmund Freud 1873–1939* (London: Hogarth, 1961). *British Journal of Psychology*, 1962, 53. Also published in C. Winnicott, R. Shepherd & M. Davis (Eds.), *Psycho-analytic explorations* (pp. 474–477). Cambridge, MA: Harvard University Press, 1989. [CW 6:3:15]

Review: Jones, E., *Papers on psycho-analysis* (5th ed., London: Ballière, 1948). *British Journal of Medical Psychology*, June 1951, 24(2). [CW 3:6:17]

Review: Jung, C. G., *Memories, dreams, reflections* (London: Collins and Routledge, 1963). *International Journal of Psychoanalysis*, 1964, 45, 450–454. Also published in C. Winnicott, R. Shepherd & M. Davis (Eds.), *Psycho-analytic explorations* (pp. 482–492). Cambridge, MA: Harvard University Press, 1989. [CW 7:1:16]

Review: Kanner, L., *Child psychiatry* (Springfield, IL: Charles C. Thomas, 1935; London: Ballière, Tindall & Cox, 1937). *International Journal of Psychoanalysis*, 1938, 19, 362–363. Also published in R. Shepherd, J. Johns & H. Taylor Robinson (Eds.), *Thinking about children* (pp. 191–193, as part of 'Three reviews of books on autism'). London: Karnac, 1996. [CW 1:4:15]

Review: Kirk, H. D., *Shared fate: A theory of adoption and mental health* (New York: The Free Press of Glencoe; London: Collier-Macmillan, 1964). *New Society*, September 1965, 6(154), 29, 9. [CW 7:2:26]

Review: Klein, M., *Envy and gratitude* (London: Tavistock, 1957). *Case Conference*, 1959, 5, as 'On envy'. Also published in C. Winnicott, R. Shepherd & M. Davis (Eds.), *Psycho-analytic explorations* (pp. 443–446). Cambridge, MA: Harvard University Press, 1989. [CW 5:5:1]

Review: Lask, A., *Asthma: Attitude & milieu* (London: Tavistock, 1966). *New Society*, November 1966, 8(216), 771, 17. [CW 7:3:26]

Review: Lebovici, S. & McDougall, J., *Un cas de psychose infantile* (Paris: Presses universitaires de France, 1960). *Journal of Child Psychology and Psychiatry*, 1962, 3(1), 63–64. [CW 6:3:17]

Review: LeShan, E. J., *How to survive parenthood* (Harmondsworth: Penguin, 1965). *New Society*, 26 October 1967, 10(265), 601. [CW 8:1:28]

Review: Middlemore, M. P., *The nursing couple* (London: Hamish Hamilton, 1941). *International Journal of Psychoanalysis*, 1942, 23, 179–180. [CW 2:4:5]

Review: Milner, M., *On not being able to paint* (London: Heinemann, 1950). *British Journal of Medical Psychology*, March 1951, 24, as 'Critical notice'. Also published in C. Winnicott, R. Shepherd & M. Davis (Eds.), *Psycho-analytic explorations* (pp. 390–392). Cambridge, MA: Harvard University Press, 1989. [CW 3:6:15]

Review: *Problems of infancy and childhood: Transactions of the third conference* (New York: Josiah Macy Jr. Foundation, 1949). *British Journal of Medical Psychology*, June 1951, 24(2). [CW 3:6:16]

Review: Rickman, J. (Ed.), *On the bringing up of children* (London: Kegan Paul, 1936). *British Journal of Medical Psychology*, 1936, 16(2), 151–152. [CW 1:4:13]

Review: Riese, H., *Heal the hurt child* (Chicago: Chicago University Press, 1963). *New Society*, 30 January 1964, 3(70), 27. [CW 7:1:2]

Review: Rimland, B., *Infantile autism* (New York: Appleton-Century-Crofts, 1964) [1966]. *British Medical Journal*, 10 September 1966, 2(5514), 634. Also published in R. Shepherd, J. Johns & H. Taylor Robinson (Eds.), *Thinking about children* (pp. 195–196, part of 'Three reviews of books on autism'). London: Karnac, 1996. [CW 7:3:18]

Review: Robertson, J., *Going to hospital with mother* [film]. (London: Tavistock Institute of Human Relations, 1958). *International Journal of Psychoanalysis*, 1959, 40, 62–63. [CW 5:5:23]

Review: Rosen, J. N., *Direct analysis* (New York: Grune & Stratton, 1953). *British Journal of Psychology*, 1953, *44*, 384. [CW 4:2:17]

Review: Sandström, C. I., *The psychology of childhood and adolescence* (Harmondsworth: Penguin Books, 1968; originally published as 'Barn och ungdomspsykologi'. Almqvist & Wiksell, 1961). *National Marriage Guidance Council Journal*, 1968, *11*. [CW 8:2:46]

Review: Searles, H. F., *The non-human environment* (New York: International Universities Press, 1960). *International Journal of Psychoanalysis*, 1963, *44*, 237–238. Also published in C. Winnicott, R. Shepherd & M. Davis (Eds.), *Psycho-analytic explorations* (pp. 478–481). Cambridge, MA: Harvard University Press, 1989. [CW 6:4:16]

Review: Senn, M. (Ed.), *Problems of infancy and childhood: Transactions of the sixth conference* (New York: Josiah Macy Jr. Foundation, 1953). *British Medical Journal*, 19 September 1953, *2*(4837), 664. [CW 4:2:12]

Review: Simey, T. S., *The concept of love in child care* (Oxford University Press, 1961). *New Statesman*, 5 May 1961. [CW 6:2:8]

Review: Slavson, S. R., *Child psychotherapy* (New York: Columbia University Press, 1952). *British Medical Journal*, 15 May 1953, *1*(4871), 1135. [CW 4:3:12]

Review: Soddy, K., *Clinical child psychiatry* (London: Baillière, Tindall and Cox. 1960). *British Medical Journal*, 1961, *1*, 1443. [CW 6:2:10]

Review: Stein, L., *The infancy of speech and the speech of infancy* (London: Methuen, 1949). *British Journal of Medical Psychology*, 1950, *23*, 120–121. [CW 3:5:8]

Review: Stewart, S., *A home from home* (London: Longmans, Green & Co., 1967). *New Society*, 25 May 1967, *9*(243), 772–773. Also published in C. Winnicott, R. Shepherd & M. Davis (Eds.), *Deprivation and delinquency* (pp. 200–201). London: Tavistock, 1984, as 'The persecution that wasn't'. [CW 8:1:10]

Review: Storr, C. A., *Human aggression* (Harmondsworth: Penguin, 1968). *New Statesman*, 5 July 1968, *76*, 15–18. [CW 8:2:18]

Review: Thomson, H., *The successful stepparent* (London: W. H. Allen, 1966). *New Society*, 13 April 1967, *9*(237), 545–546. [CW 8:1:7]

Review: Watson, J. A. F., *The child and the magistrate* (London: Jonathan Cape, 1950). *British Medical Journal*, January 6 1951, *1*(4696), 22. [CW 3:6:1]

Review: Wickes, F., *The inner world of man: With psychological drawings and paintings* (London: Methuen, 1950). *Lancet*, 14 July 1951, *258*(6672), 66. [CW 3:6:7]

Review (with M. M. R. Khan): Fairbairn, W. R. D., *Psychoanalytic studies of the personality*. (London: Tavistock, 1952). *International Journal of Psycho-Analysis*, 1953, *34*, 329–332. Also published in C. Winnicott, R. Shepherd & M. Davis (Eds.), *Psycho-analytic explorations* (pp. 413–422). Cambridge, MA: Harvard University Press, 1989. [CW 4:2:18]

Review: Wolff, W., *The personality of the preschool child* (New York: Grune & Stratton, 1946). *British Medical Journal*, October 23 1948, *2*, 747. [CW 3:3:10]

Review: Ziman, E., *Jealousy in children* (London: Victor Gollancz, 1951). *British Medical Journal*, 1 September 1951, *2*, 532. [CW 3:6:10]

The rheumatic clinic. In *Clinical notes on disorders of childhood* (pp. 64–68). London: Heinemann, 1931. [CW 1:3:7]

Rheumatic fever. In *Clinical notes on disorders of childhood* (pp. 58–63). London: Heinemann, 1931. [CW 1:3:6]

Rheumatism in children [1928]. In *Annual report of the London County Council*: Vol. 3. *Report of the school medical officer for the year 1928*. London: P. S. King and Son, 1928. [CW 1:2:12]

'Robert' aet 9 years. In *Therapeutic consultation in child psychiatry* (pp. 89–104). London: Hogarth, 1971. [CW 10:1:5]

'Robin' aet 5 years. In *Therapeutic consultations in child psychiatry* (pp. 28–41). London: Hogarth, 1971. [CW 10:1:2]

Roots of aggression. In *The child, the family, and the outside world* (pp. 232–239). Harmondsworth: Penguin Books, 1964; and C. Winnicott, R. Shepherd & M. Davis (Eds.), *Deprivation and delinquency* (pp. 92–99, part of 'Aggression and its roots'). London: Tavistock, 1984. [CW 7:1:18]

Roots of aggression [1968]. In C. Winnicott, R. Shepherd & M. Davis (Eds.), *Psycho-analytic explorations* (pp. 458–461, part of the chapter 'Melanie Klein: On her concept of envy'). Cambridge, MA: Harvard University Press, 1989. [CW 8:2:21]

'Rosemary' aet 10 years. In *Therapeutic consultations in child psychiatry* (pp. 105–109). London: Hogarth, 1971. [CW 10:1:6]. See also 'A child psychiatry interview'.

'Ruth' aet 8 years. In *Therapeutic consultations in child psychiatry* (pp. 315–330). London: Hogarth, 1971. [CW 10:3:17]. See also 'Becoming deprived as a fact: A psychotherapeutic consultation'.

Sakari: A therapeutic consultation [1961]. [CW 6:2:16]

Saying 'No' [1960]. In C. Winnicott, C. Bollas, M. Davis & R. Shepherd (Eds.), *Talking to parents* (pp. 21–39). Reading, MA: Addison-Wesley, 1993. Also published in *Winnicott on the child* (pp. 108–121). Cambridge, MA: Perseus, 2002. Broadcast as parts 1–3 of 'The ordinary devoted mother and her children', 25 January, 1 and 8 February 1960. I. Benzie & E. Brewer (Producers), *Parents and children*. Network Three. London: British Broadcasting Corporation. [CW 6:1:1]

Security. In C. Winnicott, C. Bollas, M. Davis & R. Shepherd (Eds.), *Talking to parents* (pp. 87–93). Reading, MA: Addison-Wesley, 1993; and *Winnicott on the child* (pp. 155–159). Cambridge, MA: Perseus, 2002. Published here as 'On security'. [CW 6:1:9]

Sex education in schools. *Medical Press*, 1949, 222. Also published in *The child and the outside world: Studies in developing relationships* (pp. 40–44). London: Tavistock, 1957; and *The child, the family, and the outside world* (pp. 216–220). Harmondsworth: Penguin, 1964. [CW 3:4:35]

Short communication on enuresis. *St Bartholomew's Hospital Journal*, April 1930, 125–127. Also published in R. Shepherd, J. Johns & H. Taylor Robinson (Eds.), *Thinking about children* (pp. 170–175). London: Karnac, 1996. [CW 1:2:18]

A Shropshire surgeon (Poem). *St Bartholomew's Hospital Journal*, 1920, 27. [CW 1:1:12]

Shyness and nervous disorders in children. *New Era in Home and School*, 1938, 19. Also published in *The child and the outside world: Studies in developing relationships* (pp. 35–39). London: Tavistock, 1957; and *The child, the family, and the outside world* (pp. 211–215). Harmondsworth: Penguin, 1964. [CW 1:4:17]

Skin changes in relation to emotional disorder. *St John's Hospital Dermatological Society Report*, 1938, 27, 62–73. [CW 1:4:18]

Sleep (Poem). In C. Winnicott, 'D. W. W.: A reflection'. [CW 12:Afterword]

Sleep refusal in children. *Medical News Magazine* (Suppl. *Paediatrics*, pp. 8–9), July 1968. Also published in R. Shepherd, J. Johns & H. Taylor Robinson (Eds.), *Thinking about children* (pp. 42–45). London: Karnac, 1996. [CW 8:2:19]

Small things for small people. *New Society*, 7 December 1967, *10*(271), 835. Published here as 'Review: *A collection of children's books*'. [CW 8:1:35]

Smith. *The Fortnightly* (The Leys School, Cambridge), 3 October 1913. [CW 1:1:3]

The snag. *St Bartholomew's Hospital Journal*, 1921, 28, 188. [CW 1:1:15]

Social aspects of autism [1966]. [CW 7:3:7]

Some principles of child analysis [1969]. [CW 9:1:9]

Some psychological aspects of juvenile delinquency. *New Era in Home and School*, 1946, 27(10), 295. Also published in *Delinquency Research*, 1946, 24(5); and *The child and the outside world: Studies in developing relationships* (pp. 181–187). London: Tavistock, 1957; and C. Winnicott, R. Shepherd & M. Davis (Eds.), *Deprivation and delinquency* (pp. 113–119). London: Tavistock, 1984. [CW 3:1:7]. See also 'Aspects of juvenile delinquency'.

Some thoughts on the meaning of the word democracy. *Human Relations*, 1950, 3. Also published in *The family and individual development* (pp. 155–169). London: Tavistock, 1965; and C. Winnicott, R. Shepherd & M. Davis (Eds.), *Home is where we start from: Essays by a psychoanalyst* (pp. 239–259). Harmondsworth: Penguin, 1986. [CW 3:5:17]

Spoken comments on obsessional neurosis and 'Frankie' [1965]. [CW 7:2:11]

Speech disorders. In *Clinical notes on disorders of childhood* (pp. 191–200). London: Heinemann, 1931. [CW 1:3:20]

The split-off male and female elements to be found in men and women [1966]. In *Playing and reality* (pp. 72–85, part of the chapter 'Creativity and its origins'). London: Tavistock, 1971. Also published in C. Winnicott, R. Shepherd & M. Davis (Eds.), *Psycho-analytic explorations* (pp. 169–183). Cambridge, MA: Harvard University Press, 1989. [CW 7:3:2]. Also published here as part of 'Creativity and its origins'. [CW 9:3:7]

The spontaneous gesture: Selected letters (F. R. Rodman, Ed.). Cambridge, MA: Harvard University Press, 1987. [Not printed in this form in the *Collected Works*]

The squiggle game [1964, 1968]. In C. Winnicott, R. Shepherd & M. Davis (Eds.), *Psycho-analytic explorations* (pp. 299–317). Cambridge, MA: Harvard University Press, 1989. Published, in part, in *Voices: The Art and Science of Psycho-therapy*, 1968, 4, 98–112. Also published, in part, as 'Die volle Nutzung der ersten Behandlungsstunde. Beitrag zu Problemen der Kinderanalyse' or 'Meeting the challenge of the case'. In G. Biermann (Ed.), *Handbuch der Kinderpsychotherapie* (pp. 269–277). München/Basel: Ernst Reinhardt Verlag, 1968. Includes 'Case of L'. Also published in *Therapeutic consultations in child psychiatry* (pp. 42–63, as '"Eliza" aet 7½ years'). London: Hogarth, 1971. [CW 8:2:47]

Squiggles [1968]. *Voices: The Art and Science of Psycho-therapy*, 1968, 4, 98–112. Published here as part of 'The squiggle game'. [CW 8:2:47]

St Bartholomew's Hospital amateur dramatic club. *St Bartholomew's Hospital Journal*, 1920, 27, 152–154. [CW 1:1:13]

Stealing and telling lies [1949]. In *The child and the family*. London: Tavistock, 1957 (pp. 117–120). Also published in *The child, the family, and the outside world* (pp. 161–166). Harmondsworth: Penguin, 1964. [CW 3:4:33]

Strength out of misery. *The Observer*, 31 May 1964. Published here as 'The value of depression'. [CW 6:4:10]

String: A technique of communication. *Journal of Child Psychology and Psychiatry*, 1960, *1*(1), 49–52, as 'String'. Also published in *The maturational processes and the facilitating environment: Studies in the theory of emotional development* (pp. 153–157). London: Hogarth, 1965; and *Playing and reality* (pp. 15–20, as part of 'Transitional objects and transitional phenomena'). London: Tavistock, 1971. [CW 6:1:20]

Struggling through the doldrums. *New Society*, 25 April 1963, *1*(30), 8–11. Also published in C. Winnicott, R. Shepherd & M. Davis (Eds.), *Deprivation and delinquency* (pp. 145–155). London: Tavistock, 1984. [CW 6:4:7] See also 'Adolescence: Struggling through the doldrums' [CW 6:2:4]

A study of envy and gratitude [1956]. [CW 5:2:5]

Sum, I am [1968]. *Mathematics teaching*, March 1984. Also published in C. Winnicott, R. Shepherd & M. Davis (Eds.), *Home is where we start from: Essays by a psychoanalyst* (pp. 55–64). Harmondsworth: Penguin, 1986. [CW 8:2:10]

Support for normal parents [1944]. First published in *New Era in Home and School*, 1945, 26. Also published in *Getting to know your baby* (pp. 25–27, 'Postscript'). London: Heinemann, 1945; and *The child and the family: First relationships* (pp. 137–140). London: Tavistock, 1957; and *The child, the family, and the outside world* (pp. 173–176). Harmondsworth: Penguin, 1964. [CW 2:6:11]

Symptoms suggesting post-encephalitis. In *Proceedings of the Royal Society of Medicine*, 1929, 22(9), 1248–1249. [CW 1:2:15]

Symptom tolerance in paediatrics: A case history. *Proceedings of the Royal Society of Medicine*, 1953, 46. Also published in *Collected papers: Through paediatrics to psychoanalysis* (pp. 101–117). London: Tavistock, 1958. [CW 4:2:4]

Tailpiece. In *Playing and reality* (p. 151). London: Tavistock, 1971. [CW 9:3:10]

Talking about psychology. *New Era in Home and School*, 1945, 26. Published here as 'Towards an objective study of human nature'. [CW 2:7:11] See also 'What is psychoanalysis?

Talking to parents (C. Winnicott, C. Bollas, M. Davis & R. Shepherd, Eds.). [Introduction by T. Berry Brazelton] Reading, MA: Addison-Wesley, 1993. Also published as Part Two of *Winnicott on the child*. Cambridge, MA: Perseus, 2002. [Not reprinted in this form in the *Collected Works*]

The teacher, the parent and the doctor. [1936]. In R. Shepherd, J. Johns & H. Taylor Robinson (Eds.), *Thinking about children* (pp. 77–93). London: Karnac, 1996. [CW 1:4:10]

A tendency in therapeutics. *St Bartholomew's Hospital Journal*, February 1944, 7–9. [CW 2:6:5]

Their standards and yours [1944]. *New Era in Home and School*, 1945, 26. Also published in *Getting to know your baby* (pp. 21–24). London: Heinemann, 1945; and *The child and the family: First relationships* (pp. 87–91). London: Tavistock, 1957; and *The child, the family, and the outside world* (pp. 119–123). Harmondsworth: Penguin, 1964. Broadcast 12 May 1944. J. Quigley (Producer), *Happy children*. Home Service. London: British Broadcasting Corporation. [CW 2:6:9]

Theoretical statement of the field of child psychiatry. In A. Holzel & J. P. M. Tizard (Eds.), *Modern trends in paediatrics* (pp. 250–262, part of Chapter 14: 'Child psychiatry'). London: Butterworth, 1958. Also published in *The family and individual development* (pp. 97–105). London: Tavistock, 1965. [CW 5:4:25]

The theory of the parent-infant relationship. *International Journal of Psychoanalysis*, 1960, 41, 585–595. Also published in *The maturational processes and the facilitating environment: Studies in the theory of emotional development* (pp. 37–55). London: Hogarth, 1965. [CW 6:1:21]

The theory of the parent-infant relationship: Contributions to discussion. *International Journal of Psychoanalysis*, 1962, 43, 256–257. [CW 6:3:14]

The theory of the parent-infant relationship. Further remarks. *International Journal of Psychoanalysis*, 1962, 43, 238–239. Also published in C. Winnicott, R. Shepherd & M. Davis (Eds.), *Psycho-analytic explorations* (pp. 73–75). Cambridge, MA: Harvard University Press, 1989. [CW 6:3:13]

Therapeutic consultations in child psychiatry. London: Hogarth, 1971. [CW 10]

***Thinking about children* (R. Shepherd, J. Johns & H. Taylor Robinson, Eds.). London: Karnac, 1996.** [Not reprinted in this form in the *Collected Works*]

Thinking and symbol-formation [1968]. In C. Winnicott, R. Shepherd & M. Davis (Eds.), *Psycho-analytic explorations* (pp. 213–216). Cambridge, MA: Harvard University Press, 1989. [CW 8:2:48]

Thinking and the unconscious. *The Liberal Magazine*, March 1945, 125–126. Also published in C. Winnicott, R. Shepherd & M. Davis (Eds.), *Home is where we start from: Essays by a psychoanalyst* (pp. 169–171). Harmondsworth: Penguin, 1986. [CW 2:7:4]

This feminism [1964]. In C. Winnicott, R. Shepherd & M. Davis (Eds.) *Home is where we start from: Essays by a psychoanalyst* (pp. 183–194). Harmondsworth: Penguin, 1986. [CW 7:1:14]

The threat to freedom [1969]. In C. Winnicott, R. Shepherd & M. Davis (Eds.) *Home is where we start from: Essays by a psychoanalyst* (pp. 232–238). Harmondsworth: Penguin, 1986, part of 'Freedom'. [CW 9:1:17]

The toddler, the second adoption, telling children about adoption [n.d., ca. mid 1950s]. [CW 5:1:23]

Towards an objective study of human nature. *New Era in Home and School*, 1945, 26, as 'Talking about psychology'; reissued in 1952, 33(3) as 'What is psychoanalysis'? Also published in *The child and the outside world: Studies in developing relationships* (pp. 125–133). London: Tavistock, 1957; and R. Shepherd, J. Johns & H. Taylor Robinson (Eds.), *Thinking about children* (pp. 3–12). London: Karnac, 1996. [CW 2:7:11]

Training for child psychiatry [1962]. *Journal of Child Psychology and Psychiatry*, 1963, 4(2), 85–91. Also published in *The maturational processes and the facilitating environment: Studies in the theory of emotional development* (pp. 193–202). London: Hogarth, 1965. [CW 6:3:5]

Training for child psychiatry: The paediatric department of psychology [1961]. In R. Shepherd, J. Johns & H. Taylor Robinson (Eds.), *Thinking about children* (pp. 227–230). London: Karnac, 1996. Published here as 'The paediatric department of psychology'. [CW 6:2:19]

Transitional objects and transitional phenomena [1951]. *International Journal of Psychoanalysis*, 1953, 34, 89–97 [CW 4:2:21]. Also published in *Collected papers: Through paediatrics to psycho-analysis* (pp. 229–242). London: Tavistock, 1958 [CW 5:4:24]; and *Playing and reality* (pp. 1–25). London: Tavistock, 1971 [CW 9:3:5]; and *The collected works of D. W. Winnicott*. New York: Oxford University Press, 2017 [1951 version]. [CW 3:6:6]

Treatment of mental disease by induction of fits [1943]. In C. Winnicott, R. Shepherd & M. Davis (Eds.), *Psycho-analytic explorations* (pp. 516–521, in the chapter 'Physical therapy of mental disorder: Convulsion therapy'). Cambridge, MA: Harvard University Press, 1989. [CW 2:5:6]

The tree (Poem) [1963]. In F. R. Rodman, *Winnicott: Life and work* (pp. 289–291). Cambridge, MA: Perseus, 2003. [CW 6:4:14]

A tribute on the occasion of Willi Hoffer's seventieth birthday. *Psyche*, 1967, *21*, as 'Eine Kinderbeobachtung'. Also published in C. Winnicott, R. Shepherd & M. Davis (Eds.), *Psycho-analytic explorations* (pp. 499–505). Cambridge, MA: Harvard University Press, 1989. [CW 8:1:11]

Trips into partisanship [1967]. [CW 8:1:30]

Twins [1945]. In *The child and the family* (pp. 112–116). London: Tavistock, 1957. Also published in *The child, the family, and the outside world* (pp. 137–142). Harmondsworth: Penguin, 1964. Broadcast 27 April 1945. J. Quigley & D. Bridgman (Producers), *Difficult children*. Home Service. London: British Broadcasting Corporation. [CW 2:7:5]

Two adopted children [1953]. *Case Conference*, 1954, *1*. Also published in *The child and the outside world: Studies in developing relationships* (pp. 52–65). London: Tavistock, 1957; and R. Shepherd, J. Johns & H. Taylor Robinson (Eds.), *Thinking about children* (pp. 113–127). London: Karnac, 1996. [CW 4:2:19]

Two cases of post-encephalitic hyperapnœa. *Section for the Study of Disease in Children, Proceedings of the Royal Society of Medicine*, 1926, *19*, 52–53. [CW 1:2:4]

Two further clinical examples [1970]. In C. Winnicott, R. Shepherd & M. Davis (Eds.), *Psycho-analytic explorations* (pp. 272–283, in the chapter 'On the basis for self in body'). Cambridge, MA: Harvard University Press, 1989. [CW 9:2:13]

Two notes on the use of silence [1963]. In C. Winnicott, R. Shepherd & M. Davis (Eds.), *Psycho-analytic explorations* (pp. 81–86). Cambridge, MA: Harvard University Press, 1989. [CW 6:4:19]

Über die Fähigkeit, Allein zu Sein. *Psyche*, 1958, *12*. Published here as 'The capacity to be alone'. [CW 5:3:20]

The unconscious [1953]. [CW 4:2:8]

The unconscious [1966]. [CW 7:3:29]

The use of an object and relating through identifications [1968]. *International Journal of Psychoanalysis*, 1969, *50*, 711–716, as 'The use of an object'. Also published in *Playing and reality* (pp. 86–94). London: Tavistock, 1971; and C. Winnicott, R. Shepherd & M. Davis (Eds.), *Psycho-analytic explorations* (pp. 218–227). Cambridge, MA: Harvard University Press, 1989. [CW 8:2:28]

The use of an object in the context of *Moses and Monotheism* [1969]. In C. Winnicott, R. Shepherd & M. Davis (Eds.), *Psycho-analytic explorations* (pp. 240–246, in the chapter 'The use of an object'). Cambridge, MA: Harvard University Press, 1989. [CW 9:1:4]

The use of the word 'use' [1968]. In C. Winnicott, R. Shepherd & M. Davis (Eds.), *Psycho-analytic explorations* (pp. 233–235, in the chapter 'The use of an object'). Cambridge, MA: Harvard University Press, 1989. [CW 8:2:5]

The value of breastfeeding (psychological) [abstract]. *Archives of Disease in Childhood*, 1945, *20*(104), 186. Published here as a footnote in 'Breast feeding'. [CW 2:7:12 (footnote *i*)]

The value of depression [1963]. *British Journal of Psychiatric Social Work*, 1964, *7*(3), 123–127; and *The Observer*, 31 May 1964 as 'Strength out of misery'. Also published in

C. Winnicott, R. Shepherd & M. Davis (Eds.), *Home is where we start from: Essays by a psychoanalyst* (pp. 71–79). Harmondsworth: Penguin, 1986. [CW 6:4:10]

The value of the therapeutic consultation [1965]. In C. Winnicott, R. Shepherd & M. Davis (Eds.), *Psycho-analytic explorations* (pp. 318–324). Cambridge, MA: Harvard University Press, 1989. First published, together with '"Ashton" aet 12 years', in E. Miller (Ed.), *Foundations of child psychiatry* (pp. 593–608, as 'The value of the therapeutic consultation'). Oxford, UK: Pergamon Press, 1968. [CW 7:2:22]

Varicella encephalitis and vaccinia encephalitis (with N. Gibbs). *British Journal of Children's Diseases*, 1926, 23, 107–127. [CW 1:2:1]

Varieties of psychotherapy [1961]. In C. Winnicott, R. Shepherd & M. Davis (Eds.), *Deprivation and delinquency* (pp. 232–240). London: Tavistock, 1984. Also published in C. Winnicott, R. Shepherd & M. Davis (Eds.), *Home is where we start from: Essays by a psychoanalyst* (pp. 101–111). Harmondsworth: Penguin, 1986. [CW 6:2:5]

Visiting children in hospital [1951]. *Child-Family Digest*, October 1952; and *New Era in Home and School*, 1952, 33. Also published in *The child and the family: First relationships* (pp. 121–126). London: Tavistock, 1957; and *The child, the family, and the outside world* (pp. 221–226). Harmondsworth: Penguin, 1964. Broadcast in two parts, 16 and 23 May 1951, under the same title. Benzie, I. (Producer) *Woman's hour* Light Programme. London: British Broadcasting Corporation. [CW 3:6:5]

Walking. In *Clinical notes on disorders of childhood* (pp. 143–151). London: Heinemann, 1931. [CW 1:3:15]

Weaning. In *The ordinary devoted mother and her baby* (pp. 43–47). London: C. A. Brock, 1949. Also published in *The child and the family: First relationships* (pp. 64–68). London: Tavistock, 1957; and *The child, the family, and the outside world* (pp. 80–84). Harmondsworth: Penguin, 1964. Broadcast 30 November 1949. I. Benzie (Producer), *How's the baby?* Home Service. London: British Broadcasting Corporation. [CW 3:4:31]

The wearing of masks in the nursing of premature and older infants [abstract] [1943]. *Archives of Disease in Childhood*, 1944, 19(97), 38. [CW 2:5:9]

What about father? [1944]. *New Era in Home and School*, 1945, 26. Also published in *Getting to know your baby* (pp. 16–21). London: Heinemann, 1945; and *The child and the family: First relationships* (pp. 81–86). London: Tavistock, 1957; and *The child, the family, and the outside world* (pp. 113–118). Harmondsworth: Penguin, 1964. Broadcast 17 March 1944, as 'Where does Dad come in?' J. Quigley (Producer), *Happy children*. Home Service. London: British Broadcasting Corporation. [CW 2:6:8]

What do we know about babies as cloth suckers? [1956]. In C. Winnicott, C. Bollas, M. Davis & R. Shepherd (Eds.), *Talking to parents* (pp. 15–20). Reading, MA: Addison-Wesley, 1993. Also published in *Winnicott on the child* (pp. 104–107). Cambridge, MA: Perseus, 2002. Broadcast 31 January 1956. I. Benzie (Producer), *Woman's hour*. Light Programme. London: British Broadcasting Corporation. [CW 5:2:1]

What do we mean by a normal child? *New Era in Home and School*, 1946, 27. Also published in *The child and the family: First relationships* (pp. 100–106). London: Tavistock, 1957; and *The child, the family, and the outside world* (pp. 124–130). Harmondsworth: Penguin, 1964. Broadcast 23 June 1944. J. Quigley (Producer), *Happy children*. Home Service. London: British Broadcasting Corporation. [CW 2:6:10]

What irks? [1960]. In C. Winnicott, C. Bollas, M. Davis & R. Shepherd (Eds.), *Talking to parents* (pp. 65–86). Reading, MA: Addison-Wesley, 1993. Also published in *Winnicott on the child* (pp. 139–154). Cambridge, MA: Perseus, 2002. Broadcast as parts 8–9 of 'The ordinary devoted mother and her children', 14 and 21 March 1960. I. Benzie & E. Brewer (Producers), *Parents and children*. Network Three. London: British Broadcasting Corporation. [CW 6:1:7]

What is psychoanalysis? *New Era in Home and School*, 1952, 33(3). Published here as 'Towards an objective study of human nature'. [CW 2:7:11] See also 'Talking about psychology'.

What is worthwhile in medicine [ca. 1917–1923]. [CW 1:1:16]

Where angels fear to tread, or, a comment on generic teaching [1958]. [CW 5:4:9]

Where the food goes. In *The ordinary devoted mother and her baby* (pp. 12–16). London: C. A. Brock, 1949. Also published in *The child and the family: First relationships* (pp. 23–27). London: Tavistock, 1957; and *The child, the family, and the outside world* (pp. 35–39). Harmondsworth: Penguin, 1964. Broadcast 19 October 1949, as 'The baby and its food'. I. Benzie (Producer), *How's the baby?* Home Service. London: British Broadcasting Corporation. [CW 3:4:25]

Why children play. *New Era in Home and School*, 1942, 23. Also published in *The child and the outside world: Studies in developing relationships* (pp. 149–152). London: Tavistock, 1957; and *The child, the family, and the outside world* (pp. 143–146). Harmondsworth: Penguin, 1964. [revised 1968] [CW 2:4:4]

Why do babies cry? [1944]. *New Era in Home and School*, 1945, 26. Also published in *The child and the family: First relationships* (pp. 43–52). London: Tavistock, 1957; and *The child, the family, and the outside world* (pp. 58–68). Harmondsworth: Penguin, 1964; and *Parents*, 1967, 22(8), as 'Winnicott's wisdom: Why do babies cry?' Broadcast in two parts, 4 and 11 February 1944, as 'Why does your baby cry?' J. Quigley (Producer), *Happy children*. Home Service. London: British Broadcasting Corporation. [CW 2:6:2]

Winnicott on the child. Cambridge, MA: Perseus, 2002. Part One first published as *Babies and their mothers* (C. Winnicott, R. Shepherd & M. Davis, Eds.). Reading, MA: Addison-Wesley, 1987; Part Two first published as *Talking to parents* (C. Winnicott, C. Bollas, M. Davis & R. Shepherd, Eds.). Reading, MA: Addison-Wesley, 1993. [Not reprinted in this form in the *Collected Works*]

Winnicott's wisdom: Hobgoblins and good habits. *Parents*, 1967, 22(9), 63–65. [CW 8:1:22]

Winnicott's wisdom: How a baby begins to feel sorry and to make amends. *Parents*, 1967, 22(7), 32–35. [CW 8:1:16]

Winnicott's wisdom: The meaning of mother love. *Parents*, 1967, 22(6), 22–23. [CW 8:1:13]

Winnicott's wisdom: Why do babies cry? *Parents*, 1967, 22(8), 22–23. [CW 8:1:17]

Withdrawal and regression. *Revue Française de Psychanalyse*, 1955, 19, 1–2, as 'Repli et régression'. Also published in *Psyche*, 10, 1956–1957; and *Collected papers: Through paediatrics to psycho-analysis* (pp. 255–261). London: Tavistock, 1958; and *Holding and interpretation: Fragment of an analysis* [1954] (pp. 187–192, as 'Appendix: Withdrawal and regression'). London: Karnac, 1986. [CW 4:3:29]

The world in small doses. In *The ordinary devoted mother and her baby* (pp. 32–37). London: C. A. Brock, 1949. Also published in *The child and the family: First relationships* (pp. 53–58). London: Tavistock, 1957; and *The child, the family, and the outside world* (pp. 69–74). Harmondsworth: Penguin, 1964. Broadcast 16 November 1949, as

'Presenting the world to a baby'. I. Benzie (Producer), *How's the baby?* Home Service. London: British Broadcasting Corporation. [CW 3:4:29]

'Yes, but how do we know it's true?' [1950]. In R. Shepherd, J. Johns & H. Taylor Robinson (Eds.), *Thinking about children* (pp. 13–18). London: Karnac, 1996. [CW 3:5:18]

Young children and other people. *Young Children*, 1949, 1. Also published *The child and the family: First relationships* (pp. 92–99). London: Tavistock, 1957; and *The child, the family, and the outside world* (pp. 103–110). Harmondsworth: Penguin, 1964. [CW 3:4:32]

Youth will not sleep. *New Society*, 28 May 1964, 3(87), 5. Also published in C. Winnicott, R. Shepherd & M. Davis (Eds.), *Deprivation and delinquency* (pp. 156–158). London: Tavistock, 1984. [CW 7:1:7]

Complete Back Catalogue of the Published Books of D. W. Winnicott

Clinical Notes on Disorders of Childhood

Practioner's Aid Series

By D. W. Winnicott MA (Cantab.), MRCP (London)

    Physician, Paddington Green Children's Hospital; Asst. Physician, The Queen's Hospital for Children; in charge of the LCC Rehumatism Clinic at the Queen's Hospital for Children.

London: William Heinemann (Medical Books), 1931

Preface [CW 1:3:Preface]		v
Introduction [CW 1:3:Introduction]		1
1.	History-taking [CW 1:3:1]	7
2.	Physical Examination [CW 1:3:2]	22
3.	A Note on Temperature and the Importance of Charts [CW 1:3:3]	32
4.	The Nose and Throat [CW 1:3:4]	38
5.	The Heart, with Special Reference to Rheumatic Carditis [CW 1:3:5]	42
6.	Rheumatic Fever [CW 1:3:6]	58
7.	The Rheumatic Clinic [CW 1:3:7]	64
8.	Active Heart Disease [CW 1:3:8]	69
9.	Growing Pains [CW 1:3:9]	76
10.	Arthritis Associated with Emotional Disturbance [CW 1:3:10]	81
11.	Fidgetiness [CW 1:3:11]	87
	Chorea	89
12.	A Note on Normality and Anxiety [CW 1:3:12]	98
13.	Anxiety (continued), Treatment [CW 1:3:13]	122
	The Parents' Part	125
	Sexual Enlightenment	127
14.	Disease of the Nervous System [CW 1:3:14]	129
15.	Walking [CW 1:3:15]	143

	Posture, Movement	148
16.	Mental Defect [CW 1:3:16]	152
17.	Convulsions, Fits [CW 1:3:17]	157
18.	Micturition Disturbances [CW 1:3:18]	172
	Enuresis	177
19.	Masturbation [CW 1:3:19]	183
20.	Speech Disorders [CW 1:3:20]	191
	Stuttering	195

Index   201

Getting to Know Your Baby

London: William Heinemann, 1945

Preface [CW 1:3:Preface]
1. Getting to Know Your Baby [CW 2:5:8]
2. Why Do Babies Cry? [CW 2:6:2]
3. Infant Feeding [CW 2:6:13]
4. What About Father? [CW 2:6:8]
5. Their Standards and Yours [CW 2:6:9]
6. Postscript ['Support for Normal Parents' CW 2:6:11]

The Ordinary Devoted Mother and Her Baby

Nine Broadcast Talks (Autumn 1949)
London: C. A. Brock, 1950

1.	Introduction ['A Man Looks at Motherhood' CW 3:4:23]	3
2.	The Baby as a Going Concern [CW 3:4:24]	7
3.	Where the Food Goes [CW 3:4:25]	12
4.	The End of the Digestive Process [CW 3:4:26]	17
5.	The Baby as a Person [CW 3:4:27]	22
6.	Close-up of Mother Feeding Baby [CW 3:4:28]	27
7.	The World in Small Doses [CW 3:4:29]	32
8.	The Innate Morality of the Baby [Training Babies: Problems of Management [CW 12:3:4c]; revised as CW 3:4:30]	38
9.	Weaning [CW 3:4:31]	43

The Child and the Family: First Relationships

EDITED BY JANET HARDENBERG

First published London: Tavistock, 1957

Editor's Note	vii
Preface [CW 7:1:17]	xi

Part I. The Ordinary Devoted Mother and Her Baby

1.	A Man Looks at Motherhood [CW 3:4:23]	3
2.	Getting to Know Your Baby [CW 2:5:8]	7
3.	The Baby as a Going Concern [CW 3:4:24]	13
4.	Infant Feeding [CW 2:6:13]	18
5.	Where the Food Goes [CW 3:4:25]	23
6.	The End of the Digestive Process [CW 3:4:26]	28
7.	The Baby as a Person [CW 3:4:27]	33
8.	Close-up of Mother Feeding Baby [CW 3:4:28]	38
9.	Why Do Babies Cry? [CW 2:6:2]	43
10.	The World in Small Doses [CW 3:4:29]	53
11.	The Innate Morality of the Baby [CW 3:4:30]	59
12.	Weaning [CW 3:4:31]	64
13.	Knowing and Learning [CW 3:5:14]	69
14.	Instincts and Normal Difficulties [CW 3:5:15]	74

Part II. Family Affairs

1.	What About Father? [CW 2:6:8]	81
2.	Their Standards and Yours [CW 2:6:9]	87
3.	Young Children and Other People [CW 3:4:32]	92
4.	What Do We Mean by a Normal Child? [CW 3:4:32]	100
5.	The Only Child [CW 2:7:1]	107
6.	Twins [CW 2:7:5]	112
7.	Stealing and Telling Lies [CW 3:4:33]	117
8.	Visiting Children in Hospital [CW 3:6:5]	121
9.	On Adoption [CW 5:1:2]	127
10.	First Experiments in Independence [CW 5:1:20]	131
11.	Support for Normal Parents [CW 2:6:11]	137

Postscript: The Mother's Contribution to Society [CW 5:3:30]	141
Index	147

The Child and the Outside World: Studies in Developing Relationships

EDITED BY JANET HARDENBERG

First published London: Tavistock, 1957

Editor's Note	vii
Acknowledgements	viii

Part I. The Care of Growing Children

1. Needs of the Under-Fives in a Changing Society [CW 4:3:18] — 3
2. The Child's Needs and the Role of the Mother in the Early Stages ['Mother, Teacher, and the Child's Needs' CW 4:2:20] — 14
3. On Influencing and Being Influenced [CW 2:3:3] — 24
4. Educational Diagnosis [CW 3:1:2] — 29
5. Shyness and Nervous Disorders in Children [CW 1:4:17] — 35
6. Sex Education in Schools [CW 3:4:35] — 40
7. Pitfalls in Adoption [CW 4:3:30] — 45
8. Two Adopted Children [CW 4:2:19] — 52

Part II. Children Under Stress
(Including Wartime Broadcasts)

9. Children in the War [CW 2:2:4] — 69
10. The Deprived Mother [CW 2:1:4] — 75
11. The Evacuated Child [CW 2:7:2] — 83
12. The Return of the Evacuated Child [CW 2:7:3] — 88
13. Home Again [CW 2:7:7] — 93
14. Residential Management as Treatment for Difficult Children [CW 3:2:3] — 98
15. Children's Hostels in War and Peace [CW 3:1:1] — 117

Part III. Reflections on Impulse in Children

16. Towards an Objective Study of Human Nature [CW 2:7:11] — 125
17. Further Thoughts on Babies as Persons [CW 3:2:4] — 134
18. Breast Feeding [CW 2:7:12] — 141
19. Why Children Play [CW 2:4:4] — 149
20. The Child and Sex [CW 3:2:5] — 153
21. Aggression [CW 2:1:8] — 167
22. The Impulse to Steal [CW 3:4:34] — 176
23. Some Psychological Aspects of Juvenile Delinquency [CW 3:1:7] — 181

Index — 188

Collected Papers: Through Paediatrics to Psychoanalysis

First published London: Hogarth and the Institute of Psychoanalysis, 1958.

Second edition, with an Introduction by M. M. R. Khan, published London: Hogarth, 1975; reprinted 1977, 1978, 1982 and 1987 by Hogarth.

Reprinted (with permission of Hogarth) London: Karnac, 1984. Reprinted 2003, 2004, 2007.

Preface [CW 5:3:32]	ix
Acknowledgements [CW 5:3:32]	x
Introduction by M. Masud R. Khan (2nd ed.)	xi

Part 1

1.	A Note on Normality and Anxiety [CW 1:3:12]	3
2.	Fidgetiness [CW 1:3:11]	22

Part 2

3.	Appetite and Emotional Disorder [CW 1:4:11]	33
4.	The Observation of Infants in a Set Situation [CW 2:3:6]	52
5.	Child Department Consultations [CW 2:4:2]	70
6.	Ocular Psychoneuroses of Childhood [CW 2:6:15]	85
7.	Reparation in Respect of Mother's Organized Defence Against Depression [CW 3:3:1]	91
8.	Anxiety Associated with Insecurity [CW 4:1:11]	97
9.	Symptom Tolerance in Paediatrics: A Case History [CW 4:2:4]	101
10.	A Case Managed at Home [CW 5:1:18]	118

Part 3

11.	The Manic Defence [CW 1:4:6]	129
12.	Primitive Emotional Development [CW 2:7:8]	145
13.	Paediatrics and Psychiatry [CW 3:3:2]	157
14.	Birth Memories, Birth Trauma, and Anxiety [CW 3:4:8]	174
15.	Hate in the Countertransference [CW 3:2:1]	194
16.	Aggression in Relation to Emotional Development [CW 3:5:2]	204
17.	Psychoses and Child Care [CW 4:1:5]	219
18.	Transitional Objects and Transitional Phenomena [CW 5:4:24]	229
19.	Mind and Its Relation to the Psyche-Soma [CW 3:4:20]	243
20.	Withdrawal and Regression [CW 4:3:29]	255
21.	The Depressive Position in Normal Emotional Development [CW 4:3:5]	262
22.	Metapsychological and Clinical Aspects of Regression Within the Psycho-Analytical Set-Up [CW 4:3:6]	278
23.	Clinical Varieties of Transference [CW 5:1:11]	295
24.	Primary Maternal Preoccupation [CW 5:2:16]	300

25. The Antisocial Tendency [CW 5:2:8]	306
26. Paediatrics and Childhood Neurosis [CW 5:2:11]	316

Bibliography [CW 12:1:4a]	322
Index	326

The Child, the Family and the Outside World

First published London: Pelican, 1964

Reprinted London: Penguin, 1991

A large part of the material in this book was originally published in two volumes: *The Child and the Family* and *The Child and the Outside World* (both Tavistock, 1957).

Reprinted with an Introduction by Marshall H. Klaus, Reading, MA: Addison-Wesley, 1987.

Page numbers here are given for the Penguin editions.

Introduction [CW 7:1:17]	9

Part I. Mother and Child

1. A Man Looks at Motherhood [CW 3:4:23]	15
2. Getting to Know Your Baby [CW 2:5:8]	19
3. The Baby as a Going Concern [CW 3:4:24]	25
4. Infant Feeding [CW 2:6:13]	30
5. Where the Food Goes [CW 3:4:25]	35
6. The End of the Digestive Process [CW 3:4:26]	40
7. Close-up of Mother Feeding Baby [CW 3:4:28]	45
8. Breast Feeding [CW 2:7:12]	50
9. Why Do Babies Cry? [CW 2:6:2]	58
10. The World in Small Doses [CW 3:4:29]	69
11. The Baby as a Person [CW 3:4:27]	75
12. Weaning [CW 3:4:31]	80
13. Further Thoughts on Babies as Persons [CW 3:2:4]	85
14. The Innate Morality of the Baby [CW 3:4:30]	93
15. Instincts and Normal Difficulties [CW 3:5:15]	98
16. Young Children and Other People [CW 3:4:32]	103

Part II. The Family

17. What About Father? [CW 2:6:8]	113
18. Their Standards and Yours [CW 2:6:9]	119
19. What Do We Mean by a Normal Child? [CW 3:4:32]	124

20. The Only Child [CW 2:7:1] — 131
21. Twins [CW 2:7:5] — 137
22. Why Children Play [CW 2:4:4] — 143
23. The Child and Sex [CW 3:2:5] — 147
24. Stealing and Telling Lies [CW 3:4:33] — 161
25. First Experiments in Independence [CW 5:1:20] — 167
26. Support for Normal Parents [CW 2:6:11] — 173

Part III. The Outside World

27. Needs of the Under-Fives [CW 4:3:18] — 179
28. Mother, Teacher and the Child's Needs [CW 4:2:20] — 189
29. On Influencing and Being Influenced [CW 2:3:3] — 199
30. Educational Diagnosis [CW 3:1:2] — 205
31. Shyness and Nervous Disorders in Children [CW 1:4:17] — 211
32. Sex Education in Schools [CW 3:4:35] — 216
33. Visiting Children in Hospital [CW 3:6:5] — 221
34. Aspects of Juvenile Delinquency [CW 3:1:7] — 227
35. Roots of Aggression [CW 7:1:18] — 232

The Family and Individual Development

First published London: Tavistock, 1965. Reprinted six times.

Issued as a Tavistock Social Science Paperback in 1968.

Reprinted by Routledge in 1989, 1993, 1999. Reprinted by Brunner-Routledge, 2001. Reprinted, with an Introduction by Martha Nussbaum, by Routledge Classics, 2006.

Page numbers here are given for the Tavistock editions.

To Clare

Preface [CW 7:2:25] — vii
Acknowledgements [CW 7:2:25] — vii

Part 1

· 1. The First Year of Life: Modern Views on the Emotional Development [CW 5:4:6] — 3
2. The Relationship of a Mother to Her Baby at the Beginning [CW 6:1:8] — 15
3. Growth and Development in Immaturity [CW 3:5:16] — 21
4. On Security [CW 6:1:9] — 30
5. The Five-Year-Old [CW 6:3:6] — 34
6. Integrative and Disruptive Factors in Family Life [CW 5:3:26] — 40

7.	The Family Affected by Depressive Illness in One or Both Parents [CW 5:4:17]	50
8.	The Effect of Psychosis on Family Life [CW 6:1:6]	61
9.	The Effect of Psychotic Parents on the Emotional Development of the Child [CW 5:5:21]	69
10.	Adolescence: Struggling Through the Doldrums [CW 6:2:4]	79
11.	The Family and Emotional Maturity [CW 6:1:17]	88

Part 2

12.	Theoretical Statement of the Field of Child Psychiatry [CW 5:4:25]	97
13.	The Contribution of Psycho-Analysis to Midwifery [CW 5:3:15]	106
14.	Advising Parents [CW 5:3:27]	114
15.	Casework with Mentally Ill Children [CW 5:5:15]	121
16.	The Deprived Child and How He Can Be Compensated for Loss of Family Life [CW 3:5:10]	132
17.	Group Influences and the Maladjusted Child: The School Aspect [CW 5:1:9]	146
18.	Some Thoughts on the Meaning of the Word Democracy [CW 3:5:17]	155

Index 171

The Maturational Process and the Facilitating Environment

First published London: Hogarth, and the Institute of Psychoanalysis, 1965.

Reprinted London: Karnac, 1990 (with permission from Hogarth). Reprinted 2002, 2003, 2004, 2005, 2006, 2007.

Editorial Note 7
Introduction [CW 7:2:24] 9

Part I: Papers on Development

1.	Psycho-Analysis and the Sense of Guilt (1958) [CW 5:2:7]	15
2.	The Capacity to Be Alone (1958) [CW 5:3:20]	29
3.	The Theory of the Parent-Infant Relationship (1960) [CW 6:1:21]	37
4.	Ego Integration in Child Development (1962) [CW 6:3:19]	56
5.	Providing for the Child in Health and Crisis (1962) [CW 6:3:10]	64
6.	The Development of the Capacity for Concern (1963) [CW 6:3:11]	73

7. From Dependence Towards Independence in the Development
   of the Individual (1963) [CW 6:4:11]   83
8. Morals and Education (1963) [CW 6:3:18]   93

Part II: Theory and Technique

9. On the Contribution of Direct Child Observation
   to Psycho-Analysis (1957) [CW 5:3:21]   109
10. Child Analysis in the Latency Period (1958) [CW 5:4:13]   115
11. Classification: Is There a Psycho-Analytic Contribution to
    Psychiatric Classification? (1959–64) [CW 5:5:5]   124
12. Ego Distortion in Terms of True and False Self (1960)
    [CW 6:1:22]   140
13. String: A Technique of Communication (1960) [CW 6:1:20]   153
14. Countertransference (1960) [CW 5:5:20]   158
15. The Aims of Psycho-Analytical Treatment (1962) [CW 6:3:3]   166
16. A Personal View of the Kleinian Contribution (1962) [CW 6:3:8]   171
17. Communicating and Not Communicating Leading to a
    Study of Certain Opposites (1963) [CW 6:4:8]   179
18. Training for Child Psychiatry (1963) [CW 6:3:5]   193
19. Psychotherapy of Character Disorders (1963) [CW 6:4:9]   203
20. The Mentally Ill in Your Caseload (1963) [CW 6:4:5]   217
21. Psychiatric Disorder in Terms of Infantile Maturational
    Processes (1963) [CW 6:4:12]   230
22. Hospital Care Supplementing Intensive Psychotherapy in
    Adolescence (1963) [CW 6:4:13]   242
23. Dependence in Infant-Care, in Child-Care and in the
    Psycho-Analytic Setting (1963) [CW 6:3:9]   249

Bibliography I: Books and Papers Referred to in the Text
    [CW 12:1:4c]   261
Bibliography II: Editor's List of Author's Publications (1926–1964)   264
Index   277

Playing and Reality

First published London: Tavistock, 1971.

Published by Pelican, 1974. Reprinted by Penguin Education, 1980.

Published by Routledge, 1991; reprinted 1992, 1993, 1994, 1996, 1997, 1999. Reprinted by Brunner-Routledge, 2002.

Published, with a Preface by F. R. Rodman, by Routledge Classics, Oxford, and Routledge, New York, 2005; reprinted 2006 (twice), 2007, 2008 (twice), 2009 (twice), 2010.

Page numbers here are given for the Tavistock editions.

To my patients
who have paid to teach me

Acknowledgements [CW 9:3:4]   ix
Introduction [CW 9:3:4]   xi

1. Transitional Objects and Transitional Phenomena [CW 9:3:5]   1
2. Dreaming, Fantasying and Living: A Case-History Describing a Primary Dissociation [CW 9:3:6]   26
3. Playing: A Theoretical Statement [CW 8:2:15]   38
4. Playing: Creative Activity and the Search for the Self [CW 8:1:27]   53
5. Creativity and Its Origins [CW 9:3:7]   65
6. The Use of an Object and Relating Through Identifications [CW 8:2:28]   86
7. The Location of Cultural Experience [CW 7:3:31]   95
8. The Place Where We Live [CW 8:2:1]   104
9. Mirror-role of Mother and Family in Child Development [CW 8:1:38]   111
10. Interrelating Apart from Instinctual Drive and in Terms of Cross-Identifications [CW 9:3:8]   119
11. Contemporary Concepts of Adolescent Development and Their Implications for Higher Education [CW 9:3:9]   138

Tailpiece [CW 9:3:10]   151
References [CW 12:1:4d]   153
Index   157

Therapeutic Consultations in Child Psychiatry

Published by The International Psychoanalytical Library (M. Masud R. Khan, Ed.), No. 87. Published London: Hogarth and the Institute of Psychoanalysis, 1971. Reprinted by Karnac, London (with the permission of Hogarth), 1996.

Published in the United States by Basic Books, 1990.

Part 1

Introduction [CW 10:1:Introduction]   1

1. 'Iiro' *aet* 9 Years 9 Months [CW 10:1:1]   12
2. 'Robin' *aet* 5 Years [CW 10:1:2]   28
3. 'Eliza' *aet* 7½ Years [CW 10:1:3]   42
4. 'Bob' *aet* 6 Years [CW 10:1:4]   64

Back Catalogue of Winnicott's Published Books   133

   5. 'Robert' *aet* 9 Years [CW 10:1:5]   89
   6. 'Rosemary' *aet* 10 Years [CW 10:1:6]   105
   7. 'Alfred' *aet* 10 Years [CW 10:1:7]   110

Part 2

Introduction [CW 10:2:Introduction]   127
   8. 'Charles' *aet* 9 Years [CW 10:2:8]   129
   9. 'Ashton' *aet* 12 Years [CW 10:2:9]   147
 10. 'Albert' *aet* 7 Years 9 Months [CW 10:2:10]   161
 11. 'Hesta' *aet* 16 Years [CW 10:2:11]   176
 12. 'Milton' *aet* 8 Years [CW 10:2:12]   194

Part 3

Introduction [CW 10:3:Introduction]   216
 13. 'Ada' *aet* 8 Years [CW 10:3:13]   220
 14. 'Cecil' *aet* 21 Months at First Consultation [CW 10:3:14]   240
 15. 'Mark' *aet* 12 Years [CW 10:3:15]   270
 16. 'Peter' *aet* 13 Years [CW 10:3:16]   296
 17. 'Ruth' *aet* 8 Years [CW 10:3:17]   315
 18. 'Mrs X' *aet* 30 Years [CW 10:3:18]   332
 19. 'Lily' *aet* 5 Years [CW 10:3:19]   342
 20. 'Jason' *aet* 8 Years 9 Months [CW 10:3:20]   344
 21. 'George' *aet* 13 Years [CW 10:3:21]   380

Bibliographical Note by Masud R. Khan   397
Index   399

The Piggle: An Account of the Psycho-Analytic Treatment of a Little Girl

EDITED BY ISHAK RAMZY

First published London: Hogarth, 1977.

Published by Penguin, Harmondsworth, UK, 1980. Reprinted by Pelican, 1989. Reprinted by Penguin, 1991.

Appearing here as [CW 11:2]

Preface – Clare Winnicott and R. D. Shepherd   vii
Editor's Foreword – Ishak Ramzy   xi

Introduction   1
The Patient [CW11:2:1]   5
First Consultation [CW 11:2:2]   9
Second Consultation [CW 11:2:3]   25

Third Consultation [CW 11:2:4]	39
Fourth Consultation [CW 11:2:5]	55
Fifth Consultation [CW 11:2:6]	67
Sixth Consultation [CW 11:2:7]	77
Seventh Consultation [CW 11:2:8]	89
Eighth Consultation [CW 11:2:9]	99
Ninth Consultation [CW 11:2:10]	111
Tenth Consultation [CW 11:2:11]	123
Eleventh Consultation [CW 11:2:12]	135
Twelfth Consultation [CW 11:2:13]	149
Thirteenth Consultation [CW 11:2:14]	165
Fourteenth Consultation [CW 11:2:15]	179
Fifteenth Consultation [CW 11:2:16]	185
Sixteenth Consultation [CW 11:2:17]	195
Afterword – By the Parents of the Piggle	199

Deprivation and Delinquency

EDITED BY CLARE WINNICOTT, RAY SHEPHERD
AND MADELEINE DAVIS

London: Tavistock, 1984.

Published by Routledge, 1990. Republished, with a Foreword by Jan Abram, by Routledge Classics, Oxford, and Routledge, New York, 2012.

Page numbers here are for the Tavistock editions.

Acknowledgements	vii
Editors' Preface	viii
Introduction by Clare Winnicott	1

Part I. Children Under Stress: Wartime Experience
Editors' Introduction — 9

1. Evacuation of Small Children (1939/1940)
    - Letter to the *British Medical Journal* (1939) [CW 2:1:6] — 13
    - Children and Their Mothers (1940) [CW 2:2:2] — 14
2. Review of *The Cambridge Evacuation Survey* (1941) [CW 2:3:5] — 22
3. Children in the War (1940) [CW 2:2:4] — 25
4. The Deprived Mother (1939) [CW 2:1:4] — 31
5. The Evacuated Child (1945) [CW 2:7:2] — 39
6. The Return of the Evacuated Child (1945) [CW 2:7:3] — 44
7. Home Again (1945) [CW 2:7:7] — 49
8. Residential Management as Treatment for Difficult Children (1947) [CW 3:2:3] — 54
9. Children's Hostels in War and Peace (1948) [CW 3:1:1] — 73

Part II. The Nature and Origins of the Antisocial Tendency

Editors' Introduction   81

10. Aggression and Its Roots (1939–64)
    Aggression (ca. 1939) [CW 2:1:8]   84
    Roots of Aggression (1964) [CW 7:1:18]   92
11. The Development of the Capacity for Concern (1963) [CW 6:3:11]   100
12. The Absence of a Sense of Guilt (1966) [CW 7:3:32]   106
13. Some Psychological Aspects of Juvenile Delinquency (1946) [CW 3:1:7]   113
14. The Antisocial Tendency (1956) [CW 5:2:8]   120
15. The Psychology of Separation (1958) [CW 5:4:7]   132
16. Aggression, Guilt and Reparation (1960) [CW 6:1:10]   136
17. Struggling Through the Doldrums (1963) [CW 6:4:7]   145
18. Youth Will Not Sleep (1964) [CW 7:1:7]   156

Part III. The Social Provision

Editors' Introduction   161

19. Correspondence with a Magistrate (1944) ['Letter to Roger North' CW 2:6:1]   163
20. The Foundation of Mental Health (1951) [CW 3:6:4]   168
21. The Deprived Child and How He Can Be Compensated for Loss of Family Life (1950) [CW 3:5:10]   172
22. Group Influences and the Maladjusted Child: The School Aspect (1955) [CW 5:1:9]   189
23. The Persecution That Wasn't (1967) ['Review: *A Home from Home*' CW 8:1:10]   200
24. Comments on the *Report of the Committee on Punishment in Prisons and Borstals* (1961) [CW 6:2:22]   202
25. Do Progressive Schools Give Too Much Freedom to the Child? (1965)
    Contribution to Conference at Dartington Hall [CW 7:2:5]   209
    Notes Made in the Train [CW 7:2:6]   214
26. Residential Care as Therapy (1970) [CW 9:2:9]   220

Part IV. Individual Therapy

Editors' Introduction   231

27. Varieties of Psychotherapy (1961) [CW 6:2:5]   232
28. The Psychotherapy of Character Disorders (1963) [CW 6:4:9]   241

29. Dissociation Revealed in a Therapeutic Consultation
    (1965) [CW 7:2:21]   256
    Sources of the Papers in this Volume   283

Name Index   285
Subject Index   286

Holding and Interpretation: Fragment of an Analysis

First published London: Hogarth and the Institute of Psychoanalysis, 1986.

Reprinted with permission by Karnac, London, 1989.

Introduction by M. Masud R. Khan   1
Fragment of an Analysis [CW 4:4:1]   19
Appendix: Withdrawal and Regression [CW 4:3:29]   187
References [CW 12:1:4b]   193
Index   195

Home Is Where We Start From: Essays by a Psychoanalyst

EDITED BY CLARE WINNICOTT, RAY SHEPHERD AND MADELEINE DAVIS

First published in the United Kingdom by Pelican Books, 1986.

First published in the United States by W. W. Norton & Company, 1986.

Reprinted by Penguin, 1990.

Preface   9
Acknowledgements   10

Psychoanalysis and Science: Friends or Relations? [CW 6:2:9]   13

Part 1. Health and Illness

The Concept of a Healthy Individual [CW 8:1:4]   21
Living Creatively [CW 9:2:11]   39
Sum, I Am [CW 8:2:10]   55
The Concept of the False Self [CW 7:1:1]   65
The Value of Depression [CW 6:4:10]   71
Aggression, Guilt and Reparation [CW 6:1:10]   80
Delinquency as a Sign of Hope [CW 8:1:8]   90
Varieties of Psychotherapy [CW 6:2:5]   101
Cure [CW 9:2:8]   112

Part 2. The Family

The Mother's Contribution to Society [CW 5:3:30]   123
The Child in the Family Group [CW 7:3:17]   128
Children Learning [CW 8:2:16]   142
Adolescent Immaturity [CW 9:3:9]   150

Part 3. Reflections on Society

Thinking and the Unconscious [CW 2:7:4]   169
The Price of Disregarding Psychoanalytic Research [CW 7:2:4]   172
This Feminism [CW 7:1:14]   183
The Pill and the Moon [CW 9:1:23] & [CW 9:1:18]   195
Discussion of War Aims [CW 2:2:3]   210
Berlin Walls [CW 9:1:25]   221
Freedom [CW 9:1:16] & [CW 9:1:17]   228
Some Thoughts on the Meaning of the Word Democracy [CW 3:5:17]   239
The Place of the Monarchy [CW 9:2:6]   260

Index   269

Babies and Their Mothers

EDITED BY CLARE WINNICOTT, RAY SHEPHERD AND
MADELEINE DAVIS

First published by Addison-Wesley, 'A Merloyd Lawrence Book', 1987.

Published, with a Foreword by Sir Peter Tizard, by Free Association Books in 1988. Reprinted, with an Introduction by Benjamin Spock, M.D., as Part 1 of *Winnicott on the Child* by Perseus, 2002.

Editors' Preface   xiii

1. The Ordinary Devoted Mother [CW 7:3:3]   3
2. Knowing and Learning [CW 3:5:14]   15
3. Breast-feeding as Communication [CW 8:2:26]   23
4. The Newborn and His Mother [CW 7:1:4]   35
5. The Beginning of the Individual [CW 7:3:34]   51
6. Environmental Health in Infancy [CW 8:1:6]   59
7. The Contribution of Psychoanalysis to Midwifery [CW 5:3:15]   69
8. Dependence in Child Care [CW 9:2:15]   83
9. Communication Between Infant and Mother, and Mother and Infant, Compared and Contrasted [CW 8:2:2]   89

Original Source of Each Chapter   105
Bibliographical Note: The works of D. W. Winnicott   111
Index   113

The Spontaneous Gesture: Selected Letters

EDITED BY F. R. RODMAN

Cambridge, MA/London: Harvard University Press, 1987

Preface	ix
Acknowledgements	xi
Introduction	xiii
Letters 1-126	1
Winnicott's Correspondents	199
Index	205

Human Nature

EDITED BY CHRISTOPHER BOLLAS, MADELEINE DAVIS AND RAY SHEPHERD

London: Free Association Books, 1988

Appearing here as [CW 11:1]

Preface	ix
Editorial Note	xi
Acknowledgements	xiii
INTRODUCTION	1

Part I. The Human Child Examined: Soma, Psyche, Mind

INTRODUCTION	7
Chapter 1 THE PSYCHE-SOMA AND THE MIND	11
Somatic Health	11
Psyche Health	12
Intellect and Health	12
Chapter 2 ILL-HEALTH	15
Somatic Ill-health	15
Psyche Ill-health	16
Chapter 3 INTER-RELATIONSHIP OF BODY DISEASE AND PSYCHOLOGICAL DISORDER	19
The Effect of the Body and Its Health on the Psyche	19
Heredity	19
Congenital Disorder	20
Deficiencies of Intake	21
Elimination Defects	22

Accidents	22
A Category for the Not-Yet-Known	23
Allergy	23
The Effect of the Psyche on the Body and Its Functioning	24

Chapter 4 THE PSYCHO-SOMATIC FIELD — 26

Part II. The Emotional Development of the Human Being — 33

INTRODUCTION — 33

Chapter 1 INTERPERSONAL RELATIONSHIPS — 36

First Part of the Statement	36
The Family	39
Instinct	39
Love Relationships	48

Chapter 2 THE CONCEPT OF HEALTH USING INSTINCT THEORY — 51

Imaginative Elaboration of Function	51
The Psyche	52
The Soul	52
Excited and Quiet States	53
The Oedipus Complex	54
Restatement	56
Infantile Sexuality	58
Reality and Fantasy	58
The Unconscious	60
Summary	62
Chart Showing Psychology of Small Boy in Terms of Instinct Theory	63
Defences Against Anxiety – Castration Threat	63
Breakdown of Defences	64

Part III. Establishment of Unit Status — 65

INTRODUCTION: Emotional Development Characteristic of Infancy — 67

Chapter 1 THE DEPRESSIVE POSITION — 69

Concern, Guilt and Inner Personal Psychic Reality	69
The Depressive Position: Recapitulation	78
Repression Reconsidered	80
The Management of Bad Forces and Objects	81
Inner Richness and Complexity	82

Chapter 2 DEVELOPMENT OF THE THEME OF THE INNER WORLD — 84

Introduction	84
Paranoid Way of Life	84

Depression and the 'Depressive Position'	85
The Manic Defence	86
Chapter 3 VARIOUS TYPES OF PSYCHO-THERAPY MATERIAL	88
Chapter 4 HYPOCHONDRIACAL ANXIETY	94

Part IV From Instinct Theory to Ego Theory — 97

INTRODUCTION: Primitive Emotional Development	99
Chapter 1 ESTABLISHMENT OF RELATIONSHIP WITH EXTERNAL REALITY	100
Excited and Quiet Relationships	100
The Value of Illusion and Transitional States	106
Failure in Initial Contact	107
Primary Creativity	110
The Mother's Importance	112
The Baby at Birth	113
The Philosophy of 'Real'	114
Chapter 2 INTEGRATION	116
Chapter 3 DWELLING OF PSYCHE IN BODY	122
Body Experience	122
Paranoia and Naiveté	124
Chapter 4 THE EARLIEST STATES	126
Diagram of the Environment Individual Set-Up	126
Action of Gravity	130
Chapter 5 A PRIMARY STATE OF BEING: PRE-PRIMITIVE STAGES	131
Chapter 6 CHAOS	135
Chapter 7 THE INTELLECTUAL FUNCTION	139
Chapter 8 WITHDRAWAL AND REGRESSION	141
Chapter 9 THE BIRTH EXPERIENCE	143
Chapter 10 ENVIRONMENT	152
Chapter 11 PSYCHO-SOMATIC DISORDER RECONSIDERED	160
Asthma	160
Gastric Ulcer	162
APPENDIX	165
Synopsis I	165
Synopsis II	168
Bibliography	171
Index	173

Psycho-Analytic Explorations

EDITED BY CLARE WINNICOTT, RAY SHEPHERD
AND MADELEINE DAVIS

Cambridge, MA: Harvard University Press, 1989

Preface — xi
D. W. W.: A Reflection by Clare Winnicott — 1

Part 1: Psycho-Analysis: Theory and Practice

1. Early Disillusion *1939* [CW 2:1:5] — 21
2. Knowing and Not Knowing: A Clinical Example *Undated* [CW 9:4:4] — 24
3. A Point in Technique *Undated* [CW 9:4:5] — 26
4. Play in the Analytic Situation *1954* [CW 4:3:28] — 28
5. Fragments Concerning Varieties of Clinical Confusion *1956* [CW 5:2:4] — 30
6. Excitement in the Aetiology of Coronary Thrombosis *1957* [CW 5:3:29] — 34
7. Hallucination and Dehallucination *1957* [CW 5:3:23] — 39
8. Ideas and Definitions *1950s* [CW 9:4:1] — 43
9. Psychogenesis of a Beating Fantasy *1958* [CW 5:4:4] — 45
10. Nothing at the Centre *1959* [CW 5:5:10] — 49
11. The Fate of the Transitional Object *1959* [CW 5:5:22] — 53
11. Notes on Play *Undated* [CW 9:4:8] — 59
13. Psycho-Neurosis in Childhood *1961* [CW 6:2:17] — 64
14. Further Remarks on the Theory of the Parent-Infant Relationship *1961* [CW 6:3:14] — 73
15. A Note on a Case Involving Envy *1963* [CW 6:4:3] — 76
16. Perversions and Pregenital Fantasy *1963* [CW 6:4:18] — 79
17. Two Notes on the Use of Silence *1963* [CW 6:4:19] — 81
18. Fear of Breakdown *1963–64* [CW 6:4:21] — 87
19. The Importance of the Setting in Meeting Regression in Psycho-Analysis *1964* [CW 7:1:9] — 96
20. Psycho-Somatic Disorder — 103
    I. Psycho-Somatic Illness in Its Positive and Negative Aspects *1964* [CW 7:1:6] — 103
    II. Additional Note on Psycho-Somatic Disorder *1969* [CW 9:1:21] — 115
21. The Psychology of Madness: A Contribution from Psycho-Analysis *1965* [CW 7:2:18] — 119

22. The Concept of Trauma in Relation to the Development of the
    Individual Within the Family *1965* [CW 7:2:7] — 130
23. Notes on Withdrawal and Regression *1965* [CW 7:2:19] — 149
24. New Light on Children's Thinking *1965* [CW 7:2:1] — 152
25. Comment on Obsessional Neurosis and 'Frankie' *1965*
    [CW 7:2:10] — 158
26. A Note on the Mother-Foetus Relationship *1960s*
    [CW 9:4:11] — 161
27. Absence and Presence of a Sense of Guilt Illustrated in
    Two Patients *1966* [CW 7:3:32] — 163
28. On the Split-off Male and Female Elements — 168
    I.   The Split-off Male and Female Elements to Be
         Found in Men and Women *1966* [CW 7:3:2] — 169
    II. Clinical Material *1959–1963* [CW 5:5:26] & [CW 6:4:21] — 183
    III. Answer to Comments *1968–1969* [CW 9:1:30] — 189
29. The Concept of Clinical Regression Compared with
    that of Defence Organisation *1967* [CW 8:1:29] — 193
30. Addendum to 'The Location of Cultural Experience' *1967*
    [CW 8:1:37] — 200
31. Playing and Culture *1968* [CW 8:2:9] — 203
32. Interpretation in Psycho-Analysis *1968* [CW 8:2:6] — 207
33. Thinking and Symbol-Formation *1968* [CW 8:2:48] — 213
34. On 'The Use of an Object' — 217
    I.   The Use of an Object and Relating Through
         Identifications *1968* [CW 8:2:38] — 218
    II. D. W. W.'s Dream Related to Reviewing Jung *1963*
         [CW 6:4:15] — 228
    III. Notes Made on the Train *1965* [CW 7:2:6] — 231
    IV. The Use of the Word 'Use' *1968* [CW 8:2:5] — 233
    V.   Clinical Illustration of 'The Use of an Object' *1968*
         [CW 8:2:29] — 235
    VI. Comments on My Paper 'The Use of an Object' *1968*
         [CW 8:2:38] — 238
    VII. The Use of an Object in the Context of *Moses and
         Monotheism* *1969* [CW 9:1:4] — 240
35. Development of the Theme of the Mother's Unconscious as
    Discovered in Psycho-Analytic Practice *1969* [CW 9:1:15] — 247
36. The Mother-Infant Experience of Mutuality *1969* [CW 9:1:28] — 251
37. On the Basis for Self in Body — 261
    I.   Basis for Self in Body *1970* [CW 9:2:12] — 261
    II. Two Further Clinical Examples *1970* [CW 9:2:13] — 272
38. Individuation *1970* [CW 9:2:10] — 284

Part 2: Psycho-Analytic Psychotherapy with Children and Adolescents

39. Private Practice *1955* [CW 5:1:7]	291
40. The Squiggle Game *1964–68* [CW 8:2:47]	299
41. The Value of the Therapeutic Consultation *1965* [CW 7:2:22]	318
42. Deductions Drawn from a Psychotherapeutic Interview with an Adolescent *1964* [CW 7:1:5]	325
43. A Child Psychiatry Case Illustrating Delayed Reaction to Loss *1965* [CW 7:2:23]	341
44. Physical and Emotional Disturbances in an Adolescent Girl *1968* [CW 8:2:3]	369
45. Mother's Madness Appearing in the Clinical Material as an Ego-Alien Factor *1969* [CW 9:1:29]	375

Part 3: On the Work of Other Analysts

46. Susan Isaacs
 - I. Obituary *1948* [CW 3:3:11] — 385
 - II. Foreword to *Susan Isaacs*, by D. E. M. Gardner [CW 8:2:22] — 387
47. Marion Milner
 - Critical Notice of *On Not Being Able to Paint 1951* [CW 3:6:15] — 390
48. Ernest Jones
 - I. Obituary *1958* [CW 5:4:21] — 393
 - II. Funeral Address *1958* [CW 5:4:3] — 405
49. Dorothy Burlingham
 - Review of Twins: *A Study of Three Pairs of Identical Twins 1953* [CW 4:2:6] — 408
50. W. R. D. Fairbairn
 - Review of *Psycho-Analytic Studies of the Personality 1953* [CW 4:2:18] — 413
51. John Bowlby
 - I. Review of *Maternal Care and Mental Health 1953* [CW 4:2:10] — 423
 - II. Discussion of 'Grief and Mourning in Infancy' *1959* [CW 5:5:17] — 426
52. Michael Balint
 - I. Character Types: The Foolhardy and the Cautious *1954* [CW 4:3:26] — 433
 - II. Review of *The Doctor, His Patient and the Illness 1958* [CW 5:4:23] — 438
53. Melanie Klein: On Her Concept of Envy

I.	Review of *Envy and Gratitude* 1959 [CW 5:5:1]	443
II.	The Beginnings of a Formulation of an Appreciation and Criticism of Klein's Envy Statement 1962 [CW 6:3:7]	447
III.	Roots of Aggression 1968 [CW 8:2:21]	458
IV.	Contribution to a Symposium on Envy and Jealousy 1969 [CW 9:1:8]	462

54. Joseph Sandler
    Comments on 'On the Concept of the Superego' 1960
    [CW 6:1:19] 465
55. Sigmund Freud
    Review of *Letters of Sigmund Freud, 1873–1939* 1962
    [CW 6:3:15] 474
56. Harold F. Searles
    Review of *The Non-Human Environmental in Normal Development and in Schizophrenia* 1963 [CW 6:4:16] ... 478
57. C. J. Jung
    Review of *Memories, Dreams, Reflections* 1964 [CW 7:1:16] ... 482
58. Erik H. Erikson
    Review of *Childhood and Society* 1965 [CW 4:2:16] 493
59. Virginia Axline
    A Commentary on *Play Therapy* 1960s [CW 9:1:32] 495
60. Willi Hoffer
    A Tribute on the Occasion of Hoffer's Seventieth Birthday 1967 [CW 8:1:11] 499
61. James Strachey
    Obituary 1969 [CW 8:1:14] 506
62. Anna Freud
    Review of *Indications for Child Analysis and Other Papers* 1969 [CW 9:1:20] 511

Part 4: On Other Forms of Treatment

63. Physical Therapy of Mental Disorder: Convulsion Therapy ... 515

I.	Treatment of Mental Disease by Induction of Fits 1943 [CW 2:5:6]	516
II.	Shock Treatment of Mental Disorder 1943 [CW 2:5:20]	522
III.	Shock Therapy 1944 [CW 2:6:4]	523
IV.	Introduction to a Symposium on the Psycho-Analytic Contribution to the Theory of Shock Therapy 1944 [CW 2:6:6]	525
V.	Kinds of Psychological Effect of Shock Therapy 1944 [CW 2:6:7]	529
VI.	Physical Therapy of Mental Disorder 1947 [CW 3:2:2]	534

Back Catalogue of Winnicott's Published Books   145

    64. Physical Therapy of Mental Disorder: Leucotomy   542
        I.   Prefrontal Leucotomy *1943* [CW 2:5:4]   542
        II. Leucotomy *1949* [CW 3:4:21]   543
        III. Notes on the General Implications of Leucotomy *1951*
             [CW 3:6:14]   548
        IV. Prefrontal Leucotomy *1956* [CW 5:2:2]   553
    65. Occupational Therapy
        Review of Adrian Hill's Book *Art Versus Illness 1949*
        [CW 3:4:22]   555
    66. Behaviour Therapy *1969* [CW 9:1:13]   558
    67. Physiotherapy and Human Relations *1969* [CW 9:1:14]   561

Postscript: D. W. W. on D. W. W. [CW 8:1:2]   569
Acknowledgements   585
Index   586

Talking to Parents

EDITED BY CLARE WINNICOTT, CHRISTOPHER BOLLAS,
MADELEINE DAVIS AND RAY SHEPHERD

Reading, MA: Addison-Wesley, 1993. With an introduction by T. Berry Brazelton M.D.

Reprinted as Part 2 of *Winnicott on the Child*, Perseus, 2002.

Acknowledgement   v
On Reading Winnicott by T. Berry Brazelton, M.D.   ix
Editors' Preface   xiii

    1. Health Education Through Broadcasting [CW 5:3:31]   1
    2. For Stepparents [CW 5:1:10]   7
    3. What Do We Know About Babies as Cloth Suckers? [CW 5:2:1]   15
    4. Saying 'No' [CW 6:1:1]   21
    5. Jealousy [CW 6:1:4]   41
    6. What Irks? [CW 6:1:7]   65
    7. Security [CW 6:1:9]   87
    8. Feeling Guilty [CW 6:2:6]   95
    9. The Development of a Child's Sense of Right and
       Wrong [CW 6:3:4]   105
  10. Now They Are Five [CW 6:3:6]   111
  11. The Building Up of Trust [CW 9:1:26]   121

Original Source of Each Chapter   135
Bibliographical Note: The Works of D. W. Winnicott   137
Index   139
About the Author   143

Thinking About Children

EDITED BY RAY SHEPHERD, JENNIFER JOHNS AND
HELEN TAYLOR ROBINSON

London: Karnac, 1996

Acknowledgements	xiii
Preface	xv
Introduction	xix

Part 1: Observation, Intuition and Empathy

1. Towards an Objective Study of Human Nature [CW 2:7:11]   3
2. 'Yes, But How Do We Know It's True?' [CW 3:5:18]   13

Part 2: Early Infant Development

3. Primary Introduction to External Reality: The Early Stages [CW 3:3:12]   21
4. Environmental Needs; the Early Stages; Dependence and Essential Independence [CW 3:3:13]   29

Part 3: The Family

5. The Bearing of Emotional Development on Feeding Problems [Part of CW 8:1:6]   39
6. Sleep Refusal in Children [CW 8:2:19]   42
7. The Effect of Loss on the Young [CW 8:2:12]   46
8. Out of the Mouths of Adolescents ['Review: *Adolescents and Morality*' CW 7:3:20]   48
9. The Delinquent and Habitual Offender [CW 2:1:3]   51
10. A Clinical Approach to Family Problems: The Family [CW 5:5:27]   54

Part 4: Starting School

11. Mental Hygiene of the Pre-school Child [CW 1:4:9]   59
12. The Teacher, the Parent and the Doctor [CW 1:4:10]   77

Part 5: Case Studies and Observations

Back Catalogue of Winnicott's Published Books

13. A Clinical Example of Symptomatology Following the Birth of a Sibling [CW 1:2:22]	97
14. Notes on a Little Boy [CW 1:4:16]	102
15. The Niffle [CW 9:4:10]	104

Part 6: Adoption

16. Two Adopted Children [CW 4:2:19]	113
17. Pitfalls in Adoption [CW 4:3:30]	128
18. Adopted Children in Adolescence [CW 5:1:12]	136

Part 7: Psychosomatic Problems

19. Contribution to a Discussion on Enuresis [CW 1:4:9]	151
20. Papular Urticaria and the Dynamics of Skin Sensation [CW 1:4:3]	157
21. Short Communication on Enuresis [CW 1:2:18]	170
22. Child Psychiatry: The Body as Affected by Psychological Factors [CW 1:2:23]	176
23. On Cardiac Neurosis in Children [CW 7:3:16]	179

Part 8: Autism and Schizophrenia

24. Three Reviews of Books on Autism [CW 1:4:15] [CW 7:3:18] & [CW 6:4:16]	191
25. Autism [CW 7:3:8]	197
26. The Aetiology of Infantile Schizophrenia in Terms of Adaptive Failure [CW 8:1:25]	218

Part 9: Professional Care of the Growing Child

27. Training for Child Psychiatry: The Paediatric Department of Psychology [CW 6:2:19]	227
28. Notes on the Time Factor in Treatment [CW 6:2:11]	231
29. The Association for Child Psychology and Psychiatry Observed as a Group Phenomenon [CW 8:1:3]	235
30. A Link Between Paediatrics and Child Psychology: Clinical Observations [CW 8:2:14]	255
31. Child Psychiatry, Social Work and Alternative Care [CW 9:2:3]	277

Glossary of Medical Terms	283
Original Source of Each Chapter	287
Bibliography of Winnicott's Works Compiled by Harry Karnac	291
List of Volumes	291
Alphabetical List	293
Chronological List	311

Winnicott on the Child

Cambridge, MA: Perseus, 2002

With introductions to his works by T. Berry Brazelton, Stanley I. Greenspan and Benjamin Spock. Part 1 previously published as *Babies and Their Mothers* (C. Winnicott, R. Shepherd, & M. Davis, Eds.), Reading, MA: Addison-Wesley, 1987; Part 2 previously published as *Talking to Parents* (C. Winnicott, C. Bollas, M. Davis & R. Shepherd, Eds.), Reading, MA: Addison-Wesley, 1993.

Part 1: Babies and Their Mothers

Introduction by Benjamin Spock, M.D.	3
Editors' Preface	9
1. The Ordinary Devoted Mother [CW 7:3:3]	11
2. Knowing and Learning [CW 3:5:14]	19
3. Breast-feeding as Communication [CW 8:2:26]	24
4. The Newborn and His Mother [CW 7:1:4]	32
5. The Beginning of the Individual [CW 7:3:34]	43
6. Environmental Health in Infancy [CW 8:1:6]	49
7. The Contribution of Psycho-analysis to Midwifery [CW 5:3:15]	56
8. Dependence in Child Care [CW 9:2:15]	65
9. Communication Between Infant and Mother, and Mother and Infant, Compared and Contrasted [CW 8:2:2]	70

Part 2: Talking to Parents

On Reading Winnicott by T. Berry Brazelton, M.D.	85
Editors' Preface	89
10. Health Education Through Broadcasting [CW 5:3:31]	95
11. For Stepparents [CW 5:1:10]	99
12. What Do We Know About Babies as Cloth Suckers? [CW 5:2:1]	104
13. Saying 'No' [CW 6:1:1]	108
14. Jealousy [CW 6:1:4]	122
15. What Irks? [CW 6:1:7]	139
16. Security [CW 6:1:9]	155
17. Feeling Guilty [CW 6:2:6]	160
18. The Development of a Child's Sense of Right and Wrong [CW 6:3:4]	167
19. Now They Are Five [CW 6:3:6]	171

20. The Building Up of Trust [CW 9:1:26]   178

Part 3: The Child in the Family

Introduction by Stanley I. Greenspan, M.D.   191

21. Advising Parents [CW 5:3:27]   193
22. The Mother's Contribution to Society [CW 5:3:30]   202
23. The Family and Emotional Maturity [CW 6:1:17]   207
24. The Development of the Capacity for Concern [CW 6:3:11]   215
25. The Child in the Family Group [CW 7:3:17]   221
26. Children Learning [CW 8:2:16]   232

Original Source of Each Chapter   239
The Works of D. W. Winnicott   245
Index   247
Biographical Note   265

Winnicott's Plans for Books

Contents

1. Plan for Two Books: Tavistock A, Tavistock B
2. Plan for Two Books (ca. 1968)
3. Plan for a Book (1968 or early 1969)
4. Suggestions for the Proposed Transitional Book

1. Plan for Two Books: Tavistock A, Tavistock B

BOOK A

Mother-Infant Experience of Mutuality [CW 9:1:28]
Gerber [Environmental Health in Infancy; CW 8:1:6]
Breast-Feeding as Communication [CW 8:2:26]
Winter Lecture 1968 [Communication between infant and mother, and mother and infant, compared and contrasted; CW 8:2:2]
Sleep Refusal [CW 8:2:19]
Mirror Role of Mum [CW 8:1:38]
Social Aspects of Autism [CW 7:3:7]
Autism (Recherches) 1967 [The aetiology of infantile schizophrenia in terms of adaptive failure; CW 8:1:25]
Physio-therapy [CW 9:1:14]
Children Learning + Thinking [CW 8:2:16] and [CW 7:2:1]
Progressive Schools [CW 7:2:5]

Place Where We Live [CW 8:2:1]
Sum, I Am [CW 8:2:10]
Absence of Guilt [CW 7:3:32]
Psychoneurosis, Helsinki 1961 [CW 6:2:17]
Ast.
   Borstal
Trauma Concept [CW 7:2:7]

Youth Won't Sleep [CW 7:1:7]
Newcastle Symposium [Adolescent process and the need for personal confrontation; CW 9:3:9]

Adop. Adolesc [CW 5:1:12]
Adolesc. and Menopause [see CW 8:2:3]
Price of (1965) [The price of disregarding psychoanalytic research; CW 7:2:4]
War Aims Discussion [CW 2:2:3]

BOOK B

Beginning of Individual [CW 7:3:34]
Neonate and Mum [CW 7:1:4]
Link = Chisholm [A link between paediatrics and child psychology; CW 8:2:14]
Ped. Dept of Psych. [CW 6:2:19]
Split-off Male and Female Elements [CW 7:3:2]
Regr. as a Defense [CW 8:1:29]
Concept of Healthy [CW 8:1:4]
Madness [CW 7:2:18]
Psycho-somatics 1964 [CW 7:1:6]
Cross Identifications [CW 9:3:8]
ACPP as Group [CW 8:1:3]
Creative Activity – Search for Self [CW 8:1:27]
False Self Concept [CW 7:1:1]
Play
Location of [CW 7:3:31]
Use of Word Use [CW 8:2:5]
Use of Object [CW 8:2:28]

2. Plan for Two Books (ca. 1968)

BOOK I

1964	The Neonate & His Mother [CW 7:1:4]	Lecture, Rome, 1.4.64. *Acta Paediatrica Latina*, Vol. XVII
1964	Psycho-Somatic Illness in Its Positive and Negative Aspects [CW 7:1:6]	Lecture, Society for Psycho-somatic Research, 21.5.64. *Int. J. Psycho-Anal.* (1966) 47, 510
1965	The Psychology of Madness [CW 7:2:18]	Written only
1966	The Split-off Male and Female Elements to Be Found Clinically in Men and Women: Theoretical Inferences [CW 7:3:2 and CW 9:1:30]	Lecture, BPAS, 2.2.66. Revised 11.6.68 for publication in *FORUM*

1966	Lessons Learned in a London County Council Rheumatism Supervisory Clinic. Symposium on Cardiac Neurosis in Children	Lecture, The Association of European Paediatric Cardiologists, Helsinki, 30.6.66
1966	The Location of Cultural Experience [CW 7:3:31]	Lecture, BPAS, 7.12.66 *Int. J. Psycho-Anal.* (1966) 48, 368
1967	The Concept of a Healthy Individual [CW 8:1:4]	Lecture, RMPA, 8.3.67
1967	The Concept of Clinical Regression Compared with that of Defence Organization [CW 8:1:29]	Lecture, McLean Hospital, Boston. Symposium on the nature of psychotherapy with schizophrenic patients, 27.10.67
1967	Creative Activity & the Search for the Self: Added Observation on Psychotherapy in this Area [CW 8:1:27]	Lecture, BPS, 25.10.67
1967	Playing Between Patient & Therapist: The Clinical Aspects of Transitional Objects & Phenomena [CW 8:2:15]	Lecture, BPAS, 18.10.67, under the title 'Towards a Theory of Psychotherapy: The Link with Playing'. *Int. J. Psycho-Anal.* Also given in Rome, 1968
1967	The A.C.P.P. Observed as Group Phenomenon [CW 8:1:3]	Lecture, 17.2.67
1967	The Etiology of Infantile Schizophrenia in Terms of Adaptive Failure [CW 8:1:25]	Lecture given in Dr. W's absence, at Journées d'études sur les psychoses chez l'enfant. 21.10.67, Paris. Published in *Recherches* in French
1968	Inter-Relating in Terms of Cross Identifications [CW 9:3:8]	Written for 25th anniversary of *Revista de Psicoanalisis*
1968	The Mother-Infant Experience of Mutuality [CW 9:1:28]	Written for *Parenthood: Its Psychology & Psychopathology*. Not yet published
1968	The Location of Cultural Exp. [Playing and Culture; CW 8:2:9]	Rewritten as a lecture for the Imago Group, 12.3.68
1968	The Use of the Word Use [CW 8:2:5]	Written

1968	Clinical Regression Compared with Defense Organization [CW 8:1:29]	Written for *Psychotherapy in the Designed Therapeutic Milieu*. Little, Brown & Co. I.P.C. 5, No. 1, 1968
1968	A Link Between Paediatrics & Child Psychology – Clinical Observations [CW 8:2:14]	Lecture, Catherine Chisholm Memorial, Manchester, 24.5.68 To be published in *Dynamische Psychiatrie*
1968	The Use of an Object [CW 8:2:28]	Lecture, NY Psycho-Anal. Soc., 12.11.68

BOOK II

1955	Adopted Children in Adolescence [CW 5:1:12]	Standing Conference of Societies Registered for Adoption, Roehampton, 13.7.55. Published 1966
1961	Psycho-neurosis in Childhood [CW 6:2:17]	Scandinavian orthopsychiatric congress, 8.9.61
1961	Paediatric Dept. of Psychology [CW 6:2:19]	*St Mary's Hospital Gazette*, Vol. LXVII. No. 6, Sept. 1961
1963	The Value of Depression [CW 6:4:10]	A.P.S.W. Sept. 1963 and pub. *Brit. J. Psychiatric Social Work*, Vol. VII, 1964, No. 3
1964	The Concept of the False Self [CW 7:1:1]	Crime – A Challenge, All Souls College, Oxford, 29.1.64
1964	Background to War Aims Discussion [see CW 2:2:3]	Revised January 1964
1964	Youth Will Not Sleep [CW 7:1:7]	*New Society*, May 1964 *Atlas*, Sept. 1964
1964	The Positive Aspect of Antisocial Behaviour with Illustrative Case	Summer school of the Davidson Clinic, 30.7.64
1965	Do Progressive Schools Give Too Much Freedom to the Child? [CW 7:2:5] Routledge Kegan Paul 1969, *Who Are the Progressives Now?*	Conf. on the Future for Progressive Educations, Dartington Hall, 12.4.65 In a book by Maurice Ash
1965	Introductory Lecture to New Light on Children's Thinking [CW 7:2:1]	Devon Centre for Further Education, 3.1.65

1965	The Price of Disregarding Psycho-analytical Research Findings [CW 7:2:4]	NAMH Annual Conf. at Church House, Westminster, on The Price of Mental Health. Public report of the conf. 1965
1965	The Concept of Trauma [CW 7:2:7]	May 1965
1966	A Psychoanalytic View of the Anti-social Tendency [CW 7:2:21]	In: *Crime, Law, & Corrections*, Slovenko. Charles Thomas, U.S.A., 1966
1966	The Beginning of the Individual [CW 7:3:34]	1966
1966	Social Aspects of Autism [CW 7:3:7]	Soc. for Autistic Children. Conf. Leicester, 26.3.66
1966	The Absence of a Sense of Guilt [CW 7:3:32]	Devon & Exeter Assoc. for Mental Health, 10.12.66
1967	The Bearing of Emotional Development on Feeding Problems [CW 8:1:6]	Symposium: Environmental Health in Infancy. Gerber Baby Council, 17.3.67. Pub. in *Maternal & Child Care*, Jan. 1968, Vol. IV, No. 33, under title: Infant Feeding & Emotional Development
1967	Mirror-role of Mother and Family in Child Development [CW 8:1:38]	Chapter in I.P.A. family book, *The Family Predicament*. 1967
1967	Delinquency as a Sign of Hope [CW 8:1:8]	Borstal assistant governors' Conf. Winchester, 18.4.67. Pub. in *Prison Service J*. April 1968, Vol. VII, No. 27
1968	Communication Between Infant & Mother, & Mother and Infant: Compared and Contrasted [CW 8:2:2]	The Winter Lectures, 1968. Pub. in special booklet, 1969
1968	Breast-feeding as a Communication [CW 8:2:26]	Conf. National Childbirth Trust. Westminster, 28.11.68
1968	The Place Where We Live [CW 8:2:1]	The Geigy Bequest Lecture, (Sussex Postgraduate Federation). Brighton, 19.1.68
1968	Symposium on Contemporary Concepts in Adolescent Development and Their Implications in Higher Education [CW 9:3:9]	Brit. Student Health Associ. 21st Annual meeting, Newcastle, 18.7.68. Rewritten as Death & Murder in the Adolescent Process

1968	Sum, I Am [CW 8:2:10]	Conf. of Association of Teachers of Mathematics, 17.4.68
1968	Children Learning [CW 8:2:16]	Conf. on Family Evangelism Christian Teamwork Int. of Education, 5.6.68 Pub. in *The Human Family and God*, a report
1968	Sleep Refusal in Children [CW 8:2:19]	*Medical News Magazine*, July 1968
	A chapter for: *Physiotherapy* [CW 9:1:14]	
	The Psychology of the Adolescent and the Menopausal Woman [see CW 8:2:3]	A chapter in *Scientific Foundations of Obstetrics and Gynaecology*

3. Plan for a Book (undated, 1968 or early 1969)

AS ONE BOOK

A.C.P.P. as group [CW 8:1:3] (add chapter on Psychology) [CW 9:1:31]
Concept of Healthy [CW 8:1:4]   Psychoneurosis – Helsinki [CW 6:2:17]
Cross Identifications [CW 9:3:8]
Split-off Male Female Elements [CW 7:3:2]
Regression of Defence [CW 8:1:29]   Absence of Guilt [CW 7:3:32]
False Self Concept [CW 7:1:1]
Madness [CW 7:2:18]   Ast and Borstal
Psychosomatics of 1964 [CW 7:1:6]
Trauma concept [CW 7:2:7]
Creative activity – search for self [CW 8:1:27]
   Play
   Location, etc. – Use of Word Use [CW 8:2:5]
   Place Where We Live [CW 8:2:1]
   Use of Object [CW 8:2:28]

Sum, I Am [CW 8:2:10]
Youth Won't Sleep [CW 7:1:7]
Newcastle Symp. [CW 9:3:9]
Adopt Adolesc [CW 5:1:12]
Adolesc. Menopause [see CW 8:2:3]
War Aims Discussion [CW 2:2:3]

Price of (1965) [The price of disregarding psychoanalytic research; CW 7:2:4]
Mother Infant Experience of Mutuality [CW 9:1:28]
Gerber Lecture: Emotional Development and Feeding Problems [CW 8:1:6]
Breast Feeding as Communication Nat. Childbirth Trust [CW 8:2:26]
The Beginning of the Individual [CW 7:3:34]
Neonate and Mother [CW 7:1:4]
Winter Lecture 1968 [Communication between infant and mother, and mother and infant, compared and contrasted; CW 8:2:2]
Sleep Refusal [CW 8:2:19]
Mirror Role of Mother (Lomas) [CW 8:1:38]
Physiology
Autism (Recherches) [CW 8:1:25]
Social Aspects of Autism [CW 7:3:7]
Link Psychiatry and Pediatrics (Chisholm) [CW 8:2:14]
Paed. Dept. of Psychiatry – Psychology [CW 6:2:19]
Children Learning [CW 8:2:16]
      Thinking [CW 7:2:1]
Progressive Schools [CW 7:2:5]

4. Suggestions for the Proposed Transitional Book

TO MR MASUD KHAN   FROM DR D. W. WINNICOTT

7th May 1968

Suggestions relative to the proposed transitional book. Winnicott, D. W.

(1) Original paper modified [CW 9:3:5]

(2) Chapter 25 of the Pelican [First Experiments in Independence; CW 5:1:20]

(3) String [CW 6:1:20]

(4) Location of Cultural Experience [CW 7:3:31]

(5) Play 1

(6) Play 2

(7) Squiggles as an example of the use of the concept

(8) The transitional object relative to dolls

(9) Transitional phenomena relative to hallucinating

(10) Dream, fantasy, and fantasying compared and contrasted

Hoffer. 1949.	Mouth, hand, ego, etc.
Greenacre.	An invited critical survey of the concept relative to fetishism
? Wulff.	On fetishism
? James, Martin. 1960.	
Fraser, A.W. 1963.	A relation between transitional objects and preconscious mental processes
Fintzy, Robert T.	q.v.
Gaddini, Professor Renata.	Original researches now in progress
Moore, Terence. Institute of Education.	Invited critical statement. (His team has watched these phenomena over a period of ten years and I believe is critical of the concept.)
Segal, Hanna.	An invited critical comment
Modell. 1961.	See Fintzy page 3.
Bastiaans.	(Who uses the concept in teaching medical students, encouraging observation thereby.)
? Spock.	
? Spitz.	
Hacker, of Los Angeles.	(Who I believe sponsored an investigation into transitional phenomena.)
? Bradley.	On the doll (I.J.P.A. 1961.)
? Freud, Anna.	On lack of phase dominance in borderline cases. See Fintzy page 10, bottom.

What about a reference to Karen Stephen who referred to an intermediate area of experience in her book?

I am rather hoping that you will find this group of ideas the sort of stimulus that you want when you are thinking out the possibilities.

Reference Lists from Books in Winnicott's Back Catalogue

Collected Papers: Through Paediatrics to Psychoanalysis (1958)

Abraham, K. (1916). The first pregenital stage of the libido. In *Selected papers on psycho-analysis*. London: Hogarth.
Abraham, K. (1927). *Selected papers on psycho-analysis*. London: Hogarth.
Abraham, K. (1955). *Clinical papers and essays on psycho-analysis*. London: Hogarth.
Aichhorn, A. (1925). *Wayward youth*. London: Imago.
Balint, M. (1955). Friendly expanses—Horrid empty spaces. *International Journal of Psycho-Analysis*, 36(4–5), 225–241.
Bender, L. (1947). Childhood schizophrenia. *American Journal of Orthopsychiatry*, 17(1), 40–56.
Bowlby, J. (1951). *Maternal care and mental health*. Geneva: World Health Organization.
Bowlby, J., Robertson, J., & Rosenbluth, D. (1952). A two-year-old goes to hospital. In R. S. Eisler, A. Freud, H. Hartmann, & E. Kris (Eds.), *The psychoanalytic study of the child*, 7 (pp. 82–94). London: Imago.
Brierley, M. (1951). *Trends in psycho-analysis*. London: Hogarth.
Britton, C. (1955). Casework techniques in the child care services. *Case Conference*, 1(9), 3–15.
Burlingham, D., & Freud, Anna. (1942). *Young children in wartime: A years work in a residential war nursery*. London: Allen & Unwin.
Casteret, N. (1947). *My caves*. London: Dent.
Creak, M. (1951). Psychoses in childhood. *Journal of Mental Science*, 97(408), 545–554.
Creak, M. (1952). Discussion: Psychoses in childhood. *Proceedings of the Royal Society of Medicine*, 45(11), 797–800.
Fairbairn, W. R. D. (1952). *Psychoanalytic studies of the personality*. London: Tavistock.
Freud, A. (1937). *The ego and the mechanisms of defence*. London: Hogarth.
Freud, A. (1947). Aggression in relation to emotional development; normal and pathological. In A. Freud, H. Hartmann, & E. Kris (Eds.), *The psychoanalytic study of the child*, 3/4 (pp. 37–42). London: Imago.
Freud, A. (1947). Emotional and instinctive development. In R. W. B. Ellis (Ed.), *Child health and development*. London: John Churchill.
Freud, A. (1952). A connection between the states of negativism and of emotional surrender (Hörigkeit) (Author's abstract). *International Journal of Psycho-Analysis*, 33, 265.

Freud, A. (1952). The role of bodily illness in the mental life of children. In R. S. Eisler, A. Freud, H. Hartmann, & E. Kris (Eds.), *The psychoanalytic study of the child*, 7 (pp. 69–81). London: Imago.

Freud, A. (1953). Some remarks on infant observation. In R. S. Eisler, A. Freud, H. Hartmann, E. Kris (Eds.), *The psychoanalytic study of the child*, 8 (pp. 9–19). London: Imago.

Freud, A., Greenacre, P., Kris, E., Hartmann, H., Lewin, B.D., Spitz, R., Loewenstein, R. et al. (1954). Problems of infantile neurosis: A discussion. In R. S. Eisler, A. Freud, H. Hartmann, E. Kris (Eds.), *The psychoanalytic study of the child*, 9 (pp. 16–75). London: Imago.

Freud, A. (1954). The widening scope of indications for psycho-analysis. *Journal of the American Psychoanalytic Association*, 2(4), 607–620.

Freud, A., & Burlingham, D. (1942). *Young children in wartime: A years work in a residential war nursery*. London: Allen & Unwin.

Freud, S. (1905). Fragment of an analysis of a case of hysteria. In J. Strachey (Ed.), *Standard edition of the complete psychological works of Sigmund Freud* (vol. 7). London: Hogarth.

Freud, S. (1905). Three essays on the theory of sexuality. In J. Strachey (Ed.), *Standard edition of the complete psychological works of Sigmund Freud* (vol. 7). London: Hogarth.

Freud, S. (1909). Notes upon a case of obsessional neurosis. In J. Strachey (Ed.), *Standard edition of the complete psychological works of Sigmund Freud* (vol. 10). London: Hogarth.

Freud, S. (1914). On narcissism: An introduction. In J. Strachey (Ed.), *Standard edition of the complete psychological works of Sigmund Freud* (vol. 14). London: Hogarth.

Freud, S. (1915). Instincts and their vicissitudes. In J. Strachey (Ed.), *Standard edition of the complete psychological works of Sigmund Freud* (vol. 14). London: Hogarth.

Freud, S. (1917). Mourning and melancholia. *Collected papers*, 4. London: Hogarth.

Freud, S. (1920). Beyond the pleasure principle. In J. Strachey (Ed.), *Standard edition of the complete psychological works of Sigmund Freud* (vol. 18). London: Hogarth.

Freud, S. (1921). Group psychology and the analysis of the ego. In J. Strachey (Ed.), *Standard edition of the complete psychological works of Sigmund Freud* (vol. 18). London: Hogarth.

Freud, S. (1923). *The ego and the id*. London: Hogarth.

Freud, S. (1926). *Inhibitions, symptoms and anxiety*. London: Hogarth.

Freud, S. (1950/1954). *The origins of psycho-analysis*. London: Imago.

Friedlander, K. (1947). *The psychoanalytical approach to juvenile delinquency*. London: Kegan Paul, Trench, Trubner.

Glover, E. (1932). A psychoanalytic approach to the classification of mental disorders. In *On the early development of mind* (pp. 161–186). London: Imago.

Glover, E. (1945). An examination of the Klein system of child psychology. In *The psychoanalytic study of the child*, 1 (pp. 75–118). London: Imago.

Glover, E. (1949). The position of psycho-analysis in Great Britain. In *On the early development of mind* (pp. 352–363). London: Imago.

Greenacre, P. (1941). The predisposition to anxiety. In *Trauma, growth and personality* (pp. 27–82). London: Hogarth.

Greenacre, P. (1945). The biological economy of birth. In *Trauma, growth and personality* (pp. 3–26). London: Hogarth.

Greenacre, P. (1954). Problems of infantile neurosis: A discussion. In R. S. Eisler, A. Freud, H. Hartmann, & E. Kris (Eds.), *The psychoanalytic study of the child*, 9 (pp. 16–71). London: Imago.

Hartmann, H. (1952). Mutual influences in the development of ego and id. In R. S. Eisler, A. Freud, H. Hartmann, & E. Kris (Eds.), *The psychoanalytic study of the child, 7* (pp. 9–30). London: Imago.

Henoch, E. (1889). *Lectures on childrens diseases*. (J. Thomson, Trans.). London: The New Sydenham Society.

Hoffer, W. (1949). Mouth, hand, and ego-integration. In A. Freud, H. Hartmann, & E. Kris (Eds.), *The psychoanalytic study of the child, 3/4* (pp. 49–56). London: Imago.

Illingworth, R. S. (1951). Sleep problems in the first three years. *British Medical Journal, 1*(4709), 722–728.

Jones, E. (1946). A valedictory address. *International Journal of Psycho-Analysis, 27*, 7–12.

Jung, C. G. *The collected works of C. G. Jung*. Herbert Read, Michael Fordham, Gerhard Adler, (Eds.) London: Routledge & Kegan Paul.

Kanner, L. (1943). Autistic disturbances of affective contact. *The Nervous Child, 2*, 217–250.

Klein, M., & Riviere, J. (1936/1937). Love, hate and reparation. In J. Rickman (Ed.), *Psychoanalytical epitomes*, No. 2, pp. 57–119. London: Hogarth.

Klein, M. (1932). *Psycho-analysis of children*. London: Hogarth.

Klein, M. (1948). *Contributions to psycho-analysis, 1921–45*. London: Hogarth.

Klein, M., Heimann, P., & Money-Kyrle, R. (1952). *Developments in psycho-analysis*. London: Hogarth.

Klein, M., Heimann, P., Isaacs, S., & Riviere, J. (1955). *New directions in psycho-analysis*. London/New York: Tavistock/Basic Books.

Lindner, S. (1879). Das saugen an den fingern, lippen, bei den kindern (Ludeln). *Jahrbuch für Kinderheilk, 14*, 68.

MacAlpine, I. (1952, February 9). Psychosomatic symptom formation. *Lancet, 259*(6702), 278–282.

Mahler, M. S. (1952). On child psychosis and schizophrenia. In R. S. Eisler, A. Freud, H. Hartmann, & E. Kris (Eds.), *The psychoanalytic study of the child, 7* (pp. 286–305). London: Imago.

Mahler, M. S. (1954). Problems of infantile neurosis: A discussion. In R. S. Eisler, A. Freud, H. Hartmann, & E. Kris (Eds.), *The psychoanalytic study of the child, 9* (pp. 16–74). London: Imago.

Marty, P. et Fain, M. (1955). La motricité dans la relation d'objet. In *Revue française de psychanalyse*. Vol 19, Nos. 1–2. Paris: Presses Universitaires de France.

Middlemore, M. P. (1941). *The nursing couple*. London: Hamish Hamilton.

Milner, M. (1952). Aspects of symbolism in comprehension of the not-self. *International Journal of Psycho-Analysis, 33*, 181–194.

Rank, O. (1924). *The trauma of birth*. London: Kegan Paul.

Read, G. D. (1942). *Revelation of childbirth*. London: Heinemann.

Read, G. D. (1950). *Introduction to motherhood*. London: Whitefriars.

Rickman, J. (1928). The development of the psycho-analytical theory of the psychoses. *Supplement No. 2 to the International Journal of Psycho-Analysis*. London: Ballière, Tindall and Cox.

Rickman, J. (1951). Methodology and research in psychopathology. *British Journal of Medical Psychology, 24*, 1–7.

Riviere, J. (1936). On the genesis of psychical conflict in earliest infancy. *International Journal of Psycho-Analysis, 17*, 395–422.

Riviere, J., & Klein, M. (1936/1937). Love, hate and reparation. In J. Rickman (Ed.), *Psycho-Analytical Epitomes*, No. 2, pp. 57–119. London: Hogarth.

Robertson, J., Bowlby, J., & Rosenbluth, D. (1952). A two-year-old goes to hospital. In R. S. Eisler, A. Freud, H. Hartmann, & E. Kris (Eds.), *The psychoanalytic study of the child*, 7 (pp. 82–94). London: Imago.

Rycroft, C. F. (1953). Some observations on a case of vertigo. *International Journal of Psycho-Analysis*, 34, 241–247.

Scott, W. C. M. (1949). The body scheme in psychotherapy. *British Journal of Medical Psychology*, 22(3–4), 139–150.

Scott, W. C. M. (1955). A note on blathering. *International Journal of Psycho-Analysis*, 36, 348–349.

Searl, N. (1929). The flight to reality. *International Journal of Psycho-Analysis*, 10, 280–291.

Sechehaye, M. A. (1951). *Symbolic realization*. New York: International Universities Press.

Spitz, R. A. (1945). Hospitalism. An inquiry into the genesis of psychiatric conditions in early childhood. In *The psychoanalytic study of the child*, 1 (pp. 53–74). London: Imago.

Spitz, R. A., & Wolf, K. M. (1946). Anaclitic depression: An inquiry into the genesis of psychiatric conditions in early childhood. In Freud, A., Hoffer W., Glover, E., et al. (Eds.), *The psychoanalytic study of the child*, 2 (pp. 313–342). London: Imago.

Spitz, R. A. (1950). Relevancy of direct infant observation. In Freud, A., Hoffer, W., Glover, E. (Eds.), *The psychoanalytic study of the child*, 5 (pp. 66–73). London: Imago.

Stevenson, O. (1954). The first treasured possession. In R. S. Eisler, A. Freud, H. Hartmann, E. Kris (Eds.), *The psychoanalytic study of the child*, 9 (pp. 199–217). London: Imago.

Whitehead, A. N. (1933). *Adventures of ideas*. Harmondsworth: Pelican.

Winnicott, D. W. (1931). *Clinical notes on disorders of childhood*. London: Heinemann.

Winnicott, D. W. (1945). *Getting to know your baby*. London: Heinemann. Republished in *The child and the family*. London/New York: Tavistock/Basic Books, 1957.

Winnicott, D. W. (1947). Physical therapy of mental disorder. [CW 3:2:2]

Winnicott, D. W. (1949). Leucotomy. [CW 3:4:21]

Winnicott, D. W. (1949). *The ordinary devoted mother and her baby*. London: C. A. Brock.

Winnicott, D. W. (1950). Some thoughts on the meaning of the word democracy. [CW 3:5:17]

Winnicott, D. W. (1957). *The child and the family*. London/New York: Tavistock/Basic Books.

Winnicott, D. W. (1957). *The child and the outside world*. London/New York: Tavistock/Basic Books.

Wolf, K. M., & Spitz, R. A. (1946). Anaclitic depression: An inquiry into the genesis of psychiatric conditions in early childhood. In Freud, A., Hoffer W., Glover, E., et al. (Eds.), *The psychoanalytic study of the child*, 2 (pp. 313–342). London: Imago.

Wulff, M. (1946). Fetishism and object choice in early childhood. *Psychoanalytic Quarterly*, 15, 450–471.

Holding and Interpretation (1986)

[The references for Masud Khan's introduction have not been included.]

Jones, E. (1955). The Dawn of Conscience. *The Observer*, p. 6, 6 February.

Winnicott, D. W. (1931). *Clinical notes on disorders of childhood*. London: Heinemann.

Winnicott, D. W. (1953). Transitional objects and transitional phenomena. [CW 4:2:21]

Winnicott, D. W. (1955). Withdrawal and regression. [CW 4:3:29]
Winnicott, D. W. (1956). Clinical varieties of transference. [CW 5:1:11]
Winnicott, D. W. (1960). The theory of the parent-infant relationship. [CW 6:1:21]
Winnicott, D. W. (1963). The development of the capacity for concern. [CW 6:3:11]
Winnicott, D. W. (1965). Ego distortion in terms of true and false self. [CW 6:1:22]
Winnicott, D. W. (1965). Psychotherapy of character disorders. [CW 6:4:9]
Wordsworth. W. (1803–06). Ode on the Intimations of Immortality from Recollections of Early Childhood. *The Complete Poetical Works*. London: Macmillan and Co., 1888.

The Maturational Processes and the Facilitating Environment (1965)

Abraham, K. (1916). The first pregenital stage of the libido. In *Selected papers of Karl Abraham*. London: Hogarth, 1927.
Abraham, K. (1924). A short study of the development of the libido, viewed in the light of mental disorders. In *Selected papers of Karl Abraham*. London: Hogarth, 1927.
Ackerman, N. (1953). Psychiatric disorders in children: Diagnosis and aetiology in our time. In Paul H. Hoch & Joseph Zubin (Eds.), *Current problems in psychiatric diagnosis*, 205–230. New York: Grune & Stratton
Aichhorn, A. (1925). *Wayward youth*. New York: Viking, 1935.
Balint, M. (1951). On love and hate. In *Primary love and psycho-analytic technique* (pp. 141–156). London: Hogarth, 1952.
Balint, M. (1958). The three areas of the mind. *International Journal of Psychoanalysis*, 39, 328–340.
Bion, W. (1959). Attacks on linking. *International Journal of Psychoanalysis*, 40, 308–315.
Bion, W. (1962a). The theory of thinking. *International Journal of Psychoanalysis*, 43, 4–5.
Bion, W. (1962b). *Learning from experience*. London: Heinemann.
Bornstein, B. (1951). On latency. In *The psychoanalytic study of the child*, 6 (pp. 279–285). London: Imago.
Bowlby, J. (1958). Psycho-analysis and child care. In J. D. Sutherland (Ed.), *Psycho-analysis and contemporary thought* (pp. 33–57). London: Hogarth
Bowlby, J. (1960). Separation anxiety. *International Journal of Psychoanalysis*, 41, 89–113.
Burlingham, D., and Freud, A. (1944). *Infants without families*. London/New York: Allen & Unwin/International UniversitiesPress.
De Monchaux, C. (1962). Thinking and negative hallucination. *International Journal of Psychoanalysis*, 43, 311–314.
Erikson, E. (1950). *Childhood and society*. London/New York: Imago/Norton.
Erikson, E. (1958). *Young man Luther*. London: Faber.
Erikson, E. (1961). The roots of virtue. In J. Huxley (Ed.), *The humanist frame* (pp. 145–165). London: Allen & Unwin.
Fenichel, O. (1945). *The theory of neurosis*. New York: Norton.
Ferenczi, S. (1931/1955). Child analysis in the analysis of adults. In M. Balint (Ed.), *Final contributions to psycho-analysis* (pp. 126–142). London: Hogarth.
Fordham, M. (1960). Contribution to symposium on counter-transference. *British Journal of Medical Psychology*, 33, 1–8.
Freud, A. (1936/1937). *The ego and the mechanisms of defence*. London: Hogarth.

Freud, A. (1946). *The psycho-analytical treatment of children*. London: Imago.
Freud, A. (1953). Some remarks on infant observations. In *The psychoanalytic study of the child*, 8 (pp. 9–19). London: Imago.
Freud, A. (1963). Regression as a principle in mental development. *Bulletin of the Menninger Clinic*, 27, 126–139.
Freud, S. (1905a). Three essays on the theory of sexuality. In J. Strachey (Ed.), *Standard edition of the complete psychological works of Sigmund Freud* (vol. 7). London: Hogarth.
Freud, S. (1905b). On psychotherapy. In J. Strachey (Ed.), *Standard edition of the complete psychological works of Sigmund Freud* (vol. 7). London: Hogarth.
Freud, S. (1909). The analysis of a phobia in a five-year-old boy. In J. Strachey (Ed.), *Standard edition of the complete psychological works of Sigmund Freud* (vol. 10). London: Hogarth.
Freud, S. (1911). Formulations on the two principles of mental functioning. In J. Strachey (Ed.), *Standard edition of the complete psychological works of Sigmund Freud* (vol. 12). London: Hogarth.
Freud, S. (1914). On narcissism. In J. Strachey (Ed.), *Standard edition of the complete psychological works of Sigmund Freud* (vol. 14). London: Hogarth.
Freud, S. (1915). Some character-types met with in psycho-analytic work. In J. Strachey (Ed.), *Standard edition of the complete psychological works of Sigmund Freud* (vol. 14). London: Hogarth.
Freud, S. (1917). Mourning and melancholia. In J. Strachey (Ed.), *Standard edition of the complete psychological works of Sigmund Freud* (vol. 14). London: Hogarth.
Freud, S. (1920). Beyond the pleasure principle. In J. Strachey (Ed.), *Standard edition of the complete psychological works of Sigmund Freud* (vol. 18). London: Hogarth.
Freud, S. (1926). Inhibitions, symptoms and anxiety. In J. Strachey (Ed.), *Standard edition of the complete psychological works of Sigmund Freud* (vol. 20). London: Hogarth.
Freud, S. (1937). Analysis terminable and interminable. In J. Strachey (Ed.), *Standard edition of the complete psychological works of Sigmund Freud* (vol. 23). London: Hogarth.
Gillespie, W. (1944). The psychoneuroses. *Journal of Mental Science*, 90, 287–306.
Glover, E. (1949). The position of psycho-analysis in Great Britain. *British Medical Bulletin*, 6(1–2), 27–31.
Glover, E. (1956). *On the early development of mind*. London: Imago.
Greenacre, P. (1958). Early physical determinants in the development of the sense of identity. *Journal of the American Psychoanalytic Association*, 6(4), 612–627.
Guntrip, H. (1961). *Personality structure and human interaction*. London: Hogarth.
Hartmann, H. (1939/1958). *Ego psychology and the problem of adaptation*. London: Imago.
Hartmann, H. (1954). Contribution to discussion of problems of infantile neurosis. In *The psychoanalytic study of the child*, 9 (pp. 16–71). London: Imago.
Hoch, P., & Zubin, J. (1953). *Current problems in psychiatric diagnosis*. New York: Grune & Stratton.
Hoffer, W. (1955). *Psychoanalysis: Practical and research aspects*. Baltimore: Williams & Wilkins.
James, H. M. (1962). Infantile narcissistic trauma. *International Journal of Psychoanalysis*, 43, 69–79.
Klein, M. (1932). *The psycho-analysis of children*. London: Hogarth.

Klein, M. (1935). Contribution to the psychogenesis of manic depressive states. In M. Klein (Ed.), *Contributions to psycho-analysis, 1921–1945*. London: Hogarth.
Klein, M. (1940). Mourning and its relation to manic depressive states. In *Contributions to psycho-analysis, 1921–1945* (pp. 282–310). London: Hogarth.
Klein, M. (1946). Notes on some schizoid mechanisms. In M. Klein, P. Heimann, S. Isaacs, & J. Riviere (Eds.), *Developments in psycho-analysis* (pp. 292–320). London: Hogarth.
Klein, M. (1948). *Contributions to psycho-analysis 1921–1945*. London: Hogarth.
Klein, M. (1961). *Narrative of a child analysis*. London: Hogarth.
Kris, E. (1950). Notes on the development and on some current problems of psychoanalytic child psychology. In *The psycho-analytic study of the child*, 5 (pp. 24–46). London: Imago.
Kris, E. (1951). Opening remarks on psychoanalytic child psychology. In *The psychoanalytic study of the child*, 6 (pp. 9–17). London: Imago.
Laing, R. D. (1960). *The divided self*. London: Tavistock.
Laing, R. D. (1961). *The self and others*. London: Tavistock.
Little, M. (1958). On delusional transference (transference psychosis). *International Journal of Psychoanalysis*, 39, 134–138.
Menninger, K., et al. (1963). *The vital balance*. New York: Basic Books.
Ribble, M. (1943). *The rights of infants*. New York: Columbia University Press.
Rickman, J. (1928). The development of the psycho-analytical theory of the psychoses, 1893–1926. *Supplement No. 2 to the International Journal of Psychoanalysis* London: Ballière, Tindall and Cox.
Searles, H. F. (1959). The effort to drive the other person crazy: An element in the aetiology and psychotherapy of schizophrenia. *British Journal of Medical Psychology*, 32, 1–19.
Searles, H. F. (1960). *The nonhuman environment*. New York: International Universities Press.
Sechehaye, M. (1951). *Symbolic realisation*. New York: International Universities Press.
Strachey, J. (1934). The nature of the therapeutic action of psycho-analysis. *International Journal of Psychoanalysis*, 15, 127–159.
Wheelis, A. (1958). *The quest for identity*. New York: Norton.
Wickes, F. G. (1938/1950). *The inner world of man*. New York/London: Farrar & Rinehart/Methuen.
Winnicott, C. (1954). Casework techniques in the child care services. In *Child Care and Social Work* (pp. 7–27). London: Codicote Press, 1964.
Winnicott, C. (1962). Casework and agency function. In *Child Care and Social Work* (pp. 59–70). London: Codicote Press, 1964.
Winnicott, D. W. (1941). The observation of infants in a set situation. [CW 2:3:6]
Winnicott, D. W. (1945). Primitive emotional development. [CW 2:7:8]
Winnicott, D. W. (1949). Hate in the countertransference. [CW 3:2:1]
Winnicott, D. W. (1949). *The ordinary devoted mother and her baby*. London: C. A. Brock.
Winnicott, D. W. (1953). Psychoses and child care. [CW 4:1:5]
Winnicott, D. W. (1953). Symptom tolerance in paediatrics: A case history. [CW 4:2:4]
Winnicott, D. W. (1953). Transitional objects and transitional phenomena. [CW 4:2:21]
Winnicott, D. W. (1954). Mind and its relation to the psyche-soma. [CW 3:4:20]
Winnicott, D. W. (1955). The depressive position in normal emotional development. [CW 4:3:5]

Winnicott, D. W. (1955). Metapsychological and clinical aspects of regression within the psycho-analytical set-up. [CW 4:3:6]
Winnicott, D. W. (1955). Withdrawal and regression. [CW 4:3:29]
Winnicott, D. W. (1958). The antisocial tendency. [CW 5:2:8]
Winnicott, D. W. (1958). Appetite and emotional disorder. [CW 1:4:11]
Winnicott, D. W. (1958). Birth memories, birth trauma, and anxiety. [CW 3:4:8]
Winnicott, D. W. (1958). *Collected papers: Through paediatrics to psycho-analysis*. London: Tavistock.
Winnicott, D. W. (1958). Primary maternal preoccupation. [CW 5:2:16]
Winnicott, D. W. (1958). Reparation in respect of mothers organized defence against depression. [CW 3:3:1]
Winnicott, D. W. (1962). Adolescence. [CW 6:2:4]
Winnicott, D. W. (1963). Regression as therapy illustrated by the case of a boy whose pathological dependence was adequately met by the parents. Published here as ' "Cecil" aet 21 months at first consultation'. [CW 10:3:14]
Zetzel, E. (1956). Current concepts of transference. *International Journal of Psychoanalysis*, 37, 369–375.

Playing and Reality (1971)

Alley, R. (1964). *Francis Bacon: Catalogue raisonné and documentation*. London: Thames & Hudson.
Axline, V. (1947). *Play therapy: The inner dynamics of childhood*. Boston, MA: Houghton Mifflin.
Balint, M. (1968). *The basic fault: Therapeutic aspects of regression*. London: Tavistock.
Bettelheim, B. (1960/1961). *The informed heart: Autonomy in a mass age*. New York/London: Free Press/Thames & Hudson.
Blake, Y. (1968). Psychotherapy with the more disturbed patient. *British Journal of Medical Psychology*, 41(2), 199–211.
Bowlby, J. (1969). *Attachment and loss. Vol. 1, Attachment*. London/New York: Hogarth and the Institute of Psychoanalysis/Basic Books.
Donne, J. (1962). *Complete poetry and selected prose*. Edited by J. Hayward. London: Nonesuch.
Erikson, E. (1956). The problem of ego identity. *Journal of the American Psychoanalytic Association*, 4, 56–121.
Fairbairn, W. R. D. (1941). A revised psychopathology of the psychoses and psychoneuroses. *International Journal of Psycho-Analysis*, 22, 250–279.
Foucault, M. (1966/1970). *Les mots et les choses*. Paris: Éditions Gallimard. Published in English under the title 'The order of things'. London/New York: Tavistock/Pantheon.
Freud, A. (1965). *Normality and pathology in childhood*. London: Hogarth/Institute of Psycho-Analysis.
Freud, S. (1900). The interpretation of dreams. In J. Strachey (Ed.), *Standard edition of the complete psychological works of Sigmund Freud* (vols. 4–5). London: Hogarth.
Freud, S. (1923). The ego and the id. In J. Strachey (Ed.), *Standard edition of the complete psychological works of Sigmund Freud* (vol. 19). London: Hogarth.

Freud, S. (1939). Moses and monotheism. In J. Strachey (Ed.), *Standard edition of the complete psychological works of Sigmund Freud* (vol. 23). London: Hogarth.

Gillespie, W. H. (1960). *The edge of objectivity: An essay in the history of scientific ideas.* Princeton, NJ: Princeton University Press.

Gough, D. (1962). The behaviour of infants in the first year of life. *Proceedings of the Royal Society of Medicine*, 55(4), 308–310.

Greenacre, P. (1960). Considerations regarding the parent-infant relationship. *International Journal of Psycho-Analysis*, 41, 571–584.

Hartmann, H. (1939/1958). *Ego psychology and the problem of adaptation.* New York/London: International Universities Press/Imago, 1958.

Hoffer, W. (1949). Mouth, hand, and ego-integration. In A. Freud, H. Hartmann, & E. Kris (Eds.), *The psychoanalytic study of the child*, 3/4 (pp. 49–56). London: Imago.

Hoffer, W. (1950). Development of the body ego. In Freud, A., Hoffer, W., Glover, E. (Eds.), *The psychoanalytic study of the child*, 5 (pp. 18–23). London: Imago.

Khan, M. M. R. (1964). The function of intimacy and acting out in perversions. In R. Slovenko (Ed.), *Sexual behavior and the law.* Springfield, IL: Thomas.

Khan, M. M. R. (1969). On the clinical provision of frustrations, recognitions and failures in the analytic situation. *International Journal of Psycho-Analysis*, 50, 237–248.

Klein, M. (1932/1949). *The psycho-analysis of children.* (Revised edition) London: Hogarth and the Institute of Psycho-Analysis.

Klein, M. (1934/1948). A contribution to the psychogenesis of manic-depressive states. In M. Klein (Ed.), *Contributions to psycho-analysis 1921–1945.* London: Hogarth and the Institute of Psycho-Analysis.

Klein, M. (1940). Mourning and its relation to manic-depressive states. In M. Klein (Ed.), *Contributions to psycho-analysis 1921–1945.* London: Hogarth and the Institute of Psycho-Analysis.

Klein, M. (1957). *Envy and gratitude.* London: Tavistock.

Knights, L. C. (1946/1964). *Explorations.* London/Harmondsworth: Chatto & Windus/Penguin (Peregrine series).

Kris, E. (1951). Some comments and observations on early autoerotic activities. In *The psychoanalytic study of the child*, 6. London: Imago.

Lacan, J. (1949/1966). Le stade du miroir comme formateur de la fonction du je, telle qu'elle nous est révélée dans l'expérience psychanalytique. In *Écrits.* Paris: Éditions du Seuil.

Lomas, P. (Ed.). (1967). *The predicament of the family.* London: Hogarth and the Institute of Psycho-Analysis.

Lowenfeld, M. (1935/1969). *Play in childhood.* Bath: Cedric Chivers.

Mahler, M. S. (1969). *On human symbiosis and the vicissitudes of individuation.* Vol. 1, Infantile Psychosis. London: Hogarth and the Institute of Psycho-Analysis.

Middlemore, M. P. (1941). *The nursing couple.* London: Hamish Hamilton Medical Books.

Miller, A. (1963). *Jane's blanket.* New York/London: Collier/Macmillan.

Milne, A. A. (1926). *Winnie the Pooh.* London: Methuen.

Milner, M. (1934/1952). *A life of one's own.* London/Harmondsworth: Chatto & Windus/Penguin.

Milner, M. (1952). Aspects of symbolism in comprehension of the not-self. *International Journal of Psycho-Analysis*, 33, 181–194.

Milner, M. (1957). *On not being able to paint.* (Revised edition) London: Heinemann.

Milner, M. (1969). *The hands of the living god.* London: Hogarth and the Institute of Psycho-Analysis.

Opie, I., & Opie, P. (Eds.) (1951). *The Oxford dictionary of nursery rhymes.* Oxford: Clarendon.

Plaut, F. (1966). Reflections about not being able to imagine. *Journal of Analytical Psychology, 11*(2), 113–133.

Riviere, J. (1936). On the genesis of psychical conflict in earliest infancy. *International Journal of Psycho-Analysis, 17,* 395–422.

Schulz, C. M. (1959). *Peanuts revisited—favorites, old and new.* New York: Holt, Rinehart & Winston.

Shakespeare, W. Hamlet, Prince of Denmark.

Solomon, J. C. (1962). Fixed idea as an internalized transitional object. *American Journal of Psychotherapy, 16,* 632–644.

Spitz, R. (1962). Autoerotism re-examined: The role of early sexual behaviour patterns in personality formation. In R. Eisler, et al. (Eds.), *The psychoanalytic study of the child, 17* (pp. 283–315). London: Imago.

Stevenson, O. (1954). The first treasured possession: A study of the part played by specially loved objects and toys in the lives of certain children. In R. S. Eisler, A. Freud, H. Hartmann, & E. Kris (Eds.), *The psychoanalytic study of the child, 9* (pp. 199–217). London: Imago.

Trilling, L. (1955/1967). Freud: Within and beyond culture. In *Beyond Culture* (pp. 89–118). Harmondsworth: Penguin (Peregrine series).

Winnicott, D. W. (1931). *Clinical notes on disorders of childhood.* London: Heinemann.

Winnicott, D. W. (1941). The observation of infants in a set situation. [CW 2:3:6]

Winnicott, D. W. (1945). Primitive emotional development. [CW 2:7:8]

Winnicott, D. W. (1948). Paediatrics and psychiatry. [CW 3:3:2]

Winnicott, D. W. (1953). Psychoses and child care. [CW 4:1:5]

Winnicott, D. W. (1954). Mind and its relation to the psyche-soma. [CW 3:4:20]

Winnicott, D. W. (1955). Metapsychological and clinical aspects of regression within the psycho-analytical set-up. [CW 4:3:6]

Winnicott, D. W. (1958). The capacity to be alone. [CW 5:3:20]

Winnicott, D. W. (1958). *Collected papers: Through paediatrics to psycho-analysis.* London: Tavistock.

Winnicott, D. W. (1958). The manic defence. [CW 1:4:6]

Winnicott, D. W. (1958). Primary maternal preoccupation. [CW 5:2:16]

Winnicott, D. W. (1958). Transitional objects and transitional phenomena. [CW 5:4:24]

Winnicott, D. W. (1960). The theory of the parent-infant relationship. [CW 6:1:21]

Winnicott, D. W. (1963). Morals and education. [CW 6:3:18]

Winnicott, D. W. (1965). Classification: Is there a psychoanalytic contribution to psychiatric classification? [CW 5:5:5]

Winnicott, D. W. (1965). Communicating and not communicating leading to a study of certain opposites. [CW 6:4:8]

Winnicott, D. W. (1965). Ego distortion in terms of true and false self. [CW 6:1:22]

Winnicott, D. W. (1965). Ego integration in child development. [CW 6:3:19]

Winnicott, D. W. (1965). *The maturational processes and the facilitating environment.* London: Hogarth.
Winnicott, D. W. (1966). Comment on obsessional neurosis and 'Frankie'. [CW 7:2:10]
Winnicott, D. W. (1967). The location of cultural experience. [CW 7:3:31]
Winnicott, D. W. (1967). Mirror-role of mother and family in child development. [CW 8:1:38]
Winnicott, D. W. (1968). Playing: Its theoretical status in the clinical situation. Published here as 'Playing: A theoretical statement.' [CW 8:2:15]
Winnicott, D. W. (1968). La schizophrénie infantile en termes d'échec d'adaptation. Published here as 'The aetiology of infantile schizophrenia in terms of adaptive failure'. [CW 8:1:25]
Winnicott, D. W. (1971). *Therapeutic consultations in child psychiatry.* London: Hogarth.
Wulff, M. (1946). Fetishism and object choice in early childhood. *Psychoanalytic Quarterly,* 15, 450–471.

PART 2

Winnicott's Correspondence

Chronological Bibliography of Letters by D. W. Winnicott

1978

C. Winnicott, 'D. W. W.: A reflection'. In S. Grolnick, L. Barkin, Muensterberger (Eds.), *Between fantasy and reality: Transitional objects and phenomena*. New York: Aronson; also published in *Psycho-analytic explorations* (1989).

1984

C. Winnicott, R. Shepherd, & M. Davis (Eds.). *Deprivation and delinquency*. London: Tavistock.

1987

Rodman, F. R. (Ed.). *The spontaneous gesture: Selected letters of D. W. Winnicott*. Cambridge, MA: Harvard University Press.

1989

Winnicott, C., Shepherd, R., Davis, M. (Eds.). *Psycho-analytic explorations*. London: Karnac.

2002

Kahr, B. (Ed.). *The legacy of Winnicott: Essays on infant and child mental health*. London: Karnac.

2003a

Rodman, F. R. *Winnicott: Life and work*. Cambridge, MA: Perseus.

2003b

Psychoanalysis and History. 2003, 5, 13–48. 'The Gaddini-Winnicott Correspondence'. Edinburgh: Edinburgh University Press.

ca. 1911–1913

Elizabeth Winnicott (Winnicott's mother). ca. 2 September 1911–1913 (1978, pp. 24–25; 1989, p. 9) [CW 1:1:1]

Stanley 'Jim' Ede. ca. 1912–1913 (1978, pp. 25–26; 1989, pp. 10–11) [CW 1:1:2]

1913

Winnicott, John Frederick, Elizabeth, Violet, & Kathleen (Winnicott's family). 3 November 1913 (2003a, p. 27) [excerpt] [CW 1:1:4]

Winnicott, John Frederick, Elizabeth, Violet, & Kathleen (Winnicott's family). ca. 23 December 1913 [excerpt] (2003a, p. 27) [CW 1:1:5]

1914

Winnicott, John Frederick, Elizabeth, Violet, & Kathleen (Winnicott's family). 9 May 1914 [excerpt] (2003a, pp. 27–28) [CW 1:1:7]

1916

Elizabeth Winnicott (mother). ca. late 1916 [excerpt] (2003a, p. 34) [CW 1:1:9]

Elizabeth Winnicott (mother). 10 September 1916 [short excerpts, 2003a, pp. 33–34] [not published in the *Collected Works*]

Winnicott, John Frederick, Elizabeth, Violet, & Kathleen (family). 9 December 1916 [excerpt] (2003a, p. 35–36) [CW 1:1:10]

1919

Violet Winnicott (sister). 15 November 1919 (1987, Letter 1, pp. 1–4) [CW 1:1:11]

1936

Robina Addis. ca. April 1936 [CW 1:4:8]

1937

Roger Money-Kyrle. 13 May 1937 [CW 1:4:15]

1938

Mrs Neville Chamberlain. 10 November 1938 (1987, Letter 2, p. 4) [CW 1:4:19]

John Bowlby. 6 December 1938 [CW 1:4:20]

1939

British Medical Journal, 'Circumcision'. (3 January) 14 January 1939, *1*(4071), 86. [CW 2:1:1]

British Medical Journal, 'Pruritus and psychology'. (10 April) 22 April 1939, 1(4085), 844. [CW 2:1:2]

British Medical Journal, 'Evacuation of small children' (with J. Bowlby & E. Miller). (6 December) 16 December 1939, 2(4119), 1202–1203 (also published in 1984, pp. 13–14). [CW 2:1:6]

1940

Kate Friedlander. 8 January 1940 (1987, Letter 3, pp. 5–6) [CW 2:2:1]

1941

British Medical Journal, 'Communal feeding in schools'. (23 August) 6 September 1941, 2(4209), 358. [CW 2:3:2]

1942

British Medical Journal, 'Loneliness in infancy'. 17 October 1942, 2(4267), 465. [CW 2:4:3]

1943

The Lancet, 'Prefrontal leucotomy'. 10 April 1943, 241(6241), 475 (also published in 1989, pp. 542–543). [CW 2:5:4]

The Lancet [not published], 'Prefrontal leucotomy'. 15 May 1943 [CW 2:5:5]

British Medical Journal, 'Responsibility and freedom'. 21 August 1943, 2 (4311), 243. [CW 2:5:7]

British Medical Journal, 'Shock treatment of mental disorder'. 25 December 1943, 2(4329), 829 (also published in 1989, pp. 522–523). [CW 2:5:10]

1944

Roger North. *New Era in Home and School*, January 1944, 25(1), 7–8 (also published in 1984 under the title 'Correspondence with a magistrate', pp. 164–167) [CW 2:6:1]

British Medical Journal, 'Shock therapy'. 12 February 1944, 1(4346), 234 (also published in 1989, pp. 523–525). [CW 2:6:4]

Marjorie Franklin. 19 October 1944 [CW 2:6:12]

1945

British Medical Journal, 'Physical therapy in mental disorder'. 22 December 1945, 2(4433), 901 (also published in 1987, Letter 4, pp. 6–7). [CW 2:7:10]

1946

British Medical Journal, 'Psychology in the child's education'. 29 June 1946, 1(4460), 998. [CW 3:1:3]

Lord Beveridge. 15 October 1946 (1987, Letter 5, p. 8) [CW 3:1:4]
The Times [not published]. 6 November 1946 (1987, Letter 6, p. 9) [CW 3:1:5]
Ella Sharpe. 13 November 1946 (1987, Letter 7, p. 10) [CW 3:1:6]

1947

British Medical Journal, 'Battle neurosis treated with leucotomy'. 13 December, 1947 2(4536), 973. [CW 3:2:6]

1948

British Medical Journal, 'Pathies in a State Service'. 14 February 1948, 1(4545), 313–314. [CW 3:3:3]
Anna Freud. 6 July 1948 (1987, Letter 8, pp. 10–12) [CW 3:3:5]

1949

Paul Federn. 3 January 1949 (1987, Letter 9, p. 12) [CW 3:4:1]
British Medical Journal [not sent for publication]. 6 January 1949 (1987, Letter 10, pp. 13–14) [CW 3:4:2]
Marjorie Stone. 14 February 1949 (1987, Letter 11, pp. 14–15) [CW 3:4:3]
Roger Money-Kyrle. 22 March 1949 [CW 3:4:5]
Roger Money-Kyrle. 31 March 1949 [CW 3:4:6]
Roger Money-Kyrle. 2 May 1949 [CW 3:4:7]
Joan Riviere. 19 May 1949 (2003a, pp. 153–155) [CW 3:4:9]
Melanie Klein. 23 May 1949 [short excerpts in 2003a, p. 155] [not published in the *Collected Works*]
Roger Money-Kyrle. 13 June 1949 [CW 3:4:10]
Roger Money-Kyrle. 22 June 1949 [CW 3:4:12]
Roger Money-Kyrle. 24 June 1949 [CW 3:4:13]
Joan Riviere. 24 June 1949 [excerpts] (2003a, pp. 155–156) [CW 3:4:14]
The Times, 'Punishment and crime: A psychologist's view'. (10 August 1949) 23 August 1949, Issue 51467, p. 6 (also published in 1987, Letter 12, pp. 15–16). [CW 3:4:16]
R. S. Hazlehurst. 1 September 1949 (1987, Letter 13, p. 17) [CW 3:4:17]
S. H. Hodge. 1 September 1949 (1987, Letter 14, pp. 17–19) [CW 3:4:18]
British Medical Journal, 'Paddington Green Children's Hospital'. 24 September 1949, 2(4629), 711. [CW 3:4:19]

1950

Clare Winnicott. Early 1950 [excerpt] (C. Winnicott, 'D. W. W.: A reflection', in 1989, p. 16–17) [CW 3:5:1]
The Times, 'Neglected children'. 31 January 1950, Issue 51603, p. 5 (also published in 1987, Letter 16, p. 21). [CW 3:5:3]
Otho W. S. Fitzgerald. 3 March 1950 (1987, Letter 15, pp. 19–20) [CW 3:5:4]
P. D. Scott. 11 May 1950 (1987, Letter 17, pp. 22–23) [CW 3:5:6]
The Times, 'Maladjusted children: Damaging effect of delay'. 13 May 1950, Issue 51690, p. 5. [CW 3:5:7]

Roger Money-Kyrle. 10 July 1950 [CW 3:5:9]
Roger Money-Kyrle. 8 August 1950 [CW 3:5:11]
Hannah ('Queen') Henry. 30 October 1950 (2003a, pp. 67–68) [CW 3:5:12]
Roger Money-Kyrle. 16 November 1950 [CW 3:5:13]

1951

Wilfred Bion. 22 January 1951 [CW 3:6:2]
James Strachey. 1 May 1951 (1987, Letter 18, p. 24) [CW 3:6:3]
The Lancet, 'Leucotomy in psychosomatic disorders'. 18 August 1951, 258(6677), 314–315. [CW 3:6:8]
British Medical Journal, 'Ethics of prefrontal leucotomy'. 25 August 1951, 2(4729), 496. [CW 3:6:9]
The Times, 'Nursery schools: A definition of functions', 8 September 1951, Issue 52101, p. 7. [CW 3:6:11]
Edward Glover. 23 October 1951 (1987, Letter 19, pp. 24–25) [CW 3:6:13]

1952

Hanna Segal. 21 February 1952 (1987, Letter 20, pp. 25–27) [CW 4:1:3]
The Lancet, 'Frontal lobes of the human brain'. 8 March 1952, 259(6706), 514. [CW 4:1:4]
Augusta Bonnard. 3 April 1952 (1987, Letter 21, p. 28) [CW 4:1:6]
Willi Hoffer. 4 April 1952 (1987, Letter 22, pp. 29–30) [CW 4:1:7]
Sonny S. Davidson. 5 May 1952 [CW 4:1:8]
Henry Ezriel. 20 June 1952 (1987, Letter 23, pp. 31–32) [CW 4:1:9]
Ernest Jones. 22 July 1952 (1987, Letter 24, p. 33) [CW 4:1:10]
Melanie Klein. 17 November 1952 (1987, Letter 25, pp. 33–38) [CW 4:1:12]
Roger Money-Kyrle. 27 November 1952 (1987, Letter 26, pp. 38–43) [CW 4:1:13]

1953

Herbert Rosenfeld. 22 January 1953 (1987, Letter 27, pp. 43–46; 2003a, pp. 187–189) [CW 4:2:2]
Hanna Segal. 22 January 1953 (1987, Letter 28, p. 47) [CW 4:2:1]
Herbert Rosenfeld. 17 February 1953 (2003a, pp. 190–191) [CW 4:2:3]
W. Clifford M. Scott. 19 March 1953 (1987, Letter 29, pp. 48–50) [CW 4:2:5]
Esther Bick. 11 June 1953 (1987, Letter 30, pp. 50–52) [CW 4:2:9]
Sylvia Payne. 7 October 1953 (1987, Letter 31, pp. 52–53) [CW 4:2:13]
David Rapaport. 9 October 1953 (1987, Letter 32, pp. 53–54) [CW 4:2:14]
Hannah Ries. 27 November 1953 (1987, Letter 33, pp. 54–55) [CW 4:2:15]

1954

W. Clifford M. Scott. 27 January 1954 (1987, Letter 34, pp. 56–57) [CW 4:3:1]
Charles F. Rycroft. 5 February 1954 (2002, pp. 156–158) [CW 4:3:2]
The Spectator, 'A psychiatrist's choice'. 12 February 1954, No. 6555, p. 13 [CW 4:3:3]
W. Clifford M. Scott. 26 February 1954 (1987, Letter 35, pp. 57–58) [CW 4:3:4]

Anna Freud. 18 March 1954 (1987, Letter 36, p. 58) [CW 4:3:7]
Betty Joseph. 13 April 1954 (1987, Letter 37, pp. 59–60) [CW 4:3:8]
W. Clifford M. Scott. 13 April 1954 (1987, Letter 38, pp. 60–63) [CW 4:3:9]
David K. Henderson. 10 May 1954 (1987, Letter 39, pp. 63–65) [CW 4:3:10]
John Bowlby. 11 May 1954 (1987, Letter 40, pp. 65–66) [CW 4:3:11]
Klara Frank. 20 May 1954 (1987, Letter 41, pp. 67–68) [CW 4:3:13]
David K. Henderson. 20 May 1954 (1987, Letter 42, pp. 68–71) [CW 4:3:14]
Anna Freud & Melanie Klein. 3 June 1954 (1987, Letter 43, pp. 71–74) [CW 4:3:15]
Michael Fordham. 11 June 1954 (1987, Letter 44, pp. 74–75) [CW 4:3:16]
Harry Guntrip. 20 July 1954 (1987, Letter 45, pp. 75–76) [CW 4:3:19]
The Times, 'Sponsored television' [not published]. 21 July 1954 (1987, Letter 46, pp. 76–77) [CW 4:3:20]
Harry Guntrip. 13 August 1954 (1987, Letter 47, pp. 77–79) [CW 4:3:21]
Thomas Stapleton. 20 September 1954 [CW 4:3:23]
Roger Money-Kyrle. 23 September 1954 (1987, Letter 48, pp. 79–80) [CW 4:3:24]
D. Chaplin. 18 October 1954 (1987, Letter 49, pp. 80–82) [CW 4:3:25]
The Times [not published]. 1 November 1954 (1987, Letter 50, pp. 82–83) [CW 4:3:27]

1955

Charles M. Schulz. 1955. [excerpt]. (2003a, p. 413) [CW 5:1:22]
Roger Money-Kyrle. 10 February 1955 (1987, Letter 51, pp. 84–85) [CW 5:1:1]
Thomas Stapleton. 3 March 1955 [CW 5:1:3]
Roger Money-Kyrle. 17 March 1955 (1987, Letter 52, p. 85) [CW 5:1:6]
Emilio Rodrigue. 17 March 1955 (1987, Letter 53, pp. 86–87) [CW 5:1:5]
Charles F. Rycroft. 21 April 1955 (1987, Letter 54, p. 87) [CW 5:1:8]
British Medical Journal, 'Comforters'. 13 August 1955, 2(4936), 437. [CW 5:1:13]
Michael Fordham. 26 September 1955 (1987, Letter 55, pp. 87–88) [CW 5:1:14]
Hanna Segal. 6 October 1955 (1987, Letter 56, p. 89) [CW 5:1:15]
Wilfred R. Bion. 7 October 1955 (1987, Letter 57, pp. 89–93) [CW 5:1:16]
Anna Freud. 18 November 1955 (1987, Letter 58, pp. 93–94) [CW 5:1:17]

1956

British Medical Journal, 'Prefrontal leucotomy'. 28 January 1956, 1(4960), 229–230 (also published in 1989, pp. 553–554). [CW 5:2:2]
Joan Riviere. 3 February 1956 (1987, Letter 59, pp. 94–97) [CW 5:2:3]
Enid Balint. 22 March 1956 (1987, Letter 60, pp. 97–98) [CW 5:2:6]
Gabriel Casuso. 4 July 1956 (1987, Letter 61, pp. 98–100) [CW 5:2:9]
Oliver H. Lowry. 5 July 1956 (1987, Letter 62, pp. 100–103) [CW 5:2:10]
Charles F. Rycroft. 7 October 1956 (2002, p. 158) [CW 5:2:12]
Charles F. Rycroft. 17 October 1956 (2002, p. 159) [CW 5:2:13]
J. Peter. M. Tizard. 23 October 1956 (1987, Letter 63, pp. 103–107) [CW 5:2:14]
Barbara Lantos. 8 November 1956 (1987, Letter 64, pp. 107–110) [CW 5:2:15]

1957

Anna M. Kulka. 15 January 1957 (1987, Letter 65, pp. 110–112) [CW 5:3:1]
Charles F. Rycroft. 17 January 1957 (2002, pp. 159–160) [CW 5:3:2]
Thomas Main. 24 January 1957 [CW 5:3:3]
Margaret Mead. 31 January 1957 [CW 5:3:5]
Thomas Main. 25 February 1957 (1987, Letter 66, pp. 112–114) [CW 5:3:6]
Melanie Klein. 7 March 1957 (1987, Letter 67, pp. 114–115) [CW 5:3:7]
Michael Balint. 27 March 1957 [CW 5:3:9]
Michael Balint. 4 April 1957 [CW 5:3:10]
Tsuicheu Cheu. 4 April 1957 [CW 5:3:11]
The Times, 'I Qant stand it' [not published]. 11 April 1957 (2003a, p. 240) [CW 5:3:12]
Martin James. 17 April 1957 (1987, Letter 68, pp. 115–116) [CW 5:3:13]
Mary Appleby. 27 May 1957 [CW 5:3:16]
Joan Riviere. 21 June 1957 [CW 5:3:18]
Prunella Briance. 15 July 1957 [CW 5:3:19]
Augusta Bonnard. 1 October 1957 (1987, Letter 69, pp. 116–117) [CW 5:3:22]
Michael Balint. 3 October 1957 [CW 5:3:24]
Francesca Bion. 3 October 1957 [CW 5:3:25]
Augusta Bonnard. 7 November 1957 (1987, Letter 70, p. 117) [CW 5:3:28]

1958

Grantly Dick-Read. 15 January 1958 [CW 5:4:1]
Marianne Baumann. 20 January 1958 [CW 5:4:2]
Anna Freud. 14 May 1958 [CW 5:4:8]
Marianne Baumann. 5 June 1958 [CW 5:4:10]
Anna Freud. 8 June 1958 [CW 5:4:11]
Joan Riviere. 13 June 1958 (1987, Letter 71, pp. 118–119) [CW 5:4:12]
R. D. Laing. 18 July 1958 (1987, Letter 72, p. 119) [CW 5:4:14]
Herbert Rosenfeld. 16 October 1958 (1987, Letter 73, p. 120) [CW 5:4:16]
Anna Freud. 7 November 1958 [CW 5:4:19]
Victor Smirnoff. 19 November 1958 (1987, Letter 74, pp. 120–124) [CW 5:4:20]

1959

Reginald Lightwood. 10 February 1959 [CW 5:5:2]
Miss Maw. 16 February 1959 [CW 5:5:3]
The Times, 'Nursery schools essential' [not published]. 25 March 1959 [CW 5:5:6]
Donald Meltzer. 21 May 1959 (1987, Letter 75, pp. 124–125) [CW 5:5:7]
Kenneth Soddy. 9 June 1959 [CW 5:5:8]
Paul Halmos. 12 June 1959 [CW 5:5:9]
Dorothy E. M. Gardner. 13 July 1959 [CW 5:5:11]
Arthur J. Metcalfe. 14 July 1959 [CW 5:5:12]

Herman Gijsbert van der Waals. 23 July 1959 [CW 5:5:13]
A. Tommy M. Wilson. 23 September 1959 [CW 5:5:14]
Elliot Jaques. 13 October 1959 (1987, Letter 76, pp. 125–126) [CW 5:5:16]
Paula Heimann. 5 November, 1959 [CW 5:5:18]
Thomas Szasz. 19 November 1959 (1987, Letter 77, pp. 126–127) [CW 5:5:19]

1960

Michael Balint. 5 February 1960 (1987, Letter 78, pp. 127–129) [CW 6:1:2]
Jacques Lacan. 11 February 1960 (1987, Letter 79, pp. 129–130) [CW 6:1:3]
Merton J. Kahne. 19 February 1960 [CW 6:1:5]
Alexander R. Luria. 7 July 1960 (1987, Letter 80, p. 130) [CW 6:1:11]
Ilse Hellman. 21 July 1960 [CW 6:1:12]
John Harvard-Watts. 28 July 1960 [CW 6:1:13]
Mr & Mrs Young. 28 July 1960 [CW 6:1:14]
Serge Lebovici. 8 November 1960 [CW 6:1:16]
Wilfred R. Bion. 17 November 1960 (1987, Letter 81, p. 131) [CW 6:1:18]

1961

Lydia James. 20 January 1961 [CW 6:2:1]
Aubrey J. Lewis. 26 January 1961 [CW 6:2:2]
Joan FitzHerbert. 25 April 1961 [CW 6:2:7]
Masud Khan. 26 June 1961 (1987, Letter 82, p. 132) [CW 6:2:13]
Pearl King. 18 July 1961 [CW 6:2:14]
Harry Guntrip. 15 September 1961 [CW 6:2:18]
Aubrey J. Lewis. 13 October 1961 [CW 6:2:20]
Wilfred R. Bion. 16 November 1961 (1987, Letter 83, p. 133) [CW 6:2:23]

1962

Benjamin Spock. 9 April 1962 (1987, Letter 84, pp. 133–138) [CW 6:3:3]

1963

Ronald MacKeith. 31 January 1963 (1987, Letter 85, pp. 138–139) [CW 6:4:2]
Timothy Raison. 9 April 1963 (1987, Letter 86, pp. 139–140) [CW 6:4:6]

1964

New Society, 'Love or skill?' (23 March) 2 April 1964, 3(79), 33 (1987, Letter 87, pp. 140–142). [CW 7:1:3]
Renata Gaddini. 26 June 1964 (2003b, 13–14) [CW 7:1:8]
The Observer, 'All of mother'. (12 October) 25 October 1964, p. 28 (1987, Letter 88, pp. 142–144). [CW 7:1:10]
John O. Wisdom 26 October 1964 (1987, Letter 89, p. 144–146) [CW 7:1:11]

The Observer, 'All of mother'. (5 November) 8 November 1964, p. 33 (1987, Letter 90, p. 146). [CW 7:1:13]

Mrs B. J. Knopf. 26 November 1964 (1987, Letter 91, p. 147) [CW 7:1:15]

1965

Michael Fordham. 2 February 1965 [CW 7:2:2]
Humberto Nagera. 15 February 1965 (1987, Letter 92, pp. 147–148) [CW 7:2:3]
Michael Fordham. 24 June 1965 (1987, Letter 93, pp. 148–150) [CW 7:2:8]
Michael Fordham. 15 July 1965 (1987, Letter 94, pp. 150–151) [CW 7:2:9]
Charles Anthony Storr. 30 September 1965 (1987, Letter 95, p. 151) [CW 7:2:15]
Martin James. 7 October 1965 [CW 7:2:17]

1966

The Times, 'George III'. 17 January 1966, Issue 56531, p. 9. [CW 7:3:1]
The Times, 'Psychiatric care' [not published]. 3 March 1966 (1987, Letter 96, pp. 152–153) [CW 7:3:4]
Herbert Rosenfeld. 17 March 1966 (1987, Letter 97, pp. 153–154) [CW 7:3:6]
Hans Thorner. 17 March 1966 (1987, Letter 98, p. 154) [CW 7:3:5]
The Times, '"Blood-tie" child: Why the courts must act swiftly' (24 March) 26 March 1966, Issue 56590, p. 11 (with J. Bowlby, M. Fordham, A. Freud, E. Miller, R. MacKeith, & K. Soddy). [CW 7:3:9]
The Times, '"Blood-tie" child'. 4 April 1966, Issue 56590, p. 11. [CW 7:3:11]
A confidant (M.). 15 April 1966 (1987, Letter 99, p. 155) [CW 7:3:12]
Lili E. Peller. 15 April 1966 (1987, Letter 100, pp. 156–157) [CW 7:3:13]
Sylvia Payne. 26 May 1966 (1987, Letter 101, p. 157) [CW 7:3:15]
Renata Gaddini. 13 September 1966 (2003b, p. 17) [CW 7:3:19]
William Gillespie (with case history). 29 September 1966 [CW 7:3:21]
Donald Meltzer. 25 October 1966 (1987, Letter 102, pp. 157–161) [CW 7:3:24]
Renata Gaddini. 21 November 1966 (2003b, p. 20) [CW 7:3:28]
A patient (Mrs N.). 13 December 1966 (1987, Letter 103, p. 162) [CW 7:3:33]
D. N. Parfitt. 22 December 1966 (1987, Letter 104, pp. 162–163) [CW 7:3:35]

1967

P. Aitken. 13 January 1967 (1987, Letter 105, pp. 163–164) [CW 8:1:1]
Renata Gaddini. 9 March 1967 (2003b, pp. 20–21) [CW 8:1:5]
A colleague (Dr P.). 4 September 1967 (1987, Letter 106, p. 165) [CW 8:1:18]
Renata Gaddini. 4 September 1967 (2003b, pp. 22–23) [CW 8:1:19]
Margaret Torrie. 4 September 1967 (1987, Letter 107, pp. 166–167) [CW 8:1:20]
Margaret Torrie. 5 September 1967 (1987, Letter 108, pp. 167–169) [CW 8:1:21]
Wilfred R. Bion. 5 October 1967 (1987, Letter 109, pp. 169–170) [CW 8:1:23]
Gillian Nelson. 6 October 1967 (1987, Letter 110, pp. 170–171) [CW 8:1:24]
Charles Clay Dahlberg. 24 October 1967 (1987, Letter 111, pp. 171–172) [CW 8:1:26]
Arthur Miller. 13 November 1967 [excerpts] (2003a, p. 316) [CW 8:1:31]

Renata Gaddini. 21 November 1967 (2003b, pp. 24–25) [CW 8:1:32]
Marjorie Spence. 23 November 1967 (1987, Letter 112, pp. 172–173) [CW 8:1:33]
Marjorie Spence. 27 November 1967 (1987, Letter 113, pp. 173–174) [CW 8:1:34]
R. S. W. Dowling. 8 December 1967 (1987, Letter 114, pp. 174–175) [CW 8:1:36]

1968

Donald Gough. 6 March 1968 (1987, Letter 115, pp. 176–177) [CW 8:2:7]
L. Joseph Stone. 18 June 1968 (1987, Letter 116, pp. 177–178) [CW 8:2:17]
Joyce Coles. 25 August 1968 [CW 12:5:caption 6]
A mother (Mrs T.). 6 September 1968 (2003b, pp. 26–27) [CW 8:2:20]
Adam Limentani. 27 September 1968 (1987, Letter 117, pp. 178–180) [CW 8:2:23]
Renata Gaddini. 21 October 1968 (2003b, p. 34) [CW 8:2:24]
Joyce Coles. 22? November 1968 [CW 8:2:31]
Joyce Coles. 25? November 1968 [CW 8:2:32]
Karl and Sheila Britton. 25 November 1968 (2003a, p. 332) [CW 8:2:33]
Joyce Coles. 26? November 1968 [CW 8:2:34]
Joyce Coles. 29 November 1968 [CW 8:2:35]
Joyce Coles. 1? December 1968 [CW 8:2:36]
Joyce Coles. 4 December 1968 [CW 8:2:37]
Karl Britton. 7? December 1968 (2003a, pp. 339–340) [CW 8:2:39]
Joyce Coles. 8 December 1968 [CW 8:2:40]
Renata Gaddini. ca. 9 December 1968 (2003b, p. 34) [CW 8:2:41]
Joyce Coles. 10? December 1968 [CW 8:2:42]
Karl and Sheila Britton. 14 December 1968 (2003a, p. 340) [CW 8:2:44]
Joyce Coles. 14 December 1968 (2003a, pp. 341–342) [CW 8:2:43]

1969

Michael Rosenbluth. 3 January 1969 [excerpt] (2003a, pp. 343–344) [CW 9:1:1]
F. Robert Rodman. 10 January 1969 (1987, Letter 118, pp. 180–182) [CW 9:1:2]
An American correspondent (Mr Q.). 14 January 1969 (1987, Letter 119, pp. 183–185) [CW 9:1:3]
Renata Gaddini. 19 January 1969 (2003b, p. 35) [CW 9:1:5]
Anna Freud. 20 January 1969 (1987, Letter 120, p. 185) [CW 9:1:6]
Michael P. Collinson. 10 March 1969 (1987, Letter 121, pp. 186–188) [CW 9:1:7]
Michael. B. Conran. 8 May 1969 (1987, Letter 122, pp. 188–191) [CW 9:1:10]
Child Care News, 'Behaviour therapy'. June 1969 (also published in 1989, pp. 558–560) [CW 9:1:13]
Agnes Wilkinson. 9 June 1969 (1987, Letter 123, p. 192) [CW 9:1:11]
William W. Sargant. 24 June 1969 (1987, Letter 124, pp. 192–194) [CW 9:1:12]
Helm Stierlin. 31 July 1969 (1987, Letter 125, pp. 195–196) [CW 9:1:19]
Robert Tod. 6 November 1969 (1987, Letter 126, pp. 196–197) [CW 9:1:22]
Renata Gaddini and her family. 15 November 1969 (2003b, pp. 36–37) [CW 9:1:24]

1970

British Journal of Psychiatry, 'Oscar Nemon's Freud Statue: An Appeal'. February 1970 [CW 12:Introduction:1]
Peter Giovacchini. 5 March 1970 [CW 9:2:1]
Michael Fordham. 10 March 1970 [CW 9:2:2]
Renata Gaddini. 31 August 1970 (2003b, pp. 43–44) [CW 9:2:7]

1971

John Davis. 1 January 1971 [CW 9:3:1]
Jeannine Kalmanovitch. 7 January 1971 (In A. Clancier & J. Kalmanovitch, *Le paradoxe de Winnicott – de la naissance à la création*. Paris: Payot, 1984.) [CW 9:3:2]
Jeannine Kalmanovitch. 19 January 1971 (*Nouvelle Revue de Psychanalyse: Lieux du corps*, Vol. 3, Spring 1971, p. 3. Paris: Gallimard) [CW 9:3:3]

Alphabetical Bibliography of Letters by D. W. Winnicott

1978

C. Winnicott, 'D. W. W.: A reflection'. In S. Grolnick, L. Barkin, Muensterberger (Eds.), *Between fantasy and reality: Transitional objects and phenomena*. New York: Aronson; also published in *Psycho-analytic explorations* (1989).

1984

C. Winnicott, R. Shepherd, & M. Davis (Eds.). *Deprivation and delinquency*. London: Tavistock.

1987

Rodman, F. R. (Ed.). *The spontaneous gesture: Selected letters of D. W. Winnicott*. Cambridge, MA: Harvard University Press.

1989

Winnicott, C., Shepherd, R., & Davis, M. (Eds.). *Psycho-analytic explorations*. London: Karnac.

2002

Kahr, B. (Ed.). *The legacy of Winnicott: Essays on infant and child mental health*. London: Karnac.

2003a

Rodman, F. R. *Winnicott: Life and work*. Cambridge, MA: Perseus.

2003b

The Gaddini-Winnicott correspondence. *Psychoanalysis and History*, 5, 13–48.

Addis, Robina. ca. April 1936 [CW 1:4:8]

Aitken, P. 13 January 1967 (1987, Letter 105, pp. 163–164) [CW 8:1:1]

An American correspondent (Mr. Q.). 14 January 1969 (1987, Letter 119, pp. 183–185) [CW 9:1:3]

Applebey, Mary. 27 May 1957 [CW 5:3:16]

Balint, Enid. 22 March 1956 (1987, Letter 60, pp. 97–98) [CW 5:2:6]

Balint, Michael. 27 March 1957 [CW 5:3:9]

Balint, Michael. 4 April 1957 [CW 5:3:10]

Balint, Michael. 3 October 1957 [CW 5:3:24]

Balint, Michael. 5 February 1960 (1987, Letter 78, pp. 127–129) [CW 6:1:2]

Baumann, Marianne. 20 January 1958 [CW 5:4:2]

Baumann, Marianne. 5 June 1958 [CW 5:4:10]

Beveridge, Lord. 15 October 1946 (1987, Letter 5, p. 8) [CW 3:1:4]

Bick, Esther. 11 June 1953 (1987, Letter 30, pp. 50–52) [CW 4:2:9]

Bion, Francesca. 3 October 1957 [CW 5:3:25]

Bion, Wilfred R. 22 January 1951 [CW 3:6:2]

Bion, Wilfred R. 7 October 1955 (1987, Letter 57, pp. 89–93) [CW 5:1:16]

Bion, Wilfred R. 17 November 1960 (1987, Letter 81, p. 131) [CW 6:1:18]

Bion, Wilfred R. 16 November 1961 (1987, Letter 83, p. 133) [CW 6:2:23]

Bion, Wilfred R. 5 October 1967 (1987, Letter 109, pp. 169–170) [CW 8:1:23]

Bonnard, Augusta. 3 April 1952 (1987, Letter 21, p. 28) [CW 4:1:6]

Bonnard, Augusta. 1 October 1957 (1987, Letter 69, pp. 116–117) [CW 5:3:22]

Bonnard, Augusta. 7 November 1957 (1987, Letter 70, p. 117) [CW 5:3:28]

Bowlby, John. 6 December 1938 [CW 1:4:20]

Bowlby, John. 11 May 1954 (1987, Letter 40, pp. 65–66) [CW 4:3:11]

Briance, Prunella. 15 July 1957 [CW 5:3:19]

British Journal of Psychiatry, 'Oscar Nemon's Freud statue: An appeal', February 1970 [CW 12:Introduction:1]

British Medical Journal [not sent for publication]. 6 January 1949 (1987, Letter 10, pp. 13–14) [CW 3:4:2]

British Medical Journal, 'Battle neurosis treated with leucotomy'. 13 December 1947, 2(4536), 973. [CW 3:2:6]

British Medical Journal, 'Circumcision'. (3 January) 14 January 1939, 1(4071), 86. [CW 2:1:1]

British Medical Journal, 'Comforters'. 13 August 1955, 2(4936), 437. [CW 5:1:13]

British Medical Journal, 'Communal feeding in schools'. 6 September 1941, 2(4209), 358. [CW 2:3:2]

British Medical Journal, 'Ethics of prefrontal leucotomy'. 25 August 1951, 2 (4729), 496. [CW 3:6:9]

British Medical Journal, 'Evacuation of small children' (with J. Bowlby & E. Miller). (6 December) 16 December 1939, 2(4119), 1202–1203 (1984, pp. 13–14). [CW 2:1:6]

British Medical Journal, 'Loneliness in infancy'. 17 October 1942, 2(4267), 465. [CW 2:4:3]

British Medical Journal, 'Paddington Green Children's Hospital'. 24 September 1949, 2(4629), 711. [CW 3:4:19]

British Medical Journal, 'Pathies in a State Service'. 14 February 1948, 1(4545), 313–314. [CW 3:3:3]

British Medical Journal, 'Physical therapy in mental disorder'. 22 December 1945, 2(4433), 901 (1987, Letter 4, pp. 6–7). [CW 2:7:10]

British Medical Journal, 'Prefrontal leucotomy'. 28 January 1956, 1(4960), 229–230 (1989, pp. 553–554). [CW 5:2:2]
British Medical Journal, 'Pruritus and psychology'. (10 April) 22 April 1939, 1(4085), 844. [CW 2:1:2]
British Medical Journal, 'Psychology in the child's education'. 29 June 1946, 1(4460), 998. [CW 3:1:3]
British Medical Journal, 'Responsibility and freedom'. 21 August 1943, 2(4311), 243. [CW 2:5:7]
British Medical Journal, 'Shock therapy'. 12 February 1944, 1(4346), 234 (1989, pp. 523–525). [CW 2:6:4]
British Medical Journal, 'Shock treatment of mental disorder'. 25 December 1943, 2(4329), 829 (1989, pp. 522–523). [CW 2:5:10]
Britton, Karl. 7? December 1968 (2003a, pp. 339–340) [CW 8:2:39]
Britton, Karl and Sheila. 25 November 1968 (2003a, p. 332) [CW 8:2:33]
Britton, Karl and Sheila. 14 December 1968 (2003a, p. 340) [CW 8:2:44]
Casuso, Gabriel. 4 July 1956 (1987, Letter 61, pp. 98–100) [CW 5:2:9]
Chamberlain, Mrs Neville. 10 November 1938 (1987, Letter 2, p. 4) [CW 1:4:19]
Chaplin, D. 18 October 1954 (1987, Letter 49, pp. 80–82) [CW 4:3:25]
Cheu, Tsuicheu. 4 April 1957 [CW 5:3:11]
Child Care News, 'Behaviour therapy'. June 1969 (1989, pp. 558–560). [CW 9:1:13]
Joyce Coles. 25 August 1968 [CW 12:5:caption 6]
Coles, Joyce. 22? November 1968 [CW 8:2:31]
Coles, Joyce. 25? November 1968 [CW 8:2:32]
Coles, Joyce. 26? November 1968 [CW 8:2:34]
Coles, Joyce. 29 November 1968 [CW 8:2:35]
Coles, Joyce. 1? December 1968 [CW 8:2:36]
Coles, Joyce. 4 December 1968 [CW 8:2:37]
Coles, Joyce. 8 December 1968 [CW 8:2:40]
Coles, Joyce. 10? December 1968 [CW 8:2:42]
Coles, Joyce. 14 December 1968 (2003a. pp. 341–342) [CW 8:2:43]
A colleague (Dr P.). 4 September 1967 (1987, Letter 106, p. 165) [CW 8:1:18]
Collinson, Michael P. 10 March 1969 (1987, Letter 121, pp. 186–188) [CW 9:1:7]
A confidant (M.). 15 April 1966 (1987, Letter 99, p. 155) [CW 7:3:12]
Conran, Michael B. 8 May 1969 (1987, Letter 122, pp. 188–191) [CW 9:1:10]
Dahlberg, Charles Clay. 24 October 1967 (1987, Letter 111, pp. 171–172) [CW 8:1:26]
Davidson, Sonny. S. 5 May 1952 [CW 4:1:8]
Davis, John. 1 January 1971 [CW 9:3:1]
Dick-Read, Grantly. 15 January 1958 [CW 5:4:1]
Dowling, R. S. W. 8 December 1967 (1987, Letter 114, pp. 174–175) [CW 8:1:36]
Ede, Stanley. ca. 1912–1913 (1978, pp. 25–26; 1989, pp. 10–11) [CW 1:1:2]
Ezriel, Henry. 20 June 1952 (1987, Letter 23, pp. 31–32) [CW 4:1:9]
Federn, Paul. 3 January 1949 (1987, Letter 9, p. 12) [CW 3:4:1]
Fitzgerald, Otho W. S. 3 March 1950 (1987, Letter 15, pp. 19–20) [CW 3:5:4]
FitzHerbert, Joan. 25 April 1961 [CW 6:2:7]
Fordham, Michael. 11 June 1954 (1987, Letter 44, pp. 74–75) [CW 4:3:16]

Fordham, Michael. 26 September 1955 (1987, Letter 55, pp. 87–88) [CW 5:1:14]
Fordham, Michael. 2 February 1965 [CW 7:2:2]
Fordham, Michael. 24 June 1965 (1987, Letter 93, pp. 148–150) [CW 7:2:8]
Fordham, Michael. 15 July 1965 (1987, Letter 94, pp. 150–151) [CW 7:2:9]
Fordham, Michael. 10 March 1970 [CW 9:2:2]
Frank, Klara. 20 May 1954 (1987, Letter 41, pp. 67–68) [CW 4:3:13]
Franklin, Marjorie. 19 October 1944 [CW 2:6:12]
Freud, Anna. 6 July 1948 (1987, Letter 8, pp. 10–12) [CW 3:3:5]
Freud, Anna. 18 March 1954 (1987, Letter 36, p. 58) [CW 4:3:7]
Freud, Anna (& Melanie Klein). 3 June 1954 (1987, Letter 43, pp. 71–74) [CW 4:3:15]
Freud, Anna. 18 November 1955 (1987, Letter 58, pp. 93–94) [CW 5:1:17]
Freud, Anna. 14 May 1958 [CW 5:4:8]
Freud, Anna. 8 June 1958 [CW 5:4:11]
Freud, Anna. 7 November 1958 [CW 5:4:19]
Freud, Anna. 20 January 1969 (1987, Letter 120, p. 185) [CW 9:1:6]
Friedlander, Kate. 8 January 1940 (1987, Letter 3, pp. 5–6) [CW 2:2:1]
Gaddini, Renata. 26 June 1964 (2003b, pp. 13–14) [CW 7:1:8]
Gaddini, Renata. 13 September 1966 (2003b, p. 17) [CW 7:3:19]
Gaddini, Renata. 21 November 1966 (2003b, p. 20) [CW 7:3:28]
Gaddini, Renata. 9 March 1967 (2003b, pp. 20–21) [CW 8:1:5]
Gaddini, Renata. 4 September 1967 (2003b, pp. 22–23) [CW 8:1:19]
Gaddini, Renata. 21 November 1967 (2003b, pp. 24–25) [CW 8:1:32]
Gaddini, Renata. 21 October 1968 (2003b, p. 34) [CW 8:2:24]
Gaddini, Renata. ca. 9 December 1968 (2003b, p. 34) [CW 8:2:41]
Gaddini, Renata. 19 January 1969 (2003b, p. 35) [CW 9:1:5]
Gaddini, Renata. 31 August 1970 (2003b, pp. 43–44) [CW 9:2:7]
Gaddini, Renata and family. 15 November 1969 (2003b, pp. 36–37) [CW 9:1:24]
Gardner, Dorothy E. M. 13 July 1959 [CW 5:5:11]
Gillespie, William (with case history). 29 September 1966 [CW 7:3:21]
Giovacchini, Peter. 5 March 1970 [CW 9:2:1]
Glover, Edward. 23 October 1951 (1987, Letter 19, pp. 24–25) [CW 3:6:13]
Gough, Donald. 6 March 1968 (1987, Letter 115, pp. 176–177) [CW 8:2:7]
Guntrip, Harry. 20 July 1954 (1987, Letter 45, pp. 75–76) [CW 4:3:19]
Guntrip, Harry. 13 August 1954 (1987, Letter 47, pp. 77–79) [CW 4:3:21]
Guntrip, Harry. 15 September 1961 [CW 6:2:18]
Halmos, Paul. 12 June 1959 [CW 5:5:9]
Harvard-Watts, John. 28 July 1960 [CW 8:1:13]
Hazlehurst, R. S. 1 September 1949 (1987, Letter 13, p. 17) [CW 3:4:17]
Heimann, Paula. 5 November 1959 [CW 5:5:18]
Hellman, Ilse. 21 July 1960 [CW 6:1:12]
Henderson, David K. 10 May 1954 (1987, Letter 39, pp. 63–65) [CW 4:3:10]
Henderson, David K. 20 May 1954 (1987, Letter 42, pp. 68–71) [CW 4:3:14]
Henry, Hannah ('Queen'). 30 Oct 1950 (2003a, pp. 67–68) [CW 3:5:12]
Hodge, S. H. 1 September 1949 (1987, Letter 14, pp. 17–19) [CW 3:4:18]
Hoffer, Willi. 4 April 1952 (1987, Letter 22, pp. 29–30) [CW 4:1:7]
James, Lydia. 20 January 1961 [CW 6:2:1]

James, Martin. 17 April 1957 (1987, Letter 68, pp. 115–116) [CW 5:3:13]
James, Martin. 7 October 1965 [CW 7:2:17]
Jaques, Elliot. 13 October 1959 (1987, Letter 76, pp. 125–126) [CW 5:5:16]
Jones, Ernest. 22 July 1952 (1987, Letter 24, p. 33) [CW 4:1:10]
Joseph, Betty. 13 April 1954 (1987, Letter 37, pp. 59–60) [CW 4:3:8]
Kahne, Merton J. 19 February 1960 [CW 6:1:5]
Kalmanovitch, Jeannine. 7 January 1971 (In A. Clancier & J. Kalmanovitch, *Le paradoxe de Winnicott–de la naissance à la création*. Paris: Payot, 1984) [CW 9:3:2]
Kalmanovitch, Jeannine. 19 January 1971 (Nouvelle Revue de Psychanalyse, *Lieux du corps*, Vol. 3, Spring 1971, p. 3. Paris: Gallimard) [CW 9:3:3]
Khan, Masud. 26 June 1961 (1987, Letter 82, p. 132) [CW 6:2:13]
King, Pearl. 18 July 1961 [CW 6:2:14]
Klein, Melanie. 23 May 1949 [short excerpts] (2003a, p. 155) [not republished in CW]
Klein, Melanie. 17 November 1952 (1987, Letter 25, pp. 33–38) [CW 4:1:12]
Klein, Melanie. 7 March 1957 (1987, Letter 67, pp. 114–115) [CW 5:3:7]
Klein, Melanie (& Anna Freud). 3 June 1954 (1987, Letter 43, pp. 71–74) [CW 4:3:15]
Knopf, Mrs B. J. 26 November 1964 (1987, Letter 91, p. 147) [CW 7:1:15]
Kulka, Anna M. 15 January 1957 (1987, Letter 65, pp. 110–112) [CW 5:3:1]
Lacan, Jacques. 11 February 1960 (1987, Letter 79, pp. 129–130) [CW 6:1:3]
Laing, R. D. 18 July 1958 (1987, Letter 72, p. 119) [CW 5:4:14]
The Lancet, 'Frontal lobes of the human brain'. 8 March 1952, 259 (6706), 514. [CW 4:1:4]
The Lancet, 'Prefrontal leucotomy' [not published]. 15 May 1943 [CW 2:5:5]
The Lancet, 'Leucotomy in psychosomatic disorders'. 18 August 1951, 258(6677) 314–315. [CW 3:6:8]
The Lancet, 'Prefrontal leucotomy'. 10 April 1943, 241(6241), 475 (1989, pp. 542–543). [CW 2:5:4]
Lantos, Barbara. 8 November 1956 (1987, Letter 64, pp. 107–110) [CW 5:2:15]
Lebovici, Serge. 8 November 1960 [CW 6:1:16]
Lewis, Aubrey J. 26 January 1961 [CW 6:2:2]
Lewis, Aubrey J. 13 October 1961 [CW 6:2:20]
Lightwood, Reginald. 10 February 1959 [CW 5:5:2]
Limentani, Adam. 27 September 1968 (1987, Letter 117, pp. 178–180) [CW 8:2:23]
Lowry, Oliver H. 5 July 1956 (1987, Letter 62, pp. 100–103) [CW 5:2:10]
Luria, Alexander R. 7 July 1960 (1987, Letter 80, p. 130) [CW 6:1:11]
MacKeith, Ronald. 31 January 1963 (1987, Letter 85, pp. 138–139) [CW 6:4:2]
Main, Thomas. 24 January 1957 [CW 5:3:3]
Main, Thomas. 25 February 1957 (1987, Letter 66, pp. 112–114) [CW 5:3:6]
Maw, Miss. 16 February 1959 [CW 5:5:3]
Mead, Margaret. 31 January 1957 [CW 5:3:5]
Meltzer, Donald. 21 May 1959 (1987, Letter 75, pp. 124–125) [CW 5:5:7]
Meltzer, Donald. 25 October 1966 (1987, Letter 102, pp. 157–161) [CW 7:3:24]
Metcalfe, Arthur J. 14 July 1959 [CW 5:5:12]
Miller, Arthur. 13 November 1967 [excerpts]. (2003a, p. 316). [CW 8:1:31]
Money-Kyrle, Roger. 13 May 1937 [CW 1:4:15]
Money-Kyrle, Roger. 22 March 1949 [CW 3:4:5]
Money-Kyrle, Roger. 31 March 1949 [CW 3:4:6]

Money-Kyrle, Roger. 2 May 1949 [CW 3:4:7]
Money-Kyrle, Roger. 13 June 1949 [CW 3:4:10]
Money-Kyrle, Roger. 22 June 1949 [CW 3:4:12]
Money-Kyrle, Roger. 24 June 1949 [CW 3:4:13]
Money-Kyrle, Roger. 10 July 1950 [CW 3:5:9]
Money-Kyrle, Roger. 8 August 1950 [CW 3:5:11]
Money-Kyrle, Roger. 16 November 1950 [CW 3:5:13]
Money-Kyrle, Roger. 27 November 1952 (1987, Letter 26, pp. 38–43) [CW 4:1:13]
Money-Kyrle, Roger. 23 September 1954 (1987, Letter 48, pp. 79–80) [CW 4:3:24]
Money-Kyrle, Roger. 10 February 1955 (1987, Letter 51, pp. 84–85) [CW 5:1:1]
Money-Kyrle, Roger. 17 March 1955 (1987, Letter 52, p. 85) [CW 5:1:6]
A mother (Mrs T.). 6 September 1968 (2003b, pp. 26–27) [CW 8:2:20]
Nagera, Humberto. 15 February 1965 (1987, Letter 92, pp. 147–148) [CW 7:2:3]
Nelson, Gillian. 6 October 1967 (1987, Letter 110, pp. 170–171) [CW 8:1:24]
New Society, 'Love or skill?' (23 March 1964) 2 April 1964, 3(79), 33 (1987, Letter 87, pp. 140–142). [CW 7:1:3]
North, Roger. *New Era in Home and School*, January 1944, 25(1), 7–8 (1984a, under the title 'Correspondence with a magistrate', pp. 164–167) [CW 2:6:1]
The Observer, 'All of mother'. (12 October) 25 October 1964, 28 (1987, Letter 88, pp. 142–144). [CW 7:1:10]
The Observer, 'All of mother'. (5 November) 8 November 1964, 33 (1987, Letter 90, p. 146). [CW 7:1:13]
Parfitt, D. N. 22 December 1966 (1987, Letter 104, pp. 162–163) [CW 7:3:35]
A patient (Mrs N.). 13 December 1966 (1987, Letter 103, p. 162) [CW 7:3:33]
Payne, Sylvia. 7 October 1953 (1987, Letter 31, pp. 52–53) [CW 4:2:13]
Payne, Sylvia. 26 May 1966 (1987, Letter 101, p. 157) [CW 7:3:15]
Peller, Lili E. 15 April 1966 (1987, Letter 100, pp. 156–157) [CW 7:3:13]
Raison, Timothy. 9 April 1963 (1987, Letter 86, pp. 139–140) [CW 6:4:6]
Rapaport, David. 9 October 1953 (1987, Letter 32, pp. 53–54) [CW 4:2:14]
Ries, Hannah. 27 November 1953 (1987, Letter 33, pp. 54–55) [CW 4:2:15]
Riviere, Joan. 19 May 1949 (2003a, p. 153–155) [CW 3:4:9]
Riviere, Joan. 24 June 1949 [excerpts] (2003a, pp. 155–156) [CW 3:4:14]
Riviere, Joan. 3 February 1956 [CW 5:2:3]
Riviere, Joan. 21 June 1957 [CW 5:3:18]
Riviere, Joan. 13 June 1958 (1987, Letter 71, pp. 118–119) [CW 5:4:12]
Rodman, F. Robert. 10 January 1969 (1987, Letter 118, pp. 180–182) [CW 9:1:2]
Rodrigue, Emilio. 17 March 1955 [CW 5:1:5]
Rosenbluth, Michael. 3 January 1969 [excerpt] (2003a, pp. 343–344) [CW 9:1:1]
Rosenfeld, Herbert. 22 January 1953 (1987, Letter 27, pp. 43–46) [CW 4:2:2]
Rosenfeld, Herbert. 17 February 1953 (2003a, pp. 190–191) [CW 4:2:3]
Rosenfeld, Herbert. 16 October 1958 (1987, Letter 73, p. 120) [CW 5:4:16]
Rosenfeld, Herbert. 17 March 1966 (1987, Letter 97, pp. 153–154) [CW 7:3:6]
Rycroft, Charles F. 5 February 1954 (2002, pp. 156–158) [CW 4:3:2]
Rycroft, Charles F. 21 April 1955 (1987, Letter 54, p. 87) [CW 5:1:8]
Rycroft, Charles F. 7 October 1956 (2002, p. 158) [CW 5:2:12]
Rycroft, Charles F. 17 October 1956 (2002, p. 159) [CW 5:2:13]

Rycroft, Charles F. 17 January 1957 (2002, pp. 159–160) [CW 5:3:2]
Sargant, William W. 24 January 1969 (1987, Letter 124, pp. 192–194) [CW 9:1:12]
Schulz, Charles M. 1955 [excerpt] (2003a, p. 413) [CW 5:1:22]
Scott, Peter. D. 11 May 1950 (1987, Letter 17, pp. 22–23) [CW 3:5:6]
Scott, W. Clifford M. 19 March 1953 (1987, Letter 29, pp. 48–50) [CW 4:2:5]
Scott, W. Clifford M. 27 January 1954 (1987, Letter 34, pp. 56–57) [CW 4:3:1]
Scott, W. Clifford M. 26 February 1954 (1987, Letter 35, pp. 57–58) [CW 4:3:4]
Scott, W. Clifford M. 13 April 1954 (1987, Letter 38, pp. 60–63) [CW 4:3:9]
Segal, Hanna. 21 February 1952 (1987, Letter 20, pp. 25–27) [CW 4:1:3]
Segal, Hanna. 22 January 1953 (1987, Letter 28, p. 47) [CW 4:2:1]
Segal, Hanna. 6 October 1955 (1987, Letter 56, p. 89) [CW 5:1:15]
Sharpe, Ella Freeman. 13 November 1946 (1987, Letter 7, p. 10) [CW 3:1:6]
Smirnoff, Victor. 19 November 1958 (1987, Letter 74, pp. 120–124) [CW 5:4:20]
Soddy, Kenneth. 9 June 1959 [CW 5:5:8]
The Spectator, 'A psychiatrist's choice'. 12 February 1954, No. 6555, 13. [CW 4:3:3]
Spence, Marjorie. 23 November 1967 (1987, Letter 112, pp. 172–173) [CW 8:1:33]
Spence, Marjorie. 27 November 1967 (1987, Letter 113, pp. 173–174) [CW 8:1:34]
Spock, Benjamin. 9 April 1962 (1987, Letter 84, pp. 133–138) [CW 6:3:3]
Stapleton, Thomas. 20 September 1954 [CW 4:3:23]
Stapleton, Thomas. 3 March 1955 [CW 5:1:3]
Stierlin, Helm. 31 July 1969 (1987, Letter 125, pp. 195–196) [CW 9:1:19]
Stone, L. Joseph. 18 June 1968 (1987, Letter 116, pp. 177–178) [CW 8:2:17]
Stone, Marjorie. 14 February 1949 (1987, Letter 11, pp. 14–15) [CW 3:4:3]
Storr, Charles Anthony. 30 September 1965 (1987, Letter 95, p. 151) [CW 7:2:15]
Strachey, James. 1 May 1951 (1987, Letter 18, p. 24) [CW 3:6:3]
Szasz, Thomas. 19 November 1959 (1987, Letter 77, pp. 126–127) [CW 5:5:19]
Thorner, Hans. 17 March 1968 [CW 7:3:5]
The Times [not published]. 6 November 1946 (1987, Letter 6, p. 9) [CW 3:1:5]
The Times [not published]. 1 November 1954 (1987, Letter 50, pp. 82–83) [CW 4:3:27]
The Times, '"Blood-tie" child'. 4 April 1966, Issue 56590, 1. [CW 7:3:11]
The Times, '"Blood-tie" child: Why the courts must act swiftly' (with J. Bowlby, M. Fordham, A. Freud, E. Miller, R. MacKeith, & K. Soddy). (24 March) 26 March 1966, Issue 56590, 11. [CW 7:3:9]
The Times, 'George III'. 17 January 1966, Issue 56531, 9. [CW 7:3:1]
The Times, 'I Qant stand it' [not published]. 11 April 1957 [CW 5:3:12]
The Times, 'Maladjusted children: Damaging effect of delay'. 13 May 1950, Issue 51690, 5. [CW 3:5:7]
The Times, 'Neglected children'. 31 January 1950, Issue 51603, 5 (1987, Letter 16, p. 21) [CW 3:5:3]
The Times, 'Nursery schools: A definition of functions'. 8 September 1951, Issue 52101, 7. [CW 3:6:11]
The Times, 'Nursery schools essential' [not published]. 25 March 1959 [CW 5:5:6]
The Times, 'Psychiatric care' [not published]. 3 March 1966 (1987, Letter 96, pp. 152–153) [CW 7:3:4]
The Times, 'Punishment and crime: A psychologist's view'. (10 August 1949) 23 August 1949, Issue 51467, 6 (1987, Letter 12, pp. 15–16). [CW 3:4:16]

The Times, 'Sponsored television' [not published]. 21 July 1954 (1987, Letter 46, pp. 76–77) [CW 4:3:20]
Tizard, J. Peter M. 23 October 1956 (1987, Letter 63, pp. 103–107) [CW 5:2:14]
Tod, Robert. 6 November 1969 (1987, Letter 126, pp. 196–197) [CW 9:1:22]
Torrie, Margaret. 4 September 1967 (1987, Letter 107, pp. 166–167) [CW 8:1:20]
Torrie, Margaret. 5 September 1967 (1987, Letter 108, pp. 167–169) [CW 8:1:21]
van der Waals, Herman Gijsbert. 23 July 1959 [CW 5:5:13]
Wilkinson, Agnes. 9 June 1969 (1987, Letter 123, p. 192) [CW 9:1:11]
Wilson, A. Tommy M. 23 September 1959 [CW 5:5:14]
Winnicott, Clare. Early 1950. [excerpt] (1978, p.31; 1989, p. 16-17). [CW 3:5:1]
Winnicott, Elizabeth (mother). ca. 2 September 1911-1913 (1978, pp. 24-25; 1989, p. 9) [CW 1:1:1]
Winnicott, Elizabeth (mother). ca. late 1916 [excerpt] (2003a, p. 34). [CW 1:1:9]
Winnicott, Elizabeth (mother). 10 September 1916 [short excerpts] (2003a, pp. 33–34). [Not published in the *Collected Works*]
Winnicott, John Frederick, Elizabeth, Violet, & Kathleen (family). 3 November 1913 [excerpt] (2003a, p. 27). [CW 1:1:4]
Winnicott, John Frederick, Elizabeth, Violet, & Kathleen (family). 9 May 1914 [excerpt] (2003a, pp. 27–28) [CW 1:1:7]
Winnicott, John Frederick, Elizabeth, Violet, & Kathleen (family). 9 December 1916 [excerpt] (2003a, pp. 35–36) [CW 1:1:10]
Winnicott, John Frederick, Elizabeth, Violet, & Kathleen (family). ca. 23 December 1913 [excerpt] (2003a, p. 27) [CW 1:1:5]
Winnicott, Violet (sister). 15 November 1919 (1987, Letter 1, pp. 1–4) [CW 1:1:11]
Wisdom, John O. 26 October 1964 [CW 7:1:11]
Young, Mr & Mrs. 28 July 1960 [CW 6:1:14]

Winnicott's Correspondents

Addis, Robina
(1900–86) One of the first professionally trained Psychiatric Social Workers in Britain, Addis also worked in the child guidance movement and extensively for the National Association for Mental Health.
ca. April 1936 [CW 1:4:8]

Aitken, Mrs P.
A reader of Winnicott's *The Child, the Family, and the Outside World*.
13 January 1967 [CW 8:1:1]

An American Correspondent (Mr Q.)
A man who had written to Winnicott about his personal problems.
14 January 1969 [CW 9:1:3]

Applebey, Mary
(1916–2012) The General Secretary of the National Association for Mental Health (1951–74), publisher of a monograph called 'The Case as the Patient Sees It', for which Winnicott wrote the preface.
27 May 1957 [CW 5:3:16]

Balint, Enid
(1903–84) Psychoanalyst and welfare worker, organiser of the Citizens' Advice Bureau in London on behalf of the Family Welfare Association.
22 March 1956 [CW 5:2:6]

Balint, Michael
(1896–1970) Hungarian-born psychoanalyst, member of the Middle Group, President of the British Psychoanalytic Society (1969–70) and President of the Medical Section of the British Psychological Society. He was author of *The Basic Fault, The Doctor, His Patient, and the Illness* and founder of 'Balint-groups' for the training of medical doctors and general practitioners in the psychological aspects of illness.
27 March 1957 [CW 5:3:9]
4 April 1957 [CW 5:3:10]
3 October 1957 [CW 5:3:24]
5 February 1960 [CW 6:1:2]

Baumann, Marianne
Swiss psychoanalyst.
20 January 1958 [CW 5:4:2]
5 June 1958 [CW 5:4:10]

Beveridge, Lord
William Beveridge (1879–1963), economist and social reformer, author of a report on the state of the health services in the United Kingdom which led to the introduction of a National Health Service.
15 October 1946 [CW 3:1:4]

Bick, Esther
(1902–93) Viennese-born psychoanalyst and member of the Kleinian group. In 1948, Bick was appointed head of the first child psychotherapy training at the Tavistock Clinic and is widely credited with recognising the value and defining the method of direct infant observation to psychotherapeutic training.
11 June 1953 [CW 4:2:9]

Bion, Francesca
(1922–2015) (née McCallum) Researcher at the Tavistock Clinic, wife of Wilfred Bion.
3 October 1957 [CW 5:3:25]

Bion, Wilfred R.
(1897–1979) Psychoanalyst and President of the British Psychoanalytic Society (1962–65). Recipient of a Distinguished Service Order during World War I, Bion read History at Oxford and subsequently trained in medicine, winning the gold medal for surgery from University College Hospital, London, in 1930. He was encouraged by Melanie Klein to train in psychoanalysis, becoming an analysand of the Kleinian John Rickman with whom he later developed the use of groups in military psychiatry during the 'Northfield experiments'. Bion's earlier works, *Second Thoughts* and *Learning from Experience*, and his work after moving to Los Angeles in 1968, have been extremely influential in different schools of contemporary psychoanalytic and psychological thought.
22 January 1951 [CW 3:6:2]
7 October 1955 [CW 5:1:16]
17 November 1960 [CW 6:1:18]
16 November 1961 [CW 6:2:23]
5 October 1967 [CW 8:1:23]

Bonnard, Augusta
(1903–74) Consultant physician at Paddington Green Children's Hospital with Winnicott in the 1930s, trained as a psychoanalyst with Anna Freud, founder and director of the East London Child Guidance Clinic after the war.
3 April 1952 [CW 4:1:6]

1 October 1957 [CW 5:3:22]
7 November 1957 [CW 5:3:28]

Bowlby, John
(1907–90) Psychiatrist, psychologist, psychoanalyst, and director of the Department for Children and Parents at the Tavistock Clinic for two decades, during which time he published his influential work on juvenile delinquency, *Forty-Four Juvenile Thieves*. Bowlby was instrumental in establishing the effects of separation between mother and infant as a subject of scientific research, and his three classic works *Attachment, Separation* and *Loss* form the foundation of Attachment Theory.
6 December 1938 [CW 1:4:20]
16 December 1939 (co-author of a letter to the *British Medical Journal*) [CW 2:1:6]
11 May 1954 [CW 4:3:11]
26 March 1966 (co-author of a letter to *The Times*) [CW 7:3:9]

Briance, Prunella
(b. 1926) The author of the book *Childbirth with Confidence*, published by the Natural Childbirth Association of Great Britain, for which Winnicott wrote the preface. Briance established the Association in 1956 to promote and understand the Dick-Read system of natural childbirth. The charity later became the Natural Childbirth Trust.
15 July 1957 [CW 5:3:19]

Britton, Clare
(1906–84) Social worker and psychoanalyst. Britton worked on the Oxfordshire evacuation programme during the war and was appointed the head of the first training course for social works at the London School of Economics. She was Director of Child Care Studies at the Home Office 1964–71. She married Donald Winnicott in 1951.
Early 1950 [CW 3:5:1]

Britton, Karl and Sheila
Karl (1909–83), older brother of Clare Winnicott (*née* Britton), chair of philosophy at Newcastle University and author of *Philosophy and the Meaning of Life*, and his wife Sheila.
25 November 1968 [CW 8:2:33]
7? December 1968 [CW 8:2:39]
14 December 1968 [CW 8:2:44]

Casuso, Gabriel
Cuban-born American psychoanalyst. In the early 1970s, Casuso was appointed the first Training and Supervising Analyst at the Florida Psychoanalytic Society.
4 July 1956 [CW 5:2:9]

Chamberlain, Anne
(1883–1967) Anne, wife of Neville Chamberlain, British Prime Minister (1937–40).
10 November 1938 [CW 1:4:19]

Chaplin, D.
Child psychotherapist.
18 October 1954 [CW 4:3:25]

Cheu, Tsuicheu
Paediatrician from Shanghai whom Winnicott met at the International Paediatric Congress in Copenhagen, 1956.
4 April 1957 [CW 5:3:11]

Coles, Joyce
Winnicott's secretary from 1948 until his death. Coles was married to Arthur Coles.
25 August 1968 [CW 12:5: caption 6]
22? November 1968 [CW 8:2:31]
25? November 1968 [CW 8:2:32]
26? November 1968 [CW 8:2:34]
29 November 1968 [CW 8:2:35]
1? December 1968 [CW 8:2:36]
4 December 1968 [CW 8:2:37]
8 December 1968 [CW 8:2:40]
10? December 1968 [CW 8:2:42]
14 December 1968 [CW 8:2:43]

Collinson, Michael P.
(Active from 1960s, retired 1996) British social scientist and farm economist working in Tanzania.
10 March 1969 [CW 9:1:7]

Conran, M. B.
(1923–2001) Psychoanalyst of the Middle Group and psychiatric registrar at Shenley Hospital from the late 1960s, at that time a progressive mental hospital near St Albans, UK.
8 May 1969 [CW 9:1:10]

Dahlberg, Charles Clay.
Research psychologist, physician and President (1967) of the William Alanson White Institute of Psychiatry, Psychoanalysis and Psychology, New York.
24 October 1967 [CW 8:1:26]

Davidson, S. S.
(1911–61) Sonny Davidson, physician and psychoanalyst who worked at the Cassel Hospital, UK.
5 May 1952 [CW 4:1:8]

Davis, John
Paediatrician at St Mary's, Paddington, colleague and friend of Winnicott, and later Foundation Professor of Paediatrics, Cambridge University.
1 January 1971 [CW 9:3:1]

Dick-Read, Grantly
(1890–1959) Obstetrician, promoter of natural childbirth and author of the books *Natural Childbirth* and *Revelation of Childbirth* (USA: *Childbirth Without Fear*).
15 January 1958 [CW 5:4:1]

Dowling, R. S. W.
Editor of the periodical *The Family Doctor*.
8 December 1967 [CW 8:1:36].

Ezriel, Henry
(1909–85) Psychoanalyst and member of the Tavistock Clinic.
20 June 1952 [CW 4:1:9]

Federn, Paul
(1871–1950) Viennese-born American psychologist, early contributor to the psychoanalytic literature on psychosis, most famous for his many papers in the field of ego psychology.
3 January 1949 [CW 3:4:1]

Fitzgerald, Otho
(1908–2000) Medical superintendent at Shenley hospital, St Albans, UK, and secretary of the International Conference on Psychotherapy, 1948.
3 March 1950 [CW 3:5:4]

FitzHerbert, Joan
Psychiatrist in the Child Guidance Service of the Kent Education Committee.
25 April 1961 [CW 6:2:7]

Fordham, Michael
(1905–95) Jungian analyst, founder of the Society of Analytical Psychology and co-editor of the Collected Works of Jung. A personal friend of Winnicott.
11 June 1954 [CW 4:3:16]
26 September 1955 [CW 5:1:14]
2 February 1965 [CW 7:2:2]
24 June 1965 [CW 7:2:8]
15 July 1965 [CW 7:2:9]
26 March 1966 (co-author of a letter to *The Times*) [CW 7:3:9]
10 March 1970 [CW 9:2:2]

Frank, Klara
Viennese psychoanalyst and associate of Anna Freud.
20 May 1954 [CW 4:3:13]

Franklin, Marjorie

(1877–1975) Psychoanalyst and psychiatrist, founder of the Planned Environment Therapy Trust and a co-founder of the Institute for the Scientific Treatment of Delinquency. Franklin introduced Winnicott to the Q Camps therapeutic community experiment, and to David and Ruth Wills, with whom he worked briefly at the Bicester Q Camp.

19 October 1944 [CW 2:6:12]

Freud, Anna

(1895–1982) Daughter of Sigmund Freud and one of the founders of child psychoanalysis. Anna Freud, along with other German and Austrian analysts, came to London at the invitation of Ernest Jones and the British Psychoanalytic Society in the 1930s. In London, she was founder of the Hampstead Child-Therapy Course and Clinic (now the Anna Freud Centre), the 'Hampstead war nurseries', and co-editor of *The Psychoanalytic Study of the Child*. The theoretical disagreements between Anna Freud and Melanie Klein formed the backdrop of psychoanalytic life and training in Britain throughout the middle of the twentieth century.

6 July 1948 [CW 3:3:5]
18 March 1954 [CW 4:3:7]
(and Melanie Klein) 3 June 1954 [CW 4:3:15]
18 November 1955 [CW 5:1:17]
14 May 1958 [CW 5:4:8]
8 June 1958 [CW 5:4:11]
7 November 1958 [CW 5:4:19]
26 March 1966 (co-author of a letter to *The Times*) [CW 7:3:9]
20 January 1969 [CW 9:1:6]

Friedlander, Kate

(1902–49) Viennese psychoanalyst and associate of Anna Freud.
8 January 1940 [CW 2:2:1]

Gaddini, Renata

(1919–2013) Italian psychoanalyst, Professor of Psychopathology of Development, La Sapienza University, Rome, and a foremost proponent of Winnicott in Italy. Gaddini worked on a translation of *The Family and Individual Development* which was not ultimately published.

26 June 1964 [CW 7:1:8]
13 September 1966 [CW 7:3:19]
21 November 1966 [CW 7:3:28]
9 March 1967 [CW 8:1:5]
4 September 1967 [CW 8:1:19]
21 November 1967 [CW 8:1:32]
21 October 1968 [CW 8:2:24]
ca. 9 December 1968 [CW 8:2:41]

(and family) 15 November 1969 [CW 9:1:24]
19 January 1969 [CW 9:1:5]
31 August 1970 [CW 9:2:7]

Gardner, Dorothy E. M.
(1900–92) A colleague of Susan Isaacs at the progressive Maltings House School, and Isaacs's successor at the Child Development Department of the Institute of Education, University of London, where Winnicott gave a regular lecture courses. Gardner was Susan Isaacs' first biographer, a book for which Winnicott wrote the Preface [CW 8:2:22].
13 July 1959 [CW 5:5:11]

Gillespie, William
(1901–2001) Psychoanalyst, President of the British Psychoanalytic Society (1950–53) and the International Psychoanalytic Association (1961–64).
29 September 1966 [CW 7:3:21]

Giovacchini, Peter
(1922–2004) Psychiatrist and psychoanalyst based in Chicago. Editor of the volume *Tactics and Techniques in Psychoanalytic Therapy* (1972), which included the first publication of Winnicott's *Holding and Interpretation*.
5 March 1970 [CW 9:2:1]

Glover, Edward
(1888–1972) Psychoanalyst and founding member of the British Psychoanalytical Society alongside Ernest Jones, with whom he fought for the recognition of psychoanalysis as a medical and scientific discipline. Glover resigned from the BPAS in 1944.
23 October 1951 [CW 3:6:13]

Gough, Donald
(b. 1925) Psychoanalyst and child psychiatrist at the Tavistock Clinic.
6 March 1968 [CW 8:2:7]

Guntrip, Harry
(1901–75) Psychoanalytic psychotherapist and analysand of both Fairbairn and Winnicott. Guntrip was formerly a Congregational minister and the author of several papers on the origin and treatment of schizoid phenomena.
20 July 1954 [CW 4:3:19]
13 August 1954 [CW 4:3:21]
15 September 1961 [CW 6:2:18]

Halmos, Paul
Lecturer in Psychology and Education at the University College of North Staffordshire, where Winnicott lectured in November 1959.
12 June 1959 [CW 5:5:9]

Harvard-Watts, John
(d. 1979) The founder of Tavistock Publications, publisher of several of Winnicott's books, including *The Child, the Family and the Outside World*.
28 July 1960 [CW 8:1:13]

Hazlehurst, R. S.
British Minister who responded to Winnicott's letter to *The Times*, 10 August 1949: 'Punishment and Crime, A Psychologist's View' [CW 3:4:16].
1 September 1949 [CW 3:4:17]

Heimann, Paula
(1899–1982) Psychoanalyst who emigrated from Berlin to London in 1933. An analysand and close associate of Klein until the mid-1940s, Heimann's important theory on countertransference precipitated a rift with Klein, and, in 1955, Heimann resigned from the Melanie Klein Trust to become a member of the independent Middle Group.
5 November 1959 [CW 5:5:18]

Hellman, Ilse
(1908–98) Psychoanalyst who had trained in juvenile delinquency and child development in Vienna and Paris before coming to London at the invitation of Anna Freud in 1942. Hellman qualified in London as a psychoanalyst while working with Anna Freud and Dorothy Burlingham at the Hampstead War Nurseries and Hampstead Child Therapy Clinic.
21 July 1960 [CW 6:1:12]

Henderson, Sir David
(1884–1965) Professor of psychiatry at Edinburgh University and co-author of the influential *Textbook of Psychiatry*.
10 May 1954 [CW 4:3:10]
20 May 1954 [CW 4:3:14]

Henry, Hannah
Known as 'Queen', Hannah Henry was a close friend of Winnicott from 1926 until his death. Winnicott stayed with Henry in Suffolk on his separation from his first wife Alice Taylor in 1949.
30 October 1950 [CW 3:5:12]

Hodge, S. H.
British Minister who responded to Winnicott's letter to *The Times*, 10 August 1949: 'Punishment and Crime, A Psychologist's View' [CW 3:4:16]
1 September 1949 [CW 3:4:18]

Hoffer, Willi
(1897–1967) Psychoanalyst and associate of Anna Freud.
4 April 1952 [CW 4:1:7]

James, Lydia
(d. 2001) Founder of *The Observer* newspaper column 'Within the family' in January 1960, under the pseudonym Bridget Colgan, which served as a model for the introduction of parenting and childcare advice columns in national newspapers in the UK.
20 January 1961 [CW 6:2:1]

James, Martin
(1914–92) British psychiatrist and psychoanalyst, member of the Middle Group and friend of Winnicott.
17 April 1957 [CW 5:3:13]
7 October 1965 [CW 7:2:17]

Jaques, Elliot
(1917–2003) Canadian-born London-based psychoanalyst and member of the Kleinian group. Founding member of the Tavistock Institute of Human Relations; founder of the School of Social Sciences at Brunel University, London; and an anonymous doctor on BBC *Woman's Hour* in the late 1940s. Jaques was a specialist in social and organizational development, and is perhaps best known for having coined the term 'mid-life crisis'.
13 October 1959 [CW 5:5:16]

Jones, Ernest
(1879–1958) Founder of the British Psychoanalytical Society and its President from 1913 to 1944. Jones, a member of Freud's original circle, was the central figure in British psychoanalysis for five decades. He was instrumental in bringing Melanie Klein, and later, the Freuds, to London.
22 July 1952 [CW 4:1:10]

Joseph, Betty
(1917–2013) Psychoanalyst and leading member of the Kleinian group, chairman of the Klein Trust for fifteen years and author of the influential paper 'Transference: The Total Situation'.
13 April 1954 [CW 4:3:8]

Kahne, Merton J.
(b. 1924) A doctor at McLean Hospital, Belmont, Massachusetts, where Winnicott gave two lectures during his US tour in October 1963.
19 February 1960 [CW 6:1:5]

Kalmanovitch, Jeannine
(1919–93) A friend of Winnicott and a translator of his work into French.
7 January 1971 [CW 9:3:2]
19 January 1971 [CW 9:3:3]

Khan, Masud

(1924–89) Editor of the International Psychoanalytical Library, controversial psychoanalyst, analysand and colleague of Winnicott, and one of his most persuasive proponents.
26 June 1961 [CW 6:2:13]

King, Pearl

(1918–2015) Psychoanalyst, member of the Middle Group, and the British Society's first non-medical President (1982–84).
18 July 1961 [CW 6:2:14]

Klein, Melanie

(1882–1960) Viennese psychoanalyst who trained with Ferenczi and Abraham before moving to London at the invitation of Ernest Jones in 1926. Klein supervised Winnicott during his training in child analysis and referred him for analysis to her follower Joan Riviere. Her theories of the depressive and paranoid-schizoid position, object relations, the good and bad breast, the pre-eminence of envy and guilt have become central to the British School of psychoanalysis. The theoretical disagreements between Melanie Klein and her followers and other groups in the BPAS formed the backdrop of psychoanalytic life and training in Britain throughout the middle of the twentieth century.
17 November 1952 [CW 4:1:12]
(and Anna Freud) 3 June 1954 [CW 4:3:15]
7 March 1957 [CW 5:3:7]

Knopf, Mrs B. J.

A mother who had written to Winnicott after the publication of his two letters to *The Observer* on autism in October and November 1964.
26 November 1964 [CW 7:1:15]

Kulka, Anna M.

(b. 1896) Child psychiatrist, Assistant Clinical Professor of Psychiatry, UCLA.
15 January 1957 [CW 5:3:1]

Lacan, Jacques

(1901–81) Influential French psychiatrist, psychoanalyst and intellectual, founder of the Société Française de Psychanalyse and, after his expulsion from this, the École Freudienne de Paris. Lacan commissioned the translation into French of Winnicott's 'Transitional Objects and Transitional Phenomena' for the journal *La Psychanlyse*.
11 February 1960 [CW 6:1:3]

Laing, R. D.

(1927–89) Scottish psychiatrist and psychoanalyst who trained in London at the BPAS while working at the Tavistock Clinic.
18 July 1958 [CW 5:4:14]

Lantos, Barbara
(1894–1962) Hungarian-born psychoanalyst. Lantos lectured on the Hampstead Child Therapy course and represented the Anna Freudian Group in the training committee of the British Society.
8 November 1956 [CW 5:2:15]

Lebovici, Serge
(1915–2000) French psychoanalyst, Professor Emeritus of Child Psychiatry and President of the International Psychoanalytic Association (1973–77).
8 November 1960 [CW 6:1:16]

Lewis, Sir Aubrey J.
(1900–75) Professor of Psychiatry and clinical director at the Maudsley Hospital, London, for more than twenty years.
26 January 1961 [CW 6:2:2]
13 October 1961 [CW 6:2:20]

Lightwood, Reginald
(1898–1985) Director of the Paediatric Unit of St Mary's Hospital Medical School, London. Lightwood would later become President of the British Paediatric Association.
10 February 1959 [CW 5:5:2]

Limentani, Adam
(1913–94) Psychiatrist, psychoanalyst, President of the British Psychoanalytical Society (1974–77) and the International Psychoanalytical Association (1981–85).
27 September 1968 [CW 8:2:23]

Lowry, Oliver H.
(1910–96) Biochemist and pharmacologist, Dean of the School of Medicine, Washington University, St Louis, Missouri.
5 July 1956 [CW 5:2:10]

Luria, Alexander
(1902–77) Renowned Soviet psychologist and neuropsychologist.
7 July 1960 [CW 6:1:11]

MacKeith, Ronald
(1908–77) British paediatrician trained at St Mary's Hospital, consultant at Guy's Hospital, the Tavistock Clinic (from 1950), and the Cassel Hospital (from 1960). Chairman of the Association of Child Psychology and Psychiatry, editor of the *Journal of Paediatric Neurology and Developmental Medicine*, and President of the Paediatrics Section of the Royal Society of Medicine.
31 January 1963 [CW 6:4:2]

Main, Thomas
(1911–90) Psychoanalyst and psychiatrist, Medical Director at the Cassel Hospital, Surrey. Author of *The Ailment*, Main coined the term 'the therapeutic community'.
24 January 1957 [CW 5:3:3]
25 February 1957 [CW 5:3:6]

Maw, Miss
An employee or stakeholder at Gisburne House, a children's home for girls in Watford, UK.
16 February 1959 [CW 5:5:3]

Mead, Margaret
(1901–77) American anthropologist and ethnologist who held the post of President of the World Federation for Mental Health as well as President of the Society for Applied Anthropology and the American Anthropological Association. Within an exceptionally wide range of research Mead published extensively on children and adolescents and popularised the term 'generation gap'.
31 January 1957 [CW 5:3:5]

Meltzer, Donald
(1922–2004) American-born London-based psychoanalyst, follower and developer of the theories of Klein and Bion.
21 May 1959 [CW 5:5:7]
25 October 1966 [CW 7:3:24]

Metcalfe, A. J.
(1895–1971) Director-General of Health, Australia (1947–60).
14 July 1959 [CW 5:5:12]

Miller, Arthur
(1915–2005) American playwright and author, second husband of Marilyn Monroe.
13 November 1967 [CW 8:1:31]

Emanuel Miller
(1893–1970) Psychiatrist at the Maudsley Hospital and founder and director of the East London Child Guidance Clinic.
16 December 1939 (co-author of a letter to the *British Medical Journal*) [CW 2:1:6]
26 March 1966 (co-author of a letter to *The Times*) [CW 7:3:9]

Money-Kyrle, Roger
(1898–1980) Psychoanalyst and follower of Melanie Klein. An analysand of Freud, Jones, and Klein, Money-Kyrle wrote widely on psychoanalysis and politics, philosophy economics, and anthropology.

13 May 1937 [CW 1:4:15]
22 March 1949 [CW 3:4:5]
31 March 1949 [CW 3:4:6]
2 May 1949 [CW 3:4:7]
13 June 1949 [CW 3:4:10]
22 June 1949 [CW 3:4:12]
24 June 1949 [CW 3:4:13]
10 July 1950 [CW 3:5:9]
8 August 1950 [CW 3:5:11]
16 November 1950 [CW 3:5:13]
27 November 1952 [CW 4:1:13]
23 September 1954 [CW 4:3:24]
10 February 1955 [CW 5:1:1]
17 March 1955 [CW 5:1:6]

Nagera, Humberto
(b. 1927) Cuban-born child psychiatrist and psychoanalyst, associate of Anna Freud at the Hampstead Clinic until the late 1960s, later Professor Emeritus of Psychiatry at the University of Michigan and the University of South Florida.
15 February 1965 [CW 7:2:3]

Nelson, Gillian
A reader of *The Child, the Family, and the Outside World.*
6 October 1967 [CW 8:1:24]

North, Roger
A magistrate and Chairman of the Quarter Sessions (later District Courts) in Norfolk, UK, who had written to Winnicott for advice on treatments for juvenile delinquency.
January 1944 [CW 2:6:1]

Parfitt, D. N.
Australian psychiatrist at Claremont Hospital, Western Australia.
22 December 1966 [CW 7:3:35]

Payne, Sylvia
(1880–1976) Psychoanalyst who held every post in the British Society, including President, twice, from 1944 to 1947 and 1954 to 1956. Payne was central to the organisation and handling of the Controversial Discussions, brokering the agreement between Anna Freud and Melanie Klein which led to the emergence of three training groups within the BPAS.
7 October 1953 [CW 4:2:13]
26 May 1966 [CW 7:3:15]

Peller, Lili E.
(1898–1966) Lay psychoanalyst and educator primarily in New York and Philadelphia, and founder of the Montessori school movement in Austria.
15 April 1966 [CW 7:3:13]

Raison, Timothy
(1929–2011) Editor of the periodical *New Society*.
9 April 1963 [CW 6:4:6]

Rapaport, David
(1911–60) Hungarian-born American clinical psychologist and psychoanalyst, working at the Menninger Clinic, Topeka, KS (1940–48) and, after that, at the Austen Riggs Center, Stockbridge, Massachusetts
9 October 1953 [CW 4:2:14]

Ries, Hannah
(ca. 1886–1970) Psychoanalyst, associate of Anna Freud in London, later emigrating to Los Angeles.
27 November 1953 [CW 4:2:15]

Riviere, Joan
(1883–1962) Psychoanalyst, supporter and follower of Melanie Klein and Winnicott's second analyst. Riviere was also a co-founder of the BPAS and an early translator of Freud.
19 May 1949 [CW 3:4:9]
24 June 1949 [CW 3:4:14]
3 February 1956 [CW 5:2:3]
21 June 1957 [CW 5:3:18]
13 June 1958 [CW 5:4:12]

Rodman, F. Robert
(1934–2004) Los Angeles-based psychoanalyst, editor of *The Spontaneous Gesture: Selected Letters of D. W. Winnicott* and author of *Winnicott: Life and Work*.
10 January 1969 [CW 9:1:2]

Rodrigue, Emilio
(1923–2008) Argentinian psychoanalyst who trained with Klein in London.
17 March 1955 [CW 5:1:5]

Rosenbluth, Michael
Winnicott's physician in the Cardiac Care Unit of Lenox Hill Hospital, New York.
3 January 1969 [CW 9:1:1]

Rosenfeld, Herbert
(1910–86) Psychoanalyst, supporter and developer of Klein's theories, Chairman of the Melanie Klein Trust, 1968–82.

22 January 1953 [CW 4:2:2]
17 February 1953 [CW 4:2:3]
16 October 1958 [CW 5:4:16]
17 March 1966 [CW 7:3:6]

Rycroft, Charles F.
(1914–98) Psychoanalyst, essayist and author, including of *A Critical Dictionary of Psychoanalysis*. Rycroft resigned from the British Society in 1968 to devote himself to a literary career.
5 February 1954 [CW 4:3:2]
21 April 1955 [CW 5:1:8]
7 October 1956 [CW 5:2:12]
17 October 1956 [CW 5:2:13]
17 January 1957 [CW 5:3:2]

Sargant, William W.
(1907–88) Psychiatrist and physician in charge of the department of psychological medicine at St Thomas's Hospital, London, and supporter of physical and organic treatments for mental disorder.
24 January 1969 [CW 9:1:12]

Schulz, Charles
(1922–2000) American cartoonist, best know for the comic strip 'Peanuts'.
1955 [CW 5:1:22]

Scott, Peter D.
(1914–77) Consultant psychiatrist at the Maudsley Hospital in London and psychiatrist in charge of a London County Council remand home.
11 May 1950 [CW 3:5:6]

Scott, W. Clifford M.
(1903–97) Canadian-born London-based psychoanalyst, analysand of Melanie Klein and friend of Winnicott. Scott worked at the Maudsley Hospital and the Cassel Hospital in London, and he was elected President of the British Psychoanalytic Society in 1953. He later returned to Canada to found the Canadian Psychoanalytic Society.
19 March 1953 [CW 4:2:5]
27 January 1954 [CW 4:3:1]
26 February 1954 [CW 4:3:4]
13 April 1954 [CW 4:3:9]

Segal, Hanna
(1918–2011) Psychoanalyst and follower of Melanie Klein.
21 February 1952 [CW 4:1:3]
22 January 1953 [CW 4:2:1]
6 October 1955 [CW 5:1:15]

Sharpe, Ella Freeman

(1857–1947) Psychoanalyst, intermediary during the Controversial Discussions and member of the Middle Group. Her 1937 work *Dream Analysis*, which linked dream work and poetic diction, influenced Lacan, among others.
13 November 1946 [CW 3:1:6]

Smirnoff, Victor

(1919–95) French psychoanalyst, friend of Masud Khan, and translator of Winnicott and Klein into French.
19 November 1958 [CW 5:4:20]

Soddy, Kenneth

(1911–86) Child psychiatrist, consultant and physician in charge of the Department of Child and Adolescent Psychiatry at University College Hospital, London, and author of the textbook *Clinical Child Psychiatry*.
9 June 1959 [CW 5:5:8]

Spence, Marjorie

A member of the public and reader of *The Child, the Family, and the Outside World*.
23 November 1967 [CW 8:1:33]
27 November 1967 [CW 8:1:34]

Spock, Benjamin

(1903–98) American paediatrician, author of the popular and influential manual *Baby and Child Care*.
9 April 1962 [CW 6:3:3]

Stapleton, Thomas

(1920–2007) Paediatrician and colleague of Winnicott at St Mary's Hospital, London during the 1950s. Professor of paediatrics at the University of Sydney, Australia from 1960.
20 September 1954 [CW 4:3:23]
3 March 1955 [CW 5:1:3]

Stierlin, Helm

(b. 1926) German psychoanalyst, psychiatrist and author, worker at the National Institute of Mental Health, Bethseda, Maryland (1965–73), later director of the Department of Psychoanalytic Research and Family Therapy in Heidelberg, Germany.
31 July 1969 [CW 9:1:19]

Stone, L. Joseph

(1912–75) Professor of Child Study at Vassar College, Poughkeepsie, New York, and early user of film recording in the study of child behaviour.
18 June 1968 [CW 8:2:17]

Stone, Marjorie
A manufacturer of children's toys.
14 February 1949 [CW 3:4:3]

Storr, Charles Anthony
(1920–2001) British psychiatrist and psychotherapist, and a prolific writer and broadcaster.
30 September 1965 [CW 7:2:15]

Strachey, James
(1887–1967) Winnicott's training analyst, translator and General Editor of *The Standard Edition of the Complete Psychological Works of Sigmund Freud*.
1 May 1951 [CW 3:6:3]

Szasz, Thomas
(1920–2012) American psychiatrist and psychoanalyst, Professor of Psychiatry at the State University of New York.
19 November 1959 [CW 5:5:19]

Mrs T.
A mother who had written to ask Winnicott for advice.
6 September 1968 [CW 8:2:20]

Thorner, Hans
(1905–91) German born physician and psychoanalyst, analysand of Klein and Bion who worked at Shenley Hospital, St Albans, during the war and later at the Cassel Hospital, London.
17 March 1968 [CW 7:3:5]

Tizard, J. Peter M.
(1916–93) Paediatrician at Paddington Green and St Mary's Hospitals, colleague and friend of Winnicott, reader and then professor at the Institute of Child Health, Royal Postgraduate Medical School, London (1954–72), first professor of paediatrics at the University of Oxford (1972–83).
23 October 1956 [CW 5:2:14]

Tod, Robert
(1915–2008) Consultant paediatrician at Alder Hey Children's Hospital and Liverpool Maternity H ospital, Liverpool. Winnicott wrote the preface for a volume of papers edited by Tod, *Disturbed Children*, to which Clare Winnicott also contributed.
6 November 1969 [CW 9:1:22]

Torrie, Margaret
(1912–99) Social worker and founder of Cruse Clubs, which later grew into Cruse Bereavement Care, the first national organisation for widows and their children.

4 September 1967 [CW 8:1:20]
5 September 1967 [CW 8:1:21]

van der Waals, Herman Gijsbert
(1894–1974) Director of the Menninger Memorial Hospital, Topeka, Kansas.
23 July 1959 [CW 5:5:13]

Wilkinson, Agnes
(1915–2005) South African-born physician and psychoanalytic psychotherapist, psychiatric advisor at the London School of Economics, President of the British Association of Health Services in Higher Education.
9 June 1969 [CW 9:1:11]

Wilson, A. Tommy M.
Psychiatrist, first Chairman of the Tavistock Clinic, London (1946–56).
23 September 1959 [CW 5:5:14]

Winnicott, Elizabeth
(1862–1925) Winnicott's mother.
ca. 2 September 1911–13 [CW 1:1:1]
ca. late 1916 [CW 1:1:9]

Winnicott, Violet
(1889–1984) The elder of Winnicott's two sisters.
15 November 1919 [CW 1:1:11]

Winnicott's family
Winnicott's father Sir John Frederick Winnicott (1855–1948), twice mayor of Plymouth; his mother Elizabeth; and his sisters Kathleen and Violet.
3 November 1913 [CW 1:1:4]
ca. 23 December 1913 [CW 1:1:5]
9 May 1914 [CW 1:1:7]
9 December 1916 [CW 1:1:10]

Wisdom, John O.
(1904–93) Professor of philosophy, London School of Economics; founding president of the Society for Psychosomatic Research; editor of the *Journal for the Philosophy of Science*; prolific contributor of articles on psychoanalysis; analysand of Ernest Jones.
26 October 1964 [CW 7:1:11]

Young, Mr and Mrs
The authors of a questionnaire sent to Winnicott.
28 July 1960 [CW 6:1:14]

PART 3

Winnicott's Lectures, Broadcasts, and Audio Recordings

Winnicott's Lectures

November 1926	The Only Child [CW 2:7:1]	Lecture to the National Society of Day Nurseries
22 November 1929	Enuresis [Abstract; CW 1:2:17]	Section for the Study of Disease in Children, Royal Society of Medicine
4 December 1935	The Manic Defence [CW 1:4:6]	Membership paper given to the British Psychoanalytical Society, London
17 April 1936	The Teacher, the Parent and the Doctor [CW 1:4:10]	Ideals in Education Conference, Lady Margaret Hall, Oxford
25 September 1936	Mental Hygiene of the Pre-school Child [CW 1:4:9]	A talk given to nursery school teachers, Conference of the Nursery School Association, Hull
1936	Appetite and Emotional Disorder [CW 1:4:11]	Medical Section, British Psychological Society, London
ca. September 1939	The Deprived Mother [CW 2:1:4]	BBC radio broadcast (uncertain)
1939	Children in the War [CW 2:2:4]	BBC radio broadcast (uncertain)
23 April 1941	Observations on Asthma in an Infant and Its Relation to Anxiety [The Observation of Infants in a Set Situation; CW 2:3:6]	British Psychoanalytical Society, London
3 June 1942	Report on Child Department Consultations [CW 2:4:2]	British Psychoanalytical Society, London
14 May 1943	Observations of Infant Behaviour During Routine Clinical Examination [Abstract in 'The Observation of Infants in a Set Situation', fn. i; CW 2:3:6]	The 15th Annual General Meeting of the British Paediatric Association, Council Chamber, Town Hall, Llandudno, Wales
10 December 1943	Getting to Know Your Baby [CW 2:5:8]	Radio broadcast, *Happy Children*, BBC Home Service
11 December 1943	The Wearing of Masks in the Nursing of Premature and Older Infants [Abstract CW 2:5:9]	Extraordinary General Meeting of the British Paediatric Association, 11 Wimpole St, London
4 February 1944	Why Does Your Baby Cry? Part 1 [Why Do Babies Cry?; CW 2:6:2]	Radio broadcast, *Happy Children*, BBC Home Service
7 February 1944	Psychological Aspects of the Birching of Children [CW 2:6:3]	Contribution to a discussion at a luncheon, Howard League for Penal Reform

11 February 1944	Why Does Your Baby Cry? Part 2 [Why Do Babies Cry?; CW 2:6:2]	Radio broadcast, *Happy Children*, BBC Home Service
15 March 1944	Kinds of Psychological Effect of Shock Therapy [CW 2:6:7]	Paper prepared for a symposium on the Psychoanalytic Contribution to the Theory of Shock Therapy, British Psychoanalytical Society, London
17 March 1944	Where Does Dad Come In? [What About Father?; CW 2:6:8]	Radio broadcast, *Happy Children*, BBC Home Service
12 May 1944	Their Standards and Yours [CW 2:6:9]	Radio broadcast, *Happy Children*, BBC Home Service
23 June 1944	What Do We Mean by a Normal Child? [CW 2:6:10]	Radio broadcast, *Happy Children*, BBC Home Service
6 December 1944	The Psychoanalytic Patient's Wish for Further Treatment	British Psychoanalytical Society, London
2 February 1945	The Only Child [CW 2:7:1]	Radio broadcast, *Difficult Children*, BBC Home Service
16 February 1945	The Evacuated Child [CW 2:7:2]	Radio broadcast, *Difficult Children*, BBC Home Service
23 February 1945	Return of the Evacuated Child [CW 2:7:3]	Radio broadcast, *Difficult Children*, BBC Home Service
27 April 1945	Twins [CW 2:7:5]	Radio broadcast, *Difficult Children*, BBC Home Service
22 June 1945	Home Again [CW 2:7:7]	Radio broadcast, *Health Magazine*, BBC Home Service
10 October 1945	Looking Forward to Your Baby's Arrival [CW 12:3:4a]	First in a series of two radio broadcasts, *The New Baby*, BBC Home Service
2 August 1945	The Value of Breast-feeding (Psychological) [Abstract in Breast-feeding, fn *ii*; CW 2:7:12]	The 16th Annual General Meeting of the British Paediatric Association, Rugby School, Warwickshire
14 November 1945	Getting to Know Your Baby [CW 12:3:4b]	Second in a series of two radio broadcasts, *The New Baby*, BBC Home Service
28 November 1945	Primitive Emotional Development [CW 2:7:8]	British Psychoanalytical Society, London
1945	What Is Psychoanalysis? [Towards an Objective Study of Human Nature; CW 2:7:11]	A talk given to the Eighth Form of St Paul's School, London, at the invitation of the Headmaster
15 January 1946	Bringing Up Children	Radio broadcast, *Home in Civvy Street*, hosted by Ruth Drew, BBC Light Programme
6 November 1946	Consultation Technique	British Psychoanalytical Society, London
27 November 1946	Physical Therapy of Mental Disorder [CW 3:2:2]	British Psychoanalytical Society, London, Medical Section
1946	Some Psychological Aspects of Juvenile Delinquency [CW 3:1:7]	An address to magistrates
ca. 1940s (n.d.)	Some Psychological Aspects of Juvenile Delinquency [CW 3:1:8]	An address to probation officers
5 February 1947	Some Observations on Hate [Hate in the Countertransference; CW 3:2:1]	British Psychoanalytical Society, London

December 1947	Aggression in Relation to Emotional Development [CW 3:5:2]	Contribution to a symposium, Royal Society of Medicine, London
7 January 1948	Reparation in Respect of the Mother's Depression [CW 3:3:1]	British Psychoanalytical Society, London
28 January 1948	Paediatrics and Psychiatry [CW 3:3:2]	Address from the Chair, British Psychological Society, Medical Section, London
ca. July 1948	Disorders of Childhood [CW 3:3:8]	Lecture given to the Institute of Public Health and Hygiene, London
Autumn 1948	Primary Introduction to External Reality [CW 3:3:12]	One of a series of talks given to students, Institute of Education, University of London
1948–49	The Infancy of Juliet [CW 3:4:4]	Manuscript dated 1 March 1949. Probably one of a series of lectures given to students, Institute of Education, University of London
1948–49	Environmental Needs; the Early Stages; Total Dependence and Essential Independence [CW 3:3:13]	Probably a lecture to students, Institute of Education, University of London
ca. 1949	Enuresis [CW 3:4:36]	Lecture at Tavistock Clinic Children's Department, London
18 May and 15 June 1949	The Present Position of Birth Trauma in Psychoanalytic Theory [CW 3:4:8]	Two lectures given at the British Psychoanalytical Society, London
5 October 1949	How's the Baby?: Caring for Children and How Babies Develop Their Personalities [A Man Looks at Motherhood; CW 3:4:23]	First in a series of nine radio broadcasts: 'The Ordinary Devoted Mother and Her Baby', *How's the baby?* BBC Home Service
12 October 1949	The Mind of a Child [The Baby as a Going Concern; CW 3:4:24]	Second in a series of nine radio broadcasts: 'The Ordinary Devoted Mother and Her Baby', *How's the baby?*, BBC Home Service
19 October 1949	The Baby and Its Food [Where the Food Goes; CW 3:4:25]	Third in a series of nine radio broadcasts: 'The Ordinary Devoted Mother and Her Baby', *How's the baby?* BBC Home Service
26 October 1949	The Passing of Excretions [The End of the Digestive Process; CW 3:4:26]	Fourth in a series of nine radio broadcasts; 'The Ordinary Devoted Mother and Her Baby', *How's the baby?* BBC Home Service
2 November 1949	No Baby Can Grow Properly Without Love [The Baby as a Person; CW 3:4:27]	Fifth series of nine radio broadcasts: 'The Ordinary Devoted Mother and Her Baby', *How's the baby?* BBC Home Service
9 November 1949	The Baby at Feeding Time [Close-up of Mother Feeding Baby; CW 3:4:28]	Sixth in a series of nine radio broadcasts: 'The Ordinary Devoted Mother and Her Baby', *How's the baby?* BBC Home Service
16 November 1949	Presenting the World to a Baby [The World in Small Doses; CW 3:4:29]	Seventh in a series of nine radio broadcasts: 'The Ordinary Devoted Mother and Her Baby', *How's the baby?* BBC Home Service

23 November 1949	Problems of Management: Training Babies [CW 12:3:4c]	Eighth in a series of nine radio broadcasts: 'The Ordinary Devoted Mother and Her Baby', *How's the baby?* BBC Home Service
30 November 1949	Weaning CW 3:4:31	Ninth in a series of nine radio broadcasts: 'The Ordinary Devoted Mother and Her Baby', *How's the baby?* BBC Home Service
22 March 1950	Management: Knowing and Learning How to Be a Mother [Knowing and Learning; CW 3:5:14]	Radio broadcast, *How's the Baby?* BBC Home Service
29 March 1950	Symptoms of Illness [Instincts and Normal Difficulties; CW 3:5:15]	Radio broadcast, *How's the Baby?* BBC Home Service
19 April 1950	A Case of Anorexia Nervosa	British Psychoanalytical Society, London
July 1950	The Deprived Child and How He Can Be Compensated for Loss of Family Life [CW 3:5:10]	Lecture to the Nursery School Association
1950	Yes, But How Do We Know It's True? [CW 3:5:18]	A talk given to students of psychology and social work, London School of Economics
16 May 1951	Visiting Children in Hospital Part 1 [CW 3:6:5]	Radio broadcast, *Woman's Hour* BBC Light Programme
23 May 1951	Visiting Children in Hospital Part 2 [CW 3:6:5]	Radio broadcast, *Woman's Hour* BBC Light Programme
30 May 1951	Children in Hospital: A Discussion of Responses to 'Visiting Children in Hospital' (with Ronald MacKeith, and two nurses, Mrs Cullen and Mrs Boote)	Radio broadcast: *Woman's Hour* BBC Light Programme
30 May 1951	Transitional Objects and Transitional Phenomena [Lecture Notes; CW 3:6:6] [Paper; CW 4:2:21, CW 5:4:24, CW 9:3:5]	British Psychoanalytical Society, London
13 November 1951	Notes on the General Implications of Leucotomy [CW 3:6:14]	Presentation given to open a discussion at London School of Economics
9 January 1952	The Baby as a Going Concern [CW 3:4:24]	Radio broadcast, *Woman's Hour*, BBC Light Programme, The Ordinary Devoted Mother and Her Baby 1
16 January 1952	The First Week [CW 4:1:1]	Radio broadcast, *Woman's Hour*, BBC Light Programme, The Ordinary Devoted Mother and Her Baby 2
23 January 1952	Breast Feeding [Close-up of Mother Feeding Baby; CW 3:4:28]	Radio broadcast, *Woman's Hour*, BBC Light Programme, The Ordinary Devoted Mother and Her Baby 3
30 January 1952	Baby Bites [CW 4:1:12]	Radio broadcast, *Woman's Hour*, BBC Light Programme, The Ordinary Devoted Mother and Her Baby 4

30 February 1952	My Fan Mail (Commenting on listeners' letters concerning the four previous talks) [CW 12:3:4d]	Radio broadcast, *Woman's Hour*, BBC Light Programme, The Ordinary Devoted Mother and Her Baby
March 1952	Psychoses and Childcare [CW 4:1:5]	Psychiatry Section of the Royal Society of Medicine, London
2 May 1952	Vivian, A Fatal Case of Anorexia Nervosa. Part II: The Analytic Work	British Psychoanalytical Society, London
5 November 1952	Anxiety Associated with Insecurity [CW 4:1:11]	British Psychoanalytical Society, London
27 February 1953	Symptom Tolerance in Paediatrics [CW 4:2:4]	Presidential address to the Section of Paediatrics, Royal Society of Medicine, London
18 March 1953	The Management of a Case of Compulsive Thieving (consideration of the bearing of the case, that was treated without psychoanalysis, on a psychoanalytic theory)	British Psychoanalytical Society, London
3 December 1953	A talk given to Child Care Officers [Two Adopted Children; CW 4:2:19]	
February 1954	The Depressive Position in Normal Emotional Development [CW 4:3:5]	Medical Section of the British Psychological Society, London
17 March 1954	Metapsychological and Clinical Aspects of Regression Within the Psychoanalytic Set-up [CW 4:3:6]	British Psychoanalytical Society, London
November 1954	Withdrawal and Regression [CW 4:3:29]	XVIIème Conférence des Psychanalystes de Langues Romanes, Paris
23 February 1955	On Adoption: Homeless Children and Childless Homes [On Adoption; CW 5:1:2]	Radio broadcast, *Woman's Hour*, BBC Light Programme
17 April 1955	Private Practice [CW 5:1:7]	Annual conference of the British Psychological Society, Durham
April 1955	Group Influences and the Maladjusted Child: The School Aspect [CW 5:1:9]	A lecture to the Association of Workers for Maladjusted Children
7 June 1955	Counterfeit and Alone: The Wicked Stepmother in the Storytelling of All Ages. Fairy Stories. [For Stepparents, part 1 CW 5:1:10]	Second in a series of four radio broadcasts, *Woman's Hour*, BBC Light Programme
8 June 1955	Counterfeit and Alone: Shall We Keep Superficial or Go Deep? Is there a Rival Even if Dead? [For Stepparents, Part 2; CW 5:1:10]	Third in a series of four radio broadcasts, *Woman's Hour*, BBC Light Programme
9 June 1955	Counterfeit and Alone: Every One of us is Unsuccessful Somewhere. Who Knows All the Answers? Who is a Stranger to Doubt? [For Stepparents, Part 3; CW 5:1:10]	Fourth in a series of four radio broadcasts, *Woman's Hour*, BBC Light Programme

29 June 1955	Withdrawal and Regression [CW 4:3:29]	British Psychoanalytical Society, London
July 1955	Clinical Varieties of the Transference [CW 5:1:11]	19th International Psychoanalytic Congress, Geneva
31 January 1956	How Much Do We Know About Babies as Cloth-Suckers? [CW 5:2:1]	Radio broadcast, *Woman's Hour*, BBC Light Programme
April 1956	Psychoanalysis and the Sense of Guilt [CW 5:2:7]	Lecture given in a series as part of the celebrations of the centenary of Freud's birth, at Friends' House, London
20 June 1956	Study of Anti-social Tendency [CW 5:2:8]	British Psychoanalytical Society, London
25 July 1956	Paediatrics and Childhood Neurosis [CW 5:2:11]	Paper read by invitation before the 8th International Congress of Paediatrics, Copenhagen, Denmark
30 January 1957	Presidential Opening Address Introducing Margaret Mead [CW 5:3:4]	8th Ernest Jones Lecture, British Psychoanalytical Society, London
May 1957	The Contribution of Psychoanalysis to Midwifery [CW 5:3:15]	Lecture given at a course organized by the Association of Supervisors of Midwives
24 July 1957	On the Capacity to Be Alone [CW 5:3:20]	British Psychoanalytical Society, London
28 July–1 August 1957	On the Contribution of Direct Child Observation to Psychoanalysis [CW 5:3:21]	20th International Psycho-Analytical Congress, Paris, France
3 October 1957	Hallucination and Dehallucination [CW 5:3:23]	Written for a seminar
3 October 1957	The Family [Integrative and Disruptive Factors in Family Life; CW 5:3:26]	The first of a series of public lectures given at Goldsmiths' College under the general title 'Children out of School'
6 November 1957	Advising Parents [CW 5:3:27]	Royal College of Midwives: Approved Refresher Course for Midwives, Brighton
November–December 1957	Course of six lectures to student nurses	Princess Louise Hospital Training School, part of St Mary's Hospital, Paddington, London
5 December 1957	Coronary Thrombosis [Excitement in the Aetiology of Coronary Thrombosis; CW 5:3:29]	The Society for Psychosomatic Research, London
14 February 1958	Funeral Address for Ernest Jones [CW 5:4:3]	Golders Green Crematorium, London
Spring 1958	Course of ten lectures	Institute of Education in Child Development Department, University of London
16 and 23 May 1958	Paediatrics	A course of four lectures for Almoner students, The Institute of Almoners
18 May 1958	What Makes a Family Tick Over? [Integrative and Disruptive Factors in Family Life; CW 5:3:26]	A lecture to The Association of Child Care Officers, Conference at Swanwick, Derbyshire

19 June 1958	Psychotherapeutic Methods: Child Analysis [Child Analysis in the Latency Period; CW 5:4:13]	4th International Congress for Child Psychiatry, Lisbon, Portugal
Summer 1958	Adult Personality Patterns	Five Lectures to the Child Care Course, London School of Economics
1 November 1958	The Family Affected by Depressive Illness of One or Both Parents [CW 5:4:17]	Family Service Units, Caseworkers' Study Weekend, The Hayes Conference Centre, Swanwick, Derbyshire
Academic Year 1958–59	A Clinical Approach to Family Problems [See CW 5:5:27]	Ten lectures on Human Growth and Development, Applied Social Studies, London School of Economics
9 February 1959	Four Doctors, Answering Listeners' Questions (as a contributor)	Radio broadcast, *Parents and Children*, BBC Network Three
Spring 1959	Series of nine lectures	Child Development Department, Institute of Education, University of London
15 March 1959	Dr Ernest Jones	Radio broadcast, Welsh Home Service and Home Service (London)
18 March 1959	Classification [CW 5:5:5]	British Psychoanalytical Society, London
3 April 1959	Problems of Adoption: The Psychiatrist's Approach	Institute for the Scientific Treatment of Delinquency conference, Bracklesham Bay, West Sussex
29 May 1959	Illegitimacy and the Broken Home	'Crime: A Challenge Society', Oxford University
2–29 August 1959	World Health Organisation Conference (as a medical consultant)	Case conferences, therapeutic supervision, and course of lectures to psychiatrists, psychologists and social workers. Helsinki, Finland
10 October 1959	Casework with Mentally Ill Children [CW 5:5:15]	The Association of London County Council Child Welfare Officers, Inter-Services Conference on the theme 'Casework Horizons', Friends' House, London
7 November 1959	Maternal Care and the Welfare State (with Dr Alice Stewart, Reader in Social Medicine at the University of Oxford)	University College of North Staffordshire, Departments of Education and Psychology
25 November 1959	Countertransference [CW 5:5:20]	Symposium on Countertransference, British Psychological Society, Medical Section, London
28 November 1959	The Effect of Psychotic Parents on the Emotional Development of the Child [CW 5:5:21]	The Association of Psychiatric Social Workers, Middlesex Hospital, Courtauld Lecture Theatre
5 December 1959	Clinical Notes Illustrating the Fate of Transitional Objects [The Fate of the Transitional Object; CW 5:5:22]	The Association for Child Psychiatry and Psychology, The Royal Hospital for Sick Children, Glasgow
12 January 1960	Adoption	Adoption Case Committee, East Sussex County Council, Children's Department, County Hall, Lewes

14 January– 11 February 1960	Series of five lectures	Child Development Department, Institute of Education, University of London
25 January 1960	Saying 'No' to Young Children 1 – Some Occasions for Saying 'No' [Part of CW 6:1:1]	First in a series of eleven radio broadcasts: 'The Ordinary Devoted Mother and Her Children', *Parents and Children*, BBC Network Three
1 February 1960	Saying 'No' to Young Children 2 – Saying 'No' isn't Just Saying 'No' [Part of CW 6:1:1]	Second in a series of eleven radio broadcasts: 'The Ordinary Devoted Mother and Her Children', *Parents and Children*, BBC Network Three
8 February 1960	Saying 'No' to Young Children 3 – The Basis of 'No' is 'Yes' [Part of CW 6:1:1]	Third in a series of eleven radio broadcasts: 'The Ordinary Devoted Mother and Her Children', *Parents and Children*, BBC Network Three
15 February 1960	Some Family Jealousies which are Only to be Expected [Part of CW 6:1:4]	Fourth in a series of eleven radio broadcasts: 'The Ordinary Devoted Mother and Her Children', *Parents and Children*, BBC Network Three
20 February 1960	The Effect of Psychosis on Family Life [CW 6:1:6]	The Association of Child Care Officers, Kingsway Hall, London
22 February 1960	The Beginnings of Jealousy [Part of CW 6:1:4]	Fifth in a series of eleven radio broadcasts: 'The Ordinary Devoted Mother and Her Children', *Parents and Children*, BBC Network Three
29 February 1960	Why Jealousy Disappears [Part of CW 6:1:4]	Sixth in a series of eleven radio broadcasts: 'The Ordinary Devoted Mother and Her Children', *Parents and Children*, BBC Network Three
5 March 1960	Clinical Material	The Child Development Society (London Group), Institute of Education, University of London
7 March 1960	Jealousy: How the Parents' Care can Help [Part of CW 6:1:4]	Seventh in a series of eleven radio broadcasts: 'The Ordinary Devoted Mother and Her Children', *Parents and Children*, BBC Network Three
12 March 1960	Lecture	Association of Adult Psychotherapists
14 March 1960	What Irks the Ordinary Mother? [Part of CW 6:1:7]	Eighth in a series of eleven radio broadcasts: 'The Ordinary Devoted Mother and Her Children', *Parents and Children*, BBC Network Three
21 March 1960	More that Irks, and Why [Part of CW 6:1:7]	Ninth in a series of eleven radio broadcasts: 'The Ordinary Devoted Mother and Her Children', *Parents and Children*, BBC Network Three
28 March 1960	What Irks a Mother – More Variations on the Theme, Discussed by Some Mothers [Part of CW 6:1:7]	Tenth in a series of eleven radio broadcasts: 'The Ordinary Devoted Mother and Her Children', *Parents and Children*, BBC Network Three

Winnicott's Lectures

10 April 1960	The Relationship of a Mother to Her Baby at the Very Beginning [CW 6:1:8]	The Association of Workers for Maladjusted Children study conference: 'Aims of Work with Maladjusted Children', Newnham College, Cambridge
18 April 1960	Too Much Security? [On Security; CW 6:1:9]	Radio broadcast, *Parents and Children*, BBC Network Three
8 May 1960	Aggression, Destruction and Reparation [Aggression, Guilt and Reparation; CW 6:1:10]	The Progressive League, Psychology Group, London
19 May 1960	The Relation of the Nursery School to the Child's Own Home	The Nursery School Association, Bradford and West Riding Branch
May 1960	Two case discussions	Informal group of child psychotherapists (ex-Tavistock Clinic)
Summer term 1960	Series of ten lectures	Course in Applied Social Studies, London School of Economics
6 October 1960	Integrating and Disintegrating Factors in Family Life [Integrative and Disruptive Factors in Family Life; CW 5:3:26]	10th Anniversary of Child Psychiatry, Montreal Children's Hospital and McGill University, Montreal, Canada
7 October 1960	The Doctor in Illness and in Health and Panel on Infant Observation	10th Anniversary of Child Psychiatry, Montreal Children's Hospital and McGill University, Montreal, Canada
10 October 1960	Parent-Infant Relationship Paper Preview [See 'The Parent-Infant Relationship'; CW 6:1:21.]	Canadian Psycho-Analytic Society, Montreal, Canada
12 November 1960	The Family and Emotional Maturity [CW 6:1:17]	Society for Psychosomatic Research, London
Academic year 1960–61	Series of fourteen lectures	Clinical Aspects of Child Development, to Mental Health Course Students, London School of Economics
26 November 1960	The Emotional Development of the Child	National Association for Mental Health, weekend course for General Practitioners on 'Psychiatry for the G.P.' The Kenilworth Hotel, London
22 February 1961	Emotionally Disturbed Adolescents [Adolescence: Struggling Through the Doldrums; CW 6:2:4]	A lecture to Senior Officers of London County Council Children's Department
February–March 1961	Series of five lectures	Course in Child Development, London University
8 March 1961	Some Varieties of Psychotherapy [CW 6:2:5]	Mental Illness Association Social and Medical Aspects (MIASMA), Newnham College, Cambridge
13 March 1961	Guilt Feelings in Young Mothers (a discussion with Claire Rayner) [Feeling Guilty; CW 6:2:6]	Radio broadcast: 'Feeling Guilty', *Parents and Children*, BBC Network Three
Summer term 1961	A Clinical Approach to Family Problems	Series of ten lectures, course in Applied Social Studies, London School of Economics

19 May 1961	Psychoanalysis and Science: Friends or Relations? [CW 6:2:9]	Oxford University Scientific Society
31 May 1961	Lecture	Tavistock Clinic group, London
4 June 1961	The Time Factor in Treatment [CW 6:2:11]	West Sussex County Council Children's Committee, 11th Annual Weekend Conference, Lodge Hill, Pulborough
26 July 1961	The Squiggle Technique in Child Psychiatry	Pre-Congress talk, Bedford College, London
July–August 1961	The Parent-Infant Relationship [CW 6:1:21]	22nd International Psychoanalytical Association Congress, Edinburgh
8 September 1961	Psycho-Neurosis in Childhood [CW 6:2:17]	Scandinavian Orthopsychiatric Congress, Helsinki
7 March 1962	The Aims of Psychoanalytic Treatment [CW 6:3:2]	British Psychoanalytical Society, London
April–July 1962	Series of ten lectures to students on 'A Clinical Approach to Family Problems' [see also CW 5:5:27]	Course in Applied Social Studies, London School of Economics
29 May 1962	An Account of an Interview with the Parent of a Child Patient	The 1952 Club, British Psychoanalytical Society, London
11 June 1962	Right and Wrong [The Development of a Child's Sense of Right and Wrong; CW 6:3:4]	Eleventh in a series of radio broadcasts: 'The First Five Years', *Parents and Children*, BBC Network Three
13 June 1962	Training for Child Psychiatry [CW 6:3:5]	Scientific Meeting of the Association for Child Psychology and Psychiatry, Royal Society of Medicine, London
20 June 1962	A Child Psychiatry Consultation	Department of Child and Family Psychiatry, Ipswich and East Suffolk Hospital
25 June 1962	Now They Are Five [The Five-Year-Old; CW 6:3:6]	Thirteenth in a series of radio broadcasts: 'The First Five Years', *Parents and Children*, BBC Network Three
3 October 1962	Didactic Statement on Child Development [A Personal View of the Kleinian Contribution; CW 6:3:8]	Lecture for candidates, Los Angeles Institute for Psychoanalysis
4 October 1962	Dependence in Infant-Care, in Child-Care, and in the Psycho-Analytic Setting [CW 6:3:9]	Los Angeles Psychoanalytical Society
6 October 1962	A Child Psychiatry Interview [CW 10:1:6]	San Francisco Psychoanalytic Institute, Curriculum Committee Colloquium for advanced students
7 October 1962	Providing for the Child in Health and Crisis [CW 6:3:10]	San Francisco Psychoanalytic Institute, Extension Division Workshop

8 October 1962	Communication Between Individuals Examined with Reference to the Development of a Capacity for Object Relationships in the Individual Infant [Communicating and Not Communicating Leading to a Study of Certain Opposites; CW 6:4:8]	San Francisco Psychoanalytic Society
12 October 1962	The Development of the Capacity for Concern [CW 6:3:11]	Topeka Psychoanalytic Society, Topeka, Kansas
15 October 1962	The Psycho-analyst and Child Psychiatry: A Matter of Economics [CW 6:3:12]	Forums Committee, Menninger School of Psychiatry, Topeka, Kansas
22 October 1962	Psychiatric staff conference	Beth Israel Hospital, Boston, Massachusetts
24 October 1962	Dependence in Infant-Care, in Child-Care, and in the Psycho-Analytic Setting [CW 6:3:9]	Boston Psychoanalytic Society
25 October 1962	Seminar with Paediatricians	Beth Israel Hospital, Boston, Massachusetts
27 October 1962	A Psychiatric Child Consultation	State University of New York, Division of Psychoanalytic Education
17 November 1962	Winnicott and Crime	National Association of Probation Officers, London branch, weekend conference: 'Aspects of Psychoanalytic Thought', Collington House, Bexhill-on-Sea
20 November 1962	The Young Child at Home and at School [Morals and Education; CW 6:3:18]	Public lecture: 'Moral Education in a Changing Society', Institute of Education, University of London
Autumn and Spring terms 1962–63	Clinical Aspects of Child Development	Series of fourteen lectures, course in Mental Health, London School of Economics
Autumn and Spring terms 1962–63	A Clinical Approach to Family Problems [see CW 5:5:27]	Series of ten lectures, course in Applied Social Studies, London School of Economics
8 February 1963	Adoption	Oxford City Children's Department committee on adoption
Spring term 1963	Series of five lectures	Child Development Department, Institute of Education, University of London
6 April 1963	The Mentally Ill in Your Caseload [CW 6:4:5]	Association of Social Workers, St Hilda's College, Oxford
26 April 1963	Seminar with Child Care Officers	Oxford
15 May 1963	Communicating and Not Communicating Leading to a Study of Certain Opposites [CW 6:4:8]	British Psychoanalytical Society, London
3 June 1963	Psychotherapy of Character Disorders [CW 6:4:9]	11th European Congress of Child Psychiatry, Rome, Italy

5 June 1963	A Child Psychiatry Interview Illustrating the Antisocial Tendency	Italian Psycho-Analytical Society, Rome
5 June 1963	A Child Psychiatry Interview Illustrating the Squiggle Technique	Child Psychiatry Department, The Children's Hospital, Rome
24 July 1963	A Psychotherapeutic Interview in Child Psychiatry	Pre-Congress Clinical Seminar, 23rd International Psychoanalytic Congress, Stockholm, Sweden
28 September 1963	The Value of Depression [CW 6:4:10]	The Association of Psychiatric Social Workers, General Meeting
30 September 1963	Hostels (discussion with a group of wardens)	The Rainer Foundation
11 October 1963	Dependence to Independence [From Dependence Towards Independence in the Development of the Individual; CW 6:4:11]	Atlanta Psychiatric Clinic, Atlanta, Georgia
12 October 1963	Psychotherapeutic Interview	Atlanta Clinic, Atlanta, Georgia
14 October 1963	Psychiatric Disorder in Terms of Infantile Maturational Processes [CW 6:4:12]	Dorothy Head Memorial Lecture, Philadelphia Psychiatric Society, The Institute of the Pennsylvania Hospital, Philadelphia
16 October 1963	Dependence to Independence [From Dependence Towards Independence in the Development of the Individual; CW 6:4:11]	Baltimore Psychiatric Society, Maryland
18 October 1963	The Individual and the Community and Hospital Care Supplementing Intensive Psychotherapy in Adolescence [CW 6:4:13]	Clinical Symposium: 'The Individual and the Community: Current Perspectives in Rehabilitation'. McLean Hospital, Belmont, Massachusetts
Weekly, October 1963–Spring 1964	Series of fourteen lectures	Course in Mental Health, London School of Economics
6 November 1963	A Child Psychiatry Case	Scientific Meeting, British Psychoanalytical Society, London
20 November 1963	A Psychotherapeutic Consultation	The Maudsley Hospital Children's Department, London
21 November 1963	Envy	The Albion Group, London
23 November 1963	The Maladjusted Child and Society	Association of Workers for Maladjusted Children
28 November 1963	The Interrelationship of Individual Growth Processes and Social Provision	Cambridge University Sociological Society
29 January 1964	The Concept of the False Self [CW 7:1:1]	'Crime: A Challenge' Society, All Souls College, Oxford
7 and 14 February 1964	Two lectures to postgraduate students	Institute of Education, London University
1 April 1964	The Neonate and His Mother [CW 7:1:4]	Symposium: Neuroclinical, neurophysiological and psychological problems of the neonate, Clinica Pediatrica dell' università di Roma, Italy

11 April 1964	Deductions Drawn from a Psychotherapeutic Interview with an Adolescent [CW 7:1:5]		Inter-Clinic Child Guidance Conference, National Association of Mental Health, London School of Economics
29 April 1964	Problems Arising out of Therapy of Individuals in Relation to Residential Care		Residential Child Care Course, Ruskin College, Oxford
29 April 1964	Report of an interview with a mother		Residential Child Care Course, Ruskin College, Oxford
8 May 1964	The Origins of Violence		Campaign for Nuclear Disarmament, Kings College, Cambridge University
21 May 1964	The Psychosomatic Dilemma [Psycho-somatic Illness in Its Positive and Negative Aspects; CW 7:1:6]		Society for Psycho-somatic Research, London
30 May 1964	The Early Mother-Child Relationship as a Contributory Factor to Psychotic Developments in the Child		One-day conference at High Wick Children's Hospital, St Albans
May 1964	Three lectures to students		Tavistock Institute of Human Relations, London
Monthly from May 1964	Monthly seminars with a group of paediatricians		87 Chester Square, London[1]
Weekly from May 1964	Series of ten lectures		Course in Applied Social Studies, London School of Economics
9 July 1964	The Importance of the Setting in Meeting Regression in Psycho-analysis [CW 7:1:9]		Written for a seminar given to third-year students, Institute of Psychoanalysis, London
12 July 1964	The Birth of the Power Complex		Progressive League, Psychology Group, London
1 August 1964	The True and the False Self [The Concept of the True and False Self; CW 7:1:1]		The Davidson Clinic Summer School, Edinburgh
2 August 1964	The Positive Aspect of Antisocial Behaviour with Illustrative Case		The Davidson Clinic Summer School, Edinburgh
3 August 1964	Special Talent Helping or Hindering Therapy		The Davidson Clinic Summer School, Edinburgh
3 weeks, September 1964	Consultations and discussions in various child psychiatry clinics		Under the auspices of the World Health Organisation, Finland
17 October 1964	Writing for Oneself or for an Audience? [part of 'The Squiggle Game'; CW 8:2:47]		The London Association for the Teaching of English, College of St Mark and St John, Chelsea
October 1964–May 1965	Series of fourteen lectures		Course in Mental Health, London School of Economics
20 or 28 November 1964	This Feminism [CW 7:1:14]		The Progressive League weekend conference on 'The Sexes Today', High Leigh, Hertfordshire

[1] Winnicott's home and consulting address.

January–March 1965	Therapeutic Consultations in Child Psychiatry	A series of ten seminars to child psychiatrists, organised by the National Association of Mental Health and the Institute of Child Health, at Great Ormond St Hospital, London
3 January 1965	New Light on Children's Thinking [CW 7:2:1]	Introductory lecture to a conference at the Devon Centre for Further Education
27 January 1965	The Psychotherapist: On Whose Side?	Medical Section of the British Psychological Society, London
25 February 1965	The Price of Disregarding Psychoanalytical Research Findings [CW 7:2:4]	National Association of Mental Health, Annual Conference: The Price of Mental Health. Church House, Westminster
12 April 1965	Do Progressive Schools Give Too Much Freedom to the Child? [CW 7:2:5]	Dartington Hall Conference: The Future for Progressive Education
May–July 1965	Series of ten lectures	Combined social studies students, London School of Economics
June 1965	Four seminars to third-year students	Institute of Psychoanalysis, London
11 June 1965	Two lectures to students at the Residential Child Care Course	Ruskin College, Oxford
18 and 25 June 1965	Some selected aspects of psychology	Two lectures to postgraduate students, Department of Child Development, Institute of Education, University of London
Academic year, 1965–1966	Bi-monthly seminars with a group of paediatricians	
7 July 1965	A Child Psychiatry Case: Description of a Psychotherapeutic Interview	Scientific Meeting, British Psychoanalytical Society, London
19 July 1965	Pre-congress seminar, Supervisory Session (with Dr E. A. Childe)	24th International Psychoanalytical Association Congress, Amsterdam, The Netherlands
October 1965–February 1966	Series of fourteen lectures	Course in Mental Health, London School of Economics
17 November 1965	Description of a Psychotherapeutic Interview with a Child, Illustrating the Point of Origin of the Antisocial Tendency	Residential Child Care Association, Winchester branch, Horseshoe Lodge, Hampshire
September–December 1965	Therapeutic Consultations in Child Psychiatry	A series of ten seminars to child psychiatrists, organised by the National Association for Mental Health and the Institute of Child Health, Mary Ward Settlement
December 1965	Seminar: Withdrawal and Regression [Case Notes for a Psychoanalytic Seminar: Withdrawal, Regression, Male Identification; CW 7:2:19]	
20 January 1966	Becoming Deprived as a Fact: Description of a Psychotherapeutic Consultation ['Ruth' aet 8 Years; CW 10:3:17]	Association of Child Psychotherapists (Non-Medical), the Tavistock Institute of Human Relations

21 and 28 January 1966	Selected Aspects of Psychology	University of London course for postgraduate teachers
2 February 1966	The Split-off Male and Female Elements to be Found Clinically in Men and Women: Theoretical Inferences [CW 7:3:2; and CW 9:3:7]	Scientific Meeting, British Psychoanalytical Society, London
16 February 1966	The Ordinary Devoted Mother [CW 7:3:3]	The Nursery School Association, Middlesex Guildhall, London
26 February 1966	Discussion of the Management of the Second Stage of the Psychoanalytic Treatment of a Case of Anorexia Nervosa	One of three papers of a workshop on the subject of co-operation, Leiden Institutes of Paediatrics and Child Psychiatry, Leiden, The Netherlands
26 February 1966	Description of a Psychotherapeutic Interview	Paediatric staff of the University Hospital Children's Department, Leiden, The Netherlands
7 March 1966	The Delusional Transference	Milan Psychoanalytical Institute, Milan, Italy
26 March 1966	Social Aspects of Autism [CW 7:3:7]	Society for Autistic Children. City of Leicester College
28 April–21 July 1966	Therapeutic Consultations in Child Psychiatry: A series of ten seminars to psychoanalysts	The Institute of Psychoanalysis, London
12 and 19 May 1966	Two lectures in the course Dynamics of Family Relationships	Tavistock Clinic students, London
21 May 1966	The Possible Significance of the Nurse Scene in Romeo and Juliet [see also 'The Infancy of Juliet'; CW 3:4:4]	Advanced course past students, Child Development Society, Institute of Education, University of London
4 June 1966	A weekend of seminars on child psychiatry (with Dr W. Granoff)	Child Guidance Clinic, Neuilly, France
21 June 1966	Description of a Psycho-therapeutic Interview	Association for Child Psychology and Psychiatry, Welsh Branch, Cardiff, Wales
30 June 1966	Lessons Learned in a London County Council Rheumatism Supervisory Clinic	Symposium on Cardiac Neurosis in Children, Association of European Paediatric Cardiologists, Annual General Meeting, Helsinki, Finland
26 July 1966	The Child and the Family [The Child in the Family Group; CW 7:3:17]	Nursery Schools Association Conference: Developments in Primary Education. New College, Oxford
19 August 1966	Every Week Has a Thursday. Interview with Jocelyn Rider-Smith on the book *Dibs: In Search of Self*, by Virginia Axline [Review: Axline, *Dibs in Search of Self*; CW 7:3:10]	Radio broadcast, *Woman's Hour*, BBC Home Service
8 October 1966	Speech on the Occasion of the Publication of the *Standard Edition* of the Psychological Works of Freud [CW 7:3:23]	Connaught Rooms, London

17 October 1966	Adolescence as a Developmental Phenomenon	Parents' day at Frensham Heights, Farnham, Surrey
25 October 1966	The Effect of Modern Life on Today's Children	Sociological Society of the College of St Mark and St John, Chelsea
5 November 1966	Creative Living in Marriage [Living Creatively; CW 9:2:11]	Progressive League Weekend Conference: 'Creativity in the Man–Woman Relationship', High Leigh, Hoddesdon, Hertfordshire
10 November 1966	Series of five seminars: The Psychotherapeutic Interview	Child Guidance Training Centre, London
29 November 1966	Maturational Processes and the Facilitating Environment	Conference for heads of schools in Surrey: 'Expanding frontiers of understanding school-children and ourselves', Moor Park College, Farnham
7 December 1966	The Location of Cultural Experience [CW 7:3:31]	Scientific Meeting, British Psychoanalytical Society, London
9 December 1966	Counseling in Schools: Its Relation to Social Work and Psychotherapy	Postgraduate teachers, University of Exeter Institute of Education
9 December 1966	Informal talk to a group of social workers	Topsham, Devon
10 December 1966	The Absence of a Sense of Guilt [CW 7:3:32]	Devon and Exeter Association for Mental Health
16 January 1967	What Is a Freudian in 1967? Interview with Penelope Leach	Radio broadcast, BBC Network Three
26 January 1967	The Relation of Dr Winnicott's Theory to Other Formulations of Early Development [see 'D. W. W. on D. W. W.'; CW 8:1:2]	The 1952 Club, British Psychoanalytical Society, London
February 1967	Series of eight lectures on 'A Clinical Approach to Family Problems'	Students of the Applied Social Studies Course, London School of Economics
17 February 1967	The A.C.P.P. Observed as a Group [CW 8:1:3]	Presidential address, A.G.M. of the Association for Child Psychology and Psychiatry, London
8 March 1967	The Concept of a Healthy Individual [CW 8:1:4]	Royal Medico-Psychological Association, Psychotherapy and Social Psychiatry Section, at the Royal Society of Medicine, London
15 March 1967	Discussion around a clinical detail	Scientific Meeting, British Psychoanalytical Society, London
17 March 1967	The Bearing of Emotional Environmental Development on Feeding Problems [Environmental Health in Infancy; CW 8:1:6]	Gerber Baby Council: 'Health in Infancy', Royal Society of Medicine, London
13 April 1967	Principles of Direct Therapy in Child Psychiatry ['Ruth' aet 8 Years; CW 10:3:17]	Judge Baker Guidance Center 50th anniversary, Boston, Massachusetts
19 April 1967	Delinquency as a Sign of Hope [CW 8:1:8]	Borstal Housemaster's Conference, King Alfred's College, Winchester, Hampshire

26 April 1967	Seminar	Hampstead Child Psychotherapy Course and Clinic, London
6 May 1967	Psychotherapy in Childhood [The Non-pharmacological Treatment of Psychosis in Childhood; CW 8:1:9]	Concilium Paedopsychiatricum. Union of European Paedopsychiatrists, European Congress of Child Psychiatry, Wiesbaden, Germany
18 May 1967	Seminar for post-graduate registrars	The Maudsley Hospital Psychotherapy Unit, London
1 and 16 June 1967	Some Selected Aspects of Psychology	Postgraduate teachers, Institute of Education, University of London
2 June 1967	Meeting the Challenge of the Case	The Bush Lecture, The Mulberry Bush School, Oxfordshire
8 June 1967	Talk at the Inaugural Meeting	Association for Mental Health, Plymouth
22 June 1967	Talk at Parents' Evening	Chelsea Open-Air School
28 June 1967 and 5 July 1967	Two lectures to the students	Tavistock Centre, London
17 and 18 July 1967	Two pre-congress seminars	University College, London
27 July 1967	Symposium: Paediatrics and Child Analysis [Note of a Contribution to Symposium on Child Analysis and Paediatrics; CW 10:1:1, see also 'Iiro' aet 9 Years 9 Months; CW 10:1:1]	25th International Psychoanalytic Association Congress, Copenhagen, Denmark
25 September 1967	Two lectures to the Residential Child Care Course	Ruskin College, Oxford
27 September 1967	Seminar with the student group	Family Welfare Association
7 October 1967	Therapeutic Consultation Illustrating Child Psychiatry Practiced by a Psycho-analyst	Association of Child Psychology and Psychiatry, Scottish Branch. David Hume Tower, Edinburgh University
From 10 October 1967	Fourteen lectures on Clinical Aspects of Child Development	Mental Health Course, London School of Economics
From 17 October 1967	Child psychiatry seminars with a group from the Tavistock Centre	Institute of Psychoanalysis, London
18 October 1967	Towards a Theory of Psychotherapy: The Link with Playing [Playing: A Theoretical Statement; CW 8:2:15]	Scientific Meeting, British Psychoanalytical Society, London
25 October 1967	Creative Activity and the Search for the Self: An Added Observation on Psychotherapy in This Area [Playing: Creative Activity and the Search for the Self; CW 8:1:27]	Medical Section, British Psychological Society, London
27 October 1967	The Concept of Clinical Regression Compared with that of Defence Organisation [CW 8:1:29]	Symposium on the nature of psychotherapy with schizophrenic patients, McLean Hospital, Boston, Massachusetts
4 December 1967	Survey of Child Development Leading up to the Concept of the Self as a Whole	Institute of Education, London University

5 December 1967	Case Material Illustrating Communication with a Child	Students' Union, College of St Mark and St John, Chelsea
13 January 1968	Ten lectures on 'A Clinical Approach to Family Problems' [see CW 5:5:27]	Course in Applied Social Studies, London School of Economics
19 January 1968	The Place Where We Live [CW 8:2:1]	The Geigy Bequest Lecture, Sussex Postgraduate Federation, Brighton General Hospital
23 January 1968	Communication Between Infant and Mother, and Mother and Infant, Compared and Contrasted [CW 8:2:2]	British Psychoanalytical Society 'Winter Lectures' on Psychoanalysis, London
24 January and 21 February 1968	Two Seminars: Psychotherapeutic Consultations	London Borough of Hammersmith Children's Service
22 February 1968	History-taking in Terms of an Interview with a Child	Folkestone Medical Society, Grand Hotel, Folkestone
26 February 1968	The Effects of Early Family Development on Personality	Bachelor of Education students, Ripon College, Yorkshire
29 February 1968	Mental Care Begins at Birth	The 59 Society of Kensington, at Kensington Central Library, London
12 March 1968	Playing and Culture [CW 8:2:9]	The Imago Group, London
22 March 1968	Towards a Theory of Psychotherapy: The Link with Playing [Playing: A Theoretical Statement; CW 8:2:15]	Rome Psycho-Analytic Society, Rome, Italy
22 March 1968	Psychotherapeutic Consultation	Clinica Pediatrica Universita di Roma (Professor Colarizi), Italy
17 April 1968	*Sum*, I Am [CW 8:2:10]	Association of Teachers of Mathematics, Whitelands College, London
30 April 1968	Psychology and Literature: The Problem of Identity	Jesus College Literary Society, Cambridge
8 May 1968	Psychotherapeutic Consultation	Association of Child Psychology and Psychiatry
13 May 1968	The Effect of Loss on the Young [CW 8:2:12]	Cruse Clubs, Annual General Meeting
14 May 1968	Psychotherapy	Psychological Society of Sussex University
24 May 1968	A Link Between Paediatrics and Child Psychology: Clinical Observations [CW 8:2:14]	The Catherine Chisholm Memorial Lecture, Institute of Child Health, Manchester University
24 May 1968	Student tutorial	Manchester University
31 May and 7 June 1968	Two lectures to post-graduate students: 'Some Selected Aspects of Psychology'	University of London Institute of Education
5 June 1968	Children Learning [CW 8:2:16]	Christian Teamwork Institute of Education, Conference on Family Evangelism
14 June 1968	Two lectures to the Residential Child Care Course	Ruskin College, Oxford
23 June 1968	Children and Death (discussion with Derek Hart)	*Meeting Point*, BBC One Television

18 July 1968	Changing Patterns: The Young Person, the Family and Society [Contemporary Concepts of Adolescent Development and Their Implications for Higher Education; CW 9:3:9]	Symposium: 'Contemporary concepts in adolescent development and their implications in higher education'. 21st annual meeting of the British Student Health Association, Newcastle
24 September 1968	The Transmission of Theory and Technique, My Own in Particular [See 'D. W. W. on D. W. W.'; CW 8:1:2]	1952 Club, British Psychoanalytical Society, London
September–November 1968	Seminars with a group mostly from the Tavistock Centre	Institute of Psychoanalysis, London
24 October 1968	Seminar	Sheffield University Psychology Society
8 November 1968	The Exploitation of the First Interview with a Child: A Study of the Dangers and the Potential Value of Such Procedure [see 'First Interview with Child May Start Resumption of Maturation'; CW 8:2:27, and '"Hesta" aet 16 Years'; CW 10:2:11]	The American Association of Psychiatric Clinics for Children, at the Waldorf Hotel, New York
11 November 1968	Seminar with graduates and candidates	William Alanson White Institute, New York
12 November 1968	The Use of an Object [The Use of an Object and Relating Through Identifications; CW 8:2:28]	New York Psychoanalytic Society
28 November 1968	Breast-feeding as Communication [CW 8:2:26]	Read in Winnicott's absence at a conference of the National Childbirth Trust, London
19 March 1969	Symposium on Envy and Jealousy [CW 9:1:8]	British Psychoanalytical Society, London. Read in Winnicott's absence by Enid Balint.
23 April 1969	Psychological Problems of the Toddler	Society of Medical Officers of Health, Manchester
From 6 May 1969	Six lectures	Course in Applied Social Studies, London School of Economics
June–July 1969	Seminars with a group mostly from the Tavistock Centre	Institute of Psychoanalysis, London
24 June 1969	Child Development and Maladjustment Course	Institute of Education, University of London
9 July 1969	Seminar with staff of the Battered Babies Department	National Society for the Protection of Cruelty to Children
~~29 September 1969~~[2]	Two seminars to students	Ruskin College, Oxford

---

[2] Some dates and lectures had been struck through on one of the source material lists in Winnicott's archive, presumably due to Winnicott's ill health at this time.

~~13 October 1969~~	Controlled and Uncontrolled Regression to Dependence	Grubb Institute of Behavioural Studies
~~23 October 1969~~	Seminars on Child Psychiatry Consultations	87 Chester Square, London
~~8 November 1969~~	Winnicott on the Pill [The Pill; CW 9:1:23]	Progressive League weekend conference: 'Men, Women and the Future'
~~8 January 1970~~	Seminar with students	The Tavistock Centre, London
~~20 April 1970~~	Child Psychiatry, Social Work and Alternative Care	A lecture to the Association of Child Psychiatry and Psychology, Newcastle
~~From 28 April 1970~~	~~Six seminars~~	~~London School of Economics~~
~~4 June 1970~~	Seminar at the Battered Babies Unit	National Society for the Protection of Cruelty to Children
~~9 July 1970~~	~~Growth and Development and Its Effect on Education~~	~~World Organisation for Early Childhood Education, International Seminar on the educational value of play, Bristol~~
2 and 9 July 1970	Two lectures	Institute of Education, University of London
14 July 1970	The Theology of Power	Post graduation training course, Bishops Stortford
28 September 1970	Two seminars	Ruskin College, Oxford University
5 October 1970	Other Sex Identifications	Society of Analytical Psychology Ltd.
8 October 1970	Interdependence of Psychoanalyst and Mental Hospital	Shenley Hospital Psychiatric Society
Fortnightly from 22 October 1970	Seminars on Psychotherapeutic Interview	87 Chester Square, London
18 October 1970	Cure: A Talk to Doctors [CW 9:2:8]	St Luke's Church, Hatfield
23 October 1970	Residential Care as Therapy [CW 9:2:9]	The David Wills Lecture, Association of Workers for Maladjusted Children
28 October 1970	Individuation [CW 9:2:10]	Medical Section, British Psychological Society
1 December 1970	The Family Today	Southlands College of Education, Wimbledon, London

Winnicott's Broadcasts

1939

[Children in the War. ca. September 1939. Uncertain] [CW 2:2:4]
[The Deprived Mother. 1939. Uncertain] [CW 2:1:4]

1943

Getting to Know Your Baby. Quigley, J. (Producer) *Happy Children*. Home Service. 10 December 1943. [CW 2:5:8]

1944

Why Does Your Baby Cry? I. Quigley, J. (Producer) *Happy Children*. Home Service. 4 February 1944. [Why Do Babies Cry?; CW 2:6:2]
Why Does Your Baby Cry? II. Quigley, J. (Producer) *Happy Children*. Home Service. 11 February 1944. [Why Do Babies Cry?; CW 2:6:2]
Where Does Dad Come In? Quigley, J. (Producer) *Happy Children*. Home Service. 17 March 1944. [What About Father?; CW 2:6:8]
Their Standards And Yours. Quigley, J. (Producer) *Happy Children*. Home Service. 12 May 1944. [CW 2:6:9]
What Do We Mean by a Normal Child? Quigley, J. (Producer) *Happy Children*. Home Service. 23 June 1944. [CW 2:6:10]

1945

The Only Child. Quigley, J. (Producer) *Difficult Children*. Home Service. 2 February 1945. [CW 2:7:1]
The Evacuated Child. Quigley, J. and Bridgman, D. (Producers) *Difficult Children*. Home Service. 16 February 1945. [CW 2:7:2]
Return of the Evacuated Child. Quigley, J. and Bridgman, D. (Producers) *Difficult Children*. Home Service. 23 February 1945. [CW 2:7:3]
Twins. Quigley, J. and Bridgman, D. (Producers) *Difficult Children*. Home Service. 27 April 1945. [CW 2:7:5]

Home Again. Quigley, J. and Bridgman, D. (Producers) *Health Magazine*. Home Service. 22 June 1945. [CW 2:7:7]

Looking Forward to Your Baby's Arrival. Benzie, I. (Producer) *The New Baby*. Home Service. 10 October 1945. [CW 12:3:4a]

Getting to Know Your Baby. Benzie, I. (Producer) *The New Baby*. Home Service. 14 November 1945. [CW 12:3:4b]

1946

Bringing Up Children. Gibbs, E. (Producer) *Home in Civvy Street*, presented by Ruth Drew. Light Programme. 15 January 1946.

1949

How's the Baby? Caring for Children and How Babies Develop Their Personalities. Benzie, I. (Producer) *How's the Baby?* Home Service. 5 October 1949. [A Man Looks at Motherhood; CW 3:4:23]

The Mind of a Child. Benzie, I. (Producer) *How's the Baby?* Home Service. 12 October 1949. [The Baby as a Going Concern; CW 3:4:24]

The Baby and Its Food. Benzie, I. (Producer) *How's the Baby?* Home Service. 19 October 1949. [Where the Food Goes; CW 3:4:25]

The Passing of Excretions. Benzie, I. (Producer) *How's the Baby?* Home Service. 26 October 1949. [The End of the Digestive Process; CW 3:4:26]

No Baby Can Grow Properly Without Love. Benzie, I. (Producer) *How's the Baby?* Home Service. 2 November 1949. [The Baby as a Person; CW 3:4:27]

The Baby at Feeding Time. Benzie, I. (Producer) *How's the Baby?* Home Service. 9 November 1949. [Close up of Mother Feeding Baby; CW 3:4:28]

Presenting the World to a Baby. Benzie, I. (Producer) *How's the Baby?* Home Service. 16 November 1949. [The World in Small Doses; CW 3:4:29]

Problems of Management: Training Babies. Benzie, I. (Producer) *How's the Baby?* Home Service. 23 November 1949. [CW 12:3:4c, see also 'The Innate Morality of the Baby'; CW 3:4:30]

Weaning. Benzie, I. (Producer) *How's the Baby?* Home Service. 30 November 1949. [CW 3:4:31]

1950

Management: Knowing and Learning How to Be a Mother. Benzie, I. (Producer) *How's the Baby?* Home Service. 22 March 1950. [Knowing and Learning; CW 3:5:14]

Symptoms of Illness. Benzie, I. (Producer) *How's the Baby?* Home Service. 29 March 1950. [Instincts and Normal Difficulties; CW 3:5:15]

1951

Visiting Children in Hospital 1. Benzie, I. (Producer) *Woman's Hour*. Light Programme. 16 May 1951. [part of CW 3:6:5]

Visiting Children in Hospital 2. Benzie, I. (Producer) *Woman's Hour*. Light Programme. 23 May 1951. [part of CW 3:6:5]

Children in Hospital (discussion, with Ronald MacKeith, and two nurses, Mrs Cullen and Mrs Boote). Benzie, I. (Producer) *Woman's Hour*. Light Programme. 30 May 1951. [see CW 3:6:5]

1952

The Ordinary Devoted Mother and Her Baby: 1. The Baby as a Going Concern. Benzie, I. (Producer) *Woman's Hour*. Light Programme. 9 January 1952. [CW 3:4:24]

The Ordinary Devoted Mother and Her Baby: 2. The First Week. Benzie, I. (Producer) *Woman's Hour*. Light Programme. 16 January 1952. [CW 4:1:1]

The Ordinary Devoted Mother and Her Baby: 3. Breast Feeding. Benzie, I. (Producer) *Woman's Hour*. Light Programme. 23 January 1952. [Close-up of Mother Feeding Baby; CW 3:4:28]

The Ordinary Devoted Mother and Her Baby: 4. Baby Bites. Benzie, I. (Producer) *Woman's Hour*. Light Programme. 30 January 1952. [CW 4:1:2]

[The Ordinary Devoted Mother and Her Baby: 5. Benzie, I. (Producer) *Woman's Hour*. Light Programme. 6 February 1952. Cancelled]

[The Ordinary Devoted Mother and Her Baby: 6. Benzie, I. (Producer) *Woman's Hour*. Light Programme. 13 February 1952. Cancelled]

The Ordinary Devoted Mother and Her Baby: 7. My Fan Mail (Commenting on Listeners' Letters Concerning the Four Previous Talks). Benzie, I. (Producer) *Woman's Hour*. Light Programme. 20 February 1952. [CW 12:3:4d]

1955

On Adoption: Homeless Children and Childless Homes. Benzie, I. (Producer) *Woman's Hour*. Light Programme. 23 February 1955. [On Adoption; CW 5:1:2]

Counterfeit and Alone: 2. The Wicked Stepmother in the Storytelling of All Ages. Fairy Stories. Benzie, I. (Producer) *Woman's Hour*. Light Programme. 7 June 1955. [For Stepparents; CW 5:1:10]

Counterfeit and Alone: 3. Shall We Keep Superficial or Go Deep? Is There a Rival Even If Dead? Benzie, I. (Producer) *Woman's Hour*. Light Programme. 8 June 1955. [For Stepparents; CW 5:1:10]

Counterfeit and Alone: 4. Every One of Us Is Unsuccessful Somewhere. Who Knows All the Answers? Who Is a Stranger to Doubt? Benzie, I. (Producer) *Woman's Hour*. Light Programme. 9 June 1955. [For Stepparents; CW 5:1:10]

1956

How Much Do We Know About Babies as Cloth Suckers? Benzie, I. (Producer) *Woman's Hour*. Light Programme. 31 January 1956. [CW 5:2:1]

1959

Four Doctors Answering Listeners' Questions. Molony, E. (Producer). *Parents and Children. Network Three.* Third Programme. 9 February 1959. [not published]

Dr Ernest Jones. Vaughn, A. (Producer). Welsh Home Service and Home Service (London). 15 March 1959.

1960

The Ordinary Devoted Mother and Her Children: 1. Saying 'No' to Young Children 1 – Some Occasions for Saying 'No'. *Parents and Children.* Benzie, I. and Brewer, E. (Producers). Network Three. 25 January 1960. [Part of 'Saying "No"'; CW 6:1:1; CW Audio 12:3:3]

The Ordinary Devoted Mother and Her Children: 2. Saying 'No' to Young Children 2 – Saying 'No' Isn't Just Saying 'No'. *Parents and Children.* Benzie, I. and Brewer, E. (Producers). Network Three. 1 February 1960. [Part of 'Saying "No"'; CW 6:1:1; CW Audio 12:3:3]

The Ordinary Devoted Mother and Her Children: 3. Saying 'No' to Young Children 3 – The Basis of 'No' Is 'Yes'. *Parents and Children.* Benzie, I. and Brewer, E. (Producers). Network Three. 8 February 1960. [Part of 'Saying "No"'; CW 6:1:1; CW Audio 12:3:3]

The Ordinary Devoted Mother and Her Children: 4. Some Family Jealousies Which Are Only To Be Expected. *Parents and Children.* Benzie, I. and Brewer, E. (Producers). Network Three. 15 February 1960. [Part of 'Jealousy'; CW 6:1:4; CW Audio 12:3:3]

The Ordinary Devoted Mother and Her Children: 5. The Beginnings of Jealousy. *Parents and Children.* Benzie, I. and Brewer, E. (Producers). Network Three. 22 February 1960. [Part of 'Jealousy'; CW 6:1:4; CW Audio 12:3:3]

The Ordinary Devoted Mother and Her Children: 6. Why Jealousy Disappears. *Parents and Children.* Benzie, I. and Brewer, E. (Producers). Network Three. 29 February 1960. [Part of 'Jealousy'; CW 6:1:4; CW Audio 12:3:3]

The Ordinary Devoted Mother and Her Children: 7. Jealousy – How the Parents' Care Can Help. *Parents and Children.* Benzie, I. and Brewer, E. (Producers). Network Three. 7 March 1960. [Part of 'Jealousy'; CW 6:1:4; CW Audio 12:3:3]

The Ordinary Devoted Mother and Her Children: 8. What Irks the Ordinary Mother? *Parents and Children.* Benzie, I. and Brewer, E. (Producers). Network Three. 14 March 1960. [Part of 'What Irks?'; CW 6:1:7; CW Audio 12:3:3]

The Ordinary Devoted Mother and Her Children: 9. More That Irks, and Why. *Parents and Children.* Benzie, I. and Brewer, E. (Producers). Network Three. 21 March 1960. [Part of 'What Irks?'; CW 6:1:7; CW Audio 12:3:3]

The Ordinary Devoted Mother and Her Children: 10. What Irks a Mother—More Variations on the Theme, Discussed by Some Mothers. *Parents and Children.* Benzie, I. and Brewer, E. (Producers). Network Three. 28 March 1960.

The Ordinary Devoted Mother and Her Children: 11. Six Mothers Discuss Their Opinions and Experiences of Bringing Up Children. *Parents and Children.* Benzie, I. and Brewer, E. (Producers). Network Three. 4 April 1960.

Too Much Security? *Parents and Children.* Benzie, I. (Producer) Network Three. 18 April 1960. [On Security; CW 6:1:9; CW Audio 12:3:3]

1961

Guilt Feelings in Young Mothers. Discussion with Claire Rayner. *Parents and Children.* Crowther, E. (Producer). Network Three. 13 March 1961. [Feeling Guilty; CW 6:2:6]

1962

The First Five Years: 11. Right and Wrong. *Parents and Children.* Waterhouse, S. (Producer). Network Three. 11 June 1962. [The Development of a Child's Sense of Right and Wrong; CW 6:3:4]

The First Five Years: 13. Now They Are Five. *Parents and Children.* Waterhouse, S. (Producer). Network Three. 25 June 1962. [The Five-Year-Old; CW 6:3:6; CW Audio 12:3:3]

1966

Every Week Has a Thursday. Interview with Jocelyn Ryder-Smith on '*Dibs: In Search of Self*', by Virginia Axline. *Woman's Hour.* Browne-Wilkinson, V. (Producer). Home Service. 19 August 1966.

1967

What Is a Freudian in 1967? Hosted by Penelope Leach. Hughes, R. (Producer) Network Three. 16 January 1967, repeated 4 April 1967.

1968

Children and Death. Hunkin, O. (Producer) *Meeting point.* Discussion with Derek Hart. BBC One (television). 23 June 1968.

Index of Available Audio Recordings

All audio material is available at www.oxfordclinicalpsych.com/winnicott

Introduction to Winnicott's Broadcasts

ANNE KARPF

This podcast can be listened to at www.oxfordclinicalpsych.com/winnicott. A longer version of this podcast can be read in *History Workshop Journal*, vol. 78, Autumn 2014.

The Ordinary Devoted Mother and Her Baby

1. A Man Looks at Motherhood [CW 3:4:23]
2. Getting to Know Your Baby [CW 2:5:8]
3. The Baby as a Going Concern [CW 3:4:24]
4. A Note on Infant Feeding [CW 2:6:13]
5. Where the Food Goes [CW 3:4:25]
6. The End of the Digestive Process [CW 3:4:26]
7. The Baby as a Person [CW 3:4:27]
8. Mother Feeding the Baby [CW 3:4:28]
9. Why Do Babies Cry? [CW 2:6:2]
10. The World in Small Doses [CW 3:4:29]
11. The Innate Morality of the Baby [CW 3:4:30]
12. On Weaning [CW 3:4:31]
13. Knowing and Learning [CW 3:5:14]
14. Instincts and Normal Difficulties [CW 3:5:15]

The Ordinary Devoted Mother and Her Children, *Parents and Children*, BBC, 1960–62

The Ordinary Devoted Mother and Her Children. *Parents and Children*. BBC Network Three, January–April 1960. (E. Brewer & I. Benzie, Producers)

1. Some Mothers Discuss when to Say No I [CW 6:1:1]
2. Some Mothers Discuss when to Say No II [CW 6:1:1]
3. Some Mothers Discuss when to Say No III [CW 6:1:1]
4. Jealousy I [CW 6:1:4]
5. Jealousy II [CW 6:1:4]
6. Jealousy III [CW 6:1:4]
7. Jealousy IV [CW 6:1:4]
8. What Irks the Ordinary Mother? [CW 6:1:7]
9. More that Irks—and Why [CW 6:1:7]
10. Too much security? *Parents and Children.* BBC Network Three, 18 April 1960. (I. Benzie, Producer) [On Security; CW 6:1:9]
11. The First Five Years. *Parents and Children.* BBC Network Three, 25 June 1962. (S. Waterhouse, Producer) [Now They Are Five; CW 6:3:6]

Further Audio Material

1. The Price of Ignoring Psychoanalytic Research Findings
   National Association for Mental Health Annual Conference: 'The Price of Mental Health'. The Assembly Hall, Church House, Westminster, 25 February 1965. [CW 7:2:4]

2. Contribution to the Discussion on 'Frankie'
   24th Congress of the International Psychoanalytical Asssociation. Amsterdam, 1965. [Spoken Comments on Obsessional Neurosis and 'Frankie'; CW 7:2:11]

3. Changing Patterns in Young People
    a. Answering questions from the floor (49.43)
    b. Further contributions to a discussion (59.16)
        21st Annual Meeting of the British Student Health Association: 'Higher Education and Modern Concepts in Adolescent and Early Adult Development'. Newcastle upon Tyne, 18 July 1968. [Contemporary Concepts of Adolescent Development and their Implications for Higher Education; CW 9:3:9]

4. The Pill: An Informal Presentation.
   The Progressive League, November 1969 [CW 9:1:23].

5. Commentary on *Play Therapy*, Virginia Axline
    Undated ca. 1969. [CW 9:1:32]

Original Broadcast Scripts

The New Baby: Looking Forward to Baby's Arrival

An incomplete broadcast script of the second talk in the series *The New Baby*. BBC Home Service, I. Benzie (Producer). Wednesday, 10 October, 1945.

Winnicott also contributed the eighth talk, 'Getting to Know Your Baby' (1945) [CW 12:3:4b], to this series of twelve broadcast talks for expectant mothers. See [CW 12:Introduction].

Presumably if I talk about preparing for the new baby I'm talking principally to expectant mothers. I've known a lot of such, and I feel very doubtful whether they want to discuss their expected babies while they are carrying them. Perhaps the last thing they want to do is to sit down in front of a wireless set and think. I don't even believe they are very good at thinking at the moment, even if at other times they like discussing problems and reading books and listening to the B.B.C.

So it seems to me that we help women who are pregnant, if we can help them at all in this way, by trying as fully as possible to understand what their position in the world is.

When I see someone who's obviously going to have a baby I feel the same as I did in the war when I met R.A.F. pilots on leave; here we were, talking about this and that over a glass of beer, but to-night or the night after one of us would be snug in bed while the other would be fighting in the dark sky overhead or flying through flak over hostile country. A sailor told me he felt odd walking the streets of Portsmouth on a rough night, watching the people in their houses drawing the curtains and preparing for their supper and bed when he was on his way back to his destroyer and due to spend the night at the mercy of the elements. In the same way we pass a woman in the street, or stand in the same queue with her in a fish shop, and we quite rightly treat her as one of ourselves, and yet we know that she is up against it in a way that we are not, and that in a few months or weeks she and not we must go through a tremendous experience.

The comparison of men's fighting with women's child-bearing is surely quite sensible. I would say that no man has a right to put a woman in the family way (as the saying is) unless he has reached that stage in his own development which enables him to risk his own life fighting. It's not a matter of chance that marriages increase when there's fighting to be done and that more babies are conceived and born during war-time than in peace-time. For it's in war especially that men discover new things about themselves including their willingness to risk life in a good cause. Without thinking things out consciously men somehow feel freed by their own bravery to give their woman the corresponding hurt which pregnancy and child-birth involve.

I can hear some people saying that these things oughtn't to be said out loud because there is a great need for more babies, and the idea of pregnancy as a hurt will frighten girls off having babies of their own altogether. I don't believe it. I think that girls need to be told that pregnancy is their war, their danger situation, their reality, and I believe that this will appeal to them because it's true.

When women are with child they say they find themselves changing and we must study these changes and remember that they are entirely natural and, for the most part temporary.

Certainly as your pregnancy establishes itself you find yourself getting heavier and standing differently, and if this is the first, you notice alterations in your shape, especially in the shape of your breasts. Also you may be a bit restless, unable to lie down for more than a certain length of time. To counteract this restlessness you are making clothes and rearranging the room and generally seeing to it that you are not left without occupation.

Every now and again you may be a bit excited about what is happening, but you can't stay excited all the time, which is perhaps a good thing.

Perhaps you yourself find yourself becoming a bit withdrawn, feeling stupid instead of your usual quick-witted self, magnificently uninterested in the coming municipal elections, in your neighbour's coal situation, or even in the future of the atomic bomb. Of course I can't talk to everyone at once, and you may easily be one of those who stride through your pregnancies without turning a hair. Some indeed feel this time to be one of particular peacefulness, so that they read books they've never had time to read and listen to music without the usual feeling that a lot of things ought to be being done. Some for the first time feel they are important, or that they're justified in eating the best food and in expecting to be looked after. But many are quite naturally and normally restless or in some other way changed, and you may well expect it to take some time after the actual birth before you will return to what you are in the ordinary way. To carry inside you six or seven pounds of heaviness which presses up against your diaphragm and heart is no joke, in fact it might be quite enough to turn a talk on the wireless to twaddle. Towards the end it must surely be usual for mothers to become mainly interested in the physical facts: burden, discomfort, limitation of movement, interference with rest.

Original Broadcast Scripts

In a physical sense it's the baby that's confined in the mother's body, but in another it's the mother who's confined in her own pregnancy, for the termination of which she can only wait, wait, wait, like a home-sick child at boarding school living with one eye on the calendar. The man who has been in the East for four years and who can't ever be sure of the date of his demobilisation, he is in the same boat.

As a matter of fact the bodily side of pregnancy's pretty well understood these days. In most localities there's efficient help for you both in prevention of mishaps and in treatment of troubles. There are of course the ordinary treatments for morning sickness and indigestion, and the other common disturbances of function, and these troubles can generally be managed by your general practitioner who in the most favourable circumstances will be able to manage the birth too. You may however welcome the ante-natal clinic which you can visit periodically and where you can be examined and be reassured when all is well, or advised as to treatment [missing text] . . . exactly right. And it must be a great relief . . . [missing text] booked a nurse for the birth in your own [missing text] . . . promised a place in a maternity ward of a hospital, so that you know what to tell people to do when the times comes.

We know that child-bearing has its grim side, and we can't expect women to do this job well unless we see that every one of them can count on getting all the help that can be given in the present state of our medical and surgical knowledge. A man from Burma told me: '. . . the army's all red tape till you get into the front line, but once you're in actual contact with the Japs you've only to ask for a pair of boots over the radio and they're thrown at you next day by parachute.' You who are bearing a child must have priority, and I think this is very largely carried out in fact. Even through the war expectant mothers have had enough food and have been able to get the best medical advice available in the district, in spite of shortage of doctors and nurses. And all this has been so *not* because the country wants more children to fight the next war, but because the recognition that men do brave things in fighting makes it easy to see the brave things women do in child-bearing. On the physical side many of you can say that you are well cared for, if you make full use of the facilities provided.

This very important thing, the management of the physical side of childbirth, is not all. Skillful care of bodies is *not* enough! I would say that every woman at this time needs a doctor whom she gets to know and to trust, and who comes to have a personal interest in her and in the baby that is expected. She will need to have such confidence in him that she will be able to lose consciousness and still feel that her cause is not neglected. This goes for the nurses too. Obviously the best thing would be for one doctor to see you through, and for one nurse to be in charge before and after the actual birth, but this state of affairs cannot often be, because there aren't enough, nor ever will be enough doctors and nurses. If in a maternity hospital you find not only modern equipment and methods but also a kind of management that is personal with someone there who believes in you, you are in clover. You'll agree that doctors and nurses are no good however much skill they practice, unless they believe in you as a whole human being. You want their care and their skill and you are quite likely to get both. You will especially need a human doctor if your husband is away and cannot even get home on compassionate leave. But wherever your husband is, home or away he too will want to know who is representing himself by looking after you. A baby's a matter of joint responsibility from the word 'go', and it's maddening for him not to be able to play his part at such an important moment of his life as the birth of his child.

For many of you, I know, the personal and wise management of your case by the doctor you know is enough to allay the anxieties that might otherwise be complicating your nine months' vigil, but you should not think it strange if you find the strain to be on the mind as well as on the body. Irrational fears and depressions may come along, and if you know they may come you'll better be able to wait for them to go, instead of adding panic to the rest of the discomfort. They tend to go when the baby is born. I know a mother who for a short time in her pregnancy had a wish to eat all sorts of things she would have scorned to eat normally. This passed. Another I spoke about just now felt convinced the world would end, but it didn't, and she now walks about with a healthy boy, and both are very much part of the world. Another was full of the fear that she would fail when it came to breast-feeding, but in the end she found this came to her easily. Another was alarmed at the degree to which she was becoming withdrawn into herself. She felt she would lose touch with reality altogether. She felt the world to be a hostile place, in which she would never be able to walk freely again. But the birth of the child enabled her to return to external reality as surely as the baby was then outside instead of inside her body. These things need not alarm if it is known that pregnancy can in some cases be a severe strain on the mind as well as on the body.

In the vast majority of cases the birth of a healthy human baby brings true relief. The physical relief is unspeakable, and if there is mental stress and strain this too is relieved, when the inside lump turns into an outside baby. Don't be surprised, though, if it takes time for relief to be complete.

So in this series of talks we come to the birth of the baby, and with it a change in the mother which I think makes her more likely than before to want to listen to discussions on infant and child care. I hope you have been able to feel from this talk that we do know you are going through it, or that you have gone through it and are by now rapidly forgetting what a strain it was. You have won our respect and we would like to help you by telling you the things we have learned by talking to mothers who have been through the experience of caring for their own children as they grow and grow up.

The New Baby: Getting to Know Your Baby

> The broadcast script of the eighth talk in the series *The New Baby*. BBC Home Service, I. Benzie (producer). Wednesday, 14 November, 1945.
>
> Winnicott contributed this talk—a summary of his first BBC series from the previous year—and 'Looking Forward to Baby's Arrival' [CW 12:3:4a], in this series of twelve broadcasts for expectant mothers. See [CW 12:Introduction].

Your baby is different from any other baby that's ever been born. Isn't that interesting!

You'd hardly think it possible, considering that just flesh and bones go to make a body, and any face has but two eyes, a nose and a mouth. How ever can there be room for millions and millions of babies each one unlike any other? Yet, it's so; even twins who look alike are never exactly alike in temperament.

Of course, people who are not used to babies find it difficult to distinguish one baby from another, but you as a mother would have no trouble if you had to pick out your baby from a number of babies, that is, once you have had the chance to hold him and to feed him. In other words, it comes naturally to you to get to know your baby, and you start right away after you have recovered from labour.

I would like to be able to help you start to get to know your baby, not so much quickly as accurately. Quickly is all right, and it's certainly fun to study the very early steps, but the really helpful thing is to be able to observe what there is to observe accurately and to keep this distinct from what you can imagine.

You can imagine all sorts of things. For instance, many newborn infants look wise, and they look as if they are lying in their cots wondering what the world will be like. There is no harm in our enjoying these ideas of ours, but we really know, don't we, that babies are not either wise or philosophical, and they have not yet the knowledge of the world which they would need in order to think out whether it's a good or a bad place to be born into. Good and bad don't begin to have any meaning for them till they are some weeks or months old.

It seems to me to be perfectly sensible to weave fantasies round babies, but as you can do this better than I can I'll leave you to it. I'm more likely to help you to see the facts, and these are quite interesting.

Babies are all the time developing, and they can be said to be developing in four ways. Firstly, they are growing physically: their bodies are using food, and in a most complex way building up bones and muscles and brains, and all other kinds of tissues. Secondly, they are developing skills, such as the ability to follow a light, to recognize a face, to smile at someone, to kick in the bath, to sit, to catch hold of objects, later on to stand, to walk, and to feed themselves. It's very interesting to compare infants with each other in these respects, because they differ greatly from each other; some walk at ten months, while others don't even sit at their first birthday, and don't walk till they are a year and a half old.

Closely bound up with this matter of skill is the development of intelligence. Here again, there are wide variations. Some babies develop obvious intelligence early, being able to learn from experience, to adapt themselves to the demands of reality, to understand mother's point of view. In contrast, other babies develop their attributes slowly, spending most of their time asleep, or apparently dreaming or thinking, and yet they can have as good a capacity for being clever eventually as have the others who show early cunning. People tend to be very pleased when babies come on fast, but I'm not one for saying that speed of development is either good or bad. I suppose the trouble is people tend to fear their child may be mentally defective until they see clear signs that [illegible text] is working well, so they like to see evidence of intelligence as soon as possible.

I've spoken of bodily development, of the development of skills, and of intelligence. The fourth kind is the development of personality. This last is by far the most interesting to watch, and it is just here that babies are especially individual and unalike. I'll go into this a little.

In this talk I can only deal with the beginnings. In the first stage of personality development, your baby is only starting to be knit together into a whole person. You're getting to know him as a human being, but he doesn't know himself yet. Let's try and see what it feels like to be a baby. It can't really be put into words, but let me say that as he lies in his cot he's a bit of skin that's itching, he's a pair of eyes watching a moving curtain, he's a colicky pain, an appetite. In the same way you are a face, a shadow, a way of handling him, a bath, a towel, a rocking movement. He's not yet become one whole person, nor are you one whole person to him. He's just a collection of feelings, bits of what will one day become himself, and you, for him are bits of what he will one day piece together and call 'mother'.

How tremendously important it must be in these first days and weeks of his life that you look after him yourself, so that he experiences no unnecessary complications! Several faces, a varying bathing technique, dissimilar toilet routine, if these complications can be avoided they are avoided with advantage. (I knew a baby who was seriously disrupted by the fact that mother was left handed while mother's mother, who also looked after him, was right handed.)

You may well ask what brings about this process, eventually, whereby the baby feels he's one whole person and feels you are a whole person too? This takes place in the course of time through the ordinary repeated experiences of infant life. Because of this mothers find themselves setting up an ordered routine, and sticking to it. There quickly comes into existence a sequence of feeding, bathing, napkin-changing and sleeping, and this is the basis of nursery life. And mothers take infinite pains to see that complications don't muddle things up. If the door bangs on two occasions just as baby is going for the nipple the baby naturally concludes that this going-for-what-you-want gives a pain in the ears, and he goes off feeding. So you shut the door carefully, and in many other ways you see that the general atmosphere round the early feeds is calm and controlled. Only against this background of monotony can you safely and usefully add your daily dose of personal richness.

These repeated experiences of your management gradually gathers him together into a person. But also there are the acute experiences which involve the whole baby, such as excitement over feeding. Just as a baby feels gathered together when you lift him up, so he comes together when he gets hungry, and goes for your breast, swallows the milk and digests it in his tummy. The feeding affects his whole body, and this helps make him feel he's one person. Even rage can be valuable in the same way, since a baby in a rage is, for the time being, pulled together into one person by his rage. When he recovers, he goes back again into a state of peace and of not minding much if he's one person or many bits. You might feel sorry for him, but on the whole he won't mind being in bits as long as from time to time he comes together; but we grown-ups get an awful feeling of madness, when through tiredness or illness we feel ourselves disintegrating, going back into the state that we were naturally in, after birth, we call 'going to pieces' and 'not being all there'.

At this early time, your baby is also discovering his own body. As he begins to become a person he begins to know that he has skin, and how nice it is to be warm. He knows that he can be hurt, and begins to distinguish pin-pricks that can be got away from, from colics that have to be endured till they go. He finds he can satisfy himself quite a lot with his own fist or finger when he suddenly wants a feed and he can't get anyone to come to the rescue quickly enough. By the age of six months he may know that what he gets rid of he has previously eaten, but by this time he is a long way on in his development, well beyond the early stages I am describing today.

In these very early stages your baby is also coming to terms with reality. In this task you have already started him off well if you and he have clicked with each other over feeding. I want to explain what I mean. Just having the will to feed your baby isn't enough, you've got to live an experience with him to bring about that human tie which is the first in the baby's life and which is so important for all his future. In fact there are two distinct things that have to be brought together. He's hungry and has ideas. You are real and have food ready. He's in need of something, and at that moment you come along with breast or bottle and good milk. But it's touch and go whether he'll feel that what you have is what he has in his mind to want. Only you can manage this tricky moment with him. Forcing is useless and harmful. But suddenly it works, the baby accepts your breast as the thing he wants to attack, and through this and its frequent repetition he gradually gains confidence in the likelihood of his being able to find in the real world the things he acutely needs.

Some babies never satisfactorily solve this problem of cooperation with mother; the two never hit it off. Perhaps they may manage with a bottle instead of the breast, but often a baby loses almost all zest for food and mechanically takes just enough to keep body and soul together. Another will take well, but in a spirit of compliance rather than of healthy greed, fitting in with mother's offer of good things, but never really feeling that what he gets is what he wants.

[Missing text] . . . holding yourself in readiness for days did you feel that you and the baby had come to terms, and that he had started to accept you as the object of his primitive greedy love.

Now what is it that I am saying? I'm trying to make it clear that very early after birth, before a baby has the ability to know you, to be pleased when you come and to be sad when you go, and before he starts to have fears and guilt feelings, he needs you terribly much. At this very early stage he needs the simplest possible environment, to be protected from complications that he cannot yet understand and allow for. You are more likely than anyone else to feel this is worth doing. To do this you don't have to be clever. You only have to be able to be natural and interested in your baby because he's yours. If you have it in you to be possessive, now's your chance.

Looking at it this way, you simply won't allow a neighbour to rush in on you when you're feeding your infant, or when you are in the middle of the routine of changing him. You simply won't allow all and sundry to have a go at bathing him. At first you will do as much as you can yourself, till the infant has had enough of you to begin to build you up as a collection of experiences with which he comes to connect your face. If you feel like yourself doing all you can you will reap a reward later on.

If you feel your baby is someone you like getting to know, you are on the right track all along. You are there with your warmth and strength and generosity, and there too is the baby with his growing needs. You and he may form a partnership which is valuable to both of you, but for this to happen you have to find each other. And as the baby is in a primitive state of development and you are mature, it must be you who at first makes the relationship possible by your patience and tolerance and your understanding of what is happening.

It is the same with training him to be clean as it is with feeding. You can train almost any baby at first by regular holding out, but this is not very valuable. Sooner or later you will have to see your baby's point of view on the subject. Sometimes he feels like cooperating, sometimes he doesn't. Sometimes he has a good reason for being in a mess. At other times he likes to please you or to give you something; and sometimes he's scared of what comes out of him and wants it taken away quickly. If you are enjoying getting to know your baby you will find out all these thing as you go along.

Some people will tell you everything depends on your starting off on the cleanliness-is-next-to-godliness principle, and they will tell you to act according to rules, and to make the baby obey these rules. Be sure these people don't know babies; and they certainly don't know your infant, for you are the only person who has had a chance to get to know him. He needs you as a person, not as a set of rules and regulations. Guiding rules are a help, but each baby needs someone who knows him and who is interested in his point of view. Gradually your infant will become interested in your point of view too, but the foundation for this is your getting to know him, and so being able to wait for what is so much more valuable than goodness and compliance, the baby's own gradually developing sense of minding what results from his actions and thoughts.

Problems of Management: Training Babies

The broadcast script of the eighth talk in the series How's the Baby? *BBC Home Service, I. Benzie (producer). Wednesday 23 November 1949, 9.30–9.45 a.m.*

This talk was published as 'The Innate Morality of the Baby' in The Child and the Family *(1957) and rewritten for republication in* The Child, the Family and the Outside World *(1964) [CW 3:4:30]. Minor alterations between the broadcast script and the publication in 1957 have been noted in square brackets. Winnicott can be heard reading this chapter in the audio material at www.oxfordclinicalpsych.com/Winnicott [CW 12:3:3]. See [CW 12:Introduction].*

The ordinary thing would be to say that this talk is about 'training'. This word 'training' certainly brings to your mind the sort of thing that I want to go into today, which is the business of how to get your baby to become nice and clean and good and obedient, sociable, moral and everything. I was going to say happy, too, but you can't teach a child to be happy.

This word 'training' always seems to me to be something that belongs to the care of dogs. Dogs do need to be trained. I suppose we can learn something from dogs in that if you know your own mind your dog is happier than if you didn't, and children, too, like you to have your own ideas about things. But a dog doesn't have to grow up eventually into a human being, so when we come to your baby we have to start again and the best thing is to see how far we can leave out the word 'training' altogether.

I have several things to get out of the way before I can get down to what I really want to say. There's the matter of your own standards. Eventually your child has either to accept your standards or else rebel against them. Your standards are deeply founded and you would be lost without them.

[But standards vary.] In one block standards are different in the different flats, because one family values physical strength or manual labour, and another puts value on cleverness, and another on cleanliness. It would be absurd for anyone to ask you to alter your standards just because you have a baby.

Another thing we have to remember is that everyone was a baby once and the way in which your parents brought you up is stored away somewhere in you, perhaps even remembered, and it isn't easy to be free from the tendency either to repeat exactly what your parents did to you, or (if an extreme attitude was adopted by them) to go to the other extreme. I am talking chiefly to parents who have standards which are not too rigid and for whom the words love and hate are more important than words like good, clean, beautiful, bad, and ugly.

And another thing I must get out of the way—I must admit that there are bound to be some children, even in the best homes, who are not developing quite satisfactorily. With a child who is in difficulties you may have to do what you rightly feel isn't good, and adopt firm training methods which definitely cramp the spontaneity of the child, simply to make life bearable. This just can't be helped, and it would be a good idea on some other occasion to discuss the management of those children who are in too much of a mess to be allowed to develop along their own lines. At present, however, I'm discussing the early stages and what an ordinary good mother does with her infant or little child who is developing satisfactorily.

Your baby is tremendously dependent on you, at the beginning almost entirely dependent on you, but this doesn't mean that the baby is dependent on you for feeling good or bad. Ideas of good and bad turn up in every infant from inside. The dependence has to do with the setting that you provide to make possible the full development of the infant into a little child and of the little child into an older child.

If I can take for granted all this about the setting you provide (bodily care, reliable behavior, active adaptation to the baby's needs, fun, etc.). I can then go on to say that there are innate tendencies in every infant towards morality and towards all the different kinds of standards of behaviour which you yourselves value. If these tendencies can be found in the infant, isn't it worthwhile waiting for them? Eventually the child will be able to adopt your standards, (in fact, your standards may prove to be too low, like when you teach him to say 'ta' when he doesn't feel gratified); but it is a complex matter, this process of development from the impulsiveness and the claim to control everyone and everything to an ability to conform. I can't tell you how complex it is. It takes time. Only if you feel it's worthwhile will you allow space and time for what has to happen.

I am still talking about infants, but it is so very difficult to describe what is happening in the first months in infant terms. To make it easier, let's look now at a boy of five or six making a picture. I shall pretend he is conscious of what is going on, though he isn't really. He's making a picture. What does he do? He knows the impulse to scribble and to make a mess. That's not a picture. These primitive pleasures have to be kept fresh but at the same time he wants to express ideas, and also to express them in such a way that they may possibly be understood. Let's look just as he makes his first picture. If he achieves a picture he has found a series of controls that satisfy him. First of all there's a piece of paper of a particular size and shape which he accepts. Then he hopes to use a certain amount of skill that has come of practice. Then he knows that the picture when it's finished must have balance—you know, the tree on either side of the house. This is an expression of the fairness which he needs and probably gets from the parents. The points of interest must balance, and so must the lights and shades and the colour scheme. The interest of the picture must be spread over the whole paper and yet there must be a central theme which knits the whole thing together. Within this system of accepted, indeed self-imposed, controls he tries to express an idea, and to keep some of the freshness of this feeling that belonged to the idea when it was born. It almost takes my breath away to describe all this, yet your children get to it quite naturally if you give them half a chance.

Of course, as I said, he doesn't know all those things in a way that would make it possible for him to talk about them. Still less does the infant know what is going on within him.

The baby is rather like this older boy only first of all it's much more obscure. The pictures don't actually get painted, in fact they aren't of course pictures at all but they are little tiny contributions to society which only the mother of the baby is sensitive enough to appreciate. A smile can contain all this, or a clumsy gesture of the arms, or a sucking noise indicating readiness for a feed. Perhaps there is a whimpering noise by which the sensitive mother knows that if she comes quickly she may be able to personally attend to a notion which otherwise just becomes a wasted mess. This is the very beginning of co-operation and social sense and is worth all the trouble it involves. How many children who wet the bed for some years after they could get out and save a lot of washing, are going back in the night to their infancy, trying to go over their experiences again, trying to find and correct something that was missing. The thing missing in that case was the mother's sensitive attention to signals of excitement or distress which would have enabled her to make personal and good what otherwise had to be wasted because there was no one there to participate in what happened.

The problem is: in order eventually to have a clean and dry child are you to *train* your baby to be clean, or are you to accept the dirtiness, not mind about it, and be contented sometimes to catch these moments which turn up in which the baby is beginning to be able to communicate with you, and is beginning to be able to let you know how to adapt with success to the baby's changing needs? You will judge according to your own inclination and according to what kind of infant you are landed with. But the first method is not so rich or rewarding as the second.

By the first method you feel your aim to implant goodness and a sense of right and wrong. But the baby is left without firm roots to the good behaviour.

[Over] here [are] the baby's spontaneity and capacity to make a contribution to society, and [over] there, quite separately, are the world's demands. It's like inviting the baby to split into two halves. By the second method the innate tendencies towards morality are being allowed. Because of the mother's sensitive behaviour [*replaced with* 'ways'], which belongs to the fact of her love, the roots of the infant's personal moral sense are preserved. The fact is the baby hates to waste an experience, and much prefers to wait and bear frustration of primitive pleasures if waiting adds the warmth of a personal relationship. Only all this doesn't become clear until you have acted in the sensitive way you love to act over a period of some months [, or years].

The mother who easily feels these things and who has the courage to act according to her feelings is actually going to have an easier time later on. She 'spoils' her infant at the beginning, except that we don't call it 'spoiling' then because it's natural and valuable at the beginning.

And then what happens? I would say that the infant builds up within the self the idea of a mother, a mother just like you. This inside mother is then a human being who (like the infant) feels it's a happy achievement to get and experience within the orbit of a human relationship. When this happens the infant is no longer completely dependent on you and your way of going to meet whatever turns up.

Because of these things building up within the infant, the mother becomes gradually released from the need to be so terribly sensitive. One could say that the infant comes to have a capacity to dream about a mother, and her loving care. A new thing happens now, for instead of presenting the mother in a crude way with a smile or a motion the baby wants to tell the mother about the dreams. The mother has to be able to be imaginative for the baby to get this across because a little playing can mean so much and who but the mother can hope to understand? But the infant will let the mother know that the dreams can be happy or frightening or sad long before talking brings the ability to tell what has been dreamed in words.

If I use again our little boy artist that I used to illustrate my meaning earlier, we see that he has gone a stage further. He is long past scribbling, and he has now got beyond drawing a picture; now he has the picture (or dream) within himself before actually attempting to put it on to paper. He now chooses the paper according to the picture he has in mind.

Very soon, therefore, if the mother has been able to be as sensitive as the infant at the beginning, she finds that the primitive gratifications which the baby needs are being experienced in the baby's own rapidly developing inner world, and therefore there is less and less dependence on her exact adaptation to the infant's needs in real life. There is less and less need in the baby, then, for actual greediness and actual messing and actual control over things.

So, civilisation has started again inside a new human being. In actual practice, then, when all goes well, you will be neither training nor neglecting your infant. You will be providing a reliable setting in which the infant can sooner or later discover an interest in co-operating with you, an interest in seeing your point of view, liking to do what you like, and being pleased to adopt your ideas of right and wrong. Such an infant will soon be playing the part of good mother with a doll. Don't be surprised if you find the doll being severely punished for making a mess. Little children are fiercely moral. It's for you to catch on to their primitive morality and to tone it down gradually to the humanity that comes from mutual understanding.

The Ordinary Devoted Mother and Her Baby: My Fan Mail

The final in a series of broadcast talks on *Woman's Hour,* BBC Light Programme, I. Benzie (producer). Wednesday, 20 February 1952. See [CW 12:Introduction].

This is the last of what has turned out to be a rather short series of talks on mothers and babies.

My fan mail consists of eight letters all of which are interesting and if I had time I would just read them out.

First I will refer to a useful letter from someone in Liverpool who says she continues to be interested in the problems of infant care although her little girl has started going to school. This mother points out that I have given the impression that books on child care are no good, whereas she gets a great deal from books, and she mentions one which happens to be by a friend of mine, and which I agree is immensely useful. I see what has happened. I have been trying to show that the management of a baby at the very beginning is something that goes deeper than book-learning, that it comes naturally under suitable conditions just because of the fact of the mother's motherhood. I do think that this that is natural *can* be disturbed by books if the mother feverishly plods away at trying to learn, when really the important thing is to get the right conditions for the development of natural processes. I am very glad to have the chance however to make it clear that books that give information and that dispel ignorance are of the greatest value, especially as the infant gets away from the very early stages, becoming gradually less dependent on a sensitive adaptation to needs.[1]

A writer from Bexleyheath, Kent, takes up this very point. She says, 'I am certain that, if left alone, the ordinary mother will establish a good relationship with her baby and will succeed in completing nature's cycle and nourishing it with her own body. But how many of us are left alone?' Here she goes off into a lurid description of the way her baby was presented to her in a nursing home, a home which I am sure she would not want to criticise on any other grounds. 'Twenty-four hours after my daughter's birth she was brought to me for her first feed, amid much hustle and bustle, and without any initial holding or fondling to enable us to accustom ourselves one to the other, her head firmly grasped in one of the nurse's hands, my breast equally firmly grasped in the other, and the two held together in a vice-like grip'. And so on.

How often I have heard this story and the sad sequel. Shall I read on? 'I am now awaiting the birth of my second baby, and if anyone' (underlined twice) 'tries to interfere in those precious moments together I shall pick up my water jug and throw it at them . . . Surely your talk is directed at the wrong people!'

I agree, but at the same time I am worried because I might be misunderstood. When we say these things, and no language is too strong, we do not forget that mothers owe a tremendous lot to those same doctors and nurses because they have been able to make child birth something that is nearly free from the awful disasters that were common fifty years ago.

And another worry: what about the effect of a discussion of these matters on a young expectant mother? For instance, someone in Devon writes: 'I go for my confinement soon; it will be to a small hospital (as I have no help at home) where I am told, the mother only sees her baby actually at feeding times. I know that in actual hours this amounts to quite a lot, but wondered how in these first two—surely all-important weeks the mother can begin to understand her baby's needs without sometimes the cradle by her. I should be most grateful for advice. . . . If you felt that this right contact with baby could not be established in such an institution I would make a great effort to arrange to have my baby at home'.

My feeling is that this mother should not change her plans just on the basis of hearing my talk, simply because there is so much else to be considered. A woman who is expecting a baby soon, especially her first, is very much in need of doctors and nurses in whom she has confidence, and it would be better to have confidence in someone on the spot (who is of course human and not perfect) than upset arrangements on account of one true thing a voice may have said over the air. Everything depends on this woman's general practitioner, who might, of course, agree with the idea of her having the baby at home, and then all would be well because he would then become the responsible person that is needed at such a special time.

On reading this letter I did at first feel that it must be altogether unwise to talk critically of established procedure, but in the end I felt that we must be able to talk, as long as we are careful to make it clear that we are talking generally and not trying to advise individuals. It's another version of the saying: 'special cases make bad laws'.

I know a young mother who had her first baby in a beautiful hospital, twilight sleep and all that, and the baby taken over and bottle fed by the most excellent nurse, but one who happened to dislike the idea of breast-feeding. The next baby she produced in the same hospital, but she achieved having the baby while fully conscious, simply by deceiving the nurses. You see she wanted to know what it was like to go through it. But this second baby's feeding was also taken over by the nurse who preferred bottle to breast. The third she had at home. She said she would take all the risks just to be able to prove she could breast-feed. She did, but she nearly lost again, because the maternity nurse was also one of those who distrust the natural processes. She only succeeded by firing the nurse, and relying on an unskilled relation, quite a brave thing to do I thought. Let me hastily add that in the last few years maternity nurses have altered, and more and more can be relied on to wish that each infant be breast fed.

Talking about relations, I said something disparaging about mothers-in-law. I'm awfully sorry. No, I do not want to qualify as a comedian as suggested in the letter from Tunbridge Wells.

I see I shan't have time to refer to all the eight letters, but I must mention an unsigned letter from Manchester. This letter is unsigned because it is fiercely critical, and it may be that the details of the relationship between a mother and her baby are strong meat for all but those actually on the job. I wonder what you think?

Note

[1] At this point the following two paragraphs were struck through, and probably not broadcast:

This letter goes on to describe the way in which the writer was able to help another young mother start her baby on breast-feeding by calmly providing the necessary setting and by giving information about facts, and how someone else produced panic in the mother by worrying about a slight loss of weight, so that immediately the milk dried up. She also points out that the mother's husband could have helped, but he was against breast-feedings, and this all the time increased the mother's doubts about her own capacity to feed the baby that way.

On a post-card a grandmother of Streatham avers that breast-feeding was the loveliest thing of her married life. She managed it with all her seven. She adds: 'Now I am a grandmother with ten grandchildren. I would very much like to know what is the difference from then and now; they are much better looked after now'. I am all the time wondering whether doctors and nurses who have become so much more skilled and clever in the promotion of bodily health have not got one more thing to learn which is that in the mothering of a new-born baby only the mother is able to do really well, since the baby needs exactly what the mother and no one else is shaped for.

PART 4

Guide to New Material in the *Collected Works*

Works Published for the First Time

Volume 1

What Is Worthwhile in Medicine [ca. 1917–23]. [CW 1:1:16]
On In-Patient Treatment for Rheumatic Fever and Chorea. [undated, ca. 1923–31]. [CW 1:2:24]

Volume 2

Delinquency: Continued [ca. 1930s]. [CW 2:1:9]
Report on Q Camps [1941]. [CW 2:3:1]
Meet to Be Stolen From. [undated, ca. 1939–45]. [CW 2:3:7]
A Doctor Looks at the Psychiatric Social Worker [1943]. [CW 2:5:1]
Memorandum on 'The Relationship Between Clinical Paediatrics and Child Psychology' [1943]. [CW 2:5:3]
Psychological Aspects of Birching [1944]. [CW 2:6:3]
Memorandum on Corporal Punishment [1945]. [CW 2:7:6]
Evidence Given to the Home Office Committee on Children's Homes (the Curtis Report) [1945]. [CW 2:7:9]

Volume 3

Enuresis: Notes for a Lecture to the Tavistock Children's Department. [undated, ca. 1949]. [CW 3:4:36]
The Gwrw Tree [1948]. [CW 3:3:4]
The Infancy of Juliet [1949]. [CW 3:4:4]

Psychological Aspects of Juvenile Delinquency (A Talk to Probation Officers) [undated, ca. 1940s]. [CW 3:1:8][i]

Notes on the Discussion Held on Dr Winnicott's Paper 'The Birth Trauma'. [CW 3:4:11]

Volume 4

The Ordinary Devoted Mother and Her Baby: The First Week [1952]. [CW 4:1:1]

The Ordinary Devoted Mother and Her Baby: Baby Bites [1952]. [CW 4:1:2]

The Unconscious [1953]. [CW 4:2:8]

Volume 5

Memorandum from Paddington Green Children's Hospital Psychology Department on Homosexuality and the Law [1955]. [CW 5:1:4]

A Note on Regression and Reassurance [1955]. [CW 5:1:21]

The Toddler, the Second Adoption, Telling Children About Adoption [undated, ca. mid 1950s]. [CW 5:1:23]

A Study of Envy and Gratitude [1956]. [CW 5:2:5]

Notes on Adolescence [ca. 1956]. [CW 5:2:17]

Address Introducing Margaret Mead, 8th Ernest Jones Lecture, British Psychoanalytical Society [1957]. [CW 5:3:4]

Remarks on a Discussion of Balint's Paper on Technique [1957]. [CW 5:3:8]

Where Angels Fear to Tread, or, a Comment on Generic Teaching [1958]. [CW 5:4:9]

On 'Separation Anxiety' by J. Bowlby [1958]. [CW 5:4:18]

Memorandum on Gisburne House [1959]. [CW 5:5:4]

Volume 6

Memorandum on Organizational Aspects of Child Care at Paddington Green Hospital [1961]. [CW 6:2:3]

Comment: J. Sandler, 'Problems of Research in Psycho-analysis' [1961]. [CW 6:2:12]

'Matti', *aet* 12 Years: A Therapeutic Consultation [1961]. [CW 6:2:15]

Sakari: A Therapeutic Consultation [1961]. [CW 6:2:16]

---

[i] See also the lecture 'Some Psychological Aspects of Juvenile Delinquency' [CW 3:1:7]

The Psychoanalyst and Child Psychiatry, a Matter of Economics [1962]. [CW 6:3:12]
Considerations in the Study of Homosexuality [1963]. [CW 6:4:4]

Volume 7

A 70th Birthday Present [1965]. [CW 7:2:20]
Clinical Material: Theme of 'Two', also Theme of 'Black' [1965]. [CW 7:2:13]
The Child, the Family and the Offender: Response to a Home Office White Paper [1965]. [CW 7:2:12]
Spoken Comments on Obsessional Neurosis and 'Frankie' [1965][ii] [CW 7:2:11]
Review: A. Freud, *Normality and Pathology in Childhood* [1965]. [CW 7:2:16]
Social Aspects of Autism [1966]. [CW 7:3:7]
On the Occasion of the Publication of the *Standard Edition* of Freud [1966]. [CW 7:3:23]
The Unconscious [1966]. [CW 7:3:29]
An Allotted Spanner in the Works [undated, ca. 1966–67]. [CW 7:3:37]

Volume 8

Trips into Partisanship [1967]. [CW 8:1:30]
Chards pil... [1968]. [CW 8:2:4]
Further Clinical Illustration of 'The Use of an Object' [1968]. [CW 8:2:30]

Volume 9

Some Principles of Child Analysis [1969]. [CW 9:1:9]
Psychologists as a Group [1969]. [CW 9:1:31]
A Personal Statement on Child Psychiatry [1970]. [CW 9:2:4]
The Day-Dreamer [undated]. [CW 9:4:2]
Notes for a Discussion on Technique in Analysis of Psychotics [undated]. [CW 9:4:3]
Note on Infant Observation [undated, after 1957]. [CW 9:4:6]
Found Objects and Waifs [undated]. [CW 9:4:7]
Cleopatra Anamnesis [undated]. [CW 9:4:9]
Outline for a Study in the Sociology of Knowledge [undated]. [CW 9:4:12]

[ii] The transcription of Winnicott's contribution which became 'Comments on Obsessional Neurosis and "Frankie"'.

Volume 12

Looking Forward to Baby's Arrival [1945]. [CW 12:3:4a]
Getting to Know Your Baby [1945]. [CW 12:3:4b]
The Ordinary Devoted Mother and Her Baby: My Fan Mail [1952]. [CW 12:3:4d]

Letters Published for the First Time

Volume 1

Robina Addis. ca. April 1936 [CW 1:4:8]
Roger Money-Kyrle. 13 May 1937 [CW 1:4:15]
John Bowlby. 6 December 1938 [CW 1:4:20]

Volume 2

The Lancet, 'Prefrontal leucotomy'. 15 May 1943 [not published] [CW 2:5:5]
Marjorie Franklin. 19 October 1944 [CW 2:6:12]

Volume 3

Roger Money-Kyrle. 22 March 1949 [CW 3:4:5]
Roger Money-Kyrle. 31 March 1949 [CW 3:4:6]
Roger Money-Kyrle. 2 May 1949 [CW 3:4:7]
Roger Money-Kyrle. 13 June 1949 [CW 3:4:10]
Roger Money-Kyrle. 22 June 1949 [CW 3:4:12]
Roger Money-Kyrle. 24 June 1949 [CW 3:4:13]
Roger Money-Kyrle. 10 July 1950 [CW 3:5:9]
Roger Money-Kyrle. 8 August 1950 [CW 3:5:11]
Roger Money-Kyrle. 16 November 1950 [CW 3:5:13]
Wilfred Bion. 22 January 1951 [CW 3:6:2]

Volume 4

Sonny S. Davidson. 5 May 1952 [CW 4:1:8]
Thomas Stapleton. 20 September 1954 [CW 4:3:23]

Volume 5

Thomas Stapleton. 3 March 1955 [CW 5:1:3]
Thomas Main. 24 January 1957 [CW 5:3:3]
Margaret Mead. 31 January 31 1957 [CW 5:3:5]
Michael Balint. 27 March 1957 [CW 5:3:9]
Michael Balint. 4 April 1957 [CW 5:3:10]
Tsuicheu Cheu. 4 April 1957 [CW 5:3:11]
Mary Appleby. 27 May 1957 [CW 5:3:16]
Joan Riviere. 21 June 1957 [CW 5:3:18]
Prunella Briance. 15 July 1957 [CW 5:3:19]
Michael Balint. 3 October 1957 [CW 5:3:24]
Francesca Bion. 3 October 1957 [CW 5:3:25]
Grantly Dick-Read. 15 January 1958 [CW 5:4:1]
Marianne Baumann. 20 January 1958 [CW 5:4:2]
Anna Freud. 14 May 1958 [CW 5:4:8]
Marianne Baumann. 5 June 1958 [CW 5:4:10]
Anna Freud. 8 June 1958 [CW 5:4:11]
Anna Freud. 7 November 1958 [CW 5:4:19]
Reginald Lightwood. 10 February 1959 [CW 5:5:2]
Miss Maw. 16 February 1959 [CW 5:5:3]
The Times, 'Nursery Schools Essential'. 25 March 1959 [not published] [CW 5:5:6]
Kenneth Soddy. 9 June 1959 [CW 5:5:8]
Paul Halmos. 12 June 1959 [CW 5:5:9]
Dorothy E. M. Gardner. 13 July 1959 [CW 5:5:11]
Arthur J. Metcalfe. 14 July 1959 [CW 5:5:12]
Herman Gijsbert van der Waals. 23 July 1959 [CW 5:5:13]
A. Tommy M. Wilson. 23 September 1959 [CW 5:5:14]
Paula Heimann. 5 November, 1959 [CW 5:5:18]

Volume 6

Merton J. Kahne. 19 February 1960 [CW 6:1:5]
Ilse Hellman. 21 July 1960 [CW 6:1:12]
John Harvard-Watts. 28 July 1960 [CW 6:1:13]
Mr and Mrs Young. 28 July 1960 [CW 6:1:14]
Serge Lebovici. 8 November 1960 [CW 6:1:16]
Lydia James. 20 January 1961 [CW 6:2:1]
Aubrey J. Lewis. 26 January 1961 [CW 6:2:2]
Joan FitzHerbert. 25 April 1961 [CW 6:2:7]

Pearl King. 18 July 1961 [CW 6:2:14]
Harry Guntrip. 15 September 1961 [CW 6:2:18]
Aubrey J. Lewis. 13 October 1961 [CW 6:2:20]

Volume 7

Michael Fordham. 2 February 1965 [CW 7:2:2]
Martin James. 7 October 1965 [CW 7:2:17]
William Gillespie (with case notes). 29 September 1966 [CW 7:3:21]

Volume 8

Joyce Coles. ca. 22 November 1968 [CW 8:2:31]
Joyce Coles. ca. 25 November 1968 [CW 8:2:32]
Joyce Coles. ca. 26 November 1968 [CW 8:2:34]
Joyce Coles. 29 November 1968 [CW 8:2:35]
Joyce Coles. ca. 1 December 1968 [CW 8:2:36]
Joyce Coles. 4 December 1968 [CW 8:2:37]
Joyce Coles. 8 December 1968 [CW 8:2:40]
Joyce Coles. ca. 10 December 1968 [CW 8:2:42]

Volume 9

Peter Giovacchini. 5 March 1970 [CW 9:2:1]
Michael Fordham. 10 March 1970 [CW 9:2:2]
John Davis. 1 January 1971 [CW 9:3:1]

Volume 12

Joyce Coles. 25 August 1968 [CW 12:5:caption 6]

Works First Published in a Winnicott Edition

Volume 1

PART 1

Smith [CW 1:1:3]
The Night Attack [CW 1:1:6]
The Best Remedy [CW 1:1:8]
A Shropshire Surgeon [CW 1:1:12]
St Bartholomew's Hospital Amateur Dramatic Club [CW 1:1:13]
A Reminder to the Binder [CW 1:1:14]
The Snag [CW 1:1:15]

PART 2

Varicella Encephalitis and Vaccinia Encephalitis (with Nancy Gibbs) [CW 1:2:1]
Case for Diagnosis (? Poliomyelitis with Some Spasticity) [CW 1:2:2]
Case for Diagnosis (? Infantile Hemiplegia) [CW 1:2:3]
Two Cases for Post-Encephalitic Hyperapnœa [CW 1:2:4]
Case of Stunted Growth [CW 1:2:5]
The Only Child [CW 1:2:6]
Facial Nerve Paralysis [CW 1:2:7]
Facial Nerve Paralysis Associated with Fits [CW 1:2:8]
Encephalitis after Measles and Chicken-pox [CW 1:2:9]
Muscle Weakness, Altered Gait and Absent Deep Reflexes After Measles [CW 1:2:10]
Abscess in Frontal Lobe (with Elisabeth O'Flynn) [CW 1:2:11]
Rheumatism in Children [CW 1:2:12]
Hemiplegia Noticed After Diphtheria [CW 1:2:13]
Measles Encephalitis [CW 1:2:14]
Symptoms Suggesting Post-Encephalitis [CW 1:2:15]
The Diagnosis of Chorea [CW 1:2:16]

Enuresis (abstract) [CW 1:2:17]
Pathological Sleeping [CW 1:2:19]
Hæmoptysis: Case for Diagnosis [CW 1:2:20]
Pre-Systolic Murmur, Possibly Not Due to Mitral Stenosis [CW 1:2:21]

PART 4

Papular Urticaria and the Dynamics of Skin Sensation [CW 1:4:3]
Skin Changes in Relation to Emotional Disorder [CW 1:4:18]
Discussion: G. A. Auden, 'The Difficult Child' [CW 1:4:4]
Abstract: F. Alexander, *Psychoanalysis and Medicine* [CW 1:4:1]
Abstract: H. Lundholm, *Repression and Rationalisation* [CW 1:4:2]
Abstract: M. Barinbaum, 'A Contribution to the Problem of Psycho-Physical Relations with Special Reference to Dermatology' [CW 1:4:5]
Review: A. Aichhorn, *Wayward Youth* [CW 1:4:12]
Review: Rickman, John (Ed.), *On the Bringing up of Children* [CW 1:4:13]

Volume 2

The Psychology of Juvenile Rheumatism [CW 2:1:7]
Delinquency Research [CW 2:5:2]
A Tendency in Therapeutics [CW 2:6:5]
Resolution K: On Scientific Aims in Psychoanalysis [CW 2:4:1]
Abstract: Observations of Infant Behaviour During Routine Clinical Examination [CW 2:3:6]
Abstract: Wearing of Masks in the Nursing of Premature and Older Infants [CW 2:5:9]
Abstract: The Value of Breastfeeding (Psychological) [CW 2:7:12]
Review: M. P. Middlemore, *The Nursing Couple* [CW 2:4:5]
Review: J. C. Flügel, *The Moral Paradox of Peace and War* [CW 2:3:4]
Letter to the *British Medical Journal*, Circumcision [CW 2:1:1]
Letter to the *British Medical Journal*, Pruritus and Psychology [CW 2:1:2]
Letter to the *British Medical Journal*, Communal Feeding in Schools [CW 2:3:2]
Letter to the *British Medical Journal*, Loneliness in Infancy [CW 2:4:3]
Letter to the *British Medical Journal*, Responsibility and Freedom [CW 2:5:7]

Volume 3

Disorders of Childhood [CW 3:3:8]
Childhood Psychosis [CW 3:5:5]
Review: A. Bowley, *The Psychology of the Unwanted Child* [CW 3:3:6]
Review: The Child Study Association of America, *Parents' Questions* [CW 3:3:7]
Review: *The Psychoanalytic Study of the Child* (Vol. 2) [CW 3:3:9]
Review: W. Wolff, *The Personality of the Pre-School Child* [CW 3:3:10]
Review: E. Harms, *Handbook of Child Guidance* [CW 3:4:15]
Review: L. Stein, *The Infancy of Speech and the Speech of Infancy* [CW 3:5:8]
Review: J. A. F. Watson, *The Child and the Magistrate* [CW 3:6:1]
Review: F. Wickes, *The Inner World of Man* [CW 3:6:7]
Review: E. Ziman, *Jealousy in Children* [CW 3:6:10]
Review: *The Psychoanalytic Study of the Child* (Vols. 3–4, Vol. 5) [CW 3:6:12]
Review: *Problems of Infancy and Childhood* [CW 3:6:16]
Review: E. Jones, *Papers on Psychoanalysis* [CW 3:6:17]
Review: P. R. Evans & R. MacKeith, *Infant Feeding and Feeding Difficulties* [CW 3:6:18]
Letter to the *British Medical Journal*, Battle Neurosis Treated with Leucotomy [CW 3:2:6]
Letter to the *British Medical Journal*, 'Pathies in a State Service [CW 3:3:3]
Letter to the *British Medical Journal*, Paddington Green Children's Hospital [CW 3:4:19]
Letter to the *British Medical Journal*, Ethics of Prefrontal Leucotomy [CW 3:6:9]
Letter to *The Times*, Maladjusted Children; Damaging Effects of Delay [CW 3:5:7]
Letter to *The Times*, Nursery Schools: A Definition of Functions [CW 3:6:11]
Letter to *The Lancet*, Leucotomy in Psychosomatic Disorders [CW 3:6:8]

Volume 4

Preface: *The First Treasured Possession* by Olive Stevenson [CW 4:3:31]
Review: D. Burlingham, *Twins: A Study of Three Pairs of Identical Twins* (in the British Medical Journal)[i] [CW 4:2:6]

---

[i] A second review of this work published in *New Era in Home and School* was reprinted in *Psychoanalytic Explorations*, 1989.

Review: E. Glover, *Psychoanalysis and Child Psychiatry* [CW 4:2:11]
Review: M. Senn (Ed.), *Problems of Infancy and Childhood* [CW 4:2:12]
Review: E. Erikson, *Childhood and Society* [CW 4:2:16]
Review: J. Rosen, *Direct Analysis* [CW 4:2:17]
Review: S. R. Slavson, *Child Psychotherapy* [CW 4:3:12]
Review: L. Jackson, *Aggression and Its Interpretation* [CW 4:3:17]
Review: H. Bakwin & R. M. Bakwin, *Clinical Management of Behaviour Disorders in Children* [CW 4:3:22]
Letter to *The Lancet*, Frontal Lobes of the Human Brain [CW 4:1:4]
Letter to *The Spectator*, A Psychiatrist's Choice [CW 4:3:3]

Volume 5

Obituary: Oscar Friedmann [CW 5:5:25]
Obituary: Ambrose Cyril Wilson [CW 5:4:22]
Foreword: *Any Wife or Any Husband* by J. Graham Malleson [CW 5:1:19]
Foreword: *Childbirth with Confidence* by Prunella Briance [CW 5:5:24]
Foreword: *The Case as the Patient Sees It: Psycho-analysis* by National Association of Mental Health [CW 5:3:17]
Review: J. Robertson, *Going to Hospital with Mother* (Film) [CW 5:5:23]
Review: E. J. Foote, *Six Children* [CW 5:3:14]
Review: *The Psychoanalytic Study of the Child* (Vol. 11) [CW 5:4:5]
Review: *The Psychoanalytic Study of the Child* (Vol. 12) [CW 5:4:15]

Volume 6

The Theory of the Parent-Infant Relationship: Contributions to Discussion [CW 6:1:21]
Obituary: Melanie Klein [CW 6:1:15]
Review: T. S. Simey, *The Concept of Love in Child Care* [CW 6:2:8]
Review: K. Soddy, *Clinical Child Psychiatry* [CW 6:2:10]
Review: M. Bergeron, *Psychologie du premier âge* [CW 6:3:16]
Review: S. Lebovici and J. McDougall, *Un Cas de Psychose Infantile* [CW 6:3:17]
Review: *The Psychoanalytic Study of the Child* (Vol. 15) [CW 6:3:1]
Review: *The Psychoanalytic Study of the Child* (Vol. 16) [CW 6:4:1]

Volume 7

Preface: R. Gaddini's Italian translation of *The Family and Individual Development* [CW 7:3:27]

Foreword: M. Torrie, *The Widow's Child* [CW 7:1:12]
Discussion: I. Alger, 'The Clinical Handling of the Analyst's Response' [CW 7:3:36]
Review: Hertha Riese, *Heal the Hurt Child* [CW 7:1:2]
Review: H. D. Kirk, *Shared Fate* [CW 7:2:26]
Review: V. Axline, *Dibs in Search of Self* [CW 7:3:10]
Review: *The Psychoanalytic Study of the Child* (Vol. 20) [CW 7:3:14]
Review: E. M. Eppel & M. Eppel, *Adolescents and Morality* [CW 7:3:20]
Review: M. Clyne, *Absent: School Refusal as an Expression of Disturbed Family Relationships* (in *New Society*) [CW 7:3:22]
Review: S. Chess, A. Thomas & H. Birch, *Your Child Is a Person* [CW 7:3:25]
Review: A. Lask, *Asthma: Attitude and Milieu* [CW 7:3:26]
Review: I. Goodacre, *Adoption Policy and Practice* [CW 7:3:30]
Letter to *The Times*, George III [CW 7:3:1]
Letter to *The Times*, 'Blood-Tie' Child: Why the Courts Must Act Swiftly [CW 7:3:9]
Letter to *The Times*, 'Blood-Tie' Child [CW 7:3:11]

Volume 8

The Non-pharmacological Treatment of Psychosis in Childhood [CW 8:1:9]
Winnicott's Wisdom: How a Baby Begins to Feel Sorry and to Make Amends [CW 8:1:16]
Winnicott's Wisdom: Why Do Babies Cry? [CW 8:1:17]
Winnicott's Wisdom: The Meaning of Mother Love [CW 8:1:13]
Winnicott's Wisdom: Hobgoblins and Good Habits[ii] [CW 8:1:22]
Foreword: *The Hands of the Living God,* by Marion Milner [CW 8:1:12]
Foreword: *Collected Papers: Vol. 3, Therapy in Child Care* by B. Dockar-Drysdale [CW 8:2:45]
Foreword: R. J. N. Tod (Ed.), *Disturbed Children* [CW 8:2:8]
Review: H. Thomson, *The Successful Stepparent* [CW 8:1:7]
Review: S. Stewart, *A Home from Home* [CW 8:1:10]
Review: Max Clyne, *Absent: School Refusal as an Expression of Disturbed Family Relationships* (in the *British Medical Journal*) [CW 8:1:15]
Review: Edna J. LeShan, *How to Survive Parenthood* [CW 8:1:28]

[ii] These four articles were reworked versions of Part 1 of *The Child, the Family and the Outside World*, for the magazine *Parents*.

Review: *A Collection of Children's Books* as 'Small Things for Small People' (in *New Society*) [CW 8:1:35]
Review: L. Burton, *Vulnerable Children. Three Studies of Children in Conflict: Accident Involved Children, Sexually Assaulted Children, and Children with Asthma* [CW 8:2:11]
Review: A. Clegg & B. Megson, *Children in Distress* [CW 8:2:25]
Review: *The Psychoanalytic Study of the Child* (Vol. 22) [CW 8:2:13]
Review: C. I. Sandström, *The Psychology of Childhood and Adolescence* [CW 8:2:46]
Review: C. A. Storr, *Human Aggression* [CW 8:2:18]

Volume 9

Contribution to the Final Number of *Case Conference*, 1970 [CW 9:2:5]
Day Dreaming [CW 9:2:14]
Dependence in Child Care [CW 9:2:15]
Preface: S. Lebovici & J. McDougall, *Dialogue with Sammy* [CW 9:1:27]

Volume 10: Therapeutic Consultations in Child Psychiatry

1.1 Note of contribution (on 'Iiro') [CW 10:Appendix 1]
1.3 A clinical study of the effect of a failure of the average expectable environment on a child's mental functioning (introductory paragraphs) [CW 10:Appendix 2]
1.7 A psychotherapeutic consultation: A case of stammering (introductory paragraphs) [CW 10:Appendix 3]
2.12 A psychotherapeutic consultation in child psychiatry: A comparative study of the dynamic processes (introductory sections) [CW 10:Appendix 4]
3.15 Child therapy: A case of anti-social behaviour (introductory paragraphs) [CW 10:Appendix 5]
3.17 Becoming deprived as a fact: A psychotherapeutic consultation [CW 10:Appendix 6]

Volume 12

Letter to *The British Journal of Psychiatry*, Oscar Nemon's Freud Statue, An Appeal [CW 12:Introduction]

Remarks on Some Chapters Revised for the *Collected Works*

Volume 2

Ocular Psychoneuroses of Childhood [CW 2:6:15]
Some sentences removed by Winnicott for the republication of this chapter in 1958 have been included here in the footnotes.

Volume 3

Aggression in Relation to Emotional Development [CW 3:5:2]
This paper was compiled from three different lectures given over the course of five years. Winnicott first composed the first section as a contribution to a pre-conference symposium in 1947, on Anna Freud's paper on the same subject. A few previously unpublished sections from this 1947 draft have been included here in the footnotes.

Volume 5

Child Analysis in the Latency Period [CW 5:4:14]
Winnicott's own hand-written annotations on his copy of the essay, made during its first reading at the Lisbon Conference of Child Psychiatry, have been included in the footnotes.

Volume 6

Envy: A Male Patient at the End of His Analysis [CW 6:2:21].
This case study, part of which is included in 'The Beginnings of a Formulation of an Appreciation and Criticism of Klein's Envy Statement', has been printed here separately and in full.

The Beginnings of a Formulation of an Appreciation and Criticism of Klein's Envy Statement [CW 6:3:7]
The final lines of the manuscript have been reinstated in this edition.

Fear of Breakdown [CW 6:4:21]
Two notes on the same subject from Winnicott's archive in the Wellcome Library London: 'On the Nature of Mental Breakdown', and 'Winnicott's Axiom', both dating from 1963, have been included as footnotes to this paper.

Volume 7

The Concept of the False Self [CW 7:1:1]
The final few incomplete paragraphs, including a brief account of a patient with an eating disorder, are reinstated at the end of this unfinished paper.

New Light on Children's Thinking [CW 7:2:1]
Winnicott included a note to himself in this lecture to present a long research case which expanded on the extract he had just quoted from D. W. Harding. Winnicott, specifying that the patient had had a trauma 'that had been retained but not experienced', draws on Harding's use (in an essay on John Donne) of a poem by Thomas Hardy to the same effect. Winnicott may have encountered Harding personally, as he was at this time Professor of Psychology at Bedford College, London.

Dissociation Revealed in a Therapeutic Consultation [CW 7:2:21]
Ralph Slovenko, the editor of the first publication of this case study, included in his edition an anonymous critique of Winnicott along with Winnicott's reply, included here in a footnote.

The Concept of Trauma in Relation to the Development of the Individual Within the Family [CW 7:2:7]
This paper is the amalgamation of two drafts of an essay on the subject of trauma. The first four pages of the second draft of the paper, comprising the sections 'The Nature of the Present Study' and 'The Good-Enough Family', have been included for the first time in the edition published here. The second draft then proceeds directly to the case of Phyllis.

Case Notes for a Psychoanalytic Seminar: Withdrawal, Regression, Male Identification [CW 7:2:19]
The complete manuscript, from which 'Notes on Withdrawal and Regression' was selected for publication in 1989, is published here for the first time.

Volume 8

Two Clinical Illustrations of the Use of an Object [CW 8:2:29 and CW 8:2:30]
The final line of the manuscript of the first clinical illustration, added by hand, has been included in this edition. A second clinical illustration prepared for the same meeting is also published here for the first time.

The Association for Child Psychology and Psychiatry Observed as a Group Phenomenon [CW 8:1:3]
The first two paragraphs of the section on 'Child Care' are published here for the first time.

The Use of an Object and Relating Through Identification [CW 8:2:28]
The summary and reading list Winnicott sent to the New York Psychoanalytic Society in advance of his presentation of this paper, and a short footnote included with the manuscript of this paper, have been included as appendices to this paper.

Volume 9

Answers to Comments on 'The Split-off Male and Female Elements' [CW 9:1:30]
Winnicott's full and specific answers to the comments by the discussants of this paper are published here, along with the generalised version of his answers as they were published in 1974 and 1989.

Commentary on Virginia Axline's Book on Play Therapy [CW 9:1:32]
Both recordings Winnicott made of himself discussing this book have been transcribed and are published here. The recordings themselves can be accessed in the Audio section [CW 12:3:3].

Child Psychiatry, Social Work and Alternative Care [CW 9:2:3]
A final paragraph from Winnicott's manuscript has been reinstated from this posthumously published chapter.

The Place of the Monarchy [CW 9:2:6]
This article exists in the form of four complete versions and was published posthumously. Several paragraphs have been added to this newly edited version, either side of the heading on *Transitional Phenomena*.

Living Creatively [CW 9:2:11]
This chapter is a posthumous amalgamation of two drafts of a lecture, one on living creatively and the other on creative living in marriage. Several paragraphs have been included for the first time in this edition.

Notes for the Vienna Congress [CW 9:3:12]
The complete set of six notes. The first four were published in *Donald Winnicott Today*;[i] the final two sections are published in the *Collected Works* for the first time.

Volume 10: Therapeutic Consultations in Child Psychiatry

Additional material from earlier publications of some of the cases in this volume has been included in Volume 10 as appendices. The shorter first version of the case of Ruth has been reprinted in full.

---

[i] J. Abram, 'D. W. W.'s Notes on the Vienna Congress 1971: A Consideration of Winnicott's Theory of Aggression and an Interpretation of the Clinical Implications'. In J. Abram (Ed.), *Donald Winnicott Today* (2013). New Library of Psychoanalysis. Hove/New York: Routledge.

PART 5

Selected Drawings and Signatures

Selected Drawings

These drawings and doodles have been selected from some of Winnicott's letters and notes, and are intended to show the easy playfulness he brought to his domestic life.

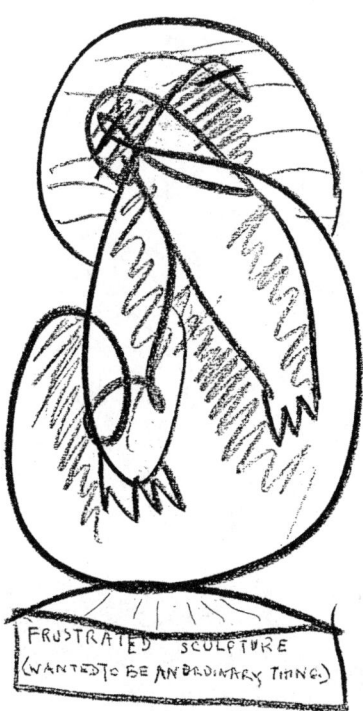

Frustrated Sculpture (Wanted to be an Ordinary Thing).

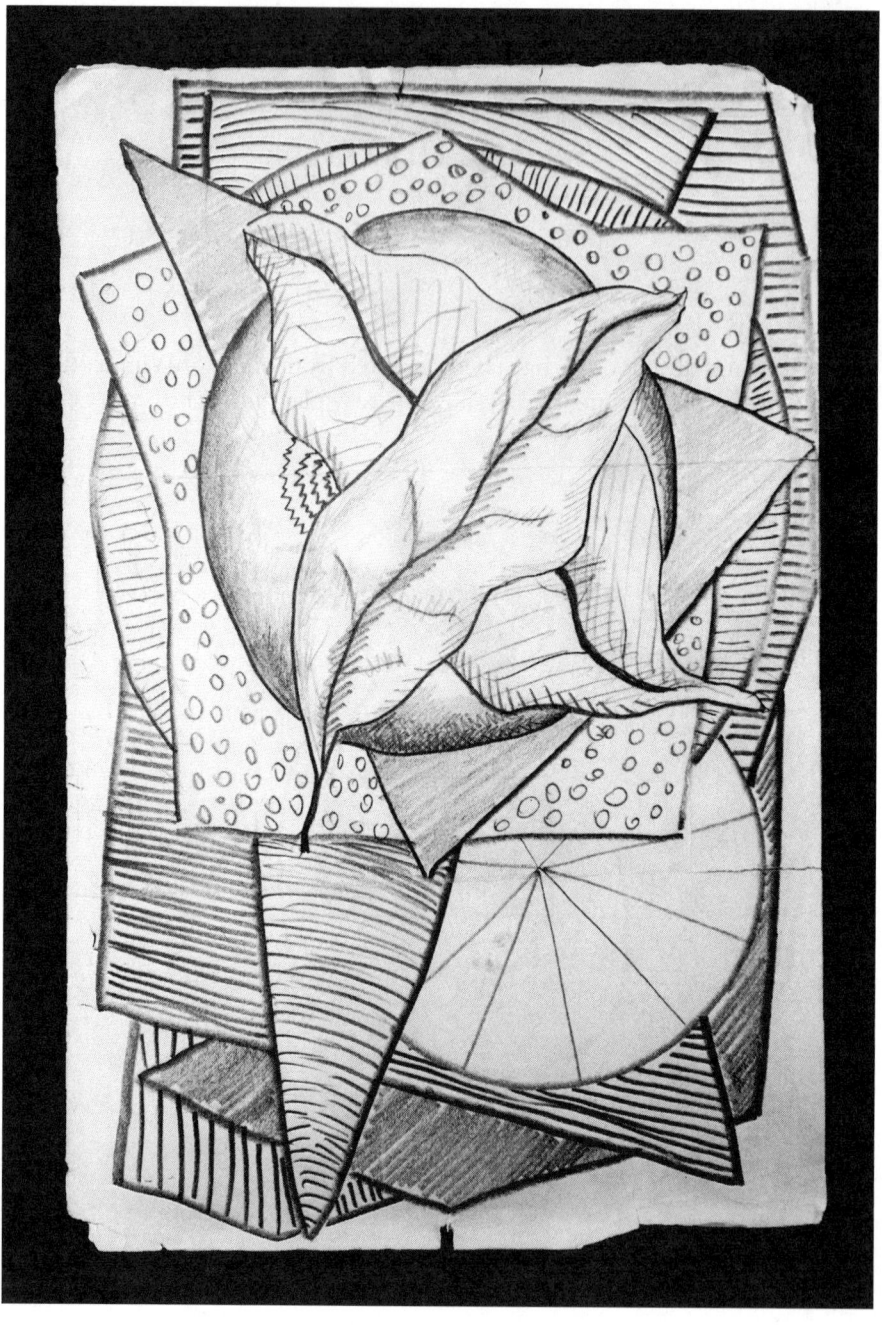

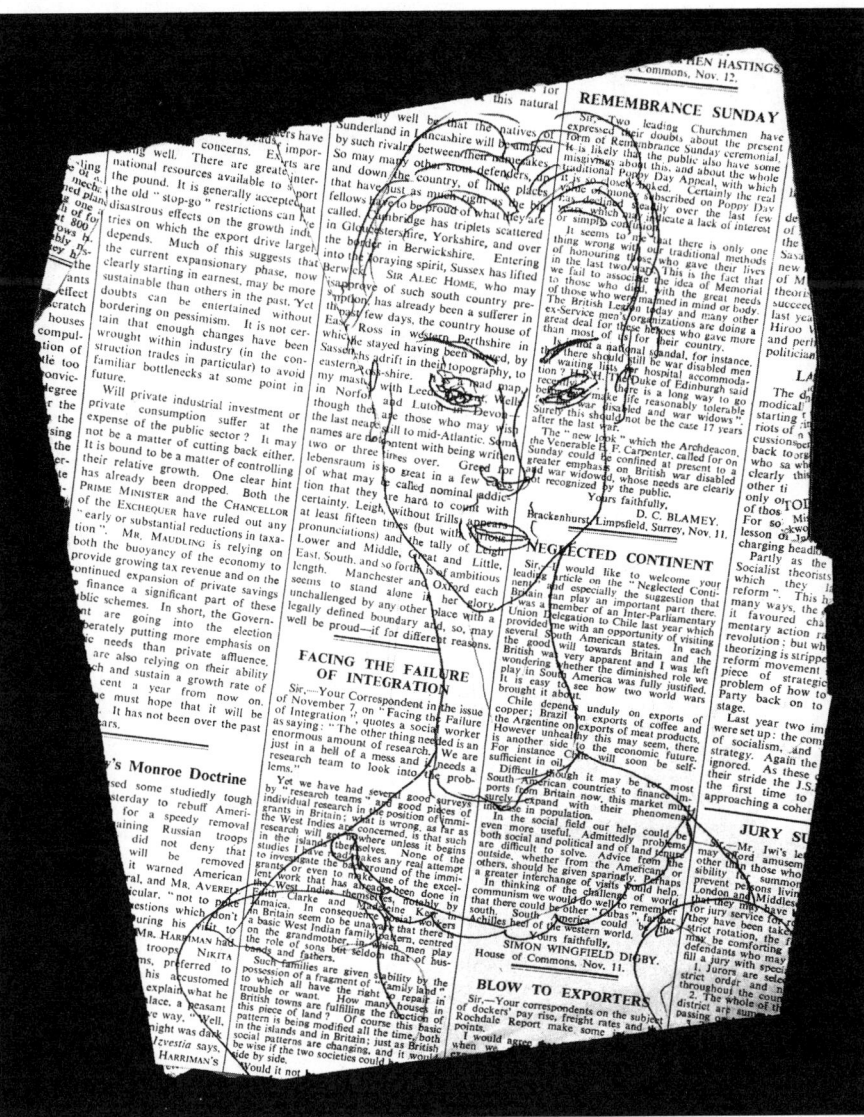

A sketch drawn inside *The Times*, 14 November, 1963.

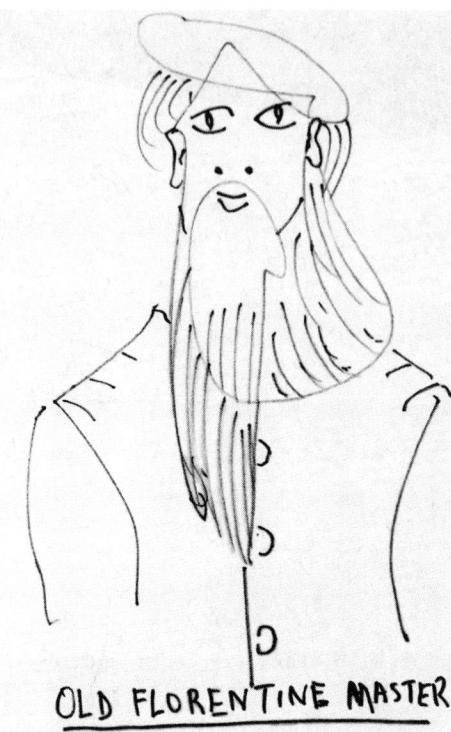

The reverse of a note Winnicott sent to his secretary Joyce Coles and her husband Arthur in May 1968 wishing them a good holiday—presumably to Italy—and asking them whether they had been caught in that spring's general strikes.

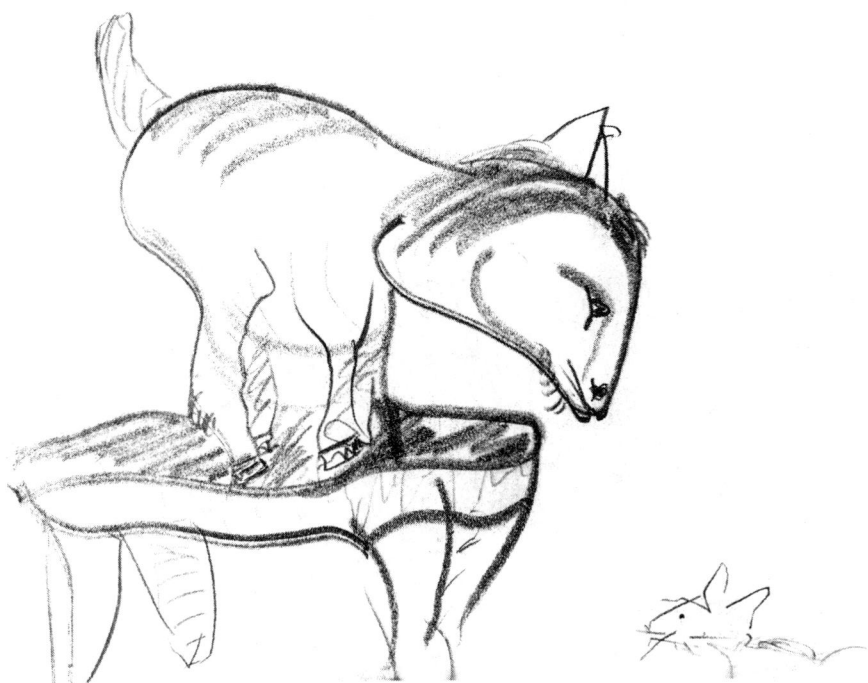

A doodle in a letter to Joyce Coles from the United States in 1968, before his illness, which Winnicott described as a 'composite made out of [a] study of my foot'.

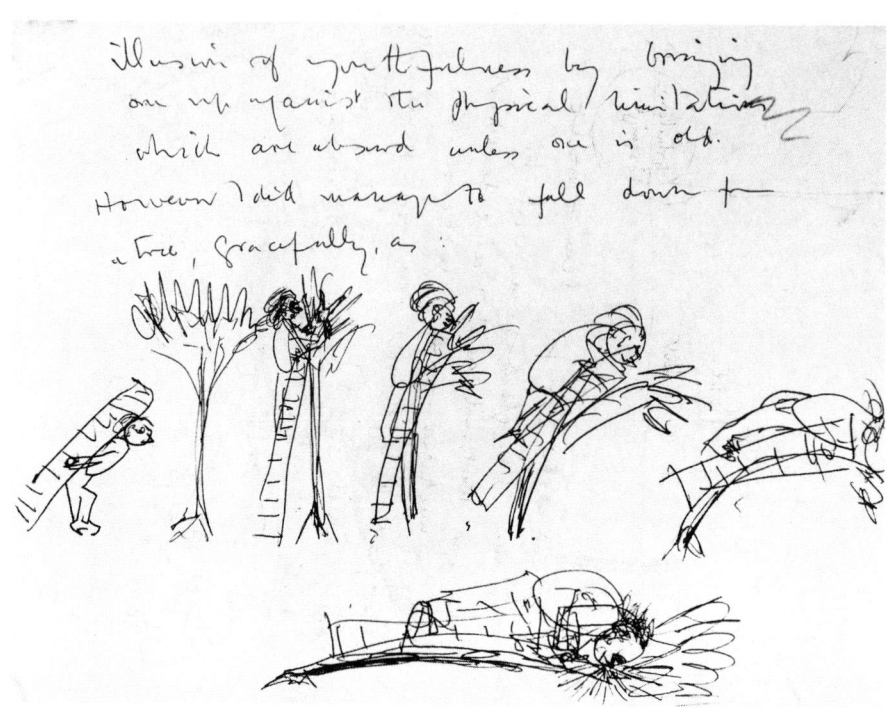

The end of a letter to Joyce Coles, 25 August 1968, from Winnicott's childhood home, Rockville, in Plymouth. The complete letter reads:

'Dear Joyce,

Thank you for your bureaucratic assistance. I'm glad you will be having a weekend next weekend which being a weekend gives a weekend to everybody except those who are permanently asleep, which might be me. I've done *nothing at all*, except suddenly drive the car out after tea for picnic suppers. The fact is that I am much older than I was, and I have only to be on holiday to realise that holiday does not restore youthfulness—in fact it can destroy the illusion of youthfulness by bringing one up against the physical limitations which are absurd unless one is old. However I did manage to fall down from a tree, gracefully, as. . .'

Winnicott was seventy-two years old. His dry self-description is movingly illuminated in a story told by Clare Winnicott to the interviewer Michael Neve in 1983 (*Free Associations*, 3:167–184):

But then he'd had about six coronaries, and recovered from them and kept himself going. And didn't stop himself doing a thing! When he went down to his home in Devon, he'd be up at the top of a tree, in the last year of his life. A few months before he died, he was at the top of a tree, cutting the top off. I said, 'What the hell are you doing up there?'

He said, 'Well, I've always wanted the top of this tree off. It spoils the view from our window'. Which it did! And he got it off.

And I thought, 'I must get him down! He's absolutely crazy'. And I thought, 'No, it's his life and he's got to live it. If he dies after this, he dies'.

But this was him. He wanted to live.

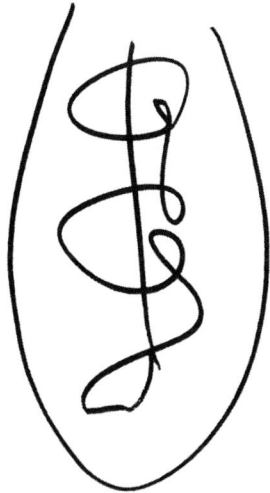

Squiggle used on the cover of *The Spontaneous Gesture: Selected Letters of D. W. Winnicott* (F. R. Rodman (Ed.), 1987).

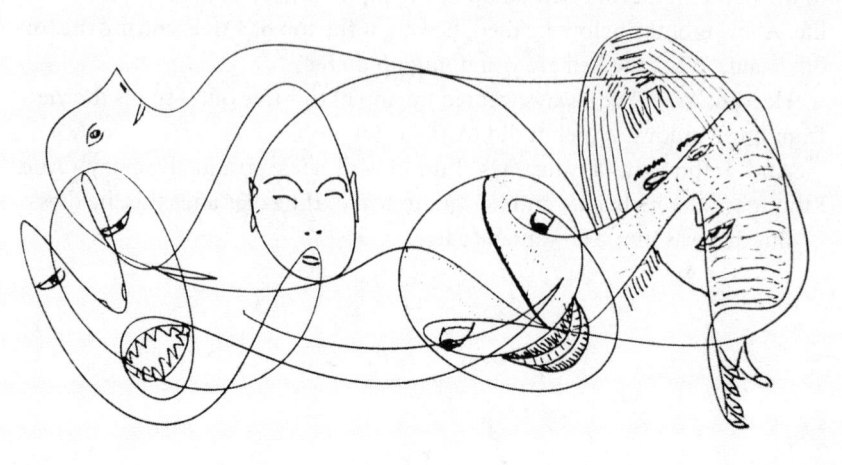

Squiggle used on the cover of *Thinking About Children* (R. Shepherd, J. Johns, H. Taylor Robinson (Eds.), 1996).

Selected Drawings

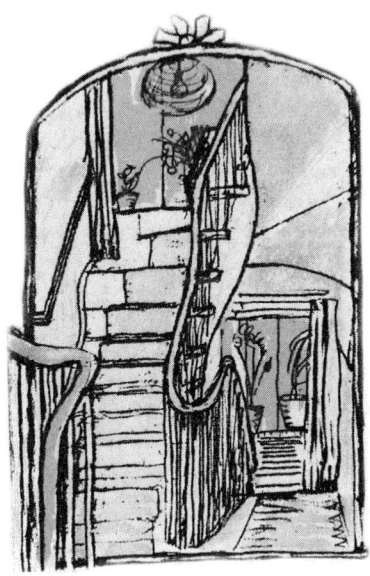

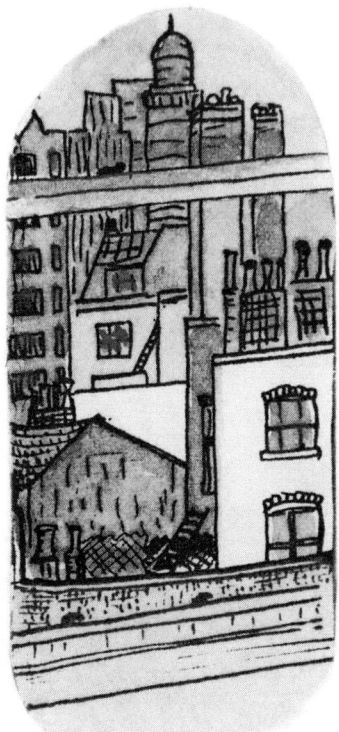

Sketches of the interior and view of Winnicott's consulting rooms at 87 Chester Square, London. Both images were sent by Donald and Clare Winnicott on Christmas cards. A few further examples of the Winnicotts' home-drawn Christmas cards can be seen in A. Clancier and J. Kalmanovitch, *Le paradoxe de Winnicott* (1984).

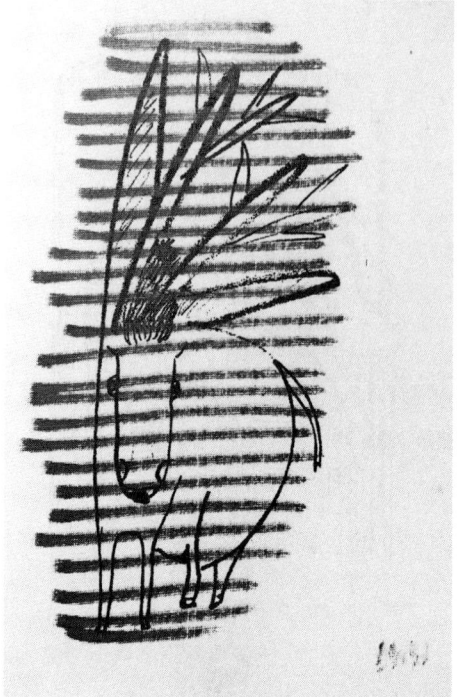

A Christmas card design.

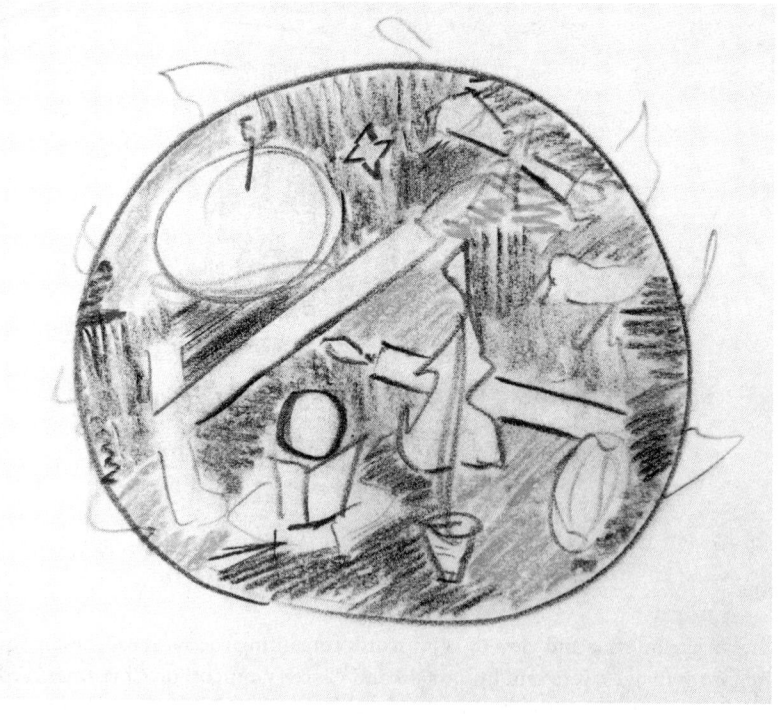

A Christmas-themed doodle.

Selected Signatures

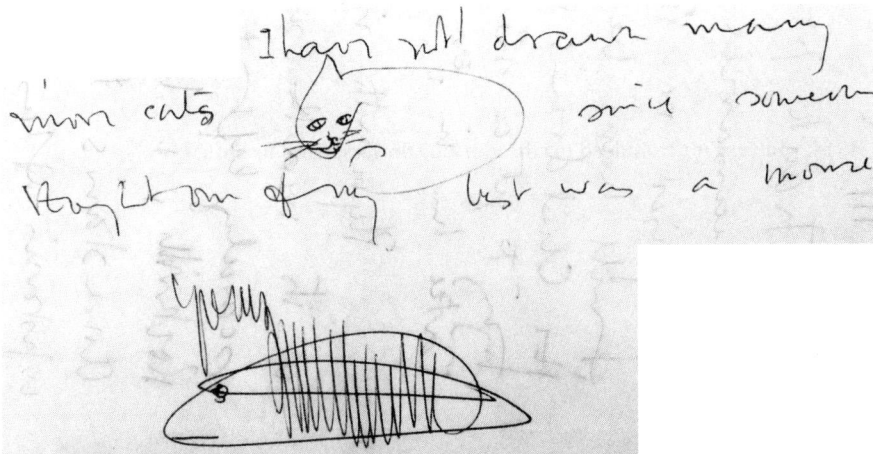

'I have not drawn many more cats since someone thought one of my best was a mouse'.

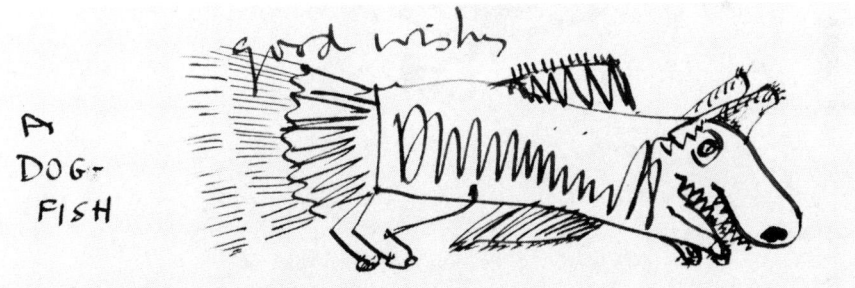

A DOG-FISH

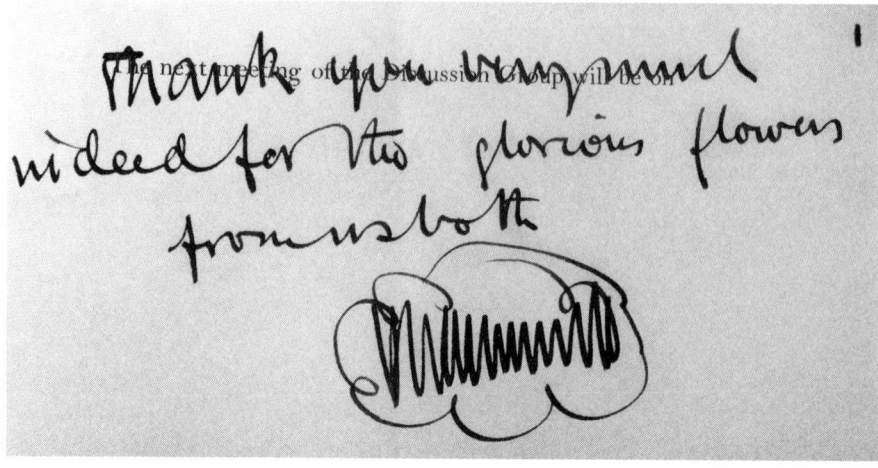

'Thank you very much indeed for the glorious flowers, from us both'.

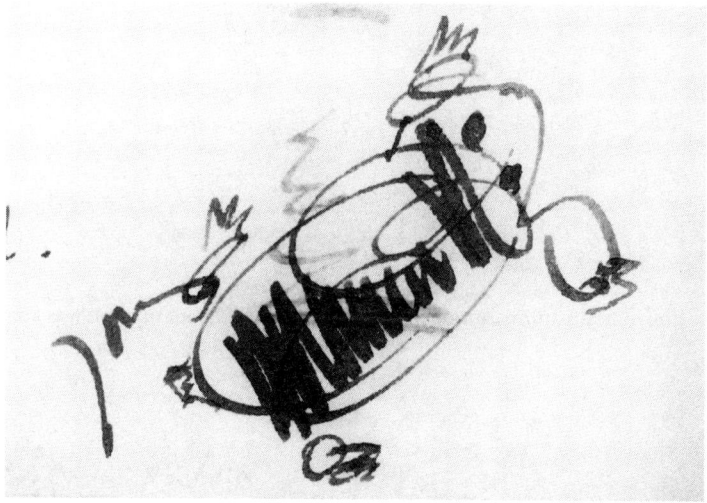

Quiet as a mouse. 'Here's for keeping Manoni quiet—at long last'.

Dr D. W. Winnicott 87 *Chester Square S W 1 Sloane 9544*

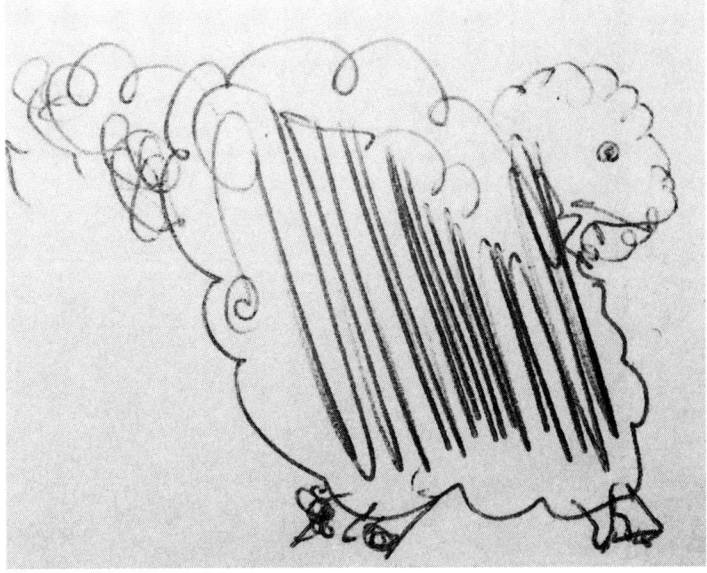

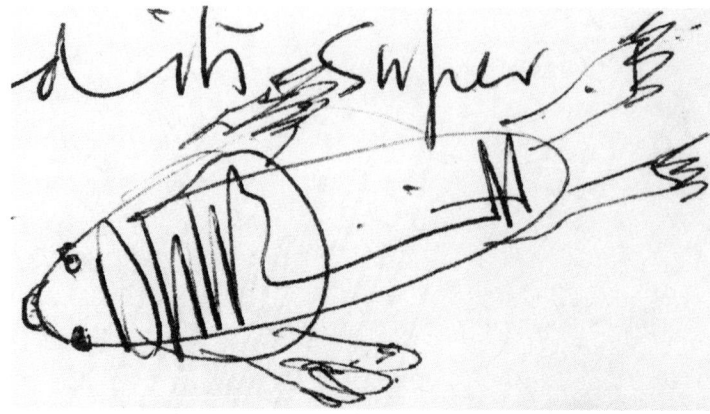

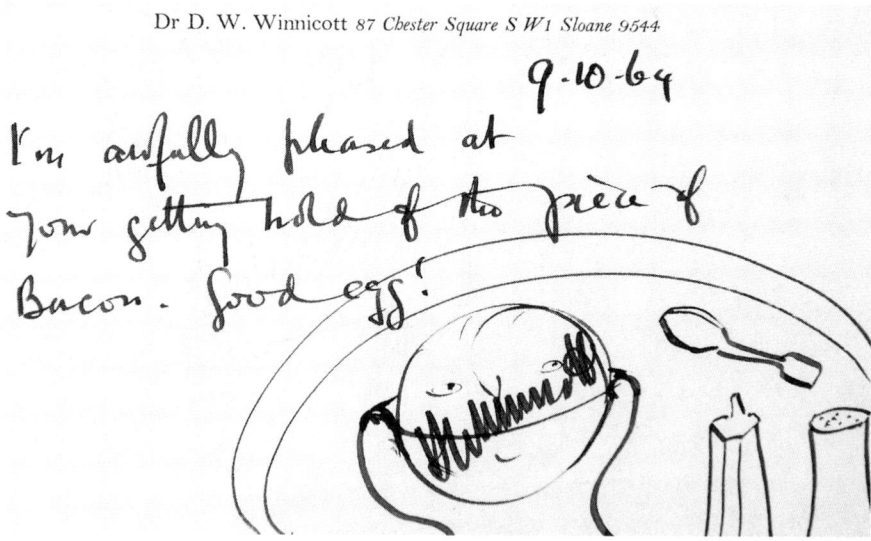

'I'm awfully pleased at your getting hold of this piece of bacon. Good egg!'

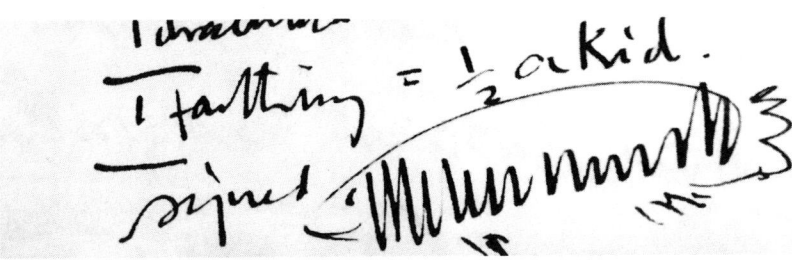

From 'Cleopatra Anamnesis Impphicough' [CW 9:4:9].

D. W. W.: A REFLECTION

Clare Winnicott

> O hours of childhood, hours when behind the figures there was more than the mere past, and when what lay before us was not the future! True, we were growing, and sometimes made haste to be grown up, half for the sake of those who'd nothing left but their grown-upness. Yet, when alone, we entertained ourselves with everlastingness: there we would stand, within the gap left between world and toy, upon a spot which, from the first beginning, had been established for a pure event.
>
> *Rainer Maria Rilke*

A few years ago the editors of a book on transitional objects and transitional phenomena[1] invited me to write something of a personal nature about D. W. W. It seems to me that what I wrote about him then, though I was naturally keeping the subject of the transitional area in the forefront of my mind, is central to the whole of his achievement.

I began with two questions: what was it about D. W. W. that made the exploration of the transitional area inevitable, and made his use of it clinically productive? It was my attempt to answer these questions that resulted in the contribution that followed, given here with a very few alterations.

I suggest that the answers have to be looked for not simply in a study of the development of D. W. W's ideas as he went along, but essentially in the kind of personality that was functioning behind them. It could seem therefore as if I were saying that these concepts arose naturally and easily out of his own way of life. In one sense this is true; but it is only half the story. The rest concerns the periods of doubt, uncertainty, and confusion, out of which form and meaning eventually emerged.

D. W. W could be excited by other people's ideas, but could use them and build on them only after they had been through the refinery of his own experience. By that time, unfortunately, he had often forgotten the source and he could, and did, alienate some people by his lack of acknowledgement. While other peoples ideas enriched him as clinician and as a person, it was the working out of ideas based on clinical practice that really absorbed him and that he grappled with to the end of his life. This was a creative process in which he was totally involved. In his clinical work D. W. W. made it his aim to enter into every situation undefended by his knowledge, so that he could be as exposed as possible to the impact of the situation itself. From his point of view this was the only way in which discovery and growth were possible, both for himself and for his patients. This approach was more than a stance; it was an essential discipline, and it added a dimension to his life as vital to him as fresh air.

The question is sometimes asked as to why D. W. W. in his writings seemed mainly concerned with exploring the area of the first two-person relationship. Strictly speaking this is not true: he wrote on a wide range of topics, including adolescence and delinquency and other matters of medical and sociological concern, and the greater part of his psychoanalytic practice was with adults. However, it could be true to say that his main contribution is likely to turn out to be in the study of the earliest relationships, and its application to the aetiology of psychosis and of the psychotic mechanisms in all of us. I suggest that his study took this direction from two sources. In the first place, he brought with him into psycho-analysis all that he had learnt and went on learning from paediatrics, and secondly, at the time he came to psycho-analysis the area of study just then opening up was that concerning the earliest experiences of life. Given his personality, his training and experience, and his urge for discovery, it seems inevitable that he would concentrate his researches on the so far comparatively unexplored area of earliest infancy and childhood. His findings however, are recognised by many as having implications far beyond the immediate area of study. It is the expressed opinion of some that they throw light on all areas of living.

As I have suggested, the essential clue to D. W. W.'s work on transitional objects and phenomena is to be found in his own personality, in his way of relating and being related to, and in his whole style of life. What I mean is that it was his *capacity to play*, which never deserted him, that led him inevitably into the area of research that he conceptualised in terms of the transitional objects and phenomena. It is not my purpose here to discuss the details of his work, but it seems important to note that in his terms the capacity to play is equated with a quality of living. In his own words, 'Playing is an experience, always a creative experience, and it is an experience in the space-time continuum, a basic form of living'.[2]

This quality of living permeates all levels and aspects of experiencing and relating, up to and including the sophisticated level described in his paper 'The Use of an Object' at which, in his own words, 'It is the destructive drive that creates the quality of externality'; and again, 'this quality of "always being destroyed" makes the reality of the surviving object felt as such, strengthens the feeling tone, and contributes to object constancy'.[3] For him, the destroying of the object in unconscious fantasy is like a cleansing process, which facilitates again and again the discovery of the object anew. It is a process of purification and renewal.

Having said that, I see my contribution as an attempt to throw some light on D. W. W.'s capacity for playing. I expect that readers will be familiar enough with his writings on this subject to know that I am not talking about playing games. I am talking about the capacity for operating in the limitless intermediate area where external and internal reality are compounded into the experience of living. I hope I do not suggest that D. W. W. lived in a state of permanent elation, because that was far from the case. He often found life hard and could be despondent and depressed and very angry, but given time he could come through and encompass these experiences in his own way and free himself from being cluttered up with resentment and prejudices. During the last years of his life the reality of his own death had to be negotiated, and this he did, again gradually and in his own way. I was always urging him to write an autobiography because I felt that his style of writing would lend itself to such a task. He started to do this, but there are only a few pages, and typically he used this exercise to deal with his immediate problem of living, which was that of dying. I know he used it in this way because he kept this notebook to himself and I did not see it until after his death.

The title of the autobiography was to be *Not Less Than Everything*, and the inner flap of the notebook reads as follows:

T. S. Eliot 'Costing not less than everything'

T. S. Eliot 'What we call the beginning is often the end

And to make an end is to make a beginning.

The end is where we start from'.

Prayer

D. W. W. Oh God! May I be alive when I die.

Following these words he started on the writing, and it begins by imaginatively describing the end of his life. I shall quote his own words:

I died.

It was not very nice, and it took quite a long time as it seemed (but it was only a moment in eternity).

There had been rehearsals (that's a difficult word to spell. I found I had left out the 'a'. The hearse was cold and unfriendly).

When the time came I knew all about the lung heavy with water that the heart could not negotiate, so that not enough blood circulated in the alveoli, and there was oxygen starvation as well as drowning. But fair enough, I had had a good innings: mustn't grumble as our old gardener used to say...

Let me see. What was happening when I died? My prayer had been answered. I was alive when I died. That was all I had asked and I had got it. (This makes me feel awful because so many of my friends and contemporaries died in the first World War, and I have never been free from the feeling that my being alive is a facet of some one thing of which their deaths can be seen as other facets: some huge crystal, a body with integrity and shape intrinsical in it.)

He then goes on to discuss the difficulty that a man has dying without a son to imaginatively kill and to survive him—'to provide the only continuity that men know. Women *are* continuous'. This dilemma is discussed in terms of King Lear and his relationship to his daughter who should have been a boy.

I hope that these quotations give some idea of D. W. W.'s capacity to come to terms with internal and external reality in a playful way, which makes reality bearable to the individual, so that denial can be avoided and the experience of living can be as fully realized as possible. In his own words, 'playing can be said to reach its own saturation point, which refers to the capacity to contain experience'.[4] He was avid for experience and would have hated to miss the inner experience of the reality of his own death, and he imaginatively achieved that experience. In conversation he would often refer to his deathday in a lighthearted way, but I knew that he was trying to get me and himself accustomed to the idea that it would come.

Having started at the end of his life, I must now go back to the beginnings and relate something about his earlier years and about the years that he and I spent together. I shall limit what I say to an attempt to illustrate the theme of playing, because that was central to his life and work.

First I must set the scene within which he grew up. It was an essentially English provincial scene in Plymouth, Devon, and it was far from London, not merely in mileage, but in custom and convention. When we drove to Plymouth from London he was always thrilled when we arrived at the place where the soil banked up at the side of the road changed color to the red soil of Devon. The richness of the soil brought back the richness of his early life which he never lost touch with. Of course on the return journey he was always equally pleased to be leaving it behind. But he was proud of being a Devonian, and that there is a village of Winnicott on the map of Devon. We never actually found the village, although we always meant to. It was enough that it was there.

The Winnicott household was a large and lively one with plenty of activity. But there was space for everyone in the large garden and house and there was no shortage of money. There were a vegetable garden, an orchard, a croquet lawn, a tennis court, and a pond, and high trees enclosed the whole garden. There was a special tree, in the branches of which Donald would do his homework in the days before he went to boarding school. Of the three children in the family Donald was the only boy, and his sisters, who still live in the house, were five and six years older than he. There is no doubt that the Winnicott parents were the centre of their children's lives, and that the vitality and stability of the entire household emanated from them. Their mother was vivacious and outgoing and was able to show and express her feelings easily. Sir Frederick Winnicott (as he later became) was slim and tallish and had an old-fashioned quiet dignity and poise about him, and a deep sense of fun. Those who knew him speak of him as a person of high intelligence and sound judgement. Both parents had a sense of humour.

Across the road was another large Winnicott household which contained Uncle Richard Winnicott (Frederick's elder brother) and his wife, and three boy cousins and two girls. The cousins were brought up almost as one family, so there was never a shortage of playmates. One of the sisters said recently that the question 'What can I do?' was never asked in their house. There was always something to do—and space to do it in, and someone to do it with if needed. But more important, there was always the vitality and imagination in the children themselves for exploits of all kinds. Donald's family, including his parents, were musical, and one sister later became a gifted painter. The household always included a nanny and a governess, but they do not seem to have hampered the natural energies of the children in any unreasonable way. Perhaps it would be more correct to say that the Winnicott children successfully evaded being hampered. As a small child Donald was certainly devoted to his nanny, and one of the first things I remember doing with him years later in London was to seek her out and ensure that she was all right and living comfortably. We discovered that the most important person in her life then (1950) was her own nephew Donald.

There is no question that from his earliest years Donald Winnicott did not doubt that he was loved, and he experienced a security in the Winnicott home which he could take for granted. In a household of this size there were plenty of chances for many kinds of relationships, and there was scope for the inevitable tensions to be isolated and resolved within the total framework. From this basic position Donald was then free to explore all the available spaces in the house and garden around him and to fill the spaces with bits of himself and so gradually to make his world his own. This capacity *to be at home* served him well throughout his life. There is a pop song which goes 'Home is in my heart'. That is certainly how Donald experienced it, and this gave him an immense freedom which enabled him to feel at home anywhere. When we were traveling in France and staying in small wayside inns, at each place I would think to myself, 'I wonder how long it will be before he's in the kitchen'—the kitchen of course being the centre of the establishment—and sure enough, he would almost always find his way there somehow. Actually, he loved kitchens, and when he was a child his mother complained that he spent more time with the cook in the kitchen than he did in the rest of the house.

Because Donald was so very much the youngest member of the Winnicott household (even the youngest boy cousin living opposite was older than he) and because he was so much loved and was in himself lovable, it seems likely that a deliberate effort was made, particularly on the part of his mother and sisters, not to spoil him. While this did not deprive him of feeling loved, it did I think deprive him of some intimacy and closeness that he needed. But as Donald possessed (as do his sisters still) a natural ability to communicate with children of almost any age, the communication between children and adults in the Winnicott home must have been of a high order. Of course they all possessed an irrepressible sense of humor, and this, together with the happiness and safety of their background, meant that there were no 'tragedies' in the Winnicott household—there were only amusing episodes. Not so many years ago, when the tank in the roof leaked, causing considerable flooding and damage, they were more excited and amused than alarmed by this unexpected happening.

At this point I should like to quote another page from Donald's autobiographical notes. Before doing so I should explain that the garden of the Winnicott home is on four levels. On the bottom level was the croquet lawn; then a steep slope (Mount Everest to a small child) leading to the pond level; next another slight slope leading to the lawn which was a tennis court; and, finally a flight of steps leading to the house level.

> Now that slope up from the croquet lawn to the flat part where there is a pond and where there was once a huge clump of pampas grass between the weeping ash trees (by the way do you know what exciting noises a pampas grass makes on a hot afternoon, when people are lying out on rugs beside the pond, reading or snoozing?) That slope up is fraught, as people say, fraught with history. It was on that slope that I took my own private croquet mallet (handle about a foot long because I was only three years old) and I bashed flat the nose of the wax doll that belonged to my sisters and that had become a source of irritation in my life because it was over that doll that my father used to tease me. She was called Rosie. Parodying some popular song he used to say (taunting me by the voice he used)
>
>> Rosie said to Donald
>> I love you
>> Donald said to Rosie
>> I don't believe you do.
>
> (Maybe the verses were the other way round, I forget) so I knew the doll had to be altered for the worse, and much of my life has been founded on the undoubted fact that I actually *did* this deed, not merely wished it and planned it.
>
> I was perhaps somewhat relieved when my father took a series of matches and, warming up the wax nose enough, remoulded it so that the face once more became a face. This early demonstration of the restitutive and reparative act certainly made an impression on me, and perhaps made me able to accept the fact that I myself, dear innocent child, had actually become violent directly with a doll, but indirectly with my good-tempered father who was just then entering my conscious life.

Again, to quote further from the notebook:

> Now my sisters were older than I, five and six years, so in a sense I was an only child with multiple mothers and with a father extremely preoccupied in my younger years with town as well as business matters. He was mayor twice and was eventually knighted, and then was made a Freeman of the City (as it has now become) of Plymouth. He was sensitive about his lack of education (he had had learning difficulties) and he always said that because of this he had not aspired to Parliament, but had kept to local politics—lively enough in those days in far away Plymouth.
>
> My father had a simple (religious) faith and once when I asked him a question that could have involved us in a long argument he just said: read the Bible and what you find there will be the true answer for you. So I was left, thank God, to get on with it myself.
>
> But when (at twelve years) I one day came home to midday dinner and said 'drat' my father looked pained as only he could look, blamed my mother for not seeing to it that I had decent friends, and from that moment he prepared himself to send me away to boarding school, which he did when I was thirteen.
>
> 'Drat' sounds very small as a swear word, but he was right; the boy who was my new friend was no good, and he and I could have got into trouble if left to our own devices.

The friendship was in fact broken up then and there, and this show of strength on the part of his father was a significant factor in Donald's development. In his own words: 'So my father was there to kill and be killed, but it is probably true that in the early years he left me too much to all my mothers. Things never quite righted themselves'.

And so Donald went away to the Leys School, Cambridge, and was in his element. To his great delight the afternoons were free, and he ran, cycled and swam, played rugger, joined the School Scouts, and made friends and sang in the choir, and each night he read a story aloud to the boys in his dormitory. He read extremely well, and years later I was to benefit from this accomplishment because we were never without a book that he was reading aloud to me. One Christmas Eve sitting on the floor (we never sat on chairs) he read all night because the book was irresistible. He read in a dramatic way, savouring the writing to the full.

Donald described to me his going away to school. The whole family would be there to see him off, and he would wave and be sorry to leave until he was taken from their sight by the train's entering quite a long tunnel just outside Plymouth. All through this tunnel he settled down to the idea of leaving, but then out again the other side he left them behind and looked forward to going on to school. He often blessed that tunnel because he could honestly manage to feel sorry to leave right up to the moment of entering it.

I have in my possession a letter which Donald wrote to his mother from school which shows the kind of interplay that existed between members of the family:

My dearest Mother,

On September 2nd all true Scouts think of their mothers, since that was the birthday of Baden Powell's mother when she was alive.

And so when you get this letter I shall be thinking of you in particular, and I only hope you will get it in the morning.

But to please me very much I must trouble you to do me a little favour. Before turning over the page I want you to go up into my bedroom and in the right-hand cupboard find a small parcel ... Now, have you opened it? Well I hope you will like it. You can change it at Pophams if you don't. Only if you do so, you must ask to see No. 1 who knows about it.

I have had a ripping holiday, and I cannot thank you enough for all you have done and for your donation to the Scouts.

My home is a beautiful home and I only wish I could live up to it. However I will do my best and work hard and that's all I can do at present.

Give my love to the others: thank Dad for his games of billiards and V and K [his sisters] for being so nice and silly so as to make me laugh. But, it being Mother's day, most love goes to you,

from your loving boy

Donald.

Some who read this abbreviated account of D. W. W.'s early life and family relationships may be inclined to think that it sounds too good to be true. But the truth is that it *was* good, and try as I will I cannot present it in any other light. Essentially he was a deeply happy person whose capacity for enjoyment never failed to triumph over the setbacks and disappointments that came his way. Moreover, there is a sense in which the quality of his early life and his appreciation of it did in itself present him with a major problem, that of freeing himself from the family, and of establishing his own separate life and identity without sacrificing the early richness. It took him a long time to do this.

It was when Donald was in the sick room at school, having broken his collarbone on the sports field, that he consolidated in his own mind the idea of becoming a doctor. Referring to that time he often said: 'I could see that for the rest of my life I should have to depend on doctors if I damaged myself or became ill, and the only way out of this position was to become a doctor myself, and from then on the idea as a real proposition was always on my mind, although I know that father expected me to enter his flourishing business and eventually take over from him'.

One of Donald's school friends, Stanley Ede (who remained a lifelong friend), had often stayed in the Winnicott household and was well known to all the family. Back at school after a visit to his home. Donald, aged sixteen, wrote the following in a letter to the friend who had not yet returned to school:

> Dear Stanley,
>
> Thank you so much for the lovely long letter you sent me in the week. It is awfully good of you to take such a lot of trouble and to want to . . .
>
> Father and I have been trying consciously and perhaps unconsciously to find out what the ambition of the other is in regard to my future. From what he had said I was *sure* that he wanted me more than anything else to go into his business. And so, again consciously and not, I have found every argument for the idea and have not thought much about anything else so that I should not be disappointed. And so I have learned to cherish the business life with all my heart, and had intended to enter it and please my father and myself.
>
> When your letter came yesterday you may have expected it to have disappointed me. But—I tell you all I feel—I was so excited that all the stored-up feelings about doctors which I have bottled up for so many years seemed to burst and bubble up at once. Do you know that—in the degree that Algy wanted to go into a monastery—I have for ever so long wanted to be a doctor. But I have always been afraid that my father did not want it, and so I have never mentioned it and—like Algy—even felt a repulsion at the thought.
>
> This afternoon I went an eight mile walk to the Roman Road with Chandler, and we told each other all we felt, and especially I told him what I have told you now. O, Stanley!
>
> Your still sober and true—
> although seemingly intoxicated—
> but never-the-less devoted
> friend.
>
>   Donald

It seems that Stanley, one year older than Donald, had offered to broach the question of Donald's future to his father, and that he did so. There is a postcard to Stanley saying, 'Thank you infinitely for having told father when and what you did. I have written Dad a letter which I think pretty nearly convinced him'.

Donald recounts that when he summoned up courage to go to the Headmaster at school and tell him that he wanted to be a doctor, the Head grunted and looked at him long and hard before replying slowly: 'Boy, not brilliant, but will do'. And so he went to Jesus College, Cambridge, and took a degree in biology. His room in College was popular as a meeting place, because he had hired a piano and played it unceasingly and had a good tenor voice for singing.

But the first World War was on, and his first year as a medical student was spent helping in the Cambridge Colleges which had been turned into military hospitals. One of the patients, who became a lifelong friend, remembers Donald in those days: 'The first time I saw him was in hospital in Cambridge in 1916 in the first war; he was a medical student who liked to sing a comic song on Saturday evenings in the ward—and sang "Apple Dumplings" and cheered us all up'.

It was a source of deep sorrow and conflict that all his friends went at once into the army, but that as a medical student Donald was exempt. Many close friends were killed early in the war, and his whole life was affected by this, because always he felt that he had a responsibility to live for those who died, as well as for himself.

The kind of relationship with friends that he had at that time in Cambridge is illustrated by a letter from a friend who had already joined up in the army and was on a course for officers in Oxford. It is written from Exeter College Oxford and dated 8 November 1915:

> What are you doing on Saturday for tea? Well, I'll tell you!! *You are going to provide a big Cambridge Tea for yourself, myself and Southwell* (of Caius) [Caius College Cambridge] whom you've met I think. He's a top-hole chap and has got a commission. If you haven't met him you ought to have, and anyway you've heard me speak of him. Can you manage it? Blow footer etc. etc. or I'll blow you next time I see you. Try and manage it will you? Good man! It's sponging on you I know, but I also know you're a silly idiot and won't mind. Silly ass! Cheer O old son of a gun and get plenty of food.

Feeling as he did Donald could not settle in Cambridge and was not satisfied until he was facing danger for himself, and, coming from Plymouth, he of course wanted to go into the navy. He applied for and was accepted as a surgeon probationer. He was drafted to a destroyer, where he was one of the youngest men on board and the only medical officer in spite of his lack of training; fortunately, there was an experienced medical orderly. He was subject to a great deal of teasing in the Officers' Mess. Most of the officers had been through one or other of the Royal Naval Colleges and came from families with a naval tradition. They were astonished that Donald's father was a *merchant*. This was a novelty, and they made the most of it, and Donald seems to have made the most of their company and of the whole experience. He has often related with amusement the banter that went on at meal times. Although the ship was involved in enemy action and there were casualties, Donald had much free time, which he seems to have spent reading the novels of Henry James.

After the war Donald went straight to St Bartholomew's Hospital in London to continue his medical training. He soaked himself in medicine and fully committed himself to the whole experience. This included writing for the hospital magazine and joining in the social life: singing sprees, dancing, occasional skiing holidays, and hurrying off at the last minute to hear operas for the first time, where he usually stood in his slippers at the back of the 'Gods'.

It is difficult to give any dates in relation to Donald's girl friends, but he had quite close attachments to friends of his sisters and later to others he met through his Cambridge friends. He came to the brink of marriage more than once but did not actually marry (for the first time) until the age of twenty-eight.

Donald had some great teachers at the hospital, and he always said that it was Lord Horder who taught him the importance of taking a careful case history, and to listen to what the patient said, rather than simply to ask questions. After qualification he stayed on at Bart's to work as casualty officer for a year. He literally worked almost all day and night, but he would not have missed the experience for the world. It contained the challenge of the unexpected and provided the stimulation that he revelled in.

During his training Donald became ill with what turned out to be an abscess on the lung and was a patient in Bart's for three months. A friend who visited him there remembers it in these words: 'It was a gigantic old ward with a high ceiling dwarfing the serried ranks of beds, patients and visitors. He was *intensely* amused and interested at being lost in a crowd and said "I am convinced that every doctor ought to have been once in his life in a hospital bed as a patient".'

Donald had always intended to become a general practitioner in a country area, but one day a friend lent him a book by Freud and so he discovered psychoanalysis; deciding that this was for him, he realized that he must therefore stay in London to undergo analysis. During his medical training he had become deeply interested in children's work, and after taking his Membership examination he set up as a consultant in children's medicine (there was no specialty in paediatrics in those days). In 1923 he obtained two hospital appointments, at The Queen's Hospital for Children and at Paddington Green Children's Hospital. The latter appointment he held for forty years. The development of his work at Paddington Green is a story in itself, and many colleagues from all over the world visited him there. Because of his own developing interests and skills over the years, his clinic gradually became a psychiatric clinic, and he used to refer to it as his 'Psychiatric Snack Bar' or his clinic for dealing with parents' hypochondria. In 1923 he also acquired a room in the Harley Street area and set up a private consultant practice.

At the beginning he found Harley Street formidable because he had few patients, so in order to impress the very dignified porter who opened the door to patients for all the doctors in the house, he tells how he used to pay the fares of some of his hospital mothers and children so that they could visit him in Harley Street. Of course this procedure was not entirely on behalf of the porter, because he selected cases in which he was particularly interested and to which he wanted to give more time so that he could begin to explore the psychological aspects of illness.

The sheer pressure of the numbers attending his hospital clinics must have been important to him as an incentive to explore as fully as he did how to use the doctor-patient *space* as economically as possible for the therapeutic task. The ways in which he did this have been described in his writing.

However, there is one detail he does not describe, and which I observed both at his Paddington Green Clinic and in his work with evacuee children in Oxfordshire during the last war. He attempted to round off and make significant a child's visit to him by giving the child something to take away which could afterwards be used and/or destroyed or thrown away. He would quickly reach for a piece of paper and fold it into some shape, usually a dart or a fan, which he might play with for a moment and then give to the child as he said goodbye. I never saw this gesture refused by any child. It could be that this simple symbolic act contained the germ of ideas he developed in the 'Use of an Object' paper written at the end of his life. There could also be a link here with the transitional object concept.

In attempting to give some idea of D. W. W's capacity to play I have somehow slipped into an historical or biographical sequence of writing without intending to do so. This is in no way meant to be a biography. What I have been trying to do is to illustrate how he related to people at different stages of his life and in different situations. But I must now abandon the historical perspective which so far protected me, and bring him briefly into focus for myself and in relation to our life together. From now on 'he' becomes 'we' and I cannot disentangle us.

Many years ago a visitor staying in our home looked round thoughtfully and said: 'You and Donald *play*'. I remember being surprised at this new light that had been thrown on us. We had certainly never *set out* to play; there was nothing self-conscious and deliberate about it. It seems just to have happened that we lived that way, but I could see what our visitor meant. We played with *things—our* possessions—rearranging, acquiring, and discarding according to our mood. We played with ideas, tossing them about at random with the freedom of knowing that we need not agree, and that we were strong enough not to be hurt by each other. In fact the question of hurting each other did not arise because we were operating in the play area where everything is permissible. We each possessed a capacity for enjoyment, and it could take over in the most unlikely places and lead us into exploits we could not have anticipated. After Donald's death an American friend described us as 'two crazy people who delighted each other and delighted their friends'. Donald would have been pleased with this accolade, so reminiscent of his words: 'We are poor indeed if we are only sane'.[5]

Early in our relationship I had to settle for the idea that Donald was, and always would be, completely unpredictable in our private life, except for his punctuality at meal times and the fact that he never failed to meet me at the station when I had been away. This unpredictability had its advantages, in that we could never settle back and take each other for granted in day-to-day living. What we could take for granted was something more basic that I can only describe as our recognition and acceptance of each other's separateness. In fact the strength of our unity lay in this recognition, and implicit in it is an acceptance of the unconscious ruthless and destructive drives which were discussed as the final development of his theories in the 'Use of an Object' paper. Our separateness left us each free to do our own thing, to think our own thoughts, and possess our own dreams, and in so doing to strengthen the capacity of each of us to experience the joys and sorrows which we shared.

There were some things that were especially important to us, like the Christmas card that Donald drew each year, and which we both painted in hundreds, staying up until 2 A.M., in the days before Christmas. I remember once suggesting to him that the drawing looked better left as it was in black and white. He said, 'Yes, I know, but I like painting'. There were his endless squiggle drawings which were part of his daily routine. He would play the game with himself and produced some very fearful and some very funny drawings, which often had a powerful integrity of their own. If I was away for a night he would send a drawing through the post for me to receive in the morning, because my part in all this was to enjoy and appreciate his productions, which I certainly did, but sometimes I could wish that there were not quite so many of them.

Donald's knowledge and appreciation of music was a joy to both of us, but it was of particular importance to me because he introduced me to much that was new. He always had a special feeling for the music of Bach, but at the end of his life it was the late Beethoven string quartets that absorbed and fascinated him. It seems as if the refinement and abstraction in the musical idiom of these works helped him to gather in and realise in himself the rich harvest of a lifetime. On quite another level he also greatly enjoyed the Beatles and bought all their recordings. Donald never had enough time to develop his own piano playing, but he would often dash up to the piano and play for a moment between patients, and invariably he celebrated the end of a day's work by a musical outburst fortissimo. He enjoyed the fact that I knew more about poets than he did, and that I could say a Shakespeare sonnet or some Dylan Thomas or T. S. Eliot to him on demand. He particularly enjoyed Edward Lear's 'The Owl and the Pussycat' and couldn't hear it often enough. In the end he memorised it himself.

Our favorite way of celebrating or simply relaxing was to dress up and go out to a long, unhurried dinner in a candle-lit dining room not so far from where we lived. In the early days sometimes we danced. I remember him looking around this room one evening and saying: 'Aren't we lucky. We still have things to say to each other'.

For years two T.V. programmes that we never missed were 'Come Dancing' (a display of all kinds of ballroom dancing) and 'Match of the Day', which was the reshowing of the best football or rugger match each Saturday, or in the summer it would be tennis.

I think that the only times when Donald actually showed that he was angry with me were on occasions when I damaged myself or became ill. He hated to have me as a patient, and not as his wife and playmate. He showed this one day when I damaged my foot and it became bruised and swollen. We had no crêpe bandage so he said he would go and buy one and I was to lie down until he returned. He was away for two hours and came back pleased with a gold expanding bracelet he had bought for me—but he had forgotten the bandage.

I was always speculating about Donald's own transitional object. He did not seem to remember one specifically, until suddenly he was able to get into touch with it. He described the experience to me in a letter written early in 1950:

> Last night I got something quite unexpected, through dreaming, out of what you said. Suddenly you joined up with the nearest thing I can get to my transition object: it was something I have always known about but I lost the memory of it, at this moment I became conscious of it. There was a very early doll called Lily belonging to my younger sister and I was fond of it, and very distressed when it fell and broke. After Lily I hated *all* dolls. But I always knew that before Lily was a *quelquechose* of my own. I knew retrospectively that it must have been a doll. But it had never occurred to me that it wasn't just like myself, a person, that is to say it was a kind of other me, and a not-me female, and part of me and yet not, and absolutely inseparable from me. I don't know what happened to it. If I love you as I loved this (must I say?) doll, I love you all out. And I believe I do. Of course I love you all sorts of other ways, but this thing came new at me. I felt enriched, and felt once more like going on writing my paper on transition objects (postponed to October). (You don't mind do you—this about you and the T.O.?)

It would not be right to give the impression that Donald and I shared only experiences that lay outside our work. It was our work that brought us together in the first place, and it remained central, and bound us inextricably together. Writing to me in December 1946 he said, 'In odd moments I have written quite a lot of the paper for the Psycho-Analytical Society in February, and I spend a lot of time working it out. My work is really quite a lot associated with you. Your effect on me is to make me keen and productive and this is all the more awful—because when I am cut off from you I feel paralyzed for all action and originality'.

In fact each of us was essential to the work of the other. During Donald's lifetime we worked in different spheres, and this was an added interest extending the boundaries of our joint existence. We were fortunate that through the years a wide circle of people came to be intimately included in our lives and work, and we in theirs. This was a strong binding force for all concerned because it provided the community of interest which is the prerequisite for creative living. How lucky we were in those who shared our lives; how much we owe to them, and how much we enjoyed their company!

Throughout his life Donald never ceased to be in touch with his dream world and to continue his own analysis. It was the deep undercurrent of his life, the orchestral accompaniment to the main theme. His poem called 'Sleep' is relevant here[6]:

> Let down your tap root
>   to the centre of your soul
> Suck up the sap
>   from the infinite source
>   of your unconscious
> and
>   be evergreen.

To conclude, I want to relate a dream about Donald which I had two and a half years after his death.

I dreamt that we were in our favorite shop in London, where there is a circular staircase to all floors. We were running up and down these stairs grabbing things here, there, and everywhere as Christmas presents for our friends. We were really having a spending spree, knowing that as usual we would end up keeping many of the things ourselves. I suddenly realized that Donald was alive after all and I thought with relief, 'Now I shan't have to worry about the Christmas card'. Then we were sitting in the restaurant having our morning coffee as usual (in fact we always went out to morning coffee on Saturday). We were facing each other, elbows on the table, and I looked at him full in the face and said: 'Donald there's something we have to say to each other, some truth that we have to say, what is it?' With his very blue eyes looking unflinchingly into mine he said: 'That this is a dream'. I replied slowly: 'Oh yes, of course, you died, you died a year ago'. He reiterated my words: 'Yes, I died a year ago'.

For me it was through this dream of playing that life and death, his and mine, could be experienced as a reality.

Notes

1. *Between Reality and Fantasy*, Simon A. Grolnick and Leonard Barkin (Eds.). New York, London: Jason Aronson, 1978.
2. From 'Playing: A Theoretical Statement' [CW 8:2:15]
3. See *Playing and Reality*; also 'The Use of an Object' [CW 8:2:28] and related papers.
4. From 'Playing: A Theoretical Statement' [CW 8:2:15].
5. From 'Primitive Emotional Development' [CW 2:7:8].
6. This poem was handwritten by Winnicott at the end of his paper 'Playing and Culture' [CW 8:2:9].

REFERENCE LIST OF THE
COLLECTED WORKS

Abel, L. (1939). Pruritus ani. *British Medical Journal*, 1(4081), 627.

Abraham, K. (1916). The first pregenital stage of the libido. In *Collected papers on psychoanalysis* (pp. 248–279). London: Hogarth.

Abraham, K. (1924). A short study of the development of the libido, viewed in the light of mental disorders. In *Selected papers of Karl Abraham* (pp. 418–501). London: Hogarth.

Abraham, K., Ferenczi, S., Freud, S., Jones, E., and Simmel, E. (1919). Zur Psychoanalyse der Kriegsneurosen. *Diskussion am 5. Internationalent Psychoanalytischen Kongress, Budapest, 1918*. Vienna: Deuticke.

Abram, J. (2012). D. W. W.'s notes on the Vienna Congress 1971: A consideration of Winnicott's theory of aggression and an interpretation of the clinical implications. *Donald Winnicott Today*, 2013, 302–330.

Ackerknecht, E. H. (1982). The history of psychosomatic medicine. *Psychological Medicine*, 12(1), 17–24.

Ackerman, A. (1953). Psychiatric disorders in children—Diagnosis and aetiology in our time. In P. Hoch & J. Zubin (Eds.), *Current problems in psychiatric diagnosis*. New York: Grune & Stratton.

Addis, R. (1936, September). Discussion on enuresis. *Proceedings of the Royal Society of Medicine*, 29. Joint Discussion No. 6: Section of Psychiatry and Section for the Study of Disease in Children.

Aichhorn, A. (1925). *Wayward youth*. London: Imago.

Aichhorn, A. (1936). *Wayward youth*. London: Putnam.

Aichhorn, A. (1949). Some remarks on the psychic structure and social care of a certain type of female juvenile delinquents. In *The psychoanalytic study of the child*, 3/4 (pp. 439–448). London: Imago.

Albee, E. (1962). *Who's afraid of Virginia Woolf?* New York: Atheneum.

Alexander, F. (1932). Psychoanalysis and medicine. *Mental Hygiene*, 16, 63.

Alger, I. (1966). The clinical handling of the analyst's response. *Psychoanalytic Forum*, 1(3), 289–302.

Allen, Clifford. (1955, 17 December). Letter: Prefrontal leucotomy. *British Medical Journal*, 2(4954), 1502.

Allen, Lady Marjory. (1959, 25 March). Letter: Freedom to thrive. *The Times*. Issue 54418, 11.

Allendy, R. (1932). A case of eczema. *Psycho-Analytic Review*, 19, 152.

Alley, R. (1964). *Francis Bacon: Catalogue raisonné and documentation*. London: Thames and Hudson.

Apley, J., Creak, M., Hubble, D. V., MacCarthy, D., MacKeith, R., Mayon-White, R., Potter, C. T. (1960). Report of the British Paediatric Association: Psychiatric services for children. *British Medical Journal*, 2, 795.

Apley, J., & MacKeith, R. (1962). *The child and his symptoms: a psychosomatic approach*. Philadelphia: F. A. Davis.

Ashdown, M. (1936). The role of the psychiatric social worker (monograph). London: The Association of Psychiatric Social Workers.

Astor, Lady Nancy. (1951, 18 August). Letter: Fewer nursery schools: Need for objective survey. *The Times*, Issue 52083.

Axline, V. (1947). *Play therapy: The inner dynamics of childhood*. Boston: Houghton Mifflin.

Axline, V. (1964). *Dibs: In search of self*. New York: Ballantine.

Bakwin, H. (1942). Loneliness in infants. *American Journal of Diseases of Children*, 63, 30–40.

Bawkin, H., & Morris, R. (1953). *Clinical management of behavior disorders in children*. Philadelphia/London: W. B. Saunders.

Balint, A. (1931/1953). *The psycho-analysis of the nursery*. London: Routledge & Kegan Paul.

Balint, A. (1933). Ber eine besondere Form der infantilen Angst (Abstract). *International Journal of Psychoanalysis*, 15, 325.

Balint, A., & Balint, M. (1939). On transference and counter-transference. *International Journal of Psychoanalysis*, 20, 223–230.

Balint, E. (1954). Three phases of a transference neurosis. In Balint 'Drei Phasen einer Übertragungsneurose'. *Psyche* 11(8), 1957, 526–542.

Balint, E. (1957). Drei phasen einer übertragungsneurose. *Psyche—Zeitschrift für Psychoanalyse*, 11(9), 526–542.

Balint, M. (1951). On love and hate. In *Primary love and psycho-analytic technique*. London: Hogarth.

Balint, M. (1955). Friendly expanses—Horrid empty spaces. *International Journal of Psychoanalysis*, 36, 225–241.

Balint, M. (1957). *The doctor, his patient and the illness*. London: Pitman Medical.

Balint, M. (1957). *Problems of human pleasure and behaviour*. London: Hogarth/Institute of Psycho-Analysis.

Balint, M. (1958). Three areas of the mind—Theoretical considerations. *International Journal of Psychoanalysis*, 39, 328–341.

Balint, M. (1959). *Thrills and regressions*. London: Hogarth.

Balint, M. (1960). Primary narcissism and primary love. *Psychoanalytic Quarterly*, 29, 1, 6–43. Reprinted in *The basic fault: Therapeutic aspects of regression*. London: Tavistock, 1968.

Balint, M. (1968). *The basic fault: Therapeutic aspects of regression*. London: Tavistock.

Banks, H. S. (1931). Intensive serum treatment of cerebro-spinal fever. *Lancet*, 2(5640), 747.

Barinbaum, M. (1934). A contribution to the problem of psycho-physical relations with special reference to dermatology. *Internationale Zeitschrift für Psychoanalyse*, 20, 241–251.

Bastiaanse. (1925). *Bulletin de l'Académie Nationale de Médecine*, 3e sér., 94, 815.

Batten, F. E. (1905). Ataxia in childhood. *Brain*, 28, 484.

Beirman, G. (Ed.). (1968). *Handbook of the psychotherapy of children*. Munich: Ernst Reinhardt.

Bender, L. (1947). Childhood schizophrenia. *American Journal of Orthopsychiatry*, 17(1), 4–56.

Bergeron, M. (1961). *Psychologie du premier âge*. Paris: Presses Universitaires de France.

Berman, L. (1949). Counter-transferences and attitudes of the analyst in the therapeutic process. *Psychiatry*, 12, 159–166.

Bettelheim, B. (1960). *The informed heart: Autonomy in a mass age*. New York/London: Free Press/Thames & Hudson.

Bettelheim, B. (1967). *The empty fortress: Infantile autism and the birth of the self*. New York/London: Free Press/Collier-Macmillan.

Bibring, E. (1954). Psychoanalysis and dynamic psychotherapies. *Journal of the American Psychoanalytical Association, 2*, 745–770.

Bick, E. (1953 [2001]). Anxiety underlying phobia of sexual intercourse in a woman. *British Journal of Psychotherapy*, 18(1), 7–21.

Bien, E. (1933). The clinical psychogenic aspects of pruritus vulvæ. *Psycho-Analytic Review, 20*, 186.

Bion, W. (1957). On arrogance. In *Second thoughts*, 86–92. London: Heinemann, 1967.

Bion, W. (1957). Differentiation of the psychotic from the non-psychotic personalities. *International Journal of Psychoanalysis, 38*, 3–4, 266–275.

Bion, W. (1959). Attacks on linking. *International Journal of Psychoanalysis, 40*, 308–341. Reprinted in *Second thoughts*, 93–109. London: Heinemann, 1967.

Bion, W. (1962). *Learning from experience*. London: Maresfield.

Bion, W. (1962). The psycho-analytic study of thinking. *International Journal of Psychoanalysis, 43*, 306–310.

Bion, W. (1967). *Second thoughts*. London: Heinemann Medical Books.

Bion, W. R. (1950). The imaginary twin. In *Second thoughts* (pp. 3–22). London: Karnac.

Birch, H. G., Chess, S., & Thomas, A. (1960). *Your child is a person*. London: Peter Davies.

Blake, W. (1793). I fear'd the fury of my wind. In *The Poetical Works* [1908].

Blake, Y. (1968). Psychotherapy with the more disturbed patient. *British Journal of Medical Psychology, 41*, 199–211.

Blanc, & Caminopetros. (1926). *Schweizerische medizinische Wochenschrif, 56*, 131.

Bonaparte, M. (1950). *Five copy-books*. London: Imago.

Bonime, W. (1957). Liking and disliking one's patients. In A. Rifkin (Ed.), *Schizophrenia in psychoanalytic office practice* (pp. 69–73). New York: Grune & Stratton.

Bonnard, A. (1958). Pre-body-ego types of (pathological) mental functioning. *Journal of the American Psychoanalytic Association, 6*, 581–611.

Bornstein, B. (1949). The analysis of a phobic child. In *The psychoanalytic study of the child*, 3 (pp. 181–226). London: Imago.

Bornstein, B. (1951). On latency. In *The psychoanalytic study of the child*, 6 (pp. 279–285). London: Imago.

Bourne, G., & Stone, G. K. (1929). *The principles of clinical pathology in practice*. London: Oxford Medical.

Bowlby, J. (1939). Hysteria in children. In R. G. Gordon (Ed.), *A survey of child psychiatry* (pp. 80–94). London: Oxford University Press.

Bowlby, J. (1940). The influence of early environment in the development of neurosis and neurotic character. *International Journal of Psychoanalysis, 21*, 154–178.

Bowlby, J. (1944). Forty-four juvenile thieves: Their characters and home-life. *International Journal of Psychoanalysis, 25*, 19–53.

Bowlby, J. (1951). *Maternal care and mental health*. Geneva: World Health Organization.

Bowlby, J. (1958). The nature of the child's tie to his mother. *International Journal of Psycho-Analysis, 39*, 350–373.

Bowlby, J. (1958). Psycho-analysis and child care. In J. D. Sutherland (Ed.), *Psycho-analysis and contemporary thought*, 33–57. London: Hogarth.

Bowlby, J. (1960). Grief and mourning in infancy and early childhood. In *The psychoanalytic study of the child*, 15. London: Imago.

Bowlby, J. (1960). Separation anxiety. *International Journal of Psychoanalysis, 41*, 89–113.

Bowlby, J. (1969). *Attachment and loss* (volume 1): *Attachment*. London/New York: Hogarth and the Institute of Psychoanalysis/Basic Books.

Bowlby, J., Robertson J., & Rosenbluth, D. (1952). A two-year-old goes to hospital. In *The psychoanalytic study of the child, 7* (pp. 82–94). London: Imago.

Bowlby, J., & Fry, M. (Eds.). (1953). *Child care and the growth of love*. Abridged version. Harmondsworth: Penguin.

Bowley, A. H. (1947). *The psychology of the unwanted child*. Edinburgh: E. and S. Livingstone.

Bowra, C. M. (1944). *Sophoclean tragedy*. Oxford: Oxford University Press.

Bradley, C. (1941). *Schizophrenia in childhood*. New York: Macmillan.

Bradley, C. (1942). Biography of a schizophrenic child. *The Nervous Child, 1*(2–3), 141.

Brain, R., & Hunter, D. (1929). Acute meningo-encephalomyelitis of childhood. *Lancet, 213*, 221–227.

Bray, G. W. (1933). Lichen urticatus or urticaria papulosa. *British Journal of Children's Diseases, 30*, 180.

Bray, G. W. (1937). Recent advances in allergy. *American Journal of the Medical Sciences, 193*.

Breasted, J. H. (1906). *A history of Egypt*. London.

Briance, P. (1982). *Childbirth with confidence*. London: Dick-Read School for Natural Birth.

Brierley, M. (1951). *Trends in psycho-analysis*. London: Hogarth.

British Medical Association Psychological Medicine Group. (1961). Report of the subcommittee on the child psychiatric service. *British Medical Journal, 1*(5229), 25 March 1961, Supplement 2931, 109–110.

British Medical Journal Leading Article. (1942, Sept. 19). Loneliness in infancy. *British Medical Journal, 2*(4263), 345.

British Medical Journal Leading Article. (1943, Apr. 24). Cutting the frontal white fibres. *British Medical Journal, 1*(4294), 510.

British Psychoanalytic Society. (1954). Minutes of the Board of the Institute of Psychoanalysis (Meeting minutes), 31 March.

British Psychoanalytic Society. (1966). Minutes of the Board of the Institute of Psychoanalysis (Meeting minutes), 7 March.

British Psychoanalytic Society. (1967). Minutes of the Board of the Institute of Psychoanalysis (Meeting minutes), 20 February.

British Psychoanalytic Society. (1967). Minutes of the Board of the Institute of Psychoanalysis (Meeting minutes), 5 June.

British Psychoanalytic Society. (1970). Minutes of the Board of the Institute of Psychoanalysis (Meeting minutes), 2 Novemeber.

British Psychoanalytic Society. (1971). Minutes of the Board of the Institute of Psychoanalysis (Meeting minutes), 15 March.

British Psychoanalytic Society. (1985). Minutes of the Board of the Institute of Psychoanalysis (Meeting minutes), 3 July.

Britton, C. (1955). Casework techniques in the child care services. *Case Conference, 1*, 9.

Britton, C., & Winnicott, D. (1944). The problem of homeless children. [CW 2:6:14]

Britton, C., & Winnicott, D. (1947). Residential management as treatment for difficult children: The evolution of a wartime hostels scheme. *Human Relations*, 1(1), 87–97. [CW 3:2:3]

Bruch, H., & Cottington, F. (1942). Diary of a psychotic child. *The Nervous Child*, 1(2–3), 232.

Bunyan, John. (1678). *The pilgrim's progress from this world to that which is to come; Delivered under the similitude of a dream*. London.

Burgess, N. (1939). Chronic urticaria. *British Medical Journal*, 1(4082), 662–665.

Burke, N. H. (1931). Stigmata of degeneration in relation to mental deficiency. *Proceedings of the Royal Society of Medicine*, 24(4), 413–428.

Burlingham, D. (1952). *Twins: A study of three pairs of identical twins*. London: Imago.

Burlingham, D., & Freud, A. (1942). *Young children in wartime: A year's work in a residential war nursery*. London: Allen & Unwin.

Burlingham, D., & Freud, A. (1944). *Infants without families*. London/New York: Allen & Unwin/International Universities Press.

Burton, L. (1968). *Vulnerable children*. London: Routledge & Kegan Paul.

Burton, R. (1621). *The anatomy of melancholy*.

Caccia, G. (1904). Contributo alla conoscenza di alcune complicanze della varicella. *Rivista di Clinica Pediatrica*, 2(2), 817.

Calverley, C. S. (1902). The cock and the bull. In *The complete works of C. S. Calverley*. London: Bell and Sons.

Campbell, M., & Warner, E. C. (1930). A study of rheumatic disease in children. *Lancet*, 215(5550), 61–66.

Carmichael, E. A., & Green, F. H. K. (1928, October). Parkinsonian rigidity. *Quarterly Journal of Medicine*, 22(85).

Carr-Saunders, A. M., Mannheim, H., & Rhodes, H. M. E. C. (1942). *Young offenders: An inquiry into juvenile delinquency*. Cambridge: Cambridge University Press.

Casteret, N. (1947). *My caves*. London: Dent.

Casuso, G. (1957). Anxiety related to the 'discovery' of the penis—An observation. In *The psychoanalytic study of the child*, 12. London: Imago.

Cheadle, W. B. (1889). *The rheumatic state in childhood*. London: Smith, Elder & Co.

Cheadle, W. B. (1889). *The various manifestations of the rheumatic state in childhood*. London: Smith, Elder & Co.

Church, R. (1955). *Over the bridge*. London: Heinemann.

Church, R. (1957). *The golden sovereign*. London: Heinemann.

Church, R. (1964). *The voyage home*. London: Heinemann.

Clancier, A., & Kalmanovitch, J. (1984). *Le Paradoxe de Winnicott—de la naissance à la création*. Paris: Payot.

Clegg, A., & Megson, B. (1968). *Children in distress*. Hammondsworth: Penguin.

Clyne, B. (1961). *Night calls: A study in general practice*. London: Tavistock.

Clyne, B. (1966). *Absent: School refusal as an expression of disturbed family relationships*. London: Tavistock.

Cohen, M. (1952). Counter-transference and anxiety. *Psychiatry*, 15, 231–243.

Committee on Homosexual Offences and Prostitution. (1963). *The Wolfenden Report: Report of the Committee on Homosexual Offences and Prostitution*. New York: Stein and Day. Originally published in 1957 as *Report of the Committee on Homosexual Offences and Prostitution*. London: H.M. Stationery Office.

Cottington, F. (1942). Treatment of schizophrenia in childhood. *The Nervous Child,* 1(2–3), 172.

Creak, E. M., & Shorting, B. J. (1944). Child psychiatry. *Journal of Mental Science,* 90, 365–381.

Creak, M. (1951). Psychoses in childhood. *Journal of Mental Science,* 97, 545–553.

Creak, M. (1952). Psychoses in childhood (Discussion). *Proceedings of the Royal Society of Medicine,* 45(11), 797–802.

Critchley, M., & Turner, W. A. (1925). Respiratory disorders in epidemic encephalitis. *Brain,* 48, 72–104.

Crothers, B., & Putnam, M. C. (1927). Obstetrical injuries of the spinal cord. *Medicine,* 6, 41–126.

Culpin, M. (1939). On pruritus and psychology. *British Medical Journal,* 1(4083), 748.

Curtis, M. (chair). (1946). *Report of the Care of Children Committee* (The Curtis Report), Cmd. 6922. London: H.M. Stationery Office.

Cuthbert, M. (1943, Nov. 20). 'Descriptive' medicine in the lay press. *British Medical Journal,* 2(4324), 660–661.

Dale, H. (1943). A prospect in therapeutics. *British Medical Journal,* 2(4317), 411–416.

Darwin, C. (1859). *On the origin of species.* London: John Murray.

Davidson, J. A., & Miller, R. (1914). The nervous complications of varicella. *British Journal of Children's Diseases,* 11, 15.

Davies, W. H. (1914). Infancy. In *The bird of paradise, and other poems.* London: Methuen.

Debré, R., Lévy-Solal, E., Netter, G., & Longchampt, J. (1925). Varicelle mortelle à forme comateuse d'emblée chez une femme enceinte. *Bulletins et Mémoires de la Société Médicale des Hôpitaux de Paris, 3e sér.,* 49, 1568–1572.

Department of Education and Science. (1968). *Psychologists in education services.* London: H. M. Stationery Office.

Despert, J. L. (1942). Prophylactic aspect of schizophrenia in childhood. *The Nervous Child,* 1(2–3), 189.

Dobinson, C. H. (1951, 3 September). Nursery schools. Letter. *The Times* Issue 52096.

Dockar-Drysdale, B. (1968). *Therapy in child care: Collected papers.* Harlow: Longmans.

Dunbar, H. F. (1935). *Emotions and bodily changes.* New York: Columbia University Press.

Dunnico, H. R. (1954). Letter: '"Pin-Up" Pictures at Approved School', *The Times,* 1 November 1954; Issue 53077, 2.

Edelston, H. (1943). 'Separation anxiety in young children: A study of hospital cases'. *Genetic Psychology Monographs,* 28, 3–95.

Editors. (1952, February). Annotation: Frontal lobes of the human brain. *Lancet,* 259(6704), 23.

Editor. (1952). Mrs. Melanie Klein—Seventieth Birthday. *International Journal of Psychoanalysis,* 33, 509.

Eissler, K. R. (1950). Ego-psychological implications of the psychoanalytic treatment of delinquents. In *The psychoanalytic study of the child,* 5 (pp. 97–121). London: Imago.

Eissler, R. S., Freud, A., & Hartmann, H. (Eds.). (1957). *The psychoanalytic study of the child,* 11. London: Imago.

Eissler, R. S., Freud, A., & Hartmann, H. (Eds.). (1958). *The psychoanalytic study of the child,* 12. London: Imago.

Eissler, R. S., Freud, A., Hartmann, H., & Kris, M. (Eds.). (1961). *The psychoanalytic study of the child,* 15. London: Imago.

Eissler, R. S., Freud, A., Hartmann, H., & Kris, M. (Eds.). (1962). In *The psychoanalytic study of the child*, 16. London: Imago.
Eissler, R. S., Freud, A., Hartmann, H., & Kris, M. (Eds.). (1966). *The psychoanalytic study of the child*, 20. London: Imago.
Eissler, R. S., Freud, A., Hartmann, H., & Kris, M. (Eds.). (1967). *The psychoanalytic study of the child*, 22. London: Hogarth.
Eliot, T. S. (1922). *The waste land*. New York: Horace Liveright.
Eliot, T. S. (1941). The dry salvages. In *Four Quartets*. New York: Harcourt.
Eliot, T. S. (1942). *Little Gidding*. London: Faber and Faber.
English, O., & Pearson, G. (1937). *Common neuroses of children and adults*. New York: W. W. Norton.
Eppel, E. M., & Eppel, M. (1966). *Adolescents and morality*. London: Routledge & Kegan Paul.
Erikson, E. (1950). *Childhood and society*. London/New York: Imago/Norton.
Erikson, E. (1956). The problem of ego identity. *Journal of the American Psychoanalytic Association, 4*.
Erikson, E. (1958). *Young man Luther*. London: Faber.
Erikson, E. (1961). The roots of virtue. In J. Huxley (Ed.), *The humanist frame* (pp. 145–166). London: Allen & Unwin.
Evans, P. R., & MacKeith, R. (1951). *Infant feeding and feeding difficulties*. London: Churchill.
Fain, M., & Marty, P. (1954). *Importance du rôle de la motricité dans la relation d'objet*. Paris: Presses universitaires de France.
Fain, M., & Marty, P. (1955). La motricité dans la relation d'objet. *Revue française de psychanalyse*. Tome XIX, Nos. 1–2. Paris: Presses Universitaires de France.
Fairbairn, W. R. D. (1941). A revised psychopathology of the psychoses and psychoneuroses. *International Journal of Psychoanalysis, 22*, 250–279.
Fairbairn, W. R. D. (1944). Endopsychic structure considered in terms of object-relationships. *International Journal of Psychoanalysis, 25*, 70–93.
Fairbairn, W. R. D. (1952). *Psychoanalytic studies of the personality*. London: Tavistock.
Fairfield, L. (1941). Communal feeding in schools. *British Medical Journal, 2*(4205), 211.
Farjeon, E. (1967). *The wonderful knight*. London: Kaye & Ward.
Farrington, B. (1953). *Greek science*. London: Pelican.
Fenichel, O. (1945). *The theory of neurosis*. New York: W. W. Norton.
Ferenczi, S. (1931). Child analysis in the analysis of adults. In M. Balint (Ed.), *Final contributions to the problems and methods of psycho-analysis*, 126–155. London: Hogarth, 1955.
FitzHerbert, J. (1960). The role of extra-sensory perception in early childhood. *British Journal of Psychiatry, 106*, 1560–1567.
Fleming, G. W. (1941). Communal feeding in schools. *British Medical Journal, 2*(4207), 282–283.
Flugel, J. C. (1941). *The moral paradox of peace and war*. London: Watts & Co.
Follett, M. P. (1924). *Creative experience*. New York: Longmans, Green, & Co.
Foote, E. J. (1956). *Six children*. Springfield, IL/Oxford: Charles C. Thomas/Blackwell Scientific.
Fordham, M. (1960). Contribution to a symposium on 'counter-transference'. *British Journal of Medical Psychology, 33*(1), 1–8.
Fordham, M. (1962). *An evaluation of Jung's work*. Lecture no. 119. London: Guild of Pastoral Psychology.

Fordham, M. (1963). The empirical foundation and theories of the self in Jung's work. *Journal of Analytic Psychology, 8*, 1–23.

Fordham, M. (1970). Reflections on training analysis. *Journal of Analytical Psychology, 15*, 59–71.

Forster, E. M. (1953). *The hill of Devi*. New York: Harcourt, Brace.

Foss, B. M. (1963). *Determinants of infant behaviour, vol. 2*. London: Methuen.

Foucault, M. (1966). *Le mots and les choses*. Paris: Éditions Gallimard. Published in English under the title *The order of things*. London/New York: Tavistock/Pantheon, 1970.

Franklin, H. W. F. (chair). (1951). Report of a Committee to Review Punishments in Prisons, Borstal Institutions, Approved Schools and Remand Homes, Parts I and II. Prisons and Borstal Institutions. Cmd. 8256. London: H.M. Stationery Office.

Fraser, J. (1926). *Surgery of childhood*. London: Arnold.

Frazer, J. G. (1911). *The golden bough: A study in magic and religion*, 3rd ed. London.

Freud, A. (1926–27). *The psycho-analytic treatment of children*. London: Imago, 1946.

Freud, A. (1936/1937). *The ego and the mechanisms of defence*. London: Hogarth.

Freud, A. (1946). *The psycho-analytical treatment of children*. London: Imago.

Freud, A. (1947). Aggression in relation to emotional development: Normal and pathological. In *The psychoanalytic study of the child, 3/4* (p. 37). London: Imago.

Freud, A. (1947). Emotional and instinctive development. In R. W. B. Ellis (Ed.), *Child health and development* (ch. 10). London: Churchill.

Freud, A. (1949). *Introduction to psycho-analysis for teachers*. London: Allen & Unwin.

Freud, A. (1952). The role of bodily illness in the mental life of children. In *The psychoanalytic study of the child, 7* (pp. 69–81). London: Imago.

Freud, A. (1953). A two-year-old goes to hospital: Scientific film by James Robertson. *International Journal of Psycho-Analysis, 34*, 284–287.

Freud, A. (1953). Some remarks on infant observation. In *The psychoanalytic study of the child, 8* (pp. 9–19). London: Imago.

Freud, A. (1954). The widening scope of indications for psycho-analysis—Discussion. *Journal of the American Psychoanalytic Association, 2*, 607–620.

Freud, A. (1954). Psychoanalysis and education. In *The psychoanalytic study of the child, 9* (pp. 9–15). London: Imago.

Freud, A. (1963). Regression as a principle in mental development. *Bulletin of the Menninger Clinic, 27*, 126–139.

Freud, A. (1965). *Normality and pathology in childhood*. London/New York: Hogarth and the Institute of Psycho-Analysis/International Universities Press.

Freud, A. (1968). *Indications for child analysis and other papers: 1945–1956*. New York: International Universities Press.

Freud, A., Hoffer W., Glover, E., et al. (Eds.). (1946). *The psychoanalytic study of the child, 2*. London: Imago.

Freud, A., Hoffer, W., & Glover, E. (Eds.). (1949). *The psychoanalytic study of the child, 3/4/5*. London: Imago.

Freud, A., Kris, E., Greenacre, P., Hartmann, H., Lewin, B. D., Escalona, S., et al. (1954). Problems of infantile neurosis: A discussion. In *The psychoanalytic study of the child, 9* (pp. 16–71). London: Imago.

Freud, S. (1895/1950). *Aus den anfängen der psychoanalyse*. London: Imago.

Freud, S. (1895). Entwurf einer Psychologie. *Aus den Anfängen der Psychoanalyse*. London: Imago, 1950. [trans: Project for a Scientific Psychology. In *The Origins of Psychoanalysis*. London: Imago, 1954.]

Freud, S. (1895). Project for a scientific psychology. In J. Strachey (Ed.), *Complete psychological works of Sigmund Freud*, 1. London: Hogarth.

Freud, S. (1900). *The interpretation of dreams*. Leipzig/Vienna: Franz Deuticke.

Freud, S. (1900/1953-73). *The interpretation of dreams*. In J. Strachey (Ed.), *Standard edition of the complete psychological works of Sigmund Freud* (vols. 4-5). London: Hogarth.

Freud, S. (1900). *The interpretation of dreams, part I*. In J. Strachey (Ed.), *Standard edition of the complete psychological works of Sigmund Freud* (vol. 4). London: Hogarth.

Freud, S. (1900). *The interpretation of dreams*. A. A. Brill (Trans.). London: George Allen & Co.

Freud, S. (1900). *The interpretation of dreams, part II*. In J. Strachey (Ed.), *Standard edition of the complete psychological works of Sigmund Freud* (vol. 5). London: Hogarth.

Freud, S. (1901). On dreams. In J. Strachey (Ed.), *Standard edition of the complete psychological works of Sigmund Freud* (vol. 5, pp. 629-686). London: Hogarth.

Freud, S. (1901). The psychopathology of everyday life. In J. Strachey (Ed.), *Standard edition of the complete psychological works of Sigmund Freud* (vol. 6). London: Hogarth.

Freud, S. (1905). Dora: Fragments of an analysis of a case of hysteria. In J. Strachey (Ed.), *Standard edition of the complete psychological works of Sigmund Freud*, 7. London: Hogarth.

Freud, S. (1905). Three essays on the theory of sexuality. In J. Strachey (Ed.), *Standard edition of the complete psychological works of Sigmund Freud* (vol. 7). London: Hogarth.

Freud, S. (1909). The analysis of a phobia in a five-year-old boy. In J. Strachey (Ed.), *Standard edition of the complete psychological works of Sigmund Freud* (vol. 10, pp. 1-149). London: Hogarth.

Freud, S. (1909). Notes upon a case of obsessional neurosis. In J. Strachey (Ed.), *Complete psychological works of Sigmund Freud*, 10. London: Hogarth.

Freud, S. (1909). The origin and development of psycho-analysis [Five lectures on Psychoanalysis]. In J. Strachey (Ed.), *Standard edition of the complete psychological works of Sigmund Freud* (vol. 11, 7-55). London: Hogarth.

Freud, S. (1910). The future prospects of psycho-analytic therapy. In *Collected papers*, 2. London: Hogarth, 1946.

Freud, S. (1911). Formulations on the two principles of mental functioning. In J. Strachey (Ed.), *Standard edition of the complete psychological works of Sigmund Freud* (vol. 12, pp. 213-226). London: Hogarth.

Freud, S. (1914). On narcissism. In J. Strachey (Ed.), *Standard edition of the complete psychological works of Sigmund Freud* (vol. 14). London: Hogarth.

Freud, S. (1915). Instincts and their vicissitudes. In J. Strachey (Ed.), *Complete psychological works of Sigmund Freud*, 14. London: Hogarth.

Freud, S. (1915). Some character-types met with in psycho-analytic work. In J. Strachey (Ed.), *Standard edition of the complete psychological works of Sigmund Freud* (vol. 14). London: Hogarth.

Freud, S. (1915). *Three essays on the theory of sexuality, 3rd ed.* Leipzig/Vienna: Deuticke.

Freud, S. (1916-1917). Introductory lectures on psycho-analysis. In J. Strachey (Ed.), *Complete psychological works of Sigmund Freud*, 15-16. London: Hogarth.

Freud, S. (1917). Mourning and melancholia. *Collected papers, 4*. London: Hogarth.
Freud, S. (1917). Mourning and melancholia. In J. Strachey (Ed.), *Standard edition of the complete psychological works of Sigmund Freud* (vol. 14). London: Hogarth.
Freud, S. (1920). Beyond the pleasure principle. In J. Strachey (Ed.), *Standard edition of the complete psychological works of Sigmund Freud* (vol. 18). London: Hogarth.
Freud, S. (1920). A child is being beaten—A contribution to the study of the origin of sexual perversions. *International Journal of Psycho-Analysis, 1*, 371–395.
Freud, S. (1921). *Group psychology and the analysis of the ego*. London/Vienna: International Psycho-Analytical Press.
Freud, S. (1921). Group psychology and the analysis of the ego. In J. Strachey (Ed.), *Standard edition of the complete psychological works of Sigmund Freud* (vol. 18). London: Hogarth.
Freud, S. (1923). The ego and the id. In J. Strachey (Ed.), *Standard edition of the complete psychological works of Sigmund Freud* (vol. 19). London: Hogarth.
Freud, S. (1925). *An autobiographical study*. London: Hogarth.
Freud, S. (1925). An autobiographical study. In J. Strachey (Ed.), *Standard edition of the complete psychological works of Sigmund Freud* (vol. 20, pp. 1–74). London: Hogarth.
Freud, S. (1925). Introduction. In A. Aichhorn, *Wayward youth*. London: Imago.
Freud, S. (1926). *Inhibitions, symptoms and anxiety*. London: Hogarth.
Freud, S. (1926). Inhibitions, symptoms and anxiety. In J. Strachey (Ed.), *Standard edition of the complete psychological works of Sigmund Freud* (vol. 20). London: Hogarth.
Freud, S. (1926). Inhibitions, symptoms and anxiety. In J. Strachey (Ed.), *Standard edition of the complete psychological works of Sigmund Freud* (vol. 20, pp. 75–175). London: Hogarth.
Freud, S. (1929). Dostoevsky and parricide. *The Realist, 1*(4), 18.
Freud, S. (1930). Civilisation and its discontents. In J. Strachey (Ed.), *Standard edition of the complete psychological works of Sigmund Freud* (vol. 21. pp. 57–145). London: Hogarth.
Freud, S. (1931). Female sexuality. In James Strachey (Ed.), *Standard edition of the complete psychological works of Sigmund Freud* (vol. 7) London: Hogarth.
Freud, S. (1933). *New introductory lectures on psycho-analysis*. New York: Norton.
Freud, S. (1937). Analysis terminable and interminable. In J. Strachey (Ed.), *Standard edition of the complete psychological works of Sigmund Freud* (vol. 23). London: Hogarth.
Freud, S. (1938). An outline of psychoanalysis. In J. Strachey (Ed.), *Standard edition of the complete psychological works of Sigmund Freud* (vol. 23, 139–207). London: Hogarth.
Freud, S. (1939). Moses and monotheism. In J. Strachey (Ed.), *Standard edition of the complete psychological works of Sigmund Freud* (vol. 23). London: Hogarth.
Freud, S. (1954). *The origins of psycho-analysis*. Kris, E., Freud, A., Bonaparte, M. (Eds.), Strachey, J., Mosbacher, E. (Trans.). London: Imago.
Freud, S., Ferenczi, S., Abraham, K., Simmel, E., & Jones, E. (1910). *Zur Psychoanalyse der Kriegsneurosen. Diskussion am 5. Internationalent Psychoanalytischen Kongress, Budapest*. Vienna: Deuticke.
Freudenberg, R. (1942). Observations on shock therapy in the psychoses. Unpublished.
Friedlander, K. (1943, June). Delinquency research. *New Era in Home and School, 24*(6), 105–108.
Friedlander, K. (1947). *The psycho-analytical approach to juvenile delinquency: Theory, case-studies, treatment*. London: K. Paul, Trench, Trübner.

Frosch, J., et al. (Eds.). (1950). *The annual survey of psychoanalysis, vol. 1*. New York: International Universities Press.

Gaddini, E. (1969). On imitation. *International Journal of Psychoanalysis, 59*, 475–484.

Galli, P. (1925). La complicazioni nervose della varicella: due casi di atassia cerebellare acuta. *La pediatria, 33*, 681.

Galsworthy, J. (1922). *The Forsythe saga*. New York: Charles Scribner's.

Gardner, D. E. M. (1969). *Susan Isaacs: The first biography*. London: Methuen.

Gibbs, N., & Winnicott, D. W. (1926). Varicella encephalitis and vaccinia encephalitis. *British Journal of Children's Diseases, 23*, 107. [CW 1:2:1]

Gilbert, W. S., & Sullivan, A. (1888). *The Yeomen of the Guard*. London: Chappell & Co.

Gillespie, W. H. (1960). *The edge of objectivity: An essay in the history of scientific ideas*. Princeton, NJ: Princeton University Press.

Gillespie, R. D., & Henderson, D. K. (1940). *A textbook of psychiatry for students and practitioners, 5th ed*. Oxford: Oxford University Medical Publications.

Gitelson, M. (1952). The emotional position of the analyst in the psycho-analytic situation. *International Journal of Psychoanalysis, 33*, 1–10.

Glover, E. (1927). Lectures on technique in psychoanalysis. *International Journal of Psychoanalysis, 8*, 311–338.

Glover, E. (1932). A psychoanalytic approach to the classification of mental disorders. In *On the early development of mind* (pp. 161–186). London: Imago.

Glover, E. (1945). An examination of the Klein system of child psychiatry. In *The psychoanalytic study of the child, 1* (pp. 75–118). London: Imago.

Glover, E. (1949). The position of psycho-analysis in Great Britain. In *On the early development of mind* (ch. 23). London: Imago.

Glover, E. (1949). The position of psycho-analysis in Great Britain. In *On the early development of mind*, 352–363. London: Imago.

Glover, E. (1953). *Psycho-analysis and child psychiatry*. London: Imago.

Glover, E. (1956). *On the early development of the mind*. London: Imago.

Glover, E. (1956). A psychoanalytic approach to the classification of mental disorders. In *On the early development of mind*, 161–186. London: Imago.

Goldsmith, W. N. (1936). Mental influences. In W. N. Goldsmith (Ed.), *Recent advances in dermatology* (p. 97). London: J. & A. Churchill.

Goodacre, I. (1966). *Adoption policy and practice: A study*. London: Allen & Unwin.

Goodenough, Sir W. (1944). *Report of inter-departmental committee on medical schools*. Ministry of Health. London: H.M. Stationery Office.

Goodhart, J. F., & Still, G. F. (1921). *Diseases of children, 11th ed*. London: J. & A. Churchill.

Gordon, M. B. (1924). Acute hemorrhagic nephritis and acute hemorrhagic encephalitis following varicella. *American Journal of Diseases of Children, 28*(5), 589–593.

Gorer, G., & Rickman, J. (1949). *The people of great Russia: A psychological study*. London: Cresset.

Gough, D. (1962). The behaviour of infants in the first year of life. *Proceedings of the Royal Society of Medicine, 55*.

Gough, D. (ca. early 1960s). *Early mother-baby relationships* [Film]. UK. 10 mins. Concord Media.

Graham, J. (1951). *Any wife or any husband*. London: Heinemann.

Graves, R. (1963/1965). *Mammon*. From his London School of Economics Annual Oration. Reprinted in *Mammon and the black goddess*. London/New York: Cassell/Doubleday.

Graves, R., & Podro, J. (1953). Nazarene gospel restored. London/New York: Cassell/Doubleday.

Greenacre, P. (1941). The predisposition to anxiety. *Psychoanalytic Quarterly, 10*, 66–94.

Greenacre, P. (1941). The predisposition to anxiety, part II. *Psychoanalytic Quarterly, 10*, 610–638.

Greenacre, P. (1945). The biological economy of birth. In *Trauma, growth and personality*. London: Hogarth.

Greenacre, P. (1958). Early physical determinants in the development of the sense of identity. *Journal of the American Psychoanalytic Association, 6*, 612–627.

Greenacre, P. (1960). Considerations regarding the parent-infant relationship. *International Journal of Psycho-Analysis, 41*, 571.

Greenacre, P. (1968). The psychoanalytic process, transference, and acting out. *International Journal of Psychoanalysis, 49*, 211–218.

Greenacre, P., Freud, A., Kris, E., Hartmann, H., Lewin, B. D., Escalona, S., et al. (1954). Problems of infantile neurosis: A discussion. In *The psychoanalytic study of the child*, 9 (pp. 16–71). London: Imago.

Greenfield, J. G. (1929). The encephalomyelitis of measles. *Proceedings of the Royal Society of Medicine, 22*, 297–300.

Griffith, G. (1895). *Valdar the oft-born*. London: C. A. Pearson.

Grinstein, A. (1957). *The index of psychoanalytic writings*. New York: International Universities Press. [Preface by Ernest Jones, vol. 2]

Grolnick, S. A., & Barkin, L. (Eds.). (1978). *Between reality and fantasy: Transitional objects and phenomena*. New York/London: Aronson.

Guntrip, H. (1961). *Personality structure and human interaction*. London: Hogarth.

Guntrip, H. (1975). My experience of analysis with Fairbairn and Winnicott. *International Journal of Psychoanalysis, 77*, 739–754.

Guthrie, L. G. (1907). *Functional nervous disorders in childhood*. Oxford: Oxford University Medical Publications.

Hallam, R. (1927). Papular urticaria. *British Journal of Dermatology and Syphilis, 39*, 95–111.

Halmos, P. (1964, 9 April). Letter to the editor, 'Love or skill?' *New Society, 3*(80), 32.

Halmos, P. (1964, 19 March). Love or skill? *New Society, 3*(77), 13.

Hambling, J. (1951). Emotions and symptoms in essential hypertension. *British Journal of Medical Psychology, 24*(4), 242–253.

Hambling, J. (1952). Psychosomatic aspects of arterial hypertension. *British Journal of Medical Psychology, 25*(1), 39–47.

Hardcastle, D. N., Donnan, L. F., & Fordham, M. (1944). Shock therapy. *British Medical Journal, 1*(4334), 159–160.

Harding, D. W. (1963). The hinterland of thought. In *Experience into words: Essays on poetry*. London: Chatto & Windus.

Harms, E. (1947). *Handbook of child guidance*. New York: Child Care Publications.

Harris, W. (1926). *Neuritis and neuralgia*. London: Oxford University Press.

Hartmann, H. (1939). *Ego psychology and the problem of adaption*. London/New York: Imago/International Universities Press.

Hartmann, H. (1952). The mutual influences in the development of ego and id. In *The psychoanalytic study of the child*, 7 (pp. 9–30). London: Imago.

Hartmann, H. (1954). Contribution to discussion of 'Problems of infantile neurosis'. In *The psychoanalytic study of the child*, 9 (pp. 31–38). London: Imago.

Hartmann, H. (1958). *Ego psychology and the problem of adaptation*. London: Imago

Hauptmann, B., Issroff, J., & Reeves, C. (2005). *Donald Winnicott and John Bowlby: personal and professional perspectives*. London: Karnac Books.

Heimann, P. (1950). On counter-transference. *International Journal of Psychoanalysis*, 31, 81–84.

Heimann, P. (1951). A contribution to the re-evaluation of the Oedipus complex: The early stages. *International Journal of Psychoanalysis*, 33, 84–92.

Heimann, P., Klein, M., & Money-Kyrle, R. (1952). *Developments in psycho-analysis*. London: Hogarth.

Heimann, P., Klein, M., & Money-Kyrle, R. (1977). *New directions in psycho-analysis*. London: Karnac.

Henderson, D. K., & Gillespie, R. D. (1940). *A textbook of psychiatry for students and practitioners*, 5th ed. Oxford: Oxford University Medical Publications.

Henderson, D. (1954). Psychiatry and General Medicine. *British Medical Journal*, 1(4867), 889.

Henoch, E. (1889). *Lectures on children's diseases: A handbook for practitioners and students*. London: New Sydenham Society. Translated by John Thomson.

Hermann, I. (1936). Sich Anklammern—auf Suche Gehen. *Internationale Zeitschrift für Psychoanalyse*, 1936, 22, 349–370. (Abstract: *International Journal of Psycho-Analysis*, 1937, 18, 475–477).

Hill, A. (1948). *Art versus illness*, 2nd ed. London: George Allen & Unwin.

Hill, D. (1963, 23 February). Letter: 'Psychiatric care', *The Times*. Issue 56563.

Hoffer, W. (1949). Mouth, hand, and ego-integration. In *The psychoanalytic study of the child*, 3/4 (pp. 49–56). London: Imago.

Hoffer, W. (1950). Development of the body ego. In *The psychoanalytic study of the child*, 5 (pp. 18–23). London: Imago.

Hoffer, W. (1952). The mutual influences in the development of ego and id: Earliest stages. In *The psychoanalytic study of the child*, 7. London: Imago.

Hoffer, W. (1955). *Psychoanalysis: Practical and research aspects*. Baltimore: Williams & Wilkins.

Hoffer, W. (1966). Infant observations and concepts relating to infancy. In W. Hoffer (Ed.), *The early development and education of the child* (pp. 75–90). London: International Psycho-Analytical Library and Hogarth.

Hoffer, W. (1981). *The early development and education of the child*. London: Hogarth.

Holder, C. (1969). Behaviour therapy. *Child Care News*, 86.

Hollowood, J. (1967). *Maggie and the chickens*. London: Chatto & Windus.

Hollowood, J. (1967). *Maggie and the roundabout*. London: Chatto & Windus.

Home Office. (1965). *The child, the family and the young offender*. (Cmnd 2742) London: H.M. Stationery Office.

Hopkins, G. M. (1918). The wreck of the Deutscheland. *Gerard Manley Hopkins* [Poems]. London: Humphrey Milford, 1918.

Hopkins, G. M. (1918/1986). Spring and fall, to a young child. In C. Phillips (Ed.), *Gerard Manley Hopkins*. New York: Oxford University Press.

Hopkins, G. M. (1960). *Gerard Manley Hopkins*. [Poems]. London: Vista Books.
Hoskyns, K., & Joseph, J. (1967). *Water*. London: Constable.
Hoskyns, K., & Joseph, J. (1967). *Wind*. London: Constable.
Horwitt, S. (1924). *Archives of Pediatrics, xli*, 476.
Housman, A. E. (1896). *A Shropshire lad*. London: K. Paul, Trench, Treubner.
Howells, J. G. (1965). Child therapy: A case of antisocial behaviour. In J. G. Howells (Ed.), *Modern perspectives in child psychiatry*. London: Oliver & Boyd.
Hurst, A. F. (1929). On asthma. *Practitioner, 1929*, 10.
Hutchison, R. (1904). *Lectures on diseases of children*. London: Edward Arnold (7th ed., 1936).
Illingworth, R. S. (1951). Sleep disturbances in young children. *British Medical Journal. 1*(4709), 722–728.
Ingram, J. T. (1933). The personality of the skin. *Lancet, 221*, 889–892.
Isaacs, S. (1929). *The nursery years*. London: Routledge.
Isaacs, S. (1930). *The intellectual growth in young children*. London: Routledge.
Isaacs, S. (1932). *The children we teach: Seven to eleven years*. London: University of London Press, Institute of Education.
Isaacs, S. (1933). *Social development in young children*. London: Routledge.
Isaacs, S., & Nunn, T. P. (1936, August 13). Nursery schools. Letter to *The Times*, Issue 47452, p. 15.
Isaacs, S. (1941). *The Cambridge evacuation survey: A wartime study in social welfare and education*. London: Methuen & Co.
Isaacs, S. (1948). *Childhood & after. Some essays and clinical studies*. London: Routledge & Kegan Paul.
Isaacs, S. (1949). *The psychological aspects of child development*. London: University of London Institute of Education.
Jackson, L. (1954). *Aggression and its interpretation*. London: Methuen & Co.
James, H. M. (1962). Infantile narcissistic trauma. *International Journal of Psycho-Analysis, 43*, 69–79.
James, M. (1964, 27 September). The mothers children need. *The Observer*.
Jaques, E. (1960). Disturbances on the capacity to work. *International Journal of Psycho-Analysis, 41*, 357.
Jones, E. (1907). Alcoholic cirrhosis of the liver in children. *British Journal of Children's Diseases, 4*, 1–14.
Jones, E. (1908). The significance of the phrictopathic sensation. *Journal of Nervous and Mental Diseases, 35*(7), 427–437.
Jones, E. (1909). Psycho-analysis in psychotherapy. *Journal of Abnormal Psychology, 4*(2), 140–150.
Jones, E. (1910). The question of the side affected in hemiplegia and in arterial lesions of the brain. *Quarterly Journal of Medicine, 3*, 233–250.
Jones, E. (1920). *Treatment of the neuroses*. London: Baillière, Tindall and Cox.
Jones, E. (1927/1950). Early development of female sexuality. In E. Jones (Ed.), *Papers on psycho-analysis* (pp. 438–451). London: Baillière, Tindall and Cox.
Jones, E. (1931). *On the nightmare*. London: Hogarth.
Jones, E. (1946). A valedictory address. *International Journal of Psycho-Analysis, 27*, 7–11.
Jones, E. (1948). *Papers on psycho-analysis, 5th ed*. London: Baillière, Tindall and Cox.

Jones, E. (1949). *What is psycho-analysis?* London: Allen & Unwin.
Jones, E. (1951). *Essays in applied psycho-analysis*, 2. London: Hogarth.
Jones, E. (1951). The symbolic significance of salt in folklore and superstition. In *Essays in applied psycho-analysis*, 2 (p. 22). London: Hogarth.
Jones, E. (1955, 6 Feb.) Morals and religion: The Dawn of Conscience. *The Observer* (p. 6).
Jones, E. (1955). A new translation of Freud. *British Medical Journal*, 2(4949), 1192.
Jones, E. (1956). *Sigmund Freud: Four centenary addresses*. New York: Basic Books.
Jones, E. (1957). Pain. *International Journal of Psycho-Analysis, 38*, 255.
Jones, E. (1957). Preface. In A. Grinstein, *The index of psychoanalytic writings*. New York: International Universities Press.
Jones, E. (1957). *Sigmund Freud: Life and work*, 3. London: Hogarth.
Jones, E. (1959). *Free association: Memories of a psycho-analyst*. London: Hogarth.
Jones, E. (Ed.). (1961). *Letters of Sigmund Freud, 1873–1939*. London: Hogarth.
Joseph, J., & Knight, D. (1967). *Judy and Jasmin*. London: Constable.
Joseph, J., & Knight, D. (1967). *Tim and Terry*. London: Constable.
Jung, C. G. (1963). *Memories, dreams, reflections*. New York: Pantheon.
Kanner, L. (1937). *Child psychiatry*. London: Baillière, Tindall and Cox.
Kanner, L. (1943). Autistic disturbances of affective contact. *The Nervous Child, 2*, 217–250.
Kaufman, G. S., & Hart, M. (1939). *The man who came to dinner*. New York: Random House
Keats, J. (1816). On first looking into Chapman's Homer. In *The Examiner*, December, 1.
Keats, J. (1818). Letter to Benjamin Bailey, 13 March, 1818. In H. E. Rollins (Ed.) *Letters of John Keats* (vol. 1). Cambridge, MA: Harvard University Press.
Kestenberg, J. S. (1958). Review: Mother and child. A primer of first relationships: By D. W. Winnicott. *Psychoanalytic Quarterly, 27*, 268–269.
Khan, M. M. R. (1964). Ego distortion, cumulative trauma, and the role of reconstruction in the analytic situation. *International Journal of Psycho-Analysis, 45*, 272–279. Also in *The privacy of the self*. London: Hogarth, 1974.
Khan, M. M. R. (1964). The function of intimacy and acting out in perversions. In R. Slovenko (Ed.), *Sexual behaviour and the law*. Springfield, IL: Thomas.
Khan, M. M. R. (1968/1979). Reparation to the self as an idolised internal object. In *Alienation in perversions*. London: Hogarth.
Khan, M. M. R. (1963). The concept of cumulative trauma. In *The psychoanalytic study of the child, 18*. London: Imago. [Reprinted in *The privacy of the self*. London: Hogarth, 1974.]
Khan, M. M. R. (1969). On the clinical provision of frustrations, recognitions and failures in the analytic situation. *International Journal of Psycho-Analysis, 50*, 237–248.
King, Allan (1967). *Warrendale* [Film]. Canada. 101 mins. The Criterion Collection.
Kinnear, J. (1933). Urticaria papulosa. *British Journal of Dermatology and Syphilis, 45*, 65–68.
Kirk, H. D. (1964). *Shared fate: A theory of adoption and mental health*. New York: Free Press of Glencoe.
Klein, M. (1930). The importance of symbol-formation in the development of the ego. *International Journal of Psycho-Analysis, 11*, 24–39.
Klein, M. (1932). *The psycho-analysis of children*. London: Hogarth.
Klein, M. (1932/1949). *The psychoanalysis of children* (Revised edition). London: Hogarth and the Institute of Psycho-Analysis.
Klein, M. (1932/1975). The psycho-analysis of children. In *Collected works*, 2. London: Hogarth.

Klein, M. (1934). A contribution to the psychogenesis of manic-depressive states. In *Collected works, 1*. London: Hogarth.

Klein, M. (1935). A contribution to the psychogenesis of manic-depressive states. *International Journal of Psycho-Analysis, 16*, 145–174.

Klein, M. (1935). Contribution to the psychogenesis of manic depressive states. In *Contributions to psycho-analysis, 1921–1945*, 282–310. London: Hogarth.

Klein, M. (1936). Weaning. In J. Rickman (Ed.), *On the bringing up of children*. London: Kegan Paul.

Klein, M. (1940). Mourning and its relation to manic-depressive states. *International Journal of Psycho-Analysis, 21*, 125–153.

Klein, M. (1940). Mourning and its relation to manic depressive states. In *Contributions to psycho-analysis, 1921–1945* (pp. 311–338). London: Hogarth.

Klein, M. (1945). The Oedipus complex in the light of early anxieties. In *Melanie Klein, contributions to psycho-analysis, 1921–1945* (pp. 339–390). London: Hogarth.

Klein, M. (1946). Notes on some schizoid mechanisms. *International Journal of Psycho-Analysis, 27*, 99–110.

Klein, M. (1948). *Contributions to psycho-analysis, 1921–1945*. London: Hogarth.

Klein, M. (1954). *The psycho-analysis of children*. London: Hogarth.

Klein, M. (1955). A study of envy and gratitude. In J. Mitchell (Ed.), *The selected Melanie Klein*. London: Penguin Books, 1986.

Klein, M. (1957). *Envy and gratitude: A study of unconscious forces*. London: Hogarth.

Klein, M. (1961). *Narrative of a child analysis*. London: Hogarth.

Klein, M., et al. (1955). *Developments in psycho-analysis*. London: Hogarth.

Klein, M., Heiman, P., & Money-Kyrle. R. E. (Eds.). (1955). *New directions in psycho-analysis*. London.

Klein, M., & Riviere, J. (1937). *Love, hate and reparation: Two lectures*. London: Hogarth.

Knights, L. C. (1946). *Explorations: Essays in criticism mainly on the literature of the seventeenth century*. London/Harmondsworth: Chatto & Windus/penguin.

Koplik, H. (1919). *Diseases of infancy and childhood, 4th ed* (p. 303). London: Henry Kimpton.

Krabbe, K. H. (1925). Varicella-myelitis. *Brain, 48*, 535–539.

Kris, E. (1950). Notes on the development and on some current problems of psychoanalytic child psychology. In *The psychoanalytic study of the child, 5*. London: Imago.

Kris, E. (1951). Opening remarks on psychoanalytic child psychology. In *The psychoanalytic study of the child, 6*. London: Imago.

Kris, E. (1951). Some comments and observations on early autoerotic activities. In *The psychoanalytic study of the child, 6*. London: Imago.

Kulka, A. Fry, C., & Goldstein, F. J. (1960). Kinesthetic needs in infancy. *American Journal of Orthopsychiatry, 30*, 562–571.

La Psychanalyses (1960). Volume 5: Essais critiques. Publication de la Société Française de Psychanalyse. Paris: Presses Universitaires de France.

Lacan, J. (1949/1966). Le Stade du Miroir comme formateur de la function du je, telle qu'elle nous est révélée dans l'expérience psychanalytique. In *Écrits*. Paris: Éditions du Seuil.

Lacan, J. (1960). A la mémoire d'Ernest Jones: sur sa théorie du symbolisme. *La Psychanalyse, 5*. Presses Universitaires de France. [In memory of Ernest Jones: On his theory of symbolism. In *Écrits*, trans. Bruce Fink 2002, 2006.]

Lacan, J. (1985). Lettre à Winnicott (5 August 1960). *Orincar?*, 33, April–June, 7–10. [Published in English as Letter to D. W. Winnicott (5 August 1960). In *October, 40*, Television (Spring), 1987, 76–68.]

Laing, R. D. (1960). *The divided self.* London: Tavistock.

Laing, R. D. (1961). *The self and others.* London: Tavistock.

Lamb, C. (1823). Dream children: A reverie. In *The Works of Charles Lamb. vol. 1. The Essays of Elia.* London/New York: Routledge/E. P. Dutton. [1905]

Lambeth, Archbishop Lord Fisher. (1966, 2 December). Reform of the abortion laws. Letter to *The Times*, Issue 56804.

Langdon-Brown, W. (1937). On getting the rash out. *Transactions of the St John's Hospital Dermatological Society, 77.*

Lask, A. (1966). *Asthma: Attitude and milieu.* London: Tavistock.

Lebovici, S., & McDougall, J. (1960). *Un cas de psychose infantile: Étude psychoanalytique.* Paris: Presses Universitaires de France.

Lebovici, S., & McDougall, J. (1969). *Dialogue with Sammy.* London: Hogarth.

Lehman, E. (Producer), & Nichols, M. (Director). (1966). *Who's afraid of Virginia Woolf?* [Motion Picture]. United States: Warner Bros.

LeShan, E. J. (1965). *How to survive parenthood.* New York: Random House.

Levaditi et Nicolau. (1926). *Comptes Rendus des séances Société de Biologie*, xciv, 114.

Lewin, B. D. (1948). Inferences from the dream screen. *International Journal of Psycho-Analysis, 29.*

Lewis, J. B. S. (1943, May 8). Prefrontal lobotomy. *Lancet, 241*(6245), 599.

Lindner, S. (1879). Das saugen an den fingern, lippen, bei den kindern (ludeln). *Jahrbuch für Kinderheilk, 14,* 68–91.

Little, H. M. (1947). The psychotic child. *Pennsylvania Medical Journal, 51,* 174.

Little, M. (1951). Counter-transference and patient's response to it. *International Journal of Psychoanalysis, 32,* 32–40.

Little, M. (1957). ' "R" - The analyst's total response to his patient's needs'. *International Journal of Psychoanalysis, 38*(3–4), 240–254.

Little, M. I. (1958). On delusional transference (transference psychosis). *International Journal of Psycho-Analysis, 39,* 134–138. [Also in M. I. Little, *Transference neurosis and transference psychosis.* New York/London: Jason Aronson, 1981].

Loach, K. (1966). Cathy come home. BBC.

Loos, A. (1935). *Gentlemen prefer blondes.* New York: Brentano.

Lovelace, R. (1642). To Althea, from prison.

Lowenfeld, M. (1935/1969). *Play in childhood.* Bath: Cedric Chivers.

Lucksch, F. (1925). Gibt es beim Menschen eine Vakzine-Encephalitis? *Centralblatt für Bakteriologie, Parasitenkunde und Infektionskrankheitin Originale, 96*(1), 309.

Lundgren, E. R. (1967). *Little Trulsa's secret.* London: Methuen.

Lundholm, H. (1933). Repression and rationalization. *British Journal of Medical Psychology, 13,* 23–50.

MacAlpine, I. (1952). Psychosomatic symptom formation. *Lancet, 259*(6702), 278–282.

MacCormac, H. (1926). Self-inflicted hysterical lesions of the skin, with special reference to the after-history. *British Journal of Dermatology, 38,* 371–375.

MacKeith, R., & Rainsford Evans, P. (1958). *Infant feeding and feeding difficulties.* London: Churchill.

MacLeod, J. M. H. (1933). Pruritus. In *Diseases of the skin* (p. 633). London: Churchill.

Mahler, M. S. (1969). *On human symbiosis and the vicissitudes of individuation. Vol. 1, Infantile psychosis.* London: Hogarth and the Institute of Psycho-Analysis.

Mahler, M. S., Freud, A., Kris, E., Greenacre, P., Hartmann, H., Lewin, B. D., et al. (1954). Problems of infantile neurosis: A discussion. In *The psychoanalytic study of the child, 9* (pp. 16–71). London: Imago.

Main, T. (1957). The ailment. *British Journal of Medical Psychology, 30*(3), 129–145.

Main, T. F. (1957). *The ailment and other psychoanalytic essays*. J. Johns (Ed.). London: Free Association Books.

Main, T. F. (1968). Psychoanalysis as a cross-bearing. *British Journal of Psychiatry, 114*, 501–507.

Malan, D. (1995). *Individual psychotherapy and the science of psychodynamics.* Oxford: Butterworth Heinemann.

Malleson, J. (1948, 18 December). Letter: Taking children's temperatures. *British Medical Journal, 2*(4589), 1078.

Marfan, A. B. (1893). *Bulletins et Mémoires de la Société Médicale des Hôpitaux de Paris, 3e sér., 10*, 183.

Marx, H., & Barber R. (1962). *Harpo speaks!*. New York: Proscenium.

McAlpine, D. (1931). Acute disseminated encephalomyelitis. *Lancet, 217*(5616), 846–852.

McKissock, W. (1943, April 17). Prefrontal lobotomy. *Lancet, 241*(6242), 511.

McWhinnie, A. M. (1967). *Adopted children.* London: Routledge & K. Paul.

Mead, M. (1957). Changing patterns of parent-child relations in an urban world. Eighth Ernest Jones lecture. *International Journal of Psycho-Analysis, 38*, 369–378.

Mead, Margaret. (1953). Discussions on child development. In J. M. Tanner & Bärbel Inhelder (Eds.), *Child development*. The International Behavioral and Social Sciences Library.

Meltzer, D. (1959). Notes on a transient inhibition of chewing. In A. Hahn (Ed.), *Sincerity and other works: Collected papers of Donald Meltzer.* London: Karnac.

Meltzer, D. (1979). The introjective basis of polymorphous tendencies in adult sexuality. In Meltzer, D. (Ed.), *Sexual states of mind*, London: Karnac.

Menko, M. L. H. S. (1899). Choreiforme bewegungen nach varicellen. *Deutsche Medizinische Wochenschrift, 25*, 745.

Menninger, K., et al. (1963). *The vital balance.* New York: Basic Books.

Middlemore, M. (1941). *The nursing couple.* London: Hamish Hamilton Medical Books.

Miller, A. (1963). *Jane's blanket.* New York/London: Collier/Macmillan.

Miller, E. (1968). The value of the therapeutic consultation. In E. Miller (Ed.), *Foundations of child psychiatry.* London: Pergamon Press.

Miller, R. (1909). Latent chorea: A contribution to the study of sydenham's chorea. *Lancet, 174*(4503), 1808–1811.

Miller, R. (1930). An address on the diagnosis of early juvenile rheumatism. *British Medical Journal, 1*(3605), 230–232.

Milne, A. A. (1926). *Winnie the Pooh.* London: Methuen.

Milner, M. (pseud. Joanna Field) (1934/1952). *A life of one's own.* London/Harmondsworth: Chatto & Windus/Penguin.

Milner, M. (pseud. Joanna Field). (1950). *On not being able to paint.* London: William Heinemann.

Milner, M. (1952). Aspects of symbolism in comprehension of the not-self. *International Journal of Psycho-Analysis, 33*.

Milner, M. (1952). Aspects of symbolism in comprehension of the not-self. *International Journal of Psycho-Analysis, 33*, 181–195.

Milner, M. (1957). *On not being able to paint*. Revised edition. London: Heinemann.

Milner, M. (1969). *The hands of the living God*. London: Hogarth and the Institute of Psycho-Analysis.

Mitchison, N. (1967). *The big surprise*. London: Kaye & Ward.

Monchaux, C. de (1962). Thinking and negative hallucination. *International Journal of Psycho-Analysis, 43*, 311–314.

Moncrieff, A., & Hussey, B. J. (1948). Temperature recording in sick children. *British Medical Journal, 2*(4587), 972–973.

Money-Kyrle, R. (1937). Primitive behaviour. *Nature, 139*(3523), 778–779.

Money-Kyrle, R. (1939). *Superstition and society*. London: Hogarth.

Money-Kyrle, R. E. (1951). *Psycho-analysts and politics: A contribution to the psychology of politics and morals*. London: Duckworth.

Myers, F. W. H. (1986). *Letters of James and Alix Strachey*. P. Meisel and W. Kendrick (Eds.). London: Chatto & Windus.

Netter, H. (1900). Beitrag zur Pathologie der Varicellen. *Archiv für Kinderheilkunde, 30*, 138. Stuttgart: Ferdinand Enke.

O'Donovan, W. J. (1927). *Dermatological neuroses*. London: Kegan Paul, Trench, Trubner.

Opie, I., & Opie, P. (Eds.). (1951). *The Oxford Dictionary of nursery rhymes*. Oxford: Clarendon Press.

Orr, D. (1954). Transference and counter-transference: A historical survey. *Journal of the American Psychoanalytic Association, 2*, 621–670.

Owen, M. (1924). *Memorial edition*. Anglo-French Music Co.

Paterson, R. (1931). Latent maxillary sinusitis. *Lancet, 218*, 117–121.

Payne, M. A. (1929). *Oliver untwisted*. London: E. Arnold & Co.

Pearson, W. J., & Wyllie, W. G. (1930). *Recent advances in diseases of children*, 2nd ed. London: J. & A. Churchill.

Pennington, Sarah. (1784). *An unfortunate mother's advice to her absent daughters in a letter to Miss Pennington*. London: printed for J. Walter.

Pennington, S. (1827). *Letter to Miss Louisa ******, on the management and education of infant children*. The Arthur and Elizabeth Schlesinger Library on the History of Women in America, Radcliffe College. New York: S. Marks.

Parfitt, D. N. (1966, 24 December). Letter: 'Treatment of anorexia nervosa'. *British Medical Journal, 2*(5529), 1595.

Pfister. O. (1917). *The psychoanalytic method*. London: Kegan Paul.

Platt, Sir H. (chair). (1959). *The welfare of children in hospital. Report of the Committee. Ministry of Health. Central Services Council*. London: H.M. Stationery Office.

Plaut, F. (1966). Reflections about not being able to imagine. *Journal of Analytical Psychology, 11*, 113–134.

Poynton, F. J. (1901). Some further investigations upon rheumatic fever. *Lancet, 157*(4053), 1260–1265.

Poynton, F. J. (1928, 22 September). Lettsomian lectures on rheumatic heart disease in childhood. *Lancet, 212*(5482), 585–589.

Poynton, F. J. (1936). *Harben lectures.* London: T. Q. Scott & Son.
Poynton, F. J. (1936). Juvenile rheumatism. *Journal of State Medicine, 44,* 655.
Poynton, F. J., & Paine, A. (1913). *Researches on rheumatism.* London: J. & A. Churchill.
Poynton, F. J., & Schlesinger, B. E. (1931). *Recent advances in the study of rheumatism.* London: Churchill.
Rickman, J. (Ed.). (1936). *On the bringing up of children. By five psycho-analysts: E. F. Sharpe, M. Klein, M. P. Middlemore, N. Searl, S. Isaacs.* London: Kegan Paul, Trench, Trubner.
Rank, O. (1929). *The trauma of birth.* London: Kegan Paul, Trench, Trubner.
Rapoport, J. (1942). Therapeutic process in case of childhood schizophrenia. *The Nervous Child,* 1(2–3), 188.
Read, G. D. (1942). *Revelation of childbirth: The principles and practice of natural childbirth.* London: Heinemann.
Ribble, M. (1943). *The rights of infants: Early psychological needs and their satisfaction.* New York: Columbia University Press.
Rickman, J. (1928). The development of the psycho-analytical theory of the psychoses, 1893–1926. (1957). *International Psycho-Analytical Library,* 52, 224–383.
Rickman, J. (1950). The factor of number in individual- and group-dynamics. *British Journal of Psychiatry,* 96(404), 770–773.
Riese, H. (1963). *Heal the hurt child: An approach through educational therapy with special reference to the extremely deprived negro child.* Chicago: University of Chicago Press.
Rimland, B. (1964). *Infantile autism.* New York: Appleton-Century-Crofts.
Rioch, J. (1943). The transference phenomenon in psychoanalytic therapy. *Psychiatry,* 6, 147–156.
Ritvo, S. (1966). Correlation of a childhood and adult neurosis: Based on the adult analysis of a reported childhood case. *International Journal of Psychoanalysis,* 47, 130–131.
Riviere, J. (1936). On the genesis of psychic conflict in earliest infancy. *International Journal of Psychoanalysis,* 17, 395–422.
Riviere, J. (Ed.). (1952). *Developments in psycho-analysis.* London: Hogarth.
Riviere, J. (1958, 22 February). Obituary of Ernest Jones. *British Medical Journal,* 1(5068), 463–465.
Robertson, James (1952). *Young children in hospital.* London: Tavistock.
Robertson, J. (1953). *A two-year-old goes to hospital* [Motion picture]. London: Concord Video and Film Council.
Robertson, Joyce (1956). 'A mother's observations on the tonsillectomy of her four-year-old daughter'. With comments by Anna Freud. In *The psychoanalytic study of the child,* 11 (pp. 410–427). London: Imago; *Nursing Times,* 15 Nov. 1957, 1395–1407.
Robertson, J. (1958). *Going to hospital with mother* [Motion picture]. London: Tavistock Child Development Research Unit.
Robertson, J. (1958). *Young children in hospital.* London: Tavistock.
Robertson, J., & Robertson, J. (1953). *A two-year-old goes to hospital* [Motion picture]. London: Concord Video and Film Council.
Robinson, K. (2015). Remembering, repeating and working through: The impact of the controversial discussions. *British Journal of Psychotherapy,* 31, 69–84.
Rocaz & Lartigout. (1921). A mixed form of primary myopathy. *Journal de Médecine de Bordeaux,* 42, 326.
Rodman, R. R. (2003). *Winnicott: Life and work.* Cambridge, MA: Da Capo Press.

Rogerson, C. H. (1944, January 15). Shock treatment of mental disorder. *British Medical Journal, 1*(4332), 94.
Rolleston, J. D. (1904). Clinical observations on diphtheritic paralysis. *The Practitioner, 73*, 597.
Rolleston, J. D. (1905). Diphtheritic hemiplegia: A case with commentary. *Review of Neurology and Psychiatry, 3*(11), 722.
Rolleston, J. D. (1909). Palpebral gangrene and other ocular complications of varicella. *Medical Chronicle, 49*, 215.
Rolleston, J. D. (1913). Diphtheritic hemiplegia. *Clinical Journal, 42*(1), 12.
Rolleston, J. D. (1916). Transient hemiplegia in diphtheria. *Review of Neurology and Psychiatry, 14*, 145.
Rolleston, J. D. (1925). *Acute infectious diseases: A handbook for practitioners and students.* London: William Heinemann.
Rolleston, J. D. (1929). *Acute infectious diseases, 2nd ed.* London: William Heinemann.
Rosen, J. N. (1953). *Direct analysis: Selected papers.* New York: Grune and Stratton.
Rosenfeld, H. (1952a). Notes on the psycho-analysis of the super-ego conflict of an acute schizophrenic patient. *International Journal of Psycho-Analysis, 33*, 111–131.
Rosenfeld, H. (1952b). Transference-phenomena and transference-analysis in an acute catatonic schizophrenic patient. *International Journal of Psycho-Analysis, 33*, 457–464.
Rosenfeld, H. (1958). Some observations on the psychopathology of hypochondriacal states. *International Journal of Psycho-Analysis, 39*, 121–124.
Rowley, J. L. (1954). Rehearsal and collusion. *International Journal of Psycho-Analysis, 35*, 421–427.
Roxburgh, A. C. (1937). On neurodermatoses. In *Common skin diseases, 4th ed.* (p. 247). London: H. K. Lewis.
Royal Medico-Psychological Association. (1961). The functions of the medical director of a child psychiatry (child guidance) clinic.
Rycroft, C. (1958). An enquiry into the function of words in the psycho-analytical situation. *International Journal of Psycho-Analysis, 39*(5), 408–415.
Rycroft, C. F. (1953). Some observations on a case of vertigo. *International Journal of Psycho-Analysis, 34*, 241–247.
Sack, W. (1927). Psycho-therapy and skin diseases. *Dermatologische Wochenschrift, 84*, 16.
Sack, W. (1928). On the psychic and nervous component of the so-called allergic skin diseases and their treatment. *British Journal of Dermatology, 40*, 441–445.
Sadger, I. (1911). Haut-, Schleimhaut- und Muskelerotik. [Skin, mucous membrane and muscle erotism.] *Jahrbuch für psychoanalytische und psychopathologische Forschungen, 3*, 525.
Sadger, I. (1913). Über den sado-masochistischen Komplex. [Regarding the sado-masochistic complex.] *Jahrbuch für psychoanalytische und psychopathologische Forschungen, 5*, 467.
Sadger, I. (1926). Contribution to the understanding of sado-masochism. *International Journal of Psychoanalysis, 7*, 484.
Sandler, J. (1960). On the concept of the superego. In *The psychoanalytic study of the child, 15* (pp. 128–162). London: Imago.
Sandler, J. (1962). Research in psycho-analysis: The Hampstead Index as an instrument of psycho-analytic research. Presented in the Symposium on Research at the 22nd International Psycho-Analytical Congress, Edinburgh, 1961. *International Journal of Psycho-Analysis, 43*, 287–291.

Sandler, J. (1987). *From safety to superego*. London/New York: Karnac/Guilford.
Sandler, J. (Ed.). (1967). Scientific Bulletin of the British Psychoanalytic Society, *10*.
Sandler, J. (Ed.). (1967). Scientific Bulletin of the British Psychoanalytic Society, *12*.
Sandler, J. (Ed.). (1967). Scientific Bulletin of the British Psychoanalytic Society, *17*.
Sargant, W. (1951). Leucotomy in psychosomatic disorders. *Lancet, 258*(6673), 87.
Sargant, W. (1951). The mechanism of 'conversion'. *British Medical Journal, 2*(4727), 311–316.
Sargant, W. (1969, May). The physiology of faith. *British Journal of Psychiatry, 115*, 505–518.
Sargant, W., & Stewart, C. M. (1947). Chronic neurosis treated with leucotomy. *British Medical Journal, 2*(4534), 866–869.
Schilder, P. (1936). Remarks on the psycho-physiology of the skin. *Psycho-Analytic Review, 23*, 274–285.
Schilder, P. (1939). The relations between clinging and equilibrium. *International Journal of Psycho-Analysis, 20*, 58–63.
Schlesinger, B., & Sheldon, W. (1931). Acute rheumatism following tonsillitis. *Lancet, 218*(5628), 97.
Schmideberg, M. (1943, March). Letter to the editor. *New Era in Home and School, 24*(3).
Schorstein, J. (1951, 28 July). Letter: Prefrontal leucotomy. *British Medical Journal, 2*(4725), 239.
Schur, M. (Ed.). (1965). A child psychiatry case illustrating delayed reaction to loss. In *Drives, affects, behavior*. New York: International University Press.
Schur, M. (Ed.). (1965). *Drives, affects, behavior: Essays in memory of Marie Bonaparte, vol. 2*. New York: International Universities Press.
Scott, W. C. M. (1949). The 'body scheme' in psychotherapy. *British Journal of Medical Psychology, 22*, 139–150.
Scott, W. C. M. (1954). A new hypothesis concerning the relationship of libidinal and aggressive instincts. *International Journal of Psycho-Analysis, 35*, 234–237.
Scott, W. C. M. (1955). A note on blathering. *International Journal of Psycho-Analysis, 36*, 348–349.
Scott, W. C. M. (1949). The body scheme in psychotherapy. *British Journal of Medical Psychology, 22*(2), 139–150.
Searl, N. (1929). The flight to reality. *International Journal of Psycho-Analysis, 10*, 280.
Searles, H. (1960). *The non-human environment in normal development and in schizophrenia*. New York: International Universities Press.
Searles, H. F. (1959). The effort to drive the other person crazy—An element in the aetiology and psychotherapy of schizophrenia. *British Journal of Medical Psychology, 32*(1), 1–18.
Sechehaye, M. A. (1951). *Symbolic realization*. New York: International Universities Press.
Segal, H. (1964). *Introduction to the work of Melanie Klein*. London: Karnac
Senn, M. (2007). Interview with John Bowlby. Retrieved from http://www.beyondthecouch.org
Senn, M. J. (Ed.) (1949). *Problems of infancy and childhood. Transactions of the Third Conference*. New York: Josiah Macy, Jr. Foundation.
Senn, M. J. E. (Ed.). (1952). *Problems of infancy and childhood*. Transactions of the sixth conference, March 17 and 18. New York: Josiah Macy Jr. Foundation.
Sequeira, J. H. (1927). *Diseases of the skin*. London: Churchill.
Sewell, A. (1877). *Black Beauty*. London: Jarold & Sons.
Shakespeare, W. *Coriolanus*.
Shakespeare, W. *Hamlet*.
Shakespeare, W. *Macbeth*.

Shakespeare, W. *Measure for Measure*.
Shakespeare, W. *Pericles*.
Shakespeare, W. *Romeo and Juliet*.
Shakespeare, W. *The Winter's Tale*.
Shakespeare, W. *Troilus and Cressida*.
Sheldon, W. (1931). On acute rheumatism following tonsillitis. *Lancet, 217*(5625), 1337–1341.
Shelley, P. B. (1824). Hymn to Mercury. In *Posthumous poems*. London: John and Henry L. Hunt.
Simey, T. S. (1961). *The concept of love in child care*. Oxford: Oxford University Press.
Slavson, S. R. (1952). *Child psychotherapy*. New York: Columbia University Press. London: Geoffrey Cumberlege, 1953.
Slovenka, R. (Ed.). (1966). A psychoanalytic view of the antisocial tendency. In *Crime, law and corrections*. Springfield, IL: Charles C. Thomas.
Smith, D. C. W. (1915). Acute myelitis following varicella. *American Journal of Diseases of Children, 10*, 445–446.
Soddy, K. (1960). *Clinical child psychiatry*. London: Baillière, Tindall and Cox.
Solomon, J. C. (1962). Fixed idea as an internalized transitional object. *American Journal of Psychotherapy, 16*, 632–644.
Sparks, R. F. (1966, 31 March). '"Blood-tie" child'. *The Times*. Issue 56594.
Spence, J. (1946/1960). The care of children in hospitals. In *The purpose and practice of medicine*. Oxford: Oxford University Press.
Spitz, R. A. (1945). Hospitalism. An inquiry into the genesis of psychiatric conditions in early childhood. In *The psych-analytic study of the child, 1* (pp. 53–74). London: Imago.
Spitz, R. A. (1949). Autoerotism. In *The psychoanalytic study of the child, 3/4* (pp. 85–120). London: Imago.
Spitz, R. A. (1950). Relevancy of direct infant observation. In *The psychoanalytic study of the child, 5* (pp. 66–73). London: Imago.
Spitz, R. A. (1962). Autoerotism re-examined: The role of early sexual behaviour patterns in personality formation. In *The psycho-analytic study of the child, 17*. London: Imago.
Spitz, R. A., & Wolf, K. M. (1946). Anaclitic depression: An inquiry into the genesis of psychiatric conditions in early childhood. In *The psychoanalytic study of the child, 2* (pp. 313–342). London: Imago.
Spock, B. (1946). *The common sense book of baby and child care*. New York: Duell, Sloan and Pearce.
Spock, B. (1955). *Baby and child care*. London: Bodley Head.
Spock, B. (1963). The striving for autonomy and some regressive object relationships. In *The psycho-analytic study of the child, 18* (pp. 361–366). London: Imago.
Standley, D. W. (1955). Letter: Prefrontal leucotomy. *British Medical Journal, 2*(4952), 1390–1391.
Steele, G. D. F. (1951). Persistent anxiety and tachycardia successfully treated by prefrontal leucotomy. *British Medical Journal, 2*(4723), 84.
Stein, L. (1949). *The infancy of speech and the speech of infancy*. London: Methuen.
Steiner, R., & King, P. (1991). *The Freud-Klein controversies 1941–1945*. London: Routledge.
Sterling, W. (1913). Ein Fall von Encephalitis nach Varicella. *Zeitschrift für die gesamte Neurologie und Psychiatrie, 8*, 536.

Stevenson, O. (1954). The first treasured possession: A study of the part played by specially loved objects and toys in the lives of certain children. In *The psychoanalytic study of the child*, 9 (pp. 199–217). London: Imago.

Stewart, S. (1967). *A home from home*. London: Longmans.

Still, G. F. (1927). *Common disorders and diseases of childhood, 5th ed*. London: Oxford Medical Press.

Stiner, O. (1925). *Schweizerische medizinische Wochenschrift*, 55, 244.

Stokes, A. (1951). *Smooth and rough*. London: Faber. Reprinted in *The critical writings of Adrian Stokes, II*. London: Thames and Hudson, 1978.

Stokes, A. (1955). Form in art. In M. Klein, P. Heiman, & R. E. Money-Kyrle (Eds.), *New directions in psycho-analysis*. London.

Storr, A. (1968). *Human aggression*. London: Allen Lane.

Strachey, J. (1930). Some unconscious factors in reading. *International Journal of Psychoanalysis*, 11, 322.

Strachey, J. (1934). The nature of the therapeutic action of psycho-analysis. *International Journal of Psycho-Analysis*, 15.

Strachey, J. (Ed.). (1953–1974). *Standard edition of the psychological works of Sigmund Freud*. London: Hogarth.

Stungo, E. (1946, 15 June). Letter: Psychology in the child's education. *British Medical Journal*, 1(4458), 930.

Summerfield (chair). (1968). *The Summerfield Report: Psychologists in education services: The report of the working party appointed by the Secretary of State for Education and Science, 20th Feb 1968*. London: H. M. Stationery Office.

Sutherland, G. A. (1929). Disorders and diseases of the heart. In F. E. Batten, A. E. Garrod, D. H. Paterson, & H. Thursfield (Eds.), *Diseases of children*. New York: William Wood & Co.

Sutherland, G. A., & Williamson, B. (1925). The treatment of purpura hæmorrhagica by splenectomy. *Lancet*, 205(5294), 323–327.

Swallow, N. (1955). Comforters. *British Medical Journal*, 2(4933), 266.

Tagore, R. (1913). On the seashore. In *The crescent moon*. London/New York: Macmillan.

Tauber, E. (1964). Exploring the therapeutic use of the counter-transference data. *Psychiatry*, 17, 331–336.

The Children's Act. (1948). London: H.M. Stationery Office.

Thomson, H. (1966). *The successful step-parent*. London: W. H. Allen.

Thomson, J. (1925). *The clinical study and treatment of sick children, 4th ed*. Edinburgh: Oliver & Boyd.

Thorner, H. (1963). Cause, reason and motif: A psychoanalytical contribution to the understanding of psychosomatic phenomena. *Psyche*, 16, 670–685.

Tod, R. J. N. (1968). *Disturbed children*. London: Longmans.

Torrie, M. (1964). *The widow's child*. London: Cruse Clubs Counselling Service for Widows and Children.

Trilling, L. (1955). Freud: Within and beyond culture. In *Beyond culture*. Harmondsworth: Penguin (Peregrine series), 1967.

Trilling, L. (1955). *Freud and the crisis of our culture*. Boston: Beacon.

van Ophuijsen, J. H. W. (1920). On the origin of the feeling of persecution. *International Journal of Psycho-Analysis*, 1, 235–239.

Walker, K. (1938). On circumcision. *British Medical Journal*, 2(4069), 1377–1378.
Watson, J. A. F. (1950). *The child and the magistrate*. London: Jonathan Cape.
Weber, F. P. (1927). Pituitary (? cystic) tumour. *Proceedings of the Royal Society of Medicine*, 20(9), 1336–1336.
Weiss, E. (1953). *Ego psychology and the psychoses*. London: Imago.
Wendell Holmes, O. (1882 [1858]). The autocrat at the breakfast table. *The 'Breakfast-table series'*. London: Routledge.
Westmacott, I. (1961). Psychiatric social work in a paediatric setting, Bristol Royal Hospital. *Case Conference*, 7.
Wheelis, A. (1958). *The quest for identity*. New York: Norton.
Whitehead, A. N. (1933). *Adventures of ideas*. Harmondsworth: Penguin.
Wickes, F. (1938). *The inner world of man*. New York/London: Farrar & Rinehart/ Methuen.
Wickes, F. (1950). *The inner world of man: With psychological drawings and paintings*. London: Methuen.
Wilde, O. (1898 [1897]). *The ballad of Reading Gaol*. London: Leonard Smithers.
Wilde, O. (1903). *The importance of being earnest*. London: Samuel French.
Willmott, P., & Young, M. (1957). *Family and kinship in East London*. London: Routledge & Kegan Paul.
Wilson, A. C. (1943). An individual point of view on shock therapy. *International Journal of Psychoanalysis*, 24, 59.
Wilson, A. C. (1946). Homosexuality. *British Medical Journal*, 1(4442), 290–291.
Wilson, A. C. (1947, 7 May). The rôle of fixation in perversion and masturbation. *Medical Press*, 217(19), 397.
Wilson, A. C. (1948). Deprivation of initiative. *British Medical Journal*, 1(4551), 614.
Winnicott, C. (1954). Casework techniques in the child care services. In *Child Care and Social Work*. Welwyn: Codicote.
Winnicott, C. (1962). Casework and agency function. In *Child care and social work*. Welwyn: Codicote.
Winnicott, C. (1964). *Child care and social work*. Welwyn: Codicote.
Winnicott, D. W. (1929). Diagnosis of chorea. [CW 1:2:16]
Winnicott, D. W. (1929). Rheumatism in children [1928]. [CW 1:2:12]
Winnicott, D. W. (1931). A note on normality and anxiety. [CW 1:3:12]
Winnicott, D. W. (1931). *Clinical notes on disorders of childhood*. [CW 1:3]
Winnicott, D. W. (1931). Convulsions, fits. [CW 1:3:17]
Winnicott, D. W. (1931). Fidgetiness. [CW 1:3:11]
Winnicott, D. W. (1934). Papular urticaria and the dynamics of skin sensation. [CW 1:4:3]
Winnicott, D. W. (1938). Notes on a little boy. [CW 1:4:16]
Winnicott, D. W. (1939). The psychology of juvenile rheumatism. [CW 2:1:7]
Winnicott, D. W. (1940). Children and their mothers. [CW 2:2:2]
Winnicott, D. W. (1941). The observation of infants in a set situation. [CW 2:3:6]
Winnicott, D. W. (1943). Delinquency research. [CW 2:5:2]
Winnicott, D. W. (1943, 21 August). Letter: Responsibility and freedom. *British Medical Journal*. [CW 2:5:7]
Winnicott, D. W. (1943, 25 December). Letter: Shock treatment of mental disorder. *British Medical Journal*. [CW 2:5:10]
Winnicott, D. W. (1945). *Getting to know your baby* [1943]. [CW 2:5:8]

Winnicott, D. W. (1945). Infant feeding [1944]. [CW 2:6:13]
Winnicott, D. W. (1945). Primitive emotional development. [CW 2:7:8]
Winnicott, D. W. (1945). Why do babies cry? [1944] [CW 2:6:2]
Winnicott, D. W. (1946). Some psychological aspects of juvenile delinquency [1944]. [CW 3:1:7]
Winnicott, D. W. (1946). What do we mean by a normal child? [1944] [CW 2:6:10]
Winnicott, D. W. (1947). Physical therapy of mental disorder. [CW 3:2:2]
Winnicott, D. W. (1948). Children's hostels in war and peace [1946]. [CW 3:1:1]
Winnicott, D. W. (1948). Pediatrics and psychiatry. [CW 3:3:2]
Winnicott, D. W. (1948). Review: *The psychoanalytic study of the child, Vol. 2*. [CW 3:3:9]
Winnicott, D. W. (1949). Baby as a going concern. [CW 3:4:24]
Winnicott, D. W. (1949). Close-up of mother feeding baby. [CW 3:4:28]
Winnicott, D. W. (1949). End of the digestive process. [CW 3:4:26]
Winnicott, D. W. (1949). Hate in the countertransference [1947]. [CW 3:2:1].
Winnicott, D. W. (1949, 23 August). Letter: Punishment and crime: A psychologist's view. *The Times*. [CW 3:4:16]
Winnicott, D. W. (1949). Leucotomy. [CW 3:4:21]
Winnicott, D. W. (1949). *The ordinary devoted mother and her baby*. Nine Broadcast Talks. Republished in *The child and the family*. London: Tavistock.
Winnicott, D. W. (1949). Weaning. [CW 3:4:31]
Winnicott, D. W. (1949). The world in small doses. [CW 3:4:29]
Winnicott, D. W. (1949). Young children and other people. [CW 3:4:32]
Winnicott, D. W. (1950). Childhood psychosis. [CW 3:5:5]
Winnicott, D. W. (1950). Some thoughts on the meaning of the word democracy. [CW 3:5:17]
Winnicott, D. W. (1951). Review: Freud, A., Hoffer, W., Glover, E. (Eds.), *The psychoanalytic study of the child* (Vols. 3-4, 5). (London: Imago, 1949). [CW 3:6:12]
Winnicott, D. W. (1951). Review: *The psychoanalytic study of the child* (Vols. 3-4, 5) [CW 3:6:12]
Winnicott, D. W. (1953). Psychoses and child care [1952]. [CW 4:1:5]
Winnicott, D. W. (1953). Symptom tolerance in paediatrics: A case history. [CW 4:2:4]
Winnicott, D. W. (1953). Transitional objects and transitional phenomena: A study of the first Not-Me possession. [CW 4:2:21]; see also CW 3:6:6, and CW 9:3:5]
Winnicott, D. W. (1954). Mind and its relation to the psyche-soma [1949]. [CW 3:4:20]
Winnicott, D. W. (1955). The depressive position in normal emotional development [1954]. [CW 4:3:5]
Winnicott, D. W. (1955). Metapsychological and clinical aspects of regression within the psychoanalytical set-up [1954]. [CW 4:3:6]
Winnicott, D. W. (1955). Withdrawal and regression [1954]. [CW 4:3:29]
Winnicott, D. W. (1956). Clinical varieties of transference [1955]. [CW 5:1:11]
Winnicott, D. W. (1957). Breast feeding [1945, revised 1954]. [CW 2:7:12]
Winnicott, D. W. (1957). *The child and the family: First relationships*. London: Tavistock.
Winnicott, D. W. (1957). *The child and the outside world*. London: Tavistock.
Winnicott, D. W. (1957). The contribution of psycho-analysis to midwifery. Part II. [CW 5:3:15]
Winnicott, D. W. (1957). First experiments in independence [1955]. [CW 5:1:20]
Winnicott, D. W. (1957). Instincts and normal difficulties [1950]. [CW 3:5:15]
Winnicott, D. W. (1957). Knowing and learning [1950]. [CW 3:5:14]

Winnicott, D. W. (1957). A man looks at motherhood [1949]. [CW 3:4:23]
Winnicott, D. W. (1957). *Mother and child: A primer of first relationships*. New York: Basic Books.
Winnicott, D. W. (1957). The mother's contribution to society. [CW 5:3:30]
Winnicott, D. W. (1957). On Adoption [1955]. (Broadcast 23 February 1995 as 'Homeless children and children's homes'.) [CW 5:1:2]
Winnicott, D. W. (1957). *The ordinary devoted mother and her baby*. Nine broadcast talks. Republished in *The child and the family*. London: Tavistock.
Winnicott, D. W. (1957). Towards an objective study of human nature. [CW 2:7:11]
Winnicott, D. W. (1958). Aggression in relation to emotional development [1950]. [CW 3:5:2]
Winnicott, D. W. (1958). The antisocial tendency [1956]. [CW 5:2:8]
Winnicott, D. W. (1958). Appetite and emotional disorder [1936]. [CW 1:4:11]
Winnicott, D. W. (1958). Anxiety associated with insecurity [1952]. [CW 4:1:11]
Winnicott, D. W. (1958). Birth memories, birth trauma, and anxiety [1949]. [CW 3:4:8]
Winnicott, D. W. (1958). The capacity to be alone [1957]. [CW 5:3:20]
Winnicott, D. W. (1958). Child analysis in the latency period. [CW 5:4:13]
Winnicott, D. W. (1958). *Collected papers: Through paediatrics to psycho-analysis*. London/New York: Tavistock/Basic Books.
Winnicott, D. W. (1958). The first year of life. [CW 5:4:6]
Winnicott, D. W. (1958). Funeral address for Ernest Jones. [CW 5:4:3]
Winnicott, D. W. (1958). The manic defence [1935]. [CW 1:4:6]
Winnicott, D. W. (1958). Obituary: Ernest Jones. [CW 5:4:21]
Winnicott, D. W. (1958). On the contribution of direct child observation to psycho-analysis [1957]. [CW 5:3:21]
Winnicott, D. W. (1958). Primary maternal preoccupation [1956]. [CW 5:2:16]
Winnicott, D. W. (1958). Psycho-analysis and the sense of guilt [1956]. [CW 5:2:7]
Winnicott, D. W. (1958). Reparation in respect of mother's organised defence against depression [1948]. [CW 3:3:1]
Winnicott, D. W. (1958). Review of *The doctor, his patient and the illness*, by M. Balint. [CW 5:4:23]
Winnicott, D. W. (1958). Theoretical statement of the field of child psychiatry. [CW 5:4:25]
Winnicott, D. W. (1958). Transitional objects and transitional phenomena. [CW 5:4:24]
Winnicott, D. W. (1960). Objets transitionels et phénomènes transitionnels. *La Psychanalyse*, volume 5. Paris: Presses Universitaires de France.
Winnicott, D. W. (1960). String: A technique of communication. [CW 6:1:20]
Winnicott, D. W. (1960). The theory of the parent-infant relationship. [CW 6:1:21]
Winnicott, D. W. (1961). The effect of psychotic parents on the emotional development of the child [1959]. [CW 5:5:21]
Winnicott, D. W. (1962). Adolescence: Struggling through the doldrums [1961]. [CW 6:2:4]
Winnicott, D. W. (1962). Review: *Un cas de psychose infantile* by S. Lebovici & J. McDougall. [CW 6:3:17]
Winnicott, D. W. (1962). The theory of the parent-infant relationship: Contributions to discussion. [CW 6:3:13]
Winnicott, D. W. (1962). The theory of the parent-infant relationship: Further remarks. [CW 6:3:14]
Winnicott, D. W. (1963). The development of the capacity for concern [1962]. [CW 6:3:11]

Winnicott, D. W. (1963). Dependence in infant-care, in child-care and in the psycho-analytic setting [1962]. [CW 6:3:9]

Winnicott, D. W. (1963). Morals and education [1962]. [CW 6:3:18]

Winnicott, D. W. (1963). The mentally ill in your caseload. [CW 6:4:5]

Winnicott, D. W. (1963). Regression as a therapy illustrated by the case of a boy whose pathological dependence was adequately met by the parents. Published here as '"Cecil" aet 21 months at first consultation'. [CW 10:3:14]

Winnicott, D. W. (1963). Struggling through the doldrums. [CW 6:4:7]

Winnicott, D. W. (1964, 25 October). 'All of mother'. Letter to the Editor, *The Observer*. [CW 7:1:10]

Winnicott, D. W. (1964, 5 November). 'All of mother'. Letter to the Editor, *The Observer*. [CW 7:1:13]

Winnicott, D. W. (1964). *The child, the family, and the outside world*. Harmondsworth: Penguin.

Winnicott, D. W. (1964). Introduction to *The child, the family, and the outside world*. [CW 7:1:17]

Winnicott, D. W. (1964). The neonate and his mother. [CW 7:1:4]

Winnicott, D. W. (1964). Roots of aggression. [CW 7:1:18]

Winnicott, D. W. (1964). Youth will not sleep. [CW 7:1:7]

Winnicott, D. W. (1965). Advising parents [1957]. [CW 5:3:27]

Winnicott, D. W. (1965). The aims of psycho-analytical treatment [1962]. [CW 6:3:2]

Winnicott, D. W. (1965). Casework with mentally ill children [1959]. [CW 5:5:15]

Winnicott, D. W. (1965). Classification: Is there a psycho-analytic contribution to psychiatric classification? [1959, 1964] [CW 5:5:5]

Winnicott, D. W. (1965). A clinical study of the effect of a failure of the average expectable environment on a child's mental functioning. Published here as '"Bob" aet 6 years'. [CW 10:1:4]

Winnicott, D. W. (1965). Communicating and not communicating leading to a study of certain opposites [1963]. [CW 6:4:8]

Winnicott, D. W. (1965). The effect of psychosis on family life [1960]. [CW 6:1:6]

Winnicott, D. W. (1965). Ego distortion in terms of true and false self [1960]. [CW 6:1:22]

Winnicott, D. W. (1965). Ego integration in child development [1962]. [CW 6:3:19]

Winnicott, D. W. (1965). The family affected by depressive illness in one or both parents [1958]. [CW 5:4:17]

Winnicott, D. W. (1965). *The family and individual development*. London: Tavistock.

Winnicott, D. W. (1965). The five-year-old [1962]. [CW 6:3:6]

Winnicott, D. W. (1965). From dependence towards independence in the development of the individual [1963]. [CW 6:4:11]

Winnicott, D. W. (1965). Hospital care supplementing intensive psychotherapy in adolescence [1963]. [CW 6:4:13]

Winnicott, D. W. (1965). *The maturational processes and the facilitating environment*. London: Hogarth and The Institute of Psycho-Analysis.

Winnicott, D. W. (1965). On security [1960]. [CW 6:1:9]

Winnicott, D. W. (1965). A personal view of the Kleinian contribution [1962]. [CW 6:3:8]

Winnicott, D. W. (1965). Preface to *The family and individual development*. [CW 7:2:25]

Winnicott, D. W. (1965). The price of disregarding psychoanalytic research. [CW 7:2:4]

Winnicott, D. W. (1965). Psychotherapy of character disorders [1963]. [CW 6:4:9]

Winnicott, D. W. (1965). The relationship of a mother to her baby at the beginning [1960]. [CW 6:1:8]

Winnicott, D. W. (1966). 'Ada' aet 8 years. [CW 10:3:13]

Winnicott, D. W. (1966). Comment on obsessional neurosis and 'Frankie' [1965]. [CW 7:2:10]

Winnicott, D. W. (1966). Psycho-somatic illness in its positive and negative aspects [1964]. [CW 7:1:6]

Winnicott. D. W. (1966). Review: *Absent: School refusal as an expression of disturbed family relationships* by Max Clyne. [CW 7:3:22]

Winnicott, D. W. (1967). The location of cultural experience [1966]. [CW 7:3:31]

Winnicott, D. W. (1967). Mirror-role of mother and family in child development. [CW 8:1:38]

Winnicott. D. W. (1967). Review: *Absent: School refusal as an expression of disturbed family relationships,* by M. B. Clyne. [CW 8:1:15]

Winnicott, D. W. (1968). The aetiology of infantile schizophrenia in terms of adaptive failure [1967]. [CW 8:1:25]

Winnicott, D. W. (1968). Communication between infant and mother, and mother and infant, compared and contrasted. [CW 8:2:2]

Winnicott, D. W. (1968). 'Eliza' aet 7½ years. [CW 10:1:3]

Winnicott, D. W. (1968). Foreword. Tod, R. J. N. (Ed.), *Disturbed children* (p.vii). [CW 8:2:8]

Winnicott, D. W. (1968). Infant feeding and emotional development [1967]. Published here as part of 'Environmental health in infancy'. [CW 8:1:6]

Winnicott, D. W. (1968). La schizophrénie infantile en termes d'échec d'adaptation [1967]. Published here as 'The aetiology of infantile schizophrenia in terms of adaptive failure' [CW 8:1:25]

Winnicott, D. W. (1968). Meeting the challenge of the case in child psychiatry [1964, 1968]. Published here as 'The squiggle game'. [CW 8:2:47]

Winnicott, D. W. (1968). Playing: Its theoretical status in the clinical situation [1967]. Published here as 'Playing: A theoretical statement'. [CW 8:2:15]

Winnicott, D. W. (1968). Review: *Human aggression,* by C. A. Storr. [CW 8:2:18]

Winnicott, D. W. (1968). The squiggle game [1964, 1968]. [CW 8:2:47]

Winnicott, D. W. (1969). A link between paediatrics and child psychology: Clinical observations [1968]. [CW 8:2:14]

Winnicott, D. W. (1969). Adolescent process and the need for personal confrontation. Published here as part of, 'Contemporary concepts of adolescent development and their implications for higher education'. [CW 9:3:9]

Winnicott, D. W. (1969). Changing patterns: The young person, the family and society. Published here as part of, 'Contemporary concepts of adolescent development and their implications for higher education'. [CW 9:3:9]

Winnicott, D. W. (1969). Preface to *A dialogue with Sammy* by S. Lebovici & J. McDougall. [CW 9:1:27]

Winnicott, D. W. (1969). The use of an object [1968]. (Published here as The use of an object and relating through identifications.) [CW 8:2:28]

Winnicott, D. W. (1971). 'Ashton' aet 12 years. [CW 10:2:9]

Winnicott, D. W. (1971). Basis for self in body [1970]. [CW 9:2:12]

Winnicott, D. W. (1971). 'Bob' aet 6 years. [CW 10:1:4]

Winnicott, D. W. (1971). Contemporary concepts of adolescent development and their implications for higher education [1968]. [CW 9:3:9]
Winnicott, D. W. (1971). Creativity and its origins. [CW 9:3:7]
Winnicott, D. W. (1971). 'Eliza' aet 7½ years. [CW 10:1:3]
Winnicott, D. W. (1971). 'Hesta' aet 16 years. [CW 10:2:11]
Winnicott, D. W. (1971). 'Iiro' aet 9 years 9 months, Case 1. [CW 10:1:1]
Winnicott, D. W. (1971). The place where we live. [CW 8:2:1]
Winnicott, D. W. (1971). Playing: Creative activity and the search for the self. [CW 8:1:27]
Winnicott, D. W. (1971). *Playing and reality*. London: Tavistock.
Winnicott, D. W. (1971). 'Ruth' aet 8 years. [CW 10:3:17]
Winnicott, D. W. (1971). The split-off male and female elements to be found in men and women [1966]. [CW 7:3:2]
Winnicott, D. W. (1971). *Therapeutic consultations in child psychiatry*. [CW 10]
Winnicott, D. W. (1972). Answers to comments on 'The split-off male and female elements' [1968–1968]. [CW 9:1:30]
Winnicott, D. W. (1974). Fear of breakdown [ca. 1963–1964]. [CW 6:4:21]
Winnicott, D. W. (1977). *The Piggle*. London: Hogarth. [CW 11:2]
Winnicott, D. W. (1984). Aggression, guilt and reparation [1960]. [CW 6:1:10]
Winnicott, D. W. (1984). Dissociation revealed in a therapeutic consultation. [CW 7:2:21]
Winnicott, D. W. (1984). Notes made in the train [1956]. [CW 7:2:6]
Winnicott, D. W. (1986). The concept of the false self [1964]. [CW 7:1:1]
Winnicott, D. W. (1986). This feminism [1964]. [CW 7:1:14]
Winnicott, D. W. (1987). The ordinary devoted mother [1966]. [CW 7:3:3]
Winnicott, D. W. (1989). The beginnings of a formulation of an appreciation and criticism of Klein's envy statement [1962]. [CW 6:3:7]
Winnicott, D. W. (1989). Clinical illustration of 'The use of an object' [1968]. [CW 8:2:29]
Winnicott, D. W. (1989). Clinical material on the theme of a male patient's exploitation of his female self [1959]. [CW 5:5:26]
Winnicott, D. W. (1989). Comments on my paper 'The use of an object' [1968]. [CW 8:2:38]
Winnicott, D. W. (1989). D. W. W.'s dream related to reviewing Jung [1963]. [CW 6:4:15]
Winnicott, D. W. (1989). D. W. W. on D. W. W. [1967]. [CW 8:1:2]
Winnicott, D. W. (1989). Hallucination and dehallucination [1957]. [CW 5:3:23]
Winnicott, D. W. (1989). The fate of the transitional object [1959]. [CW 5:5:22]
Winnicott, D. W. (1989). Kinds of psychological effects of shock therapy [1944]. [CW 2:6:7]
Winnicott, D. W. (1989). Notes on the general implications of leucotomy [1951]. [CW 3:6:14]
Winnicott, D. W. (1989). Notes on withdrawal and aggression [1965]. [Published here as 'Case notes for a psychoanalytic seminar: Withdrawal, regression, male identification'] [CW 7:2:19]
Winnicott, D. W. (1989). *Psycho-analytic explorations*. Cambridge, MA: Harvard University Press.
Winnicott, D. W. (1989). The psychology of madness: A contribution from psychoanalysis [1965]. [CW 7:2:18]
Winnicott, D. W. (1989). The split-off male and female elements to be found in men and women [1966]. [CW 7:3:2]
Winnicott, D. W. (1989). The use of an object in the context of *Moses and Monotheism* [1969]. [CW 9:1:4]

Winnicott, D. W. (1989). Use of the word 'use' [1968]. [CW 8:2:5]
Winnicott, D. W. (1991). Resolution K: On the scientific aims of psychoanalysis [1942]. [CW 2:4:1]
Winnicott, D. W. (1993). For stepparents [1955]. [CW 5:1:10]
Winnicott, D. W. (1993). *Talking to parents*. C. Winnicott, C. Bollas, M. Davis, & R. Shepherd (Eds.). Reading, MA: Harvard University Press.
Winnicott, D. W. (1996). The Association for Child Psychology and Psychiatry observed as a group phenomenon [1967]. [CW 8:1:3]
Winnicott, D. W. (1996). Autism [1966]. [CW 7:3:8]
Winnicott, D. W. (1996). The bearing of emotional development on feeding problems. Published here as part of 'Environmental health in infancy'. [CW 8:1:6]
Winnicott, D. W. (1996). On cardiac neurosis in children [1966]. [CW 7:3:16]
Winnicott, D. W. (1996). Child psychiatry, social work and alternative care [1970]. [CW 9:2:3]
Winnicott, D. W. (2003). Ditty on Enoch Powell [ca. 1968]. [CW 9:4:13]
Winnicott, D. W. (2003). Preface to Gaddini's Italian translation of *The family and individual development* [1966]. [CW 7:3:27]
Winnicott, D. W. (2017). Clinical material: Theme of 'Two', also theme of 'Black' [1965]. [CW 7:2:13]
Winnicott, D. W. (2017). Further clinical illustration of the use of an object [1968]. [CW 8:2:30]
Winnicott, D. W. (2017). The infancy of Juliet [1949]. [CW 3:4:4]
Winnicott, D. W. (2017). On the occasion of the publication of the *Standard edition of Freud* [1966]. [CW 7:3:23]
Winnicott, D. W. (2017). Report on Q Camps [1941]. [CW 2:3:1]
Winncott, D. W. (2017). Review: *Normality and pathology in childhood* [1965]. [CW 7:2:16]
Winnicott, D. W. (2017). Transitional objects and transitional phenomena [1951]. [CW 3:6:6; see also CW 4:2:21, CW 5:4:24, and CW 9:3:5]
Winnicott, D. W., & Britton, C. (1944). The problem of homeless children. [CW 2:6:14]
Winnicott, D. W., & Khan, M. R. (1953). Review: Psychoanalytic studies of the personality: By W. Ronald D. Fairbairn (London: Tavistock). *International Journal of Psycho-Analysis, 34*, 329–333.
Wolfendon, J., & Committee on Homosexual Offences and Prostitution. (1957). *Report of the Committee on Homosexual Offences and Prostitution* (The Wolfendon Report). London: H.M. Stationery Office.
Wolff, W. (1947). *The personality of the preschool child: The child's search for his self*. London: William Heinemann Medical Books.
Wolstein, B. (1959). *Counter-transference*. New York: Grune & Stratton.
Woolf, V. (1931). *The waves*. London: Hogarth.
Wordsworth, W. (1804). Ode: Intimations of immortality from recollections of early childhood. In *Poems, in two volumes*. London: Longman, Hurst, Rees, and Orme, Paternoster-Row.
Wordsworth, W. (1807). Ode: Intimations of mortality. *Poems, in Two Volumes*. London: Longman, Hurst, Rees and Orme.
World Health Organization Expert Committee on Mental Health. (1951). *Report on the second session, Geneva, 11–16 September 1950*. Technical Report Series, No. 31. Geneva: World Health Organization.

Wulff, M. (1946). Fetishism and object choice in early childhood. *Psychoanalytic Quarterly*, *15*, 450–471.

Wyllie, W. G. (1936). Diseases of muscles. In F. E. Batten, A. E. Garrod, D. H. Paterson, & H. Thursfield (Eds.), *Diseases of children, 2nd edition*. London: Edward Arnold & Co.

Zetzel, E. (1956). Current concepts of transference. *International Journal of Psycho-Analysis*, *37*, 369–376.

Zetzel, E. (1965). Additional notes on the case of obsessional neurosis: Freud 1909. *International Journal of Psychoanalysis, 47*(2), 123–129.

Zilboorg, G. (1943). *Mind, medicine and man*. New York: Harcourt, Brace.

Zilboorg, G. (1951). *Sigmund Freud*. New York: Scribner's.

Ziman, E. (1951). *Jealousy in children: A guide for parents*. London: Victor Gollancz.

CHRONOLOGY

	Biography	Significant Publications
1896	Donald Woods Winnicott born in Plymouth, Devon, England. Youngest son, with two older sisters, of Elizabeth Martha Woods Winnicott and John Frederick Winnicott, a merchant who was twice mayor of Plymouth.	
1910	Enters The Leys School, a boarding school in Cambridge.	
1914	Studies Natural Science at Jesus College, Cambridge University, in preparation to read medicine.	
1917	Enters St Bartholomew's Hospital Medical School, London. Enlists in the Royal Navy, serving during the war on H.M.S. *Lucifer* as Surgeon-Probationer.	
1920	Graduates from Barts and continues to work there as House Physician.	
1923	Appointed Assistant Physician at Paddington Green Children's Hospital, eventually becoming Physician-in-Charge. Appointed Assistant Physician at the Queen's Hospital for Children. Marries Alice Taylor. Begins his analysis with James Strachey.	
1924	Opens his own practice in Belgravia, London.	
1925	His mother, Elizabeth, dies of cardiac disease. Becomes a Fellow of the Royal Society of Medicine.	
1927	Begins his psychoanalytic training at the Institute of Psychoanalysis, London, supervised by Ella Freeman Sharpe and Nina Searl.	
1928	Appointed Physician in charge of a newly formed Rheumatism Clinic at the Queen's Hospital.	
1931		*Clinical Notes on Disorders of Childhood* [CW 1:3:1–20]
1933	Finishes his ten-year analysis with James Strachey.	
1934	Qualifies as an adult psychoanalyst and becomes an associate member of the British Psychoanalytical Society (BPAS). Resigns from the Queen's Hospital but continues to run the rheumatism clinic. Continues training as a child analyst under the supervision of Melanie Klein, Melitta Schmideberg, and Nina Searl.	
1935	Qualifies as the first male child psychoanalyst at the BPAS. Melanie Klein asks him to analyse her son Eric. Gives his membership paper, 'The Manic Defence', to the BPAS.	'The Manic Defence' [CW 1:4:6]

	Biography	Significant Publications
1936	Begins his second analysis, with Joan Riviere, lasting until 1941. Becomes a full member of the BPAS.	'Appetite and Emotional Disorder' [CW 1:4:11]
1939	Gives his first broadcasts on BBC Radio. Freud dies in London.	'Aggression' [CW 2:1:8] Letter to the *British Medical Journal*, 'The Evacuation of Small Children', with E. Miller and J. Bowlby [CW 2:1:6]
1940		'Children and Their Mothers' [CW 2:2:2]
1941	Appointed as psychiatric consultant to the scheme for evacuated children in Oxfordshire and meets Clare Britton, social worker in charge of the scheme.	'The Observation of Infants in a Set Situation' [CW 2:3:6]
1941–3	Named as one of five Kleinian training analysts and participates in the 'Controversial Discussions' in the BPAS. Becomes Director of the Child Department of the BPAS, holding the post until 1960.	'Resolution K: On Scientific Aims in Psychoanalysis' [CW 2:4:1] 'Child department consultations' [CW 2:4:2]
Mid-1940s	No longer regarded as a Kleinian. Broadcasts 'Getting to Know Your Baby' and other programmes on BBC radio, for 'the ordinary devoted mother'.	
1944	Becomes a Fellow of the Royal College of Physicians.	
1945		*Getting to Know Your Baby* 'Primitive Emotional Development' [CW 2:7:8]
1947		'Hate in the Countertransference' [CW 3:2:1] 'Residential Management as Treatment for Difficult Children' [CW 3:2:3]
1948	Chairman of the Medical Section of the British Psychological Society. His father, Sir John Frederick Winnicott, dies. Suffers his first coronary. Paddington Green Hospital is absorbed into St Mary's Hospital.	'Paediatrics and Psychiatry' [CW 3:3:2] 'Children's Hostels in War and Peace' [CW 3:1:1] 'Reparation in Respect of Mother's Organized Defence Against Depression' [CW 3:3:1]
1949	Leaves his first wife, Alice. Suffers his second coronary.	*The Ordinary Devoted Mother and Her Baby* 'Mind and Its Relation to the Psyche-Soma' [CW 3:4:20] 'Birth Memories, Birth Trauma, and Anxiety' [CW 3:4:8]
1950	Suffers a third coronary after a patient commits suicide. Named Scientific Secretary of the BPAS.	'Some Thoughts on the Meaning of the Word Democracy' [CW 3:5:17] 'Aggression in Relation to Emotional Development' [CW 3:5:2]

Chronology

	Biography	Significant Publications
1951	Divorces Alice. Marries Clare Britton. Becomes Training Secretary of the BPAS. Begins analysis of Masud Khan in October, continuing until April 1954.	'Transitional Objects and Transitional Phenomena' [CW 3:6:6; CW 4:2:21; CW 5:4:24; CW 9:3:5]
1952	President of the Paediatric Section of the Royal Society of Medicine. Broadcasts the series 'The Ordinary Devoted Mother and Her Baby' on BBC radio. Suffers his fourth coronary.	'Psychoses and Child Care' [CW 4:1:5] 'Anxiety Associated with Insecurity' [CW 4:1:11]
1953	Clare Winnicott begins analysis with Melanie Klein.	'Symptom Tolerance in Paediatrics' [CW 4:2:4] 'The Mother's Contribution to Society' [CW 5:3:30]
1954	Suffers his fifth coronary	'Withdrawal and Regression' [CW 4:3:29] 'The Depressive Position in Normal Emotional Development' [CW 4:3:5] 'Metapsychological and Clinical Aspects of Regression Within the Psycho-Analytical Set-up' [CW 4:3:6]
1955	Gives the first of many annual courses of lectures at the Child Development Department, Institute of Education, University of London.	'Clinical Varieties of Transference' [CW 5:1:11]
1956	Elected President of the BPAS for the first time, on a three-year term.	'Primary Maternal Preoccupation' [CW 5:2:16] 'The Antisocial Tendency' [CW 5:2:8] 'Paediatrics and Childhood Neurosis' [CW 5:2:11]
1957		*The Child and the Family* *The Child and the Outside World* 'On the Contribution of Direct Child Observation to Psychoanalysis' [CW 5:3:21]
1958		*Collected Papers: Through Paediatrics to Psychoanalysis* 'The Capacity to Be Alone' [CW 5:3:20] 'Child Analysis in the Latency Period' [CW 5:4:13]
1959	Spends August in Finland giving courses and lectures as part of a World Health Organisation conference.	'Classification: Is There a Psycho-analytic Contribution to Psychiatric Classification?' [CW 5:5:5]
1960	Broadcasts the series 'The Ordinary Devoted Mother and Her Children' on BBC radio. Melanie Klein dies. Steps down as Director of the Child Department of the BPAS, but remains Consultant Physician.	'The Effect of Psychosis on Family Life' [CW 6:1:6] 'The Theory of the Parent–Infant Relationship' [CW 6:1:21] 'Ego Distortion in Terms of True and False Self' [CW 6:1:22] 'String: A Technique of Communication' [CW 6:1:20] 'Counter-transference' [CW 5:5:20]

	Biography	Significant Publications
1961	Retires from St Mary's Hospital after forty years.	'Varieties of Psychotherapy' [CW 6:2:5]
1962	Undertakes a lecture tour in the United States in October, speaking in Los Angeles, San Francisco, Topeka, Boston, and New York.	'The Aims of Psycho-analytical Treatment' [CW 6:3:2] 'A Personal View of the Kleinian Contribution' [CW 6:3:8] 'Ego Integration in Child Development' [CW 6:3:19] 'Providing for the Child in Health and Crisis' [CW 6:3:10]
1962–8	Analyses Harry Guntrip 'on demand', continuing for over 150 sessions.	
1963	Undertakes a lecture tour in the United States in October, visiting Atlanta, Philadelphia, and Baltimore.	'The Development of the Capacity for Concern' [CW 6:3:11] 'Fear of Breakdown' [CW 6:4:21] 'From Dependence Towards Independence in the Development of the Individual' [CW 6:4:11] 'Morals and Education' [CW 6:3:18] 'Communicating and Not Communicating Leading to a Study of Certain Opposites' [CW 6:4:8] 'Training for Child Psychiatry' [CW 6:3:5] 'Psychotherapy of Character Disorders' [CW 6:4:9] 'The Mentally Ill in Your Caseload' [CW 6:4:5] 'Psychiatric Disorder in Terms of Infantile Maturational Processes' [CW 6:4:12] 'Dependence in Infant-Care, in Child-Care, and in the Psycho-analytic Setting' [CW 6:3:9] 'Adolescence: Struggling Through the Doldrums' [CW 6:2:4] 'The Value of Depression' [CW 6:4:10]
1964		*The Child, the Family and the Outside World* 'The Concept of the False Self' [CW 7:1:1] 'The Relationship of a Mother to Her Baby at the Beginning' [CW 6:1:8]

Chronology

	Biography	Significant Publications
1965	Elected President of the BPAS for a second three-year term	*The Family and Individual Development* *The Maturational Processes and the Facilitating Environment* 'The Value of the Therapeutic Consultation' [CW 7:2:22] 'A Clinical Study of the Effect of a Failure of the Average Expectable Environment on a Child's Mental Functioning' [CW 10:1:4]
1966		'The Absence of a Sense of Guilt' [CW 7:3:32] 'The Ordinary Devoted Mother' [CW 7:3:3] 'The Child in the Family Group' [CW 7:3:17] 'On the Split-Off Male and Female to be Found in Men and Women' [CW 7:3:2]
1967	President of the Association for Child Psychology and Psychiatry. Chair of the International Psychoanalytic Association's Sponsoring Committee for the Finnish Psychoanalytic Society, which gains status as a provisional society. Lectures in Boston, USA.	'The Location of Cultural Experience' [CW 7:3:31] 'Mirror-Role of Mother and Family in Child Development' [CW 8:1:38] 'The Concept of a Healthy Individual' [CW 8:1:4]
1968	Wins the *James Spence* Gold Medal for Paediatrics. Appointed Honorary Member of the Royal Medico-Psychological Association. Undertakes a lecture tour in the United States, speaking in New York, but suffers a serious coronary after reading 'The Use of an Object' to the New York Psychoanalytic Society.	'The Squiggle Game' [CW 8:2:47] 'Breast-Feeding as Communication' [CW 8:2:26] 'Communication Between Infant and Mother, and Mother and Infant, Compared and Contrasted' [CW 8:2:2] 'The Use of an Object and Relating Through Identifications' [CW 8:2:28] '*Sum*, I Am' [CW 8:2:10]
1969		'The Use of an Object in the Context of *Moses and Monotheism*' [CW 9:1:4] 'Mother's Madness Appearing in the Clinical Material as an Ego-Alien Factor' [CW 9:1:29]
1970	Prepares to give keynote paper to the IPA Congress in Vienna in July.	'Dependence in Child-Care' [CW 9:2:15] 'On the Basis for Self in Body' [CW 9:2:12] 'Residential Care as Therapy' [CW 9:2:9]

	Biography	Significant Publications
1971	Dies of a coronary in January.	*Playing and Reality* *Therapeutic Consultations in Child Psychiatry* [CW 10] 'Dreaming, Fantasying and Living: A Case-History Describing a Primary Dissociation' [CW 9:3:6] 'Playing: A Theoretical Statement' [CW 8:2:15] 'Playing: Creative Activity and the Search for the Self' [CW 8:1:27] 'Creativity and Its Origins' [CW 9:3:7] 'The Place Where We Live' [CW 8:2:1] 'Interrelating Apart from Instinctual Drive and in Terms of Cross-Identifications' [CW 9:3:8] 'Contemporary Concepts of Adolescent Development and Their Implications for Higher Education' [CW 9:3:9]
1977		*The Piggle: An Account of the Psychoanalytic Treatment of a Little Girl* (Ed. I. Ramzy) [CW 11:2:1–17]
1981	The Squiggle Foundation established.	
1984	Clare Winnicott dies. The Winnicott Trust founded.	*Deprivation and Delinquency* (Eds. C. Winnicott, R. Shepherd, M. Davis)
1986		*Home Is Where We Start From* (Eds. C. Winnicott, R. Shepherd, M. Davis) *Holding and Interpretation: Fragment of an Analysis*
1987		*Babies and Their Mothers* (Eds. C. Winnicott, R. Shepherd, M. Davis) *The Spontaneous Gesture: Selected Letters of D.W. Winnicott* (Ed. F. R. Rodman)
1988		*Human Nature* [CW 11:1]
1989		*Psychoanalytic Explorations* (Eds. C. Winnicott, R. Shepherd, M. Davis)
1993		*Talking to Parents* (Eds. C. Bollas, R. Shepherd, M. Davis)
1996		*Thinking About Children* (Eds. R. Shepherd, J. Johns, H. Taylor Robinson)
2002		*Winnicott on the Child*
2017		*The Collected Works of D. W. Winnicott* (Eds. L. Caldwell, H. Taylor Robinson)

CONTRIBUTORS

Lesley Caldwell, General Editor
Lesley Caldwell is a member of the British Psychoanalytic Association in private practice in London. She is an Honorary Professor in the Psychoanalysis Unit and Honorary Senior Research Associate in the Italian Department at University College, London. As Chair of the Squiggle Foundation (2000–03) and editor of the Winnicott Studies Monograph Series (2000–08), she published four edited collections on D. W. Winnicott. She has been an editor for the Winnicott Trust since 2002 and was the Chair of Trustees from 2008 to 2012. With Angela Joyce, she published *Reading Winnicott* (2011). She has a continuing interest in psychoanalysis and the arts and has also written on film and the city of Rome.

Helen Taylor Robinson, General Editor
Helen Taylor Robinson is Fellow of the Institute of Psychoanalysis, British Psychoanalytical Society, London, and was a clinical psychoanalyst with adults and children until her retirement. She was an Editor and Trustee of the Winnicott Trust for seventeen years and co-edited *Thinking about Children* with Jennifer Johns and Ray Shepherd. Her special interest is in the relationship of psychoanalysis to the arts, literature, and cinema. She has been Honorary Senior Lecturer at the Psychoanalysis Unit of University College, London. She has contributed to books and journals in the field of psychoanalysis and to the European Psychoanalysis and Film Festival.

Robert Adès
Robert Adès holds an MA (Hons) in Philosophy from Edinburgh University and an MSc in Psychoanalytic Studies from University College London. Before joining the *Collected Works*, he was Honorary Psychotherapist at the Maudsley Hospital and at Parkside Clinic, London, and was studying for a doctorate in theoretical psychoanalysis at University College London.

Clay Pearn
Clay Pearn received his MFA in creative writing from the University of Michigan and his BMus in Theory and Composition from Western University. He was previously a marketer for Caversham Productions and assistant to Elisabeth Young-Bruehl. He currently lives in Hamilton, Ontario.

Anne Karpf
Anne Karpf is a writer, journalist and sociologist. A regular broadcaster and contributor to *The Guardian*, she is the author of four books of nonfiction, including a family memoir, *The War After: Living with the Holocaust*, *The Human Voice* and *How to Age*. She is Reader in Professional Writing and Cultural Inquiry at London Metropolitan University.

Amal Treacher Kabesh

Amal Treacher Kabesh is an Associate Professor in the School of Sociology and Social Policy (University of Nottingham). She has a long-standing interest in psychoanalytic theory, especially in relation to gender and ethnicity. Her monograph *Postcolonial Masculinities: Histories, Emotions, Ethics* was published by Ashgate (2013) and *Egyptian Revolutions: Repetition, Conflict, Identification* will be published by Rowman and Littlefield (forthcoming).

CREDITS

Sources for the *Collected Works* include the published volumes of Winnicott's work, together with additional material from the Winnicott Archives, held at the Wellcome Library, London, and the Oskar Diethelm Library, Cornell Medical Center, New York; the Archives of the Institute of Psychoanalysis, London; the National Archives, Kew, UK; the British Library; the University of London Library at Senate House; the Bodleian Library, Oxford; and the archives of individual past editors of the Winnicott Trust. The *Collected Works* is as comprehensive as current sources allow; the online edition will enable the addition of any further material should it become available. The Winnicott Archives at Wellcome and Cornell contain considerable material that cannot legally be accessed for reasons of confidentiality. Unless otherwise noted, all works appear courtesy of the Winnicott Trust.

D. W. W.: A Reflection, from *Psychoanalytic Explorations* by Clare Winnicott. Originally published in Grolnick, S. and Barkin, L, (Eds.), *Between Reality and Fantasy*. London/New York: Jason Aronson, 1978. Reprinted by permission of Rowman & Littlefield.

COMPLETE INDEX OF THE *COLLECTED WORKS*

Page numbers in **bold** indicate reprinted letters and texts. Page numbers in *italics* indicate illustrations. In the index, DWW stands for Donald Woods Winnicott.

abdominal colics, 1:139, 141, 144, 231
Abel, Lawrence, 2:29
Abraham, Karl, 1:lvii, lxiii; 4:37, 133, 135; 5:10, 153, 333, 398*n*8, 419*n*5, 447, 449; 6:328, 481
    'The First Pregenital Stage of the Libido' (1916), 3:459–460; 4:177*n*7
    'A short study of the development of the libido, viewed in the light of mental disorders' (1924), 11:67
Abram, Jan, 1:lii, 14; 10:13, 17; 12:276*n*1
'Abscess in Frontal Lobe: Post-Mortem Findings' (with Elizabeth O'Flynn; 1928), 1:**119–121**; *1:120–121*
'The Absence of a Sense of Guilt' (1966), 7:**437–452**
abstracts, 12:lix
    Alexander, Franz, 'Psychoanalysis and Medicine' (1932), 1:**339**
    Barinbaum, Moses, 'A contribution to the problem of psycho-physical relations with special reference to dermatology' (1935), 1:**357**
    'Enuresis', 1:**141–142**
    Lundholm, Helge, 'Repression and Rationalisation' (1933), 1:**341**
    'Neurosis in the Child', 1:15, **15*n*vii**
    'Observation of Infant Behaviour During Routine Clinical Examination', 2:**121*n*i**
    'Psychological Aspects of Birching' (1944), 2:**247–249**
    'The Value of Breast Feeding (Psychological)', 2:**389*n*ii**
    'The Wearing of Masks in the Nursing of Premature and Older Infants' (1943), 2:**227**
abstract thinking, 4:113, 446
accidents
    Burton, Lindy, *Vulnerable Children: Three Studies of Children in Conflict* (reviewed 1968), 8:**275–276**
    car, in case study, 10:478, 492
    psychological health and, 11:50
Ackerman, A., 5:457
Ackerman, Nathan, 7:33

acne, 1:460–461; 9:244–245
ACPP. *See* Association for Child Psychology and Psychiatry
Acta Paediatrica Latina, 7:41
acting out, 4:2162, 318, 353; 6:55, 453
'Active Heart Disease', from *Clinical Notes* (1931), 1:**229–233**
'"Ada" aet 8 Years', 10:299*n*1, **307–334**
    active intervention, 10:328–329
    deprivation and, 10:329, 333
    dissociation and, 10:328, 333, 334
    drawings by Ada, 10:308–330, *308–330*
    dreams and, 10:320–324
    masturbation and, 10:313, 317, 324
    numbers as fertility symbols and, 10:330
    squiggle game not used, 10:308
    stealing as issue, 10:307, 313, 316, 324, 328–329, 333
    stock-taking, 10:317–320
    technique detail, 10:308
Adamson, Joy, 6:380
adaptation
    creativity and, 11:124, 127, 128, 130
    facilitating environment allowing, 6:487; 8:83
    failure in, 6:435; 11:127, 131–132, 153, 157, 160
    graduated adaptation, 6:349
    maladaptation and intellectual function, 11:157
    mother's adaptation to new baby, 6:5, 165, 214, 230, 381, 415, 472; 8:45, 66, 270, 313; 11:36, 120–121, 124, 130, 149, 173–174
    psychosis and, 4:42; 8:16
    regression and, 4:206
    of therapist to patient, 11:158
    transitional objects and, 4:168
'Addendum to "The Location of Cultural Experience"' (1967), 8:**207–209**
addiction to transitional objects, 5:250, 406, 410, 419; 9:112, 283–284
Addis, Robina, letter to (ca. 1936), 1:**389–390**
'Additional Note on Psycho-Somatic Disorder' (1969), 9:**95–98**
'Address Introducing Margaret Mead, VIIIth Ernest Jones Lecture' (1957), 5:**203–204**

adenoids, 1:203–204, 329
Adès, Robert, 1:xi; 12:xlix, 12:3, 5
Adler, Alfred, 3:54
adolescents and adolescence. *See also* delinquent children; puberty
   acne, 9:244–245
   'Adolescence: Struggling Through the Doldrums' (lecture 1961; published 1962; reprinted 1965), 6:18, **187–196**, 423, 493
   'Adolescent Process and the Need for Personal Confrontation' (1970), 9:167*n*i, 348*n*2
   'Adopted Children in Adolescence' (1955), 5:**67–76**
   age of DWW and work with, 9:171
   aggression in boys, 2:71
   antisocial behaviour, 6:194–195, 431
   atom bomb, effect of, 6:191, 427–428
   case studies, 6:495–497; 8:99–104, 351–352
   'Changing Patterns: The Young Person, the Family and Society' (1970), 9:57*n*i, 167*n*i
   character disorders and gender differences, 6:455–456
   compromise, toleration of, 6:192
   compulsive destructiveness, 6:103
   construction, reparation and restitution, 9:347
   'Contemporary Concepts of Adolescent Development and Their Implications for Higher Education' (1971), 8:269*n*iv; 9:57*n*i, 167*n*i, 169*n*ii, **337–348**
   contraceptive techniques, effect of, 6:191, 427
   contradictory tendencies of, 6:259
   corporal punishment of, 5:192–193
   'Death and Murder in the Adolescent Process' (1969), 9:337, **342–348**, 348*n*2
   'Deductions Drawn from a Psychotherapeutic Interview with an Adolescent' (1964), 7:6, **51–65**
   defiance-dependency paradox and, 5:190, 270; 6:189, 193, 429
   defined and described, 7:5–6, *51–52*; 6:4982–493
   doldrums of, 6:192, 194, 430, 440, 493–4958; 8:39, 43, 67
   emotional maturity in, 5:426–427, 544
   environment's importance for, 6:189
   Eppel, E. M., and M. Eppel, *Adolescents and Morality* (1966; review by DWW), 7:**401–402**
   good-enough parenting/environment and, 9:340–342
   groups and, 5:46, 50, 190–193, 427
   healthy versus ill, 6:193–194, 430–432
   and home life, 11:169
   'Hospital Care Supplementing Intensive Psychotherapy in Adolescence' (1963), 6:18, **491–497**
   idealism of, 9:347
   immaturity of, 9:338, 344–345
   isolation of, 6:189, 425–426, 443
   lack of mental hospital provision for, 7:339–340
   loyalty conflicts and, 7:395
   masturbation, 5:290–291; 6:425; 9:378
   maturational and pathological processes, 6:495
   medical histories, taking, 7:52
   mother's ability to become herself again when children reach, 6:81
   needs of, 6:193, 430
   'Notes on Adolescence' (1956), 5:**189–193**
   parents and, 5:269–270
   passage of time as solution in, 6:18, 187–188, 190, 423, 429
   'Physical and Emotional Disturbances in an Adolescent Girl' (1968), 8:**237–241**
   play and, 9:378–379
   as possible BPAS topic, 5:173
   potential at, 9:346–347
   psychoanalytic research and, 7:155
   psycho-neurosis of, 6:14
   psychotherapeutic attitude toward, 9:337–340
   resentment toward, 6:195, 423
   Romeo and Juliet, 3:185–193
   Sandström, Carl Ivar, *The Psychology of Childhood and Adolescence* (reviewed 1968), 8:10, **411–412**
   sex and, 3:324–325; 5:69; 6:189–190
   'Sex Education in Schools' (1949), 3:**323–326**
   'Struggling Through the Doldrums' (1963), 6:**423–432**, 493; 7:51*n*i; 7:439*n*ii; 9:101*n*i
   suicide and, 6:195, 431, 494; 8:68
   theoretical statement, 6:188–189, 423
   true and false self, working out, 7:30
   types of disorders, 6:493–495
   unacceptability of false solution to, 6:192–193, 428
   venereal disease and, 6:190–191, 196*n*1, 426
   wars and, 5:270
   withdrawal of authority and, 2:71
   WWII's effect on, 2:96–97
   'Youth Will Not Sleep' (1964), 7:**79–81**; 8:269*n*iv
adoption, 1:109, 173, 261–262, 278; 11:55–56, 128
   acceptance-of-difference adopters, 7:311–312
   adolescent mothers, illegitimate children of, 3:325
   'Adopted Children in Adolescence' (1955), 5:**67–76**
   age of placement, 5:75
   birth parents, adolescents researching, 5:23
   'blood-tie child' case, harm to child from delay in placement, 7:365–366; 7:369
   break-up of adoptive homes, 5:72
   breastfeeding and, 2:394; 5:75–76
   case study, 4:142–148, 293–3296

Complete Index of the Collected Works

counselling for adopted parents, 5:73
dark-skinned child in fair-skinned adoptive family, 9:243–245
effect of delay in, 4:292
deprivation/emotional disturbance and, 5:73, 74
emotional development of child affected by, 3:370
failure of, 4:291–292
fantasies of, 5:22–23
female babies, adopter preference for, 7:312
fostering compared, 5:70–72
genetics and heredity, 5:76
Goodacre, Iris, *Adoption Policy and Practice* (1966; reviewed by DWW), 7:**427–428**
illegitimacy and, 3:325; 5:74–75
Kirk's *Shared Fate*, DWW's review of, 7:311–312
'On Adoption' (1957), 5:**21–23**
'Pitfalls in Adoption' (1954), 4:**291–296**
post-adoption period, 7:428
preparation for, 7:332
private (direct and third-party), 7:428
of psychotic parent's child, 5:513–516
rejection-of-difference adopters, 7:311–312
sadness of adopted child, crying to express, 2:242–243
second adoptions, 5:111–112
sexuality, adopted children learning about, 5:68–69
spoiling, 5:74
stability and continuity, need for, 5:67–68
telling children that they are adopted, 5:21–23, 67, 111
'The Toddler, the Second Adoption, Telling Children About Adoption' (mid 1950s), 5:**111–112**
truth telling, 5:75
'Two Adopted Children' (1954), 4:**139–149**
younger child persecuted by adopted child, 9:243
'Advising Parents' (1957), 5:**277–284**; 8:34
aesthetic moment, 9:5
aetiology. *See also* mental health
 'The Aetiology of Infantile Schizophrenia in Terms of Adaptive Failure' (1967), 1:439*n*i; 8:**161–165**; 9:91, 301, 302
 of character disorders, 6:450–452
 of mental health and illness, 6:13, 163–164, 360
 of psycho-neurosis, 8:186
affection
 affectionless child, 8:264, 409
 Bowlby, 'The Making and Breaking of Affectional Bonds' (1979), 6:16
 transitional phenomena and affectionate behaviour, 5:117, 385

African Americans, population of, disturbed children in, 7:33–34. *See also* race and ethnicity
aggression. *See also* rage; hate and hatred
 'Aggression' (1939), 1:lxvi, lxvii; 2:16, **65–71**
 'Aggression' (Royal Society of Medicine paper, 1948), 3:148, 333
 'Aggression, Guilt and Reparation' (1960), 6:**97–104**; 9:77*n*i
 Aggression and Its Interpretation (Jackson 1954; reviewed 1954), 4:**247–248**
 'Aggression in Relation to Emotional Development' (1950), 1:lxvi; 3:9, 148*n*iii, **333–347**
 anger and frustration, 3:336; 6:214
 in child department consultations, 2:157
 concern and guilt, stage of, 3:335–336
 constructive activity and, 7:132–133
 correlation between DWW's concepts of transitional objects and space and, 3:9–10; 8:46
 death instinct and, 4:66
 defined, 7:129–130
 different means of expressing or dealing with, 7:131–133
 DWW and, 3:4–5; 5:4–5
 external world and, 3:344–347
 S. Freud on, 3:339; 8:331
 gender and, 8:93–94
 good breast and, 5:123, 131–132
 hate and. *See* hate and hatred
 identification with the aggressor, 3:347*n*6
 importance of, 9:30
 individuation and, 9:209–210
 inner world, growth of, 3:336–339
 at intermediate stage of emotional development, 3:335–340
 intrinsic nature of, 2:20
 Jung and, 7:122
 Klein on, 3:335, 338, 347*n*6; 4:247; 6:97, 145, 321, 324; 8:331
 lack of, in male patient, 8:365–366
 Lantos, Barbara, 'On the Problem of Aggression', 5:179*n*i
 letter to Anna Freud on (1948), 3:147–148
 life instincts and, 6:17
 love and, 7:132; 7:*133–134*
 in maturity, 3:339*n*iii
 mother-child relationship and, 3:5, 165–166, 311–312; 6:271; 8:346
 motility and, 5:328–329; 7:130–131
 object relationships and, 6:435
 organisation of, 3:334
 origins of, 2:16–17; 3:335, 340–343; 4:65; 6:145

aggression (*Cont.*)
  in *The Piggle*, 11:205, 213, 223, 233, 250, 253, 264, 269, 284, 286
  play and, 2:167–168; 7:132–133
  as primitive or magical destruction, 7:134–135
  in *Relationship between mature persons* (1947), 3:339*n*iii
  reconsideration of, 5:448; 10:17
  'Roots of Aggression' (1964), 7:9–10; **7:129–135**; 9:36
  'Roots of Aggression' (1968), 8:10, **329–332**; 9:47
  sentimentalism as denial of, 9:4–5
  separation from erotic experience, 6:148
  social value of, 3:339
  Storr, Anthony, *Human Aggression* (reviewed 1968), 8:**321–322**, 329, 329*n*i
  in therapeutic consultation, 10:473–474, 478
  violence differentiated, 7:129
  WWII's effect on children and, 2:96
agoraphobia, and DWW's concept of potential space, 3:12
Aguayo, J., 1:lxvi
Aichhorn, August, 3:473; 5:447; 11:32
  Wayward youth (1925/1936; reviewed by DWW), 1:**433–436**; 2:196; 5:149, 7:222
'The Aims of Psycho-Analytical Treatment' (1962), 6:19, **285–288**; 8:15; 11:8, 9, 10, 192
Ainsworth-Davies, Mr, 1:59
Aitken, P., letter to (1967), 8:**33–34**
Albee, Edward, *Who's Afraid of Virginia Woolf?* (1962), 9:220
'"Albert" *aet* 7 Years 9 Months', 10:**233–252**
  dreams and, 10:238, 244, 247
  drowning incident and, 10:250
  gender roles and, 10:238–240
  good and bad, preoccupation with, 10:233, 241, 250
  sea imagery and, 10:236
  sibling relationships and, 10:238, 240–241, 251–252
  squiggle game and, 10:233, 233–251, 235–240, 242–251
albuminuria, 1:317
Alcock (Leys School friend), 1:55
Alcock, Theodora, 2:119, 119*n*i
Aldrich, C. A. & Aldrich, M. M., *Babies Are Human Beings* (1938), 1:17*n*viii
Alexander, Franz, 3:147*n*i
  'Psychoanalysis and Medicine' (abstract; 1932), 1:**339**
'"Alfred" *aet* 10 Years', 10:**165–185**, **519–520**
  breathing and, 10:166, 180, 182
  defaecating and, 10:180
  dreams and, 10:176–178

father's mental breakdown and stress, 10:182, 183, 184
  squiggle game and, 10:165–181, *166–179*, *181*
  stammering, 10:165, 182, 183
Alger, Ian, 'The Clinical Handling of the Analyst's Responses' (1966), discussion of, 7:13, **457–458**
Allaire (doctor describing encephalitis case), 1:83
Allen, Clifford, 5:119
Allen, Lady Marjory, 5:461
allergies and psychological health, 11:51
Alley, R., *Francis Bacon: Catalogue raisonné and documentation* (1964), 8:218*n*3
allo-erotism, auto-erotism, and transitional objects, 3:448, 455, 456, 459, 461
'All of Mother' (letters to *The Observer*; 1964), 7:**91–93**, **101**, 101*n*i
'An Allotted Spanner in the Works' (ca.1966–67), 7:**459**, **460**
almoners, 2:177; 5:339–343
aloneness
  'The Capacity to Be Alone' (1958), 5:13–14, **241–248**; 6:11, 157*n*10; 7:430; 8:13, 310*n*3, 364
  pre-dependent aloneness of newborn, 11:149–152
Alpert, Augusta, 8:280–281
amaurotic family idiocy, 1:292
Ambache, Stella, 1:xlvii
ambivalence, 4:200*n*1; 6:353, 382, 388*n*1; 7:184; 8:102–103; 10:298; 11:73, 77, 882–83, 91
  in *The Piggle*, 11:202–204, 257–258, 267, 272
Amenophis (pharaoh), 9:36
American Association of Psychiatric Clinics for Children, 8:349; 10:253
American Correspondent, letter to (1969), 9:**29–31**
American Psychoanalytic Association, 5:391
American Psychopathological Association, 5:391
Amyotonia Congenita, 1:293
anaclitic dependence, 5:184, 241, 446
anaclitic relationship, 11:15, 92
anal erotism, 3:108, 110, 181; 9:273
anal pruritus, 1:456–458; 2:29
anal stage, 11:67–68
analysis. See psychoanalysis
analysts. See therapists
anaphasis, 11:18
Andrewes, C. H., 1:60, 89
anencephaly, 7:450
anger, 11:102*n*6, 105
  acting out and, 4:212; 6:55
  aggression and, 3:336
  baby crying due to, 2:240–241, 244
  crossing into hopelessness, 8:201
  cumulative angry experiences, 8:189

environmental failure and, 4:210–212, 2216, 224
frustration and, 3:336; 4:191; 6:214; 8:152, 237, 331, 373
healthy, 8:152, 188
Holding and Interpretation: Fragment of an Analysis (1955), 4:433–434, 450, 452
mastectomy and, 8:147
oral sadism and, 6:336
primitive love impulse and, 3:394; 8:152
of public, 4:280
therapeutic consultation, 10:444–445
angst, 3:208; 7:409
animals
  human and animal psychology compared, 4:21–22; 11:66
  playing in young animals, 9:375
  primary maternal preoccupation in, 9:173
  using transitional objects, 5:251
  wild animals analogy to babies, 4:26
Anna Freud Centre (formerly Hampstead Child Therapy Course and Clinic), 5:87, 337*n*ii, 536; 6:306; 7:147, 217, 220–221, 375; 9:41
annihilation, 6:149–150, 154, 365
Annual Report of the London County Council, 1:123
anorexia, 1:180–182, 413, 414; 2:189; 4:49*n*i; 6:343, 436, 484; 7:31, 70–72, 373–374, 455; 9:244. *See also* eating disorders
'Answers to comments on "The split-off male and female elements"' (1972), 9:14, 15, **149–154**
anti-nuclear protests, 8:192*n*i
antisocial behaviour, 11:6, 127
  of adolescents, 6:194–195, 431
  'The Antisocial Tendency' (1956), 5:5–6, 10, **149–158**; 8:17*n*2
  character disorders and, 6:448, 452
  'The Child, the Family and the Offender' (1965), 7:**203–205**
  'The Child, the Family and the Young Offender' (UK Government Home Office White Paper), 7:204
  clinical observations, 5:149–151; 10:16–17
  communication as part of cure of, 10:305
  confessed by child, 8:95
  defined and described, 5:151–153, 454; 8:43–44
  delinquency and, 2:31, 197–198; 3:46; 6:158*n*16; 8:91–97; 10:17
  denial of, 7:245, 246, 247, 250–251
  deprivation and, 3:371, 439; 5:151, 152, 156–157, 330, 333, 454; 6:255, 423, 454; 8:74, 92; 10:304, 305, 527–529; 11:6
  deprivation versus privation, 7:306
  destructiveness associated with, 10:305
  dissociation related to, 7:245–273. *See also* dissociation
  of evacuated children in WWII, 3:23–27, 79–81, 410; 5:5–6
  first signs of, 5:154–156; 6:386
  A. Freud on, 7:222–223
  masturbation and, 2:69–70
  greed and, 5:154–156
  'Group Influences and the Maladjusted Child: The School Aspect' (1955), 5:**45–54**
  guilt and, 3:241–242; 5:145–147
  hidden versus manifest, 3:410–411, 420
  Holding and Interpretation: Fragment of an Analysis (1955), 4:336–337, 400–401, 425–426
  homosexuality and, 5:29–30
  hope in, 5:152; 10:17, 304, 529
  hostels for children, 2:307–308; 3:23–27
  management of, 4:236, 279–280; 5:50–51, 145, 150, 273, 343
  minor manifestations of, 6:417
  origins of, 6:417
  playing and, 5:245
  positive elements of, 7:80, 204
  pseudologia fantastica as part of, 10:363
  psychiatric social workers and, 5:343
  psychoanalytic research and, 7:155–156
  'A Psychoanalytic View of the Antisocial Tendency', 8:319
  psychogenesis of, 10:303
  psychological aspects of juvenile delinquency and, 3:46, 49–50; 6:260
  psychosis and, 6:66
  Q principle and, 2:105
  recovery, from, 5:146, 154; 6:204
  school management of antisocial children, 4:279–280
  scope of DWW's work on, 6:17
  sheet-slashing and opening mail addressed to others, 10:403–404
  shopping, compulsive, 5:156
  social worker's role in dealing with, 6:419
  society and, 5:186
  stealing and, 5:153–154, 335; 8:93, 95, 97; 10:303, 305. *See also* stealing
  as symptom of illness, 3:239
  tendencies in course of normal development, 7:351
  theory of, 7:249–250; 10:303–306; 11:6
  therapeutic consultation and, 10:303–515, 527–529
  treatment of, 5:157–158, 424, 509; 6:204
  true and false self and, 7:30
  types of, 10:305
  war, effect on children, 2:98; 3:420
  weaning and, 6:13
Antonis, Barbie, 1:l

anxiety
    annihilation and, 4:110; 6:149–150
    'Anxiety Associated with Insecurity' (1952), 4:**55–58**, 59*n*i
    'Anxiety (continued)', in *Clinical Notes* (1931), 1:**275–280**
    apex beat, position of, 1:210
    archaic anxieties, 7:179, 221–222, 224; 10:139
    'Arthritis Associated with Emotional Disturbance', from *Clinical Notes* (1931), 1:**239–243**
    asthma and, 1:267; 2:10, 129, 135.
        See also asthma
    attachment to mother and, 9:243, 244
    birth trauma and, 3:201–202, 207, 208, 216, 217, 228
    castration, 11:73, 74, 84. *See* castration anxiety
    as cause of unwellness in children, 1:171
    chorea and, 1:246, 272; 2:50
    colic and, 1:183
    convulsions and fits due to, 1:268, 306–307
    defences against, 4:162, 164, 196–197; 5:54, 62, 64, 288, 315, 324, 408, 446; 11:45, 64, 78, 83, 84–85
    defined, 3:208
    dependence of child and, 4:154
    depressive anxiety, 4:191–194
    differential diagnosis of, 1:171, 196
    enuresis and, 1:320–321
    eyes and, 1:269–270
    fantasies and, 1:259, 260, 268, 269, 270, 273*n*2, 277; 2:132, 152–153
    fidgetiness due to, 1:245–246, 250, 266
    five-year-olds and, 6:314
    free association and, 8:171
    growing pains and, 1:235
    guilt and, 3:302, 319; 5:137–138, 141
    headaches, migraines, in anxious children, 1:139, 197, 237, 267
    holding and, 7:43
    hypochondriacal, 11:91, 154
    'Hypochondriacal Anxiety' (from *Human Nature*, 1988), 11:**113–114**
    infant experience of, 1:lxx; 2:387; 4:56, 58, 274, 276; 6:7, 354, 370, 396; 8:7
    instinct and, 4:191; 5:165; 6:145
    Klein on anxiety drive, 6:450, 511
    lack of anxiety at regression to unintegrated state, 4:58
    leucotomy and, 3:467, 481
    magical qualities in reaction to, 2:80
    masturbation and, 1:156–157, 268–269, 328; 2:199
    micturition and, 1:156–157, 246, 250, 266, 315–316
    mother's, 9:12–13; 11:122, 135, 146
    mouths causing anxiety and fear in infants, 2:227
    nasal congestion and, 1:267, 270
    neurosis and, 5:165–167
    no distinct psychology of, 11:85–86*n*2
    normal anxiety, 1:255–263, 447–448
    'A Note on Normality and Anxiety', from *Clinical Notes* (1931), 1:**255–273**
    Oedipal complex and, 11:78–79
    parents' role in treatment of, 1:277–278
    pathological sleeping, child with, 1:149–150
    persecutory, 4:66; 5:242, 251
    physical causes of, 1:265–269, 271–272
    physical disease masked by, 1:272–273
    physical examinations and, 1:189–190
    physical symptoms of, 1:262–265
    in *The Piggle*, 11:209, 214, 219, 220, 221, 229, 236, 252*n*IX, 266, 267, 274, 288
    playing, to master, 2:168
    separation anxiety. *See* separation
    sexuality and sexual knowledge affecting, 1:262, 268–269, 277–278
    shock therapy for, 2:267–268
    'Shyness and Nervous Disorders in Children' (1938), 1:17, **445–448**
    sleepiness linked with, 4:323
    speech and speaking affected by, 1:331, 334, 335
    subacute rheumatic fever and, 1:230–231
    temperature and, 1:197–198
    theories about, 5:380, 427
    transitional objects and instinct tensions, 3:449, 457
    treatment of, 1:275–276; 8:354–354
    unconscious, 3:413
    unthinkable, 9:29–30, 95, 138, 386
anxiety attacks, 1:267, 268, 273*n*2
anxiety hysteria, 1:138, 231, 263, 326, 331
aortic diastolic murmur, 1:232
aortic regurgitation, 1:214, 232
apex beat, position of, 1:209–214
aphonia, 1:270
Apley, J., *The Child and His Symptoms: A Psychosomatic Approach* (with Ronald MacKeith as co-author, 1962), 6:401*n*i
appendectomy, 1:70
appendicitis, 10:453, 469–471
apperception and perception, 6:230–231; 8:5
'Appetite and Emotional Disorder' (1936), 1:8, 14, 15, 16, **413–431**; 3:139*n*2; 6:326. *See also* eating disorders
appetite-love, 2:68
Applebey, Mary, letter to (1957), 5:**233–234**
approved schools, 5:151, 439, 441–443
archaic anxieties, 7:179, 221–222, 224

Complete Index of the Collected Works

archipelago child, 8:409
Archive[s] of Disease in Childhood, 2:227; 6:371
Arieti, S. (ed.), *The World Biennial of Psychiatry and Psychotherapy*, 10:521
Aristotle, 5:142
Armellini, Marco, 1: xlii, liii; 10:3
art. *See also* drawings by patients
   'An Allotted Spanner in the Works' (ca. 1966–67), 7:**459, 460**
   appreciation of, 8:77n1
   artistic expression, 2:363, 368n2
   Greenacre, Phyllis, 'The Childhood of the Artist', 5:363
   guilt and, 5:145
   Milner, Marion, *On Not Being Able to Paint* (1950; reviewed 1951), 3:**483–485**
   patient feeling real in relation to her painting, 7:447
   psychoanalysis as, 3:41
   Stokes, Adrian, 'Form in Art' (1955), 5:33ni
   Stokes, Adrian, *Smooth and Rough* (1951), 5:33
'Arthritis Associated with Emotional Disturbance', from *Clinical Notes* (1931), 1:**239–243**
ascensive defence, 1:364–365
Ashdown, Margaret, 2:178
'"Ashton" aet 12 Years', 7:183niv, 273, 358nii; 8:99ni; 10:210, **213–232**
   dreams and, 10:225–226, 229–230
   interpretation by DWW of painting done by Ashton, 10:227–228
   schizoid personality and, 10:213–214, 231
   squiggle game and, 10:214–228, 215–225, 227–228
   trust of DWW, 10:228
Asikainen, Helka, 6:237, 241; 10:32, 37, 53, 515
asphyxiation, erotic, 3:215
assault, homosexual, 5:28
Association for Child Psychology and Psychiatry (ACPP), 1:lix; 5:12, 523, **523–528**; 8:49
   'The Association for Child Psychology and Psychiatry Observed as a Group Phenomenon' (1967), 8:**49–64**; 9:155, 156; 10:6
   'Child Psychiatry, Social Work, and Alternative Care' (1970), 9:**171–174**
   DWW lecture (May 1968), 8:318ni
   'A Personal Statement on Child Psychiatry' (1971), 9:**175–177**
   president, DWW as, 5:9
   'Psychologists as a Group' (1969), 8:49; 9:**155–158**
   Scientific Meeting (1962), 6:299
Association for the Psychiatric Treatment of Offenders, 2:195ni
Association of Child Care Officers, 5:265
   talk to (1953), 4:139

   talk to (1960), 6:65
Association of Child Psychotherapists (Non-Medical), 10:419, 527
Association of European Paediatric Cardiologists, 7:379
Association of London County Council Child Welfare Officers, 5:481
Association of Psychiatric Social Workers, 5:513; 6:461
Association of Social Workers, 6:409
Association of Supervisors of Midwives, 5:225
Association of Teachers of Mathematics, 8:14, 267
Association of Workers for Maladjusted Children, 5:45; 6:87; 9:199
asthma
   anxiety and, 1:267; 2:10, 129, 135
   Asthma: Attitude and Milieu (1966; reviewed by DWW), 7:**417–418**
   Burton, Lindy, *Vulnerable Children: Three Studies of Children in Conflict* (reviewed 1968), 8:**275–276**
   interpretation relieving, 11:107
   as psychosomatic disorder, 11:175–177
   treatment of, 2:126–129
Astor, Lady, 3:471
ataxia, 1:81, 292, 293
Atlanta Psychiatric Clinic, 6:469
atom bomb, 6:191, 427–428; 7:152, 403
attachment theory, 6:4. *See also* Bowlby, John
attention, child demanding, 2:280
attenuation, 6:10
Auden, G. A., *The Difficult Child* (1929), discussion of (1934), 1:**353–355**
auscultation, 1:212–213
Austen, Eric, 1:59
Australian Aborigines, eating of children by, 9:107
authentic life, 6:20
autism
   'Autism' (1966), 7:7, 345, **349–363**
   Axline, Virginia A., *Dibs: In Search of Self* (reviewed 1966), 7:367
   blame and responsibility, 7:360–361
   causes of, 7:91, 93, 101, 346, 351
   clinical examples, 7:352–360, 362
   as conglomerate label, 7:346
   defining, 7:345–346
   diagnosis of, 7:346
   difficult pregnancies and, 7:352, 353–354
   'discovery' of, 7:349–350
   emotional development, as problem of, 7:351
   guilt feelings of parents and, 7:347, 349, 354, 360–362
   increasing rates, no evidence for, 7:350
   as infantile schizophrenia, 6:391; 8:161–164; 10:122, 138, 139, 518

autism (*Cont.*)
  intelligence of child and, 7:351, 358, 359
  Kanner on, 10:5
  mother-child relationship and, 7:91, 93
  not regarded as illness/disease by DWW, 7:7, 350, 351
  as 'ordinary devoted mother' failure, 7:331–332, 352–354, 355, 356, 360–363
  parental distress over medical attribution of causes of, 7:101, 113
  primary maternal preoccupation and, 5:186; 7:346; 8:187
  repetition-compulsion and, 7:190, 191–192
  Rimland, Bernard, *Infantile Autism* (1964; reviewed by DWW 1964), 7:**397–398**
  savants, 7:351, 352, 354
  schizophrenia and, 7:345–346, 356, 359, 397
  'Social Aspects of Autism' (1966), 7:**345–347**
  Society for Autistic Children (now National Autistic Society), 7:345, 349, 361–362, 363
  'specialisation' of children with, 7:354
  as universal tendency in course of normal development, 7:3520–351, 356
auto-erotism, allo-erotism, and transitional objects, 3:448, 455, 456, 459, 461; 4:168; 8:300
Axline, Virginia A.
  Dibs: In Search of Self (reviewed 1966), 7:**367–368**
  Play Therapy: The Inner Dynamics of Childhood (1947; commentary by DWW), 8:311; 9:**159–164**

babacar, in *The Piggle*, 1:200; 11:8, 198, 201, 202, 205, 206, 207, 218, 220–221, 222, 224, 228, 232, 237
Babinski's sign, 1:80, 81, 82, 85
'The Baby as a Going Concern' (1949), 3:**273–276**; 8:117
'The Baby as a Person'
  BBC radio broadcast, 2:14
  paper (1949), 3:**285–288**
Bachman, Miss, 5:307
bacilluria, 1:318
backward children, hostels for homeless children specialising in, 2:309
Bacon, Francis, 8:212, 216–217
  Francis Bacon: Catalogue Raisonné and Documentation (1964), 8:218n3
'bad breast', *see* breast
Baden Powell, Robert, 1:27, 51
'bad mother', 4:63–64, 65–66, 127–128
Bailey, Benjamin, 6:433ni
Bakwin, Harry, 2:165

Clinical Management of Behavior Disorders in Children (with Ruth Morris Bakwin 1953), 4:**265–264**
'Loneliness in Infants' (1942), 4:265
Bakwin, Ruth Morris, 3:492
  Clinical Management of Behavior Disorders in Children (with Harry Bakwin 1953), 4:**265–266**
Baldwin, James, 9:195, 195niii
Balint, Alice, 4:56; 8:35, 41; 11:32
Balint, Enid, 5:215, 401; 9:47
  letter to (1956), 5:**133–134**
  'Three Phases of a Transference Neurosis' (1957), 5:133ni
  writing to DWW during his NYC hospital stay (1968), 8:391
Balint, Michael, 1:lxixniii, lxxii; 2:15; 4:273; 5:133, 134, 500; 6:43; 7:14, 414, 417, 418; 8:129; 9:112nii
  on 'basic fault', 6:199
  The Basic Fault (1968), 4:273ni; 6:199ni; 8:171
  The Doctor, His Patients, and the Illness (1957; reviewed 1958), 5:213ni, 215ni, 261ni, **401–404**; 6:43; 7:68ni, 417
  'Funfairs, Thrills and Regressions' (1954), 4:**273–277**
  on language of psychoanalysis, 6:360; 8:46
  letters to (1957), 5:**213, 215, 261–262**
  letters to (1960), 6:**43–44**
  on manic defence, 4:276
  on primary love, 6:320
  'Primary Narcissism and Primary Love' (1960), 6:43ni
  Problems of Human Pleasure and Behaviour, 5:215; 8:77n1
  reaction to Segal, 4:30–31
  'Remarks on a Discussion of Balint's Paper on Technique' (1957), 1:lxxii; 3:215ni; 5:**211–212**; 6:43
  on teaching and student contact, 8:336
  'Three Areas of the Mind' (1958), 6:467n1
  Thrills and Regressions (1959), 4:273ni
Balogh, Lady Penelope, 12:3
Baltimore Psychiatric Society, 6:469
Banks, H. S., 1:290n5
Baranger, M. and W., 1:lxv
Barinbaum, Moses, 'A Contribution to the Problem of Psycho-physical Relations with Special Reference to Dermatology' (1935), abstract of, 1:**357**
Bartemeier, Leo H., 3:487
Bart's Hospital. *See* St Bartholomew's Hospital, London
Basic Books (publisher), 6:64, 110, 293
'basic fault', 1:lxxii; 5:212, 500

'Basis for Self in Body' (1970), 3:17; 9:**225–234**
Bastiaans, J., 1:84, 87, 88, 90; 9:262
'Battle Neurosis Treated with Leucotomy' (letter to the *British Medical Journal*; 1947), 3:**113**
Baumann, Marianne, 5:307*n*ii
　letters to (1958), 5:**307, 345**
BBC broadcasts, 2:4, 12, 21*n*iii, 221; 5; 9:179; 12:lii, 6, 8–14, 239–240, **241–255**
　'The Baby and Its Food' (Home Service; 1949), 3:277
　'The Baby as a Going Concern' (1949), 8:117
　'The Baby as a Person', 2:14
　'The Baby at Feeding Time' (Home Service; 1949), 3:289
　'Caring for Children and How Babies Develop Their Personalities' (Home Service; 1949), 3:269
　'Children in the War' (Home Service; 1939), 2:5; 12:8
　'Counterfeit and Alone' (*Woman's Hour*; 1955), 5:55
　'The Deprived Mother' (Home Service; 1939), 2:5, 35; 12:8
　'Difficult Children' (Home Service; 1945), 2:335, 343
　'Every One of Us is Unsuccessful Somewhere' (*Woman's Hour*; 1955), 5:55
　'Feeling Guilty' (1961), 6:**205–210**
　'The Five-Year-Old' (part of *Parents and children* series; 1962), 6:**309–314**
　'Getting to Know Your Baby' (1943–44), 2:21*n*iii, 221; 8:117; 12:9
　'Getting to Know Your Baby' (1945), 12:**245–249**
　'Happy Children' (1944), 2:281; 12:9
　'Health Magazine' (Home Service; 1945), 2:353
　'Homeless Children and Childless Homes' (Home Service; 1955), 5:21
　'How Much do we Know About Babies as Cloth Suckers?' (*Woman's Hour*; 1956), 5:115
　How's the Baby?, 12:9
　'Infant Feeding' (1943–44), 2:21*n*iii; 8:117; 12:9
　'The Innate Morality of the Baby' (1949), 8:151; 12:9
　'Instincts and Normal Difficulties' (1950), 8:151
　'Jealousy' (1960), 6:13, **47–61**
　'Knowing and Learning How to be a Mother' (Home Service; 1950), 3:387
　list of, 12:233–237
　'Looking Forward to Baby's Arrival', 12:**241–244**
　'A Man Looks at Motherhood' (1949), 8:117
　'The Mind of a Child' (Home Service; 1949), 3:273
　'The Mother's Contribution to Society' (1957), 5:13, **293–296**
　'No Baby Can Grow Properly Without 'Love' (Home Service; 1949), 3:285
　'The Only Child' (Home Service; 1945), 2:21*n*iii
　'The Ordinary Devoted Mother and her Baby: My Fan Mail' (1952), 12:**253–255**
　The Ordinary Devoted Mother and Her Baby (Home Service series, 1949), 6:169*n*1; 12:9, 12–13, 239
　The Ordinary Devoted Mother and Her Baby (Woman's Hour series, 1952), 12:13–14
　The Ordinary Devoted Mother and Her Baby: Baby Bites, 4:**23–26**
　The Ordinary Devoted Mother and Her Baby: The First Week, 4:**19–22**
　The Ordinary Devoted Mother and Her Children (series; 1960), 6:31, 47, 73, 293; 7:331
　original scripts of, 12:241–255
　'The Passing of Excretions' (Home Service; 1949), 3:281
　'Presenting the World to a Baby' (Home Service; 1949), 3:293
　'Problems of Management' (Home Service; 1949), 3:299, 12:**249–253**
　public recognition of DWW through, 5:3, 4, 9
　'Saying "No"' (1960) (also called 'Some occasions for saying "No"' and 'Saying "No" isn't just saying "No"'), 6:**31–42**
　'Shall We Keep Superficial or Go Deep?' (1955), 5:55
　'Support for Normal Parents' (1943–44), 2:21*n*iii; 12:9
　'Symptoms of Illness' (Home Service; 1950), 3:393
　'Their Standards and Yours' (1943–44), 2:21*n*iii
　'Twins' (1945), 2:21*n*iii
　'Unsuccess Story: Myself as Step-Mother, by a Listener in Despair' (*Woman's Hour*; 1955), 5:55
　'Weaning' (Home Service; 1949), 3:303
　'What About Father?' (1943–44), 2:21*n*iii
　'What Do We Know About Babies as Cloth Suckers?' (1956), 5:12, **115–118**
　'What Do We Mean by a Normal Child?', 12:9
　'Why Do Babies Cry?' (1943–44), 2:21*n*iii
　'The Wicked Stepmother in the Storytelling of All Ages' (*Woman's Hour*; 1955), 5:55
BBC interview style, 7:426
'The Bearing of Emotional Development on Feeding Problems' (1996), 8:81
Bearn, A. G., 1:5
beatings. *See* corporal punishment
The Beatles, 7:80
beauty, 6:507
Beckett, Samuel, 'Worstword Ho' (1983), 1:lxi

'Becoming Deprived as a Fact: A Psychotherapeutic Consultation' (1966), 10:419
Bedlam (St Mary of Bethlehem Hospital), 7:316*n*i
bed wetting. *See* enuresis
Beethoven, Ludwig van, 3:173
'The Beginning of the Individual' (1966), 7:**455–460**
'The Beginnings of a Formulation of an Appreciation and Criticism of Klein's Envy Statement' (1962), 1:lxviii; 5:11; 6:**315–324**; 9:47
behaviour. *See also* antisocial behaviour
   'Behaviour Therapy' (letter to *Child Care News*; 1969), 9:**63–65**
   'Saying "No"' (1960) (also called 'Some occasions for saying "No"' and 'Saying "No" isn't just saying "No"'), 6:**31–42**, 86
   total behaviour, described, 2:88, 91
   well-behaved toddlers, 6:31–42
being, continuity of. *See* continuity of being
being and doing
   creativity and, 9:13–15, 215
   in emotional development, 9:329
   split-off male and female elements in men and women and, 9:13–15, 150–151, 153, 314–316
Bell, Vanessa, 7:409
Bender, Loretta, 5:186
benign circle, 4:192–193, 194; 10:32, 83; 11:93–95, 98
Benzie, Isa (Mrs Royston Morley), 7:127, 331; 9:179, 12:lii, 9, 11–14,
Berenson, Bernard, 9:5
Bergeron, Marcel, *Psychologie du Premier Age* (1961; reviewed 1962), 6:**371**
Berkeley, Bishop, 11:130*n*III
'Berlin Walls' (1969), 9:**115–119**
Bernays, Martha, 6:367–369
Berry, George Packer, 6:27
'The Best Remedy' (1914), 1:**45–48**
Bethelard, F. and Young-Bruehl, E., *Cherishment* (2002), 6:16
Bettelheim, Bruno
   The Empty Fortress (1967), 8:161, 161; 9:38*n*7
   The Informed Heart: Autonomy in a Mass Age (1960), 9:302
Beveridge, William, Lord, 2:17, 18
   letter to (1946), 3:**37–38**
Bible. *See* scriptural references
Bibring, E., 7:218
Bicester Poor Law Institution. *See* Q Camps
Bick, Esther, 5:307, 345
   'Anxiety Underlying Phobia of Sexual Intercourse in a Woman' (1953), 4:109*n*i
   letter to (1953), 4:**109–110**
Bierman, G., ed., *Handbook of the Psychotherapy of Children* (1968), 8:439*n*1

binocular experiencing, Bion's concept of, 9:6, 11*n*ii
Bion, Francesca
   at banquet celebrating publication of Freud's *Standard Edition*, 7:407
   letter to (1957), 5:**263**
Bion, Wilfred R., 1:lxv, lxviii, lxxi; 3:12, 147*n*i; 5:81, 171, 262, 263; 6:12; 7:10, 17, 95–97, 407, 412; 8:6, 265
   'Arrogance', 5:263
   'Attacks on Linking' (1959), 5:263*n*i; 7:176*n*ii
   on binocular experiencing, 9:6, 11*n*ii
   'Differentiation of the Psychotic from the Non-Psychotic Personalities' (1957), 5:83*n*i
   on environment, 9:49
   'The Imaginary Twin' (1950), 3:433*n*i
   Learning from Experience (1962), 7:95*n*i
   letter to (1951), 3:**433**
   letter to (1955), 5:**83–86**
   letter to (1960), 6:**125–126**
   letter to (1961), 6:**279**
   letter to (1964), 6:12
   letter to (1967), 8:**157–158**
   'Negative Capability', 8:157*n*i
   'Personalities' (1955), 5:83–86
   Second Thoughts (1967), 8:441*n*i
   'A Theory of Functions', 6:125*n*i
   'A Theory of Thinking' (1961), 6:279*n*i, 444
   on thinking, 8:441
Birch, H. G., S. Chess, S. and A. Thomas, *Your Child Is a Person* (1960; reviewed by DWW 1966), 7:**415**
birching. *See* corporal punishment
Birksted-Breen, Dana, 6:235*n*i
birth as beginning of individual, 7:452
birth control
   adolescence and, 6:191, 427
   imaginative content of using, 9:109
   killing of children and, 9:106–108
   'The Pill' (1969), 9:**101–110**
   'The Silent Kill' (poem; 1969), 9:102, 108
birthing play, in *The Piggle*, 11:210–211, 219, 229, 307–308
birth memories
   accepting possibility of, 11:143–144, 165
   aggression, early roots of, 3:340
   analytical methodology for, 3:204
   anxiety and, 3:201–202, 207, 208, 216, 217, 228
   'Birth Memories, Birth Trauma and Anxiety' (1949), 3:16, 17, **201–220**, 221*n*i, 225–228, 340
   as break in infant's continuity of being, 3:212, 215–216, 217–218
   categorisation of, 3:207
   chest, constriction of, 3:214–215
   clinical examples of, 3:134, 204–206, 211–213
   Dick-Read on, 3:203–204

distortion between actual past and symbolism of, 7:45–46, 48–49
erotic asphyxiation and, 3:215
as experience versus trauma, 3:204, 207, 217–218
S. Freud on, 3:201–202, 207, 209, 217, 228
Greenacre on, 3:201, 202–203, 207, 217, 220n1, 222, 226, 227
head, emergence of, 3:213–214
identification of whole body with penis and, 3:214
mother-child relationship and, 3:215, 227–228
normal birth experience, 3:209–213, 216, 226
'Notes on the Discussion Held on Dr Winnicott's Paper "The Birth Trauma"' (1949), 3:**225–228**
prolonged or delayed deliveries, 11:165
pyschological disorders and, 3:217–219, 225–227
reliving, 3:226, 250–254
schizophrenics, regression of, 7:44–50
traumatic births, handling of infants after, 3:226–227
'The Birth of the Power Complex' (1964; now lost), 7:129
birth process
'The Birth Experience' (from *Human Nature*; 1988), 11:**161–167**
breathing, baby's awareness of, 11:163–164
Briance, Prunella, *Childbirth with Confidence* (foreword by DWW), 5:239, **533–534**
Caesarean section, infant experience of, 11:162
'The Contribution of Psycho-Analysis to Midwifery' (1957), 5:**225–232**, 239ni
delayed births, 11:162–163, 171
earliest stages of emotional development and, 11:143–147; 11:*144–146*
fathers and, 5:176, 226–227
gravity, effects of, 11:147–148
hospital versus home birth, 5:175–178
life of infant before, 5:116
medical histories, taking, 11:165–166
National Childbirth Trust (formerly Natural Childbirth Association), 5:13, 239, 305
natural childbirth movement, 5:12–13
bisexuality
in all human beings, 7:371; 11:72
S. Freud on, 9:14
in *Holding and Interpretation*, 4:336
mental illness and, 6:408
split-off male and female elements in men and women and, 7:317, 321, 323; 9:308–309, 310–311
biting
during breastfeeding, 2:67–68; 3:301; 4:25–27; 8:346
convulsions and fits, 1:309–312, 314n3
in love-making, 4:311

black
The Piggle, black mummy and concern with blackness in, 11:8, 198, 200–203, 205, 212–214, 218, 220–224, 228–231, 238, 245, 246, 249, 253, 257, 259, 260, 264, 265–266, 268, 289, 316
as psychiatric theme, 5:171, 258–259; 7:151–152, 207–211
black bile theory, 6:463
black people. *See* race and ethnicity
Blake, William, 'I Fear'd the Fury of my Wind', 8:366–367
Blake, Y., 'Psychotherapy with the More Disturbed Patient' (1968), 9:331
Blanc [doctor reporting case studies on encephalitis], 1:86, 88, 90
blank screen, abandonment of theory of, 7:14
blasphemy, 8:365–366
Blass, R. B., 8:18n10
Bléger, J., 1:lxv
blepharitis, 1:270
Bleuler, Eugen, 4:131
blindness
Burlingham on blind children, 8:280
creativity and, 9:216
hysterical, 1:269; 2:315
misdiagnosis of mental defect and, 1:302
'Ocular Psychoneuroses of Childhood' (1944), 2:3, **313–319**
psychological issues of blind children, 7:372
blinking, 1:136, 179, 246, 264, 270, 406–407; 10:454, 476
'blood-tie child' adoption case, letters to *The Times* on (1966), 7:**365–366**, **369**
Bloomsbury House, London, 5:536
'"Bob" aet 6 Years', 10:**113–140**, **517–518**
early history of Bob, 10:137–138
speech impediment, 10:114, 121, 140
squiggle game and, 10:114–136, *115–131*, *133–136*, 140
transference and, 10:517
body. *See also* physical deformity or difference
'Basis for Self in Body' (1970), 9:**225–234**
Bonnard, Augusta, 'Pre-Body Ego Types of Pathological Mental Functioning' (1957), 5:285ni
daydreaming, bodily accompaniment to, 9:248
'Dwelling of Psyche in Body' (from *Human Nature*, 1988), 11:**139–141**
DWW's concept of two-body relationship, 6:5
in first year of life, 5:322–323
imaginative elaboration of function, 11:75–76
Rickman's concept of three-body and two-body relationships, 5:211, 242
sense of living in, 3:129, 167, 169–170, 192
somatic health, 11:39–40
somatic ill-health, 11:43–44

body ego, 7:75
body language. *See* fidgetiness and excitability; finger-sucking; thumb-sucking
Bollas, Christopher, 1: xlvii–l, li, lxxviii, 479; 3:12; 11:3
Bonaminio, Vincenzo, 1:xxiii, xxv, xxvi; 3:3
Bonaparte, Marie, *4:17*
  Five Copy-Books (1950), 7:306*n*1
Bonham-Carter, Richard, 7:380
Bonnard, Augusta
  letters to (1957), 5:**255–256, 285**
  letter to (1952), 4:**45–46**
  'Polymorph Symptomatology', 4:45*n*i
  'Pre-Body Ego Types of Pathological Mental Functioning' (1957), 5:285*n*i
borderline cases
  absence of sense of guilt and, 7:449
  analytical process and, 8:14, 18*n*9
  atom bomb, symbolism of, 7:152
  autism, 7:354
  Bion and, 7:96
  as candidates for psychiatric treatment, 4:13
  communication between mother and infant and, 8:237
  concept of healthy individual and, 8:55
  cultural experience and, 7:433
  defined, 8:356
  dissociative phenomena associated with, 7:8, 305–306
  early developmental processes and, 6:7, 4828, 484
  environment in, 4:236
  A. Freud on, 7:223, 225
  need satisfaction and, 7:373–374
  parent-infant relationship and, 6:142–143
  psychoanalytic study of madness based on, 7:232
  regression and, 7:47
  schizophrenia, 7:44, 247, 275
  theoretical writings of DWW and, 7:4–6
boredom, 4:440; 6:82–83
Borges, Jorge Luis, 1: lxi
Bornstein, Berta, 7:197
  'The Analysis of a Phobic Child' (1949), 7:195*n*1
  'On Latency' (1951), 5:356
Borstal Assistant Governors' Conference (1967), 8:91
borstals, 5:152; 6:276–278; 8:97. *See also* delinquent children; punishment
Boston Psychoanalytic Society, 6:27, 333
bottle versus breast, 2:391–393; 3:277–278, 304; 5:419–420*n*9; 8:342, 345; 9:288*n*2
Bourne, Geoffrey, 1:88
  The Principles of Clinical Pathology in Practice (with G. K. Stone; 1929), 1:201*n*1

Bouvet (French psychiatrist), 9:130
Bowlby, John
  adoption and, 7:312
  on antisocial behaviour, 5:152, 153; 6:255; 7:222; 10:18
  Attachment and Loss (1969), 9:340–341
  attachment theory, 6:4
  British Psychoanalytical Society and, 6:116
  on children in hospital, 3:400; 5:529; 9:127, 340–341
  classification scheme of childhood abnormalities, 2:118–119
  on delinquent and habitual offenders, 2:31; 9:100
  direct observation by, 4:37
  Dowling recommended to, 8:206
  DWW compared, 2:15, 19
  DWW's rapprochement with, 2:6, 6*n*i
  DWW working with, 1:18; 10:17
  evacuation of children in WWII and, 2:6, 119; 5:5, 6
  on grief and mourning, 6:283–284
  on guilt, 5:142
  on holding, 9:204
  on individual maturational processes, 8:36
  International Psycho-Analytical Library and, 6:236
  'John Bowlby: An Interview' (1971), 10:18
  Klein, Melanie, and, 3:385; 5:10, 129, 131
  Laing, R. D., and, 5:361*n*i
  letter to (1938), 1:**465**
  letter to (1954), 4:**231–232**
  letter to *The Times* (1966) with DWW and others, 7:365–366, 371
  love of infant for mother, 6:16
  Lowry, Oliver M., put into contact with, 5:163
  reaction of DWW to papers of, 5:501
  reputation of, 2:119*n*i
  on separation and separation anxiety, 2:359; 4:254, 5:529; 7:156; 9:127, 340–341
  Spitz and, 5:255*n*i
  two-body perspective and, 2:15
  A Two-Year-Old Goes to Hospital (film), 4:113–114, 114*n*i
Bowlby, John, works of
  Child Care and Growth of Love, 6:4
  'Discussion of "Grief and Mourning in Infancy" by John Bowlby' (1959), 5:6, **495–500**; 10:18
  'Evacuation of Small Children' (*British Medical Journal* letter with DWW & Miller; 1939), 2:6, 47–48; 10:17
  'Forty-four Juvenile Thieves: Their Characters and Home-life' (1944), 2:31*n*i, 47*n*i, 222; 10:18, 528

'Grief and Mourning in Infancy' (1959),
    5:495–500; 10:18
'Hysteria in children' (1939), 1:465
'The Influence of Early Environment in the
    Development of Neurosis and Neurotic
    Character' (1939), 2:31n1
'The Making and Breaking of Affectional
    Bonds' (1979), 6:16
Maternal Care and Mental Health (1951),
    3:405n2, 437–439; 5:158n1
Maternal Care and Mental Health (1951;
    reviewed 1953), 4:**111–114**
'The Nature of the Child's Tie to His Mother'
    (1957), 5:237n1
'Separation Anxiety' (1958), 5:379–381, 383n1
'On "Separation Anxiety" by John Bowlby'
    (DWW, 1958), 5:6, **379–381**
in *The Psychoanalytic Study of the Child,
    Volume 15* (1961; reviewed 1962), 6:283–284
Bowley, Agatha H., *The Psychology of the
    Unwanted Child* (review; 1947), 3:149–150
Bowra, Cecil Maurice, 8:401
    Sophoclean Tragedy (1944), 6:517
Boxall, Helen, 7:407
Boy Scouts, 1:27, 49
BPAS. *See* British Psychoanalytical Society
brachial plexus, birth injury to, 1:295
Bradley, C., 3:354, 356
Bradshaw (train timetables), 7:354
Brain, R., 1:290n3
brain, 7:450; 11:39–41, 47, 76–77
brain disease
    'Abscess in Frontal Lobe: Post-Mortem
        Findings' (with Elizabeth O'Flynn; 1928),
        1:**119–121**; *1:120, 121*
    anxiety and, 1:272
    central nervous system disorders, 1:281,
        289–290
    cerebral tumours, 1:281, 289–290
    convulsions and fits, 1:304–305; 4:181–182
    'Frontal Lobes of the Human Brain' (letter to
        The Lancet 1943), 4:**33**
    infantile schizophrenia due to, 8:161
    mental disorders arising from, 6:409–410
    tuberculosis, intracranial, 1:119, 290
Bray, G. W., 'Lichen Urticatus or Urticaria
    Papulosa' (1933), 1:343, 352n1
breakdown
    of basic emotional development, 6:99
    definition of, 6:524–525
    environmental breakdown, 6:219, 365
    fear of, 5:458nii, 458–459; 6:466,
        523–531, 531nii
    'Fear of Breakdown' (1963), 5:458nii; 6:**523–531**
    as healthy, 6:416

'On the Nature of Mental Breakdown' (1963),
    6:523, 531nii
parent engaged in preventing, 6:364
relief from, 6:71
rhythm of breakdown-recovery, 8:7
sometimes leading to cure, 8:73
breast
    'bad breast' and 'good breast', 4:63, 198–199,
        221–222; 5:122–123, 131; 6:16, 270, 3260–324;
        7:96; 11:95–96
    creation of, by baby, 11:119, 121, 122
    idealized, 4:199
    as object, 4:63–646, 162, 164, 173n1, 174n11; 5:411,
        417n1; 9:7
    sadistic attack on, 10:296
breast cancer, 1:70; 8:372, 374
Breasted, J. H., 9:36, 303
breastfeeding. *See also* weaning
    adoption and, 5:75–76
    assistance with, 5:230–232, 280, 282
    'bad breast' and, 6:16
    biting, 2:67–68; 3:301
    in black versus white populations, 9:341
    bodily contact with mother, importance of,
        2:201; 4:131
    bottle-feeding and, 2:391–393; 3:133, 277–278,
        304; 5:419–420n9; 8:342, 345; 9:288n2
    'Breast Feeding' (1945), 2:**389–395**; 8:131
    'Breast-feeding as Communication' (1968),
        8:**341–348**, 355
    described, 3:290–291
    destruction and survival of breast,
        8:346–347, 361
    envy of the good breast, 9:314. *See also* envy
    excited relationships, setting for,
        11:119–121; *11:120*
    face masks, mothers wearing while nursing
        infants, 2:227
    failure and success in, 11:122–123
    fantasies of infant and, 2:133; 4:169, 221–222
    father's appearance in infant's life and, 4:353
    first-time management of, 3:291–292; 8:107
    'good breast', 5:123, 131–132; 6:16, 270,
        320–324; 8:342
    identity of child and object relationship of child
        and breast and, 7:324–326
    maternal knowledge about nutrition and, 3:388
    methodological approach of DWW to child
        development and, 3:6–7
    Middlemore, Merell P., *The Nursing Couple*
        (reviewed; 1942), 1: lxiv–lxv, 18; 2:12, **171–174**,
        296, 297n1
    mother, baby and, 2:223–225, 391–392; 9:390
    nurse or doctor involved in, 8:85–87, 344;
        11:122–123

breastfeeding (*Cont.*)
  nursing couple, 6:87–89
  penis envy and breast envy, 5:129
  personhood of baby and, 3:99, 100; 8:119–120
  The Piggle, breasts (yams) in, 11:8, 198, 214, 224–225, 232, 238, 276, 282, 290, 291
  positive value of, 8:344–345
  primary narcissism in, 3:10–11
  prior to giving up infant for adoption, 2:394
  reality adaptation and, 2:364
  reliving, in analysis, 4:351
  sibling's reaction to, 8:109
  social attitude to, 9:341
  split-off male and female elements in men and women and, 9:313–314
  subjective object, breast as, 9:7
  switch to bottle feeding from, 3:133
  transitional objects and, 9:271, 273
  turning away from the breast, 3:291; 8:108
  twins and, 2:345–346
breathing. *See also* asthma
  birth and baby's awareness of, 11:163–164
  infant's fears about, 2:132
  sexual intercourse and, 4:110
  therapeutic consultation and, 10:166, 180, 182
Brenner, Charles, 'The Nature and Development of the Concept of Repression in Freud's Writings', 5:363
Breuer, Josef, 6:368, 369
Briance, Prunella, 5:305
  Childbirth with Confidence (foreword by DWW), 5:239, **533–534**
  letter to (1957), 5:**239**
Brierley, Marjorie, 1: lxiv, 17, 373*n*5; 3:121; 7:408
Brill, A. A., (founder of New York Psychoanalytic Society), 5:389
Britain
  border between England and Scotland, 9:119
  Catholic-Protestant divide in Northern Ireland, 9:118
  German versus British behaviour, 2:88–89
  neurosis, English inhibited pattern of, 9:175
  place of monarchy in, 9:181–187
British Empire, 8:145
British Independents. *See* 'Middle Group' (later the Independents)
British Journal of Children's Diseases, 1:75, 343; 5:398*n*3
British Journal of Medical Psychology, 1:11, 341, 437; 3:23, 123, 245, 265, 363, 483, 487, 489, 491; 4:35, 115, 189, 249*n*i; 5:505; 10:335
British Journal of Psychiatric Social Work, 5:513; 6:461, 509
British Journal of Psychiatry, 8:149*n*i
British Journal of Psychology, 4:127; 6:367

British Medical Association, 5:8
British Medical Bulletin, 5:456
British Medical Journal
  articles by DWW first published in, 3:69, 353, 437; 4:237
  'Battle Neurosis Treated With Leucotomy' (letter; 1947), 3:**113**
  Childhood and Society (Erikson 1951; reviewed 1953), 4:**125–126**
  'Circumcision' (letter; 1939), 2:**25–27**
  Clyne, Max B., *Absent: School Refusal as an Expression of Disturbed Family Relationships* (1966; reviewed 1967), 8:**129–130**
  'Comforters' (letter; 1955), 5:12, **77**
  'Communal Feeding in Schools' (letter; 1941), 2:**107–108**
  'Ethics of Prefrontal Leucotomy' (letter; 1951), 3:**467–468**
  'Evacuation of Small Children' (letter with Bowlby & Miller; 1939), 2:6, **47–48**; 10:17
  evacuation scheme, DWW, Bowlby, and Miller paper about, 5:5
  letter of D. N. Parfitt in, 7:455
  'Loneliness in Infancy' (letter; 1942), 2:**165**
  'Paddington Green Children's Hospital' (letter; 1949), 3:**243–244**; 10:8
  ''Pathies in a State Service' (letter; 1948), 3:**141**
  'Physical Therapy in Mental Disorder' (letter; 1945), 2:**379–380**
  'Prefrontal Leucotomy' (letter; 1956), 5:10, **119–120**
  'Pruritus and Psychology' (letter; 1939), 2:**29**
  Psycho-Analysis and Child Psychiatry (Glover, reviewed 1953), 4:**115**
  The Psychoanalytic Study of the Child, Vol. 11 (1957; reviewed 1958), 5:**317–318**, 531*n*2
  The Psychoanalytic Study of the Child, Vol. 15 (1961; reviewed 1962), 6:**283–284**
  'Psychology in the Child's Education' (letter; 1946), 3:**35–36**
  'Responsibility and Freedom' (letter; 1943), 2:**217–219**
  reviews originally published in, 3:149, 151, 157, 159, 235, 431, 469, 473; 4:101, 115, 117, 125, 233; 5:223, 317, 363; 7:213, 375, 397
  'Shock Therapy' (letter; 1944), 2:207*n*i, **251–253**
  'Shock Treatment of Mental Disorder' (letter; 1943), 2:**229–230**
  Slavson, S. R., *Child Psychotherapy* (1953; reviewed 1954), 4:**233–234**
  Soddy, Kenneth, *Clinical Child Psychiatry* (1960; reviewed 1961), 6:**223**
  Spence paper on hospitalised children in (1947), 5:5

'Taking Children's Temperatures' (letter; 1949), 3:**181–182**
British Medical Student's Journal, 3:259
British Paediatric Association
  Annual General Meeting (1945), 2:389*n*ii
  'Memorandum on "The Relation Between Clinical Paediatrics and Child Psychology"' (1943), 2:7, **201–205**
  'The Wearing of Masks in the Nursing of Premature and Older Infants (abstract; 1943), 2:**227**
British Psychoanalytical Society (BPAS), 1: xlvii, lii, lix, lix, lxxviii, 13, 16, 17, 18, 359
  'The Aims of Psycho-Analytical Treatment' (1962), 6:285
  Balint's paper 'Primary Narcissism and Primary Love' (1960) delivered, 6:43*n*i
  Bion and, 5:83–84; 6:125*n*i, 229, 285*n*i
  'Birth Memories, Birth Trauma and Anxiety' (1949) presented at, 3:201, 221*n*i, 222, 225
  Bulletin of, 9:155
  candidates for membership, 3:233–234
  'Communicating and Not Communicating Leading to a Study of Certain Opposites' (1963), 6:433
  Controversial Discussions (1940s), 1: lviii, lxiii–lxv, 17; 5:8, 261*n*ii; 6:217; 7:3, 377*n*i; 11:13, 101*n*5
  discussion on 'Consultation Technique' (1946), 3:42*n*i
  DWW as member of, 11:6
  Extraordinary Business Meeting (February 1942), 2:145
  founding of, 4:53; 5:392
  A. Freud-Klein controversy in, 5:6–8, 10–11, 12, 19–20, 33, 87
  goals of, 2:147
  groups within, 4:241–243; 5:7–8, 19–20, 261, 501
  letter to Hellman on nomination, 6:107
  letter to Hoffer on papers read at Society by Associate Members, 4:48
  letter to Rycroft on possible topics for (1956), 5:171
  Medical Section, 8:169; 10:5
  'Metapsychological and Clinical Aspects of Regression within the Psychoanalytical Set-up' (1954) read before, 4:201
  'Mind and Its Relation to the Psyche-Soma' (1949) read before, 3:245
  papers of DWW presented to, 7:4, 229, 317, 429; 9:4, 47, 149, 265, 317*n*7; 11:8
  'Playing: A Theoretical Statement' (1967), 8:299
  'Playing: Its Theoretical Status in the Clinical Situation' (reading 1967), 8:12
  possibility of splitting and future of, 4:241–243
  presentation of *The Piggle*, at pre-IPA Congress program, at 1969, 11:190–191
  presidency of DWW, 5:9, 309; 7:3, 407, 411, 413; 8:8; 9:100, 169
  'Primitive Emotional Development' (lecture; 1945), 2:**357–368**
  publication of *Standard Edition of the Psychological Works of Sigmund Freud* (1966), 7:**407–410**
  Publications Committee, 6:235–236
  reparation, importance of recognising, 3:121–122
  role in DWW's life and career, 1: xlvii, lix, lxi, lxxviii, 16, 17, 18, 359; 2:4, 5, 9; 4:53
  'Roots of Aggression' (prepared 1968, but not delivered), 8:329
  Sandler's paper 'Research in Psycho-Analysis: The Hampstead Index as an Instrument of Psycho-Analytic Research' (delivered 1961), 8:229
  Scientific Bulletin (internal circulation only), 7:377
  Scientific Meeting (June 1942), 2:7
  Scientific Meeting (May 1951), 4:159
  seventieth birthday lecture series proposal by DWW, 7:243
  shock therapy, study of, 2:262
  sociology of knowledge and, 9:392–394
  statue of Freud by Nemon and, 12:4
  Strachey and, 8:126
  Training Committee, 4:179–180; 6:107
  'Transitional Objects and Transitional Phenomena' first presented to (1951), 3:435; 4:297
  'Winter Lectures on Psychoanalysis' (1968), 8:227
British Psychological Society, 1: lix, 14, 413; 2:207*n*i; 9:207
British Student Health Association, 9:57, 337
Britton, Alison, 1:xiii, 12:21
Britton, Clare. *See* Winnicott, Clare
Britton, E., *11:186*
Britton, James (brother-in-law), 6:20, 499
Britton, Karl (brother-in-law), 8:407
  letter to (1968), 8:**397**
Britton, Karl (brother-in-law) and Sheila
  letter to (November 1968), 8:12, 18*n*8, **383**
  letter to (December 1968), 8:**407**
Broadmoor Criminal Lunatic Asylum, 5:399
broken homes. *See* deprivation
bromide, 1:268, 276, 305, 306, 308, 310
bronchitis, 1:99, 100, 190, 197, 198–199, 303
Brooke, Rupert, 8:123
Bruch, H., 3:356
Bryan, Douglas, 5:392

Budd, Susan, 6:235ni
Buehler/Buhler, Charlotte, 1:15; 6:371
Buffon, Georges Louis Leclerc, Comte de, 7:432
'The Building Up of Trust' (1969), 9:**121–128**
bullying, 10:276, 293, 294
Bunyan, John, *Pilgrim's Progress*, 5:139
Bureau for Co-operation in Child Care, 8:59
Burgess, Norman, 2:29
Burke, Edmund, 5:135
Burke, N. H., 1:302n1
Burlingham, Dorothy, 3:157; 5:337, 447, 496–497; 6:399; 7:376; 10:18
   on blind children, 8:280
   A. Freud with, observations of psychoses, 4:37
   Twins: A Study of Three Pairs of Identical Twins (1952; reviewed 1953), 4:103–104, **105–108**; 10:12
   Young Children in Wartime: A Year's Work in a Residential War Nursery (with Anna Freud), 5:497; 10:18
Burt, Cyril, 9:155
Burton, Lindy, *Vulnerable Children: Three Studies of Children in Conflict* (reviewed 1968), 8:**275–276**
Burton, Robert, 2:259
   Anatomy of Melancholy (1621), 5:137, 142
Butt, Alfred, Sir, 1:59

Caccia, G., 1:78, 88
Caesarean section, infant experience of, 11:162
calamine lotion, 1:327, 344
Caldwell, Lesley, 1: xlix, li, 12:xlix
Calverley, Charles Stuart, 8:267
   Humorous Poems III. Parodies: Imitations, 8:267ni
Cambridge Evacuation Survey, 2:117–119
Cambridge University, DWW as student at, 1:xvi, 3; 12:303–304
Cameron, Dr, 1:171, 238, 355n1
Cameron, Hector, 6:301
Cameron, Kenneth, 4:228, 239
Caminopetros [doctor reporting case studies on encephalitis], 1:86, 88, 90
Camus [doctor reporting case studies on encephalitis], 1:83
Canadian Medical Association Journal, 5:265
cancer, 1:70; 8:372, 374; 11:1, 52
cannibalism, in *Holding and Interpretation*, 4:308, 309, 311, 313, 315, 349, 350
'The Capacity to Be Alone' (1958), 1: xlviii, lxxvi; 5:13–14, **241–248**; 6:11, 157n10; 7:430; 8:13, 312n3, 364; 9:298n5, 329
Capener, N. L., 1:61
Capps, F. C. W., 1:60

car accidents. *See* accidents
cardiac neurosis
   clinical observations, 7:384–386
   historical background, 7:379–3813
   medical histories, taking, 7:381–382
   'On Cardiac Neurosis in Children' (1966), 1:123ni; 7:**379–386**
   physical examinations, 7:383–384
care-cure position,
   'Cure' (1970), 9:**191–197**
   cruelty in, 9:195
   importance of, 9:197
career management, in *Holding and Interpretation*, 4:315–316, 348, 376–378, 386–387, 393, 394, 416, 442, 461–465, 464, 468–469
caretaker, mother described as, 7:221, 222
caretaker self, 6:161, 360, 391
Carmichael, E. A., 1:290n2
Carpenter, Louise, 8:387ni, 405–406, 406nvi
Carrington, Dora, 8:126
Carr-Saunders, A. M., *Young Offenders* (1942), 2:195, 200n1
The Case as the Patient Sees It: Psychoanalysis, National Association of Mental Health (foreword by DWW; 1957), 5:**235–236**
Case Conference (journal), 4:**139–149**; 5:89; 9:179–180
'A Case Managed at Home' (1955), 5:**89–97**
'Case Notes for a Psychoanalytic Seminar: Withdrawal, Regression, Male Identification' (1965), 7:**239–242**
'Case of L.' (1968), 8:413, 417–438; 10:83
case studies. *See also* clinical observations
   '"Ada" aet 8 Years', 10:299n1, **307–334**. *See also* '"Ada" aet 8 Years'
   adolescents, 6:495–497; 8:99–104, 239–243, 351–352
   adoption, 4:293–296
   aggression, 6:99–100
   '"Albert" aet 7 Years 9 Months', 10:**233–252**. *See also* '"Albert" aet 7 Years 9 Months'
   '"Alfred" aet 10 Years', 10:**165–185, 519–520**. *See also* '"Alfred" aet 10 Years'
   '"Ashton" aet 12 Years', 7:183niv, 273, 358nii; 10:210, **213–232**. *See also* '"Ashton" aet 12 Years'
   'Basis for Self in Body' (1970), 9:226–232
   '"Bob" aet 6 Years', 10:**113–140, 517–518**. *See also* '"Bob" aet 6 Years'
   'Case for Diagnosis (? Infantile Hemiplegia)' (1926), 1:**93–94**
   'Case for Diagnosis (? Poliomyelitis with Some Spasticity)' (1926), 1:**91–92**
   'Case of Stunted Growth' (1927), 1:**99–100**

'"Cecil" aet 21 Months at First Consultation', 10:18–19, **335–366**. *See also* '"Cecil" aet 21 Months at First Consultation'
character disorders, 6:456–459
'"Charles" aet 9 Years', 10:15–16, **191–212**. *See also* '"Charles" aet 9 Years'
'Clinical Illustration of "The Use of an Object"' (1968), 8:**365–368**
'Contribution to the Final Number of *Case Conference*' (1970), 9:**179–180**
'A Doctor Looks at the Psychiatric Social Worker' (1943), 2:185–190
'Dreaming, Fantasying and Living: A Case-History Describing a Primary Dissociation' (1971), 9:**289–298**
'"Eliza" aet 7½ years' (1971), 8:413; 10:9, **83–112**. *See also* '"Eliza" aet 7½ years'
enuresis, 4:81–95
envy, 6:**269–271**, 403–405
'Envy: A Male Patient Near the End of His Analysis' (1961), 6:**269–271**
on fantasies and orgiastic bodily functioning, 9:369–370
'Further Clinical Illustration of "The Use of an Object"' (1968), 8:**369–377**
futility, 6:100–101
'"George" aet 13 Years', 10:**495–514**
'Hands Case.' *See* 'Ada'
'"Hesta" aet 16 Years', 10:**253–274**. *See also* '"Hesta" aet 16 Years'
Holding and Interpretation: Fragment of an Analysis (1955), 1: lxi, lxxiii; 4:**303–474**
'"Iiro" aet 9 Years 9 Months', 8:7–8; 10:13, 15, 31–32, **37–55**, 515. *See also* '"Iiro" aet 9 Years 9 Months'
Institute of Psycho-Analysis, Child Department, 2:149–163
in 'Interrelating Apart from Instinctual Drive and in Terms of Cross-identifications' (1971), 9:**319–328**, 330–334
'"Jason" aet 8 Years 9 Months', 10:**453–493**. *See also* '"Jason" aet 8 Years 9 Months'
'Knowing and Not Knowing' (undated; first published 1989), 9:**367–368**
'"Lily" aet 5 Years', 10:17, 19, **451–452**. *See also* '"Lily" aet 5 Years'
'"Mark" aet 12 Years', 10:**369–402**, 525–526. *See also* '"Mark" aet 12 Years'
'"Matti," aet 12 1/2 years: A Therapeutic Consultation' (1961), 6:**237–239**; 10:15
'"Milton" aet 8 Years', 10:9, **275–299**, 521–523. *See also* '"Milton" aet 8 Years'
mirroring, 8:213–218
mother's death and stepmother's role to illustrate dependence, 6:474–476
'Mother's Madness Appearing in the Clinical Material as an Ego-Alien Factor' (1969), 9:**141–148**
'"Mrs X" aet 30 Years', 10:19, **441–450**. *See also* '"Mrs X" aet 30 Years'
'The Niffle' (probably before 1961; published 1996), 9:**383–387**
'A Note on a Case Involving Envy' (1963), 6:**403–405**
oversimplification of, 10:29
'"Peter" aet 13 Years', 10:**403–418**. *See also* '"Peter" aet 13 Years'
play and creativity of client, 8:172–179
psychosis, 6:66–71; 8:99–104
'"Robert" aet 9 Years', 10:**141–156**. *See also* '"Robert" aet 9 Years'
'"Robin" aet 5 Years', 10:**57–82**. *See also* '"Robin" aet 5 Years'
'"Rosemary" aet 10 Years', 10:**157–163**. *See also* '"Rosemary" aet 10 Years'
'"Ruth" aet 8 Years', 10:**419–439**, 527–533. *See also* '"Ruth" aet 8 Years'
'Sakari: A Therapeutic Consultation' (1961), 6:**241–257**; 10:15
'Two Further Clinical Examples' (undated, probably 1970), 9:**235–245**
casework
'Casework with Mentally Ill Children' (1959), 5:**481–492**; 7:399*n*iii
clinical observations, 5:483–490
holding in, 5:486, 490, 491
'The Mentally Ill in Your Caseload' (1963), 6:13, **409–420**
psychotherapy and casework, 5:481–482
teamwork and, 5:490–491
Cassel Hospital for Functional Nervous Diseases, 2:252*n*i; 3:351
Casteret, N., *My Caves* (1947), 3:213
castration, 11:18
desire of patient to castrate another person, 6:404–405
loss of ego function and, 8:442
as medical treatment, 3:479
castration anxiety, 5:352, 446, 450; 9:151, 230; 11:73, 84
brain mutilation and, 3:478
childhood sexuality and, 3:102, 104, 110
displacements of, 3:213
dreams and, 3:62, 63
Freudian concept, 4:205
and gender, 11:69, 71, 73, 74*n*,
Holding and Interpretation: Fragment of an Analysis (1955), 4:310, 323, 384, 396, 398
homosexuality and, 6:407
instinct theory and, 11:73–74, 84

castration (*Cont.*)
   loss of intellect and, 8:442
   and Oedipus complex, 11:72–73, 81, 84
   penis envy and, 3:490
   as psychological release, 11:18
   relationship with father and, 4:323
Casuso, Gabriel
   'Anxiety Related to the "Discovery" of the Penis' (1957), 5:159*n*i
   letter to (1956), 5:**159–160**
cataloguing, as thought process, 7:141–142
catarrh, 1:169, 170, 179, 184, 203, 336*n*4
cathexis
   cathected internal mother imago, 6:132–133, 165, 355
   object relation and, 8:357, 359, 362
   withdrawal of, 10:132, 135
Catholic-Protestant divide in Northern Ireland, 9:118
'Cathy Come Home' (film), 8:388*n*iv
causes of illness in children, 1:170–172
'"Cecil" *aet* 21 Months at First Consultation', 10:18–19, **335–366**
   background, 10:335
   dreams and, 10:364
   failure of Cecil to speak, 10:339, 340
   gender identity and, 10:344
   hitting his mother, 10:345
   mother's depression and, 10:339, 346, 365–366
   mother's pregnancy as trigger for symptoms, 10:336–337, 338, 362
   nursery school and, 10:345–346
   onset of symptoms, 10:336
   play capacity and, 10:340, 344
   preference of Cecil for his father over his mother, 10:341–342, 366*nn*2–3
   pseudologia fantastica as part of antisocial behaviour and, 10:363
   regression and, 10:336, 360, 361, 364, 366, 367*n*6
   sibling rivalry and, 10:344, 362
   sleeping with his parents, 10:338–339, 344–345
   squiggle game and, 10:347–359, 347–360, 363–364
   stealing as issue, 10:346, 360–363, 366*n*1
   thumb-sucking and, 10:337, 339–344, 354, 361, 366
   toilet training and, 10:336
   transitional phenomena and, 10:337
Central Hospital, Warwick, 7:455
central nervous system
   acute diseases of, 1:282–290
   'Disease of the Nervous System', from *Clinical Notes* (1931), 1:**281–290**
   medical history and physical examination, 1:281–282
   walking problems and, 1:293–294
central self. *See* true and false self
cerebral palsy, 6:391*n*i
cerebral tumours, 1:281, 289–290
Chadwick, Mary, 1:9, 11
Chair of Child Psychiatry, DWW on need for, 5:161–163
Chamberlain, Anne (Mrs. Neville), letter to (1938), 1:**463**
Chamberlain, Neville, 1:463; 2:92–93
'Changing Patterns: the Young Person, the Family and Society' (1970), 9:57*n*i, 167*n*i
'Chaos' (from *Human Nature* 1988), 11:**153–155**
Chaplin, D., letter to (1954), 4:**271–272**
character disorders, 6:447–459
   aetiology of, 6:450–452
   antisocial behaviour and, 6:448, 452
   case examples, 6:456–459
   court cases involving, 6:455
   gender differences at adolescence, 6:455–456
   indications for therapy, 6:452–455
   natural cure for, 6:450
   psycho-neurosis, 6:450
   psychosis, 6:450–451, 457–459
   'The Psychotherapy of Character Disorders' (1963), 6:13, **447–459**
   society's role in determining fate of persons with, 6:449
'Chards Pil . . .' (1968), 8:**245–247**
'"Charles" *aet* 9 Years', 10:15–16, **191–212**
   dreams and, 10:199, 205, 208–210
   mind and its division into compartments and, 10:196, 202
   penis and, 10:201
   squiggle game and, 10:*192–209*, 192–211, *211*
charts, medical, importance of, 1:195–201
Cheadle, W. B., 1:221; 2:49, 50; 7:380
Cheale, Mr. and Mrs., [superintendent at Market End House (Bicester)], 2:103–104
Chess, S., A. Thomas, and H. G. Birch, *Your Child Is a Person* (1960; reviewed by DWW 1966), 7:**415**
Chesterton, G. K., 1:32
Cheu, Tsuicheu, letter to (1957), 5:**217**
chicken pox
   encephalitis and, 1:79–81, 115–116
   papular urticaria resembling, 1:345
Child, Dr, 7:197
'The Child, the Family and the Offender' (1965), 7:**203–205**
'The Child, the Family and the Young Offender' (UK Government Home Office White Paper), 7:203–205
The Child, the Family, and the Outside World (1964), 2:293; 3:313, 323, 393, 421*n*4, 441; 5:3,

294*n*i; 7:8, (Introduction to) **125–127**, 129; 8:33, 144*n*ii, 157, 197, 197*n*i; 9:36, 44*n*i, 92, 92*n*ii; 11:102*n*9
'Child Analysis in the Latency Period' (1958), 5:**351–359**; 11:185, 186*n*5
'The Child and Sex' (1947), 3:**101–111**
The Child and the Family (1957), 2:12, 21*n*iii, 287*n*i, 293; 3:313, 387, 393; 5:3, 239, 465, 479; 6:64, 109*n*i, 293; 7:83; 8:146*n*ii, 165*n*1
The Child and the Outside World (1957), 2:21*n*iii; 3:313, 323; 5:3; 7:129; 8:146*n*ii
childbirth. *See entries at* birth
child care
  attitudes to, 4:254; 5:6, 496
  Child Care and Protection Act, 3:423
  child care workers and generic training of social workers, 5:339–344
  failure in, 4:57; 5:63, 422
  as field of study for Association for Child Psychology and Psychiatry (ACPP), 8:59–60
  good care's effect on integration, 4:56–57
  maternal care. *See* mother-child relationship
  'Psychoses and Child Care' (1953), 4:8, 9, **35–45**; 6:157*n*4
  residential child care, 8:60–61
  role of father in, 5:293
  role of medical professional in, 5:422–424
Child Care News, letter to (1969), 9:**63–65**
'Child Department Consultations' (1942), 2:3, 7, **149–163**
child development. *See also* infant development
  advice for persons seeking careers in, 9:176–177
  from being infants to four-year olds, 6:35
  continuity of development, 4:36
  emotional component of, 2:71, 203–204, 387
  environmental adaptation in, 4:214
  explanations, stage of, 6:37, 42
  of four-year-old, 4:249–250
  'Growth and Development in Immaturity' (1950), 3:**397–405**
  'The Human Child Examined' (Part 1 of *Human Nature*, 1988), 11:**25–56**
  Kleinian model of, 10:10
  'Needs of the Under-Fives' (1954), 4:**249–256**
  'The Only Child' (published & radio broadcast 1945), 2:21*n*iii, **323–327**
  opportunity, provision of, 6:386–388
  parents' role in. *See* father-child relationship; mother-child relationship; parents
  physiotherapy and, 9:69–73
  society's responsibility in, 4:254–255
  stages of, 4:233; 6:346–347; 8:67, 70–72
  'Their Standards and Yours' (published 1945 & radio broadcast 1944), 2:21*n*iii, **277–280**

thinking, 7:140. *See also* intellectual development
triangular relationship, 4:251–252
twins, 2:344, 346–347
two-person relationship, 4:252
of two-to four-year-old, 4:276
'What Do We Mean by a Normal Child?' (published & radio broadcast 1946), 2:21*n*iii, **281–286**
Child-Family Digest, 3:441
A Child Goes to Hospital (film), 4:173*n*3
Child Guidance Clinics
  access to, 8:181
  advising family to give up adopted child, 9:243
  cases described in Soddy, Kenneth, *Clinical Child Psychiatry* (1960; reviewed 1961), 6:223
  child psychiatry at Paddington Green Children's Hospital and, 6:19, 179
  children at, not representative 7:388
  defined, 6:179*n*i
  emergence of, 2:202–203; 9:63, 176
  psychiatric social workers in, 8:61
  unsatisfactory consultations in, 10:191
Child Guidance Inter-Clinic Conference, 7:51
Child Guidance movement, 10:5
Child Guidance Training Centre, 6:299
'Childhood Psychosis' (1950), 3:**353–356**
'The Child in the Family Group' (1966), 7:**387–396**
  age of DWW and work with children, 9:171
  background for, 6:301–302
  caseload of child psychiatrist versus psychoanalyst, 10:369
  Chair of Child Psychiatry, DWW on need for, 5:161–163
  'Child Psychiatry, Social Work, and Alternative Care' (1970), 9:**171–174**
  'Child Psychiatry: The Body as Affected by Psychological Factors' (ca. 1931), 1:13, **159–160**
  'A Child Psychiatry Case Illustrating Delayed Reaction to Loss' (1965), 7:11, **279–304**; 8:319
  'A Child Psychiatry Interview' (1962), 10:157
  definition of, 6:300
  development as recognised field, 10:4–7
  economics of, 10:526
  'How Little Need I Do?' as motto for, 10:183, 517, 519, 525
  paediatricians and, 2:203; 4:76, 78, 117, 228, 239; 5:423–424; 6:20, 177, 263–265, 304–305; 10:5; 11:37
  'A Personal Statement on Child Psychiatry' (1971), 9:**175–178**
  'The Psycho-analyst and Child Psychiatry: A Matter of Economics' (1962), 6:**357–358**

'The Child in the Family Group' (1966) (*Cont.*)
  relationship of adult psychiatry to, 6:302–303
  relationship of psychoanalysis to, 6:305–306, 357–358; 10:27
'Theoretical Statement of the Field of Child Psychiatry' (1958), 5:**421–429**
Therapeutic Consultations in Child Psychiatry (1971), 1: lxi, 8
'Training for Child Psychiatry' (1962), 6:**299–307**
  training in, 6:299–307; 7:419–422
Child Psychology and Psychiatry, 9:288*n*3
Children Act (1948), 2:5; 5:152, 274–275*n*1, 544; 7:33, 99
'Children and Their Mothers' (1940), 2:**81–86**; 6:158*n*16
'Children in the War'
  BBC radio broadcast (1939), 2:5; 12:8
  paper (1940), 2:**95–99**
'Children Learning' (1968), 8:**313–318**
Children's Act (1948), 3:425, 439; 8:59
'Children's Comforters' (1955), 5:12
children's homes. *See also* hostels
  evidence given to Home Office Committee on, 2:349, **369–377**
  Poor Law homes, 1:409*n*iii
'Children's Hostels in War and Peace' (1948), 3:**23–27**; 4:239*n*i
Children's Officer, role of, 2:5; 8:60
Children's services, 2:5
Child Study Association of America, *Parents' Questions* (reviewed 1947), 3:151
'Child Therapy: A Case of Antisocial Behaviour' (1965), 8:319; 10:369
Chisholm, Catherine, 8:283, 296
chorea
  anxiety and, 1:246, 272
  diagnosis of, 2:156–157
  'The Diagnosis of Chorea' (1929), 1:9, **133–140**
  DWW's early medical experience with, 1:6, 7
  encephalitis and, 1:78, 95, 133, 250
  enuresis and, 1:144
  fidgetiness and, 1:136–140, 247–253
  fright as cause of, 2:50
  'On In-Patient Treatment for Rheumatic Fever and Chorea' (ca. 1923–1931), 1:**161–163**
  physical examinations, 7:384
  psychological health and, 11:50
  rheumatic heart disease and, 1:133, 161–163; 2:50, 55–58
  seasonal variations in incidence of, 7:380–381
Christianity and the ascensive, 1:365
Christian Teamwork Institute of Education, 8:313
chronic staphylococcal infection (CSI), 1:69

chronology of DWW's life, 1:467–472; 2:397–401; 3:495–501; 4:475–481; 5:547–552; 6:533–540; 7:461–467; 8:451–457; 9:397–403; 10:535–541; 11:319–324
Church, Richard, 7:393
Churchill, Winston, 2:87, 91, 92; 7:150
cigarettes. *See* smoking
'Circumcision' (letter to *The British Medical Journal*; 1939), 2:**25–27**
citizenship, home life as basis for, 3:35
Clancier, Anne, 9:257
classification
  Bowlby, John, classification scheme for childhood abnormalities, 2:118–119
  of broken homes, 3:368–369
  of cases, 5:52–54; 6:300–301
  'Classification: Is There a Psycho-Analytic Contribution to Psychiatric Classification?' (1959/1965), 5:**445–459**; 6:14, 523; 8:357; 9:317*n*1; (1964 addendum) 7:233*n*i, 238*n*3
  countertransference, classification of phenomena of, 3:60
  depression, 6:254
  by environmental distortion, 5:457
  of environmental factors, 3:223, 381
  Glover, Edward, 'A Psycho-Analytic Approach to the Classification of Mental Disorders' (1932), 5:456
  as human, 7:449–454
  inherent conflict in life and, 5:456–457
  in *The Maturational Processes and the Facilitating Environment* (1965), 7:306
  mental breakdown, patient's fear of, 5:458–459
  mental disability, anatomical classification of, 1:299
  neurosis, 5:367–368, 450–452; 6:254, 412
  of physical versus emotional problems, 7:346
  psychopathy, 6:412
  psychosis, 5:367–368, 450–452, 455–456, 517
  true and false self, 5:445, 453–454, 458
  usefulness of, 9:172–174
claustrophobia
  infant management and, 3:135
  potential space, DWW's concept of, 3:12
cleft palate, 11:49
Clegg, Alec and Megson, Barbara, *Children in Distress* (reviewed 1968), 8:**339**
'Cleopatra Anamnesis Imphiccough' (undated; possibly ` 1960s), 9:**381**
'A Clinical Approach to Family Problems: The Family' (1959), 5:**543–545**
'A Clinical Example of Symptomatology Following the Birth of a Sibling' (ca. 1931), 1:**155–158**, 343*n*1

Complete Index of the Collected Works

'Clinical Illustration of "The Use of an Object"' (1968), 8:**365–368**
'Clinical Material: Theme of "Two," also Theme of "Black,"' 7:**207–211**
Clinical Notes on Disorders of Childhood (1931), 1: lxi, lxii, 4–8, 10, 13, 18, **165–336**, 273*n*1; 8:285; 10:5
clinical observations, 8:9–10. *See also* case studies; rheumatic clinics
  adolescents, psychotherapeutic interviews with, 7:52–65
  of antisocial tendencies, 5:149–151; 10:16–17
  autism, 7:352–360, 362
  of beating fantasy, 5:313–315
  birth memories, 3:134, 204–206, 211, 212–213
  cardiac neurosis, 7:384–386
  'A Case Managed at Home' (1955), 5:**89–97**
  'Case Notes for a Psychoanalytic Seminar: Withdrawal, Regression, Male Identification' (1965), 7:**239–242**
  'Clinical Material on the Theme of a Male Patient's Exploitation of His Female Self' (1959), 5:**539–541**; 6:519
  'Comment on Obsessional Neurosis and "Frankie"' (1966), 7:**193–195**
  consultations, 7:10–13
  depressed parents, 5:373–376
  depression and grief, mourning, sadness, and loss, relationship between, 5:127–128
  dissociation, 7:246–247, 251–272
  'Further Clinical Material on the Theme of a Male Patient's Exploitation of His Female Self' (1963), 6:**519–522**
  guilt, absence or presence of, 7:4442–446
  'Note on Infant Observation' (undated; written after Paris IPA Congress of 1957), 9:**371–372**
  'Nothing at the Centre' (1959), 5:**469–471**
  observational unit of individual–environment setup, 4:10
  'The Observation of Infants in a Set Situation' (1941), 1: lxii, 8, 310*n*ii, 431*n*5; 2:3, 10, 16, **121–139**; 4:186; 6:467*n*2; 8:11, 283*n*ii, 306, 308
  'Observations on Asthma in an Infant and Its Relations to Anxiety' (1941), 2:10, 121
  observer's language use, 4:6
  'On the Contribution of Direct Child Observation to Psycho-Analysis' (1957), 5:**249–254**, 457
  by patients, 5:233–234, 235–236
  the Pill, 9:103–106
  primitive stages of emotional development, 4:37–43
  psychosomatic disorders, 7:70–74
  of split-off male and female elements in men and women, 7:318–323; 9:305–308
  'Spoken Comments on Obsessional Neurosis and Frankie' (1965), 7:**197–201**
  of transitional objects and phenomena, 3:448, 451–455; 5:410–412; 9:112, 270–273; 9:272; 9:279–287
  on trauma and the family, 7:171–177, 178–184, 180–183
clinical regression. *See* 'The Concept of Clinical Regression Compared with that of Defence Organisation'
clinical responsibility, sharing of, 7:4035–404
'A Clinical Study of the Effect of a Failure of the Average Expectable Environment on a Child's Mental Functioning' (1965), 8:320; 9:139*n*5
'Clinical Varieties of Transference' (1955), 1: lxxii; 5:16; 5:**61–65**; 6:467*n*2
clinics
  Child Guidance. *See* Child Guidance
  compared to private practice, 5:35–38
  public clinic, 6:19–20
  rheumatic. *See* rheumatic clinics
'Close-up of Mother Feeding Baby' (1949), 3:**289–292**
Clyne, B., *Night Calls: a study in general practice* (1961), 7:417
Clyne, Max B., *Absent: School Refusal as an Expression of Disturbed Family Relationships* (1966; reviewed 1967), 7:**405–406**; 8:**129–130**
coarctation of the aorta, 1:217
cod liver oil and malt, 9:53
coffins, 7:150
Cohn, Professor, 7:407
Coker, E. C., 1:167
colds, 1:70, 184, 193, 203, 252, 267, 285, 348, 456
Cold War, 5:6
Cole, Estelle, *Three Minutes Talks About Children* (1928), 1:17–18
Coleridge, Samuel Taylor, 1:45
Coles, Arthur, 8:379, 382, 385, 387, 389, 391, 399, 403, 406
Coles, Joyce
  acknowledged in writings by DWW, 5:302; 7:306, 309; 9:263; 10:23
  on committee to erect commemorative statue of Freud, 8:381*n*i
  Human Nature, text of, 11:28
  letters to (November & December 1968), 8:12, **379–382**, **385–391**, **399–400**, **403–406**; 9:38*n*3; **394*n*ii**
  Progressive League and, 9:101
  Clare Winnicott, correspondence with (November & December 1968), 8:379, 379*nn*i–ii, 381, 385, 387, 387*n*ii, 389, 389*n*ii, 399*n*i, 399*n*iii, 403, 406*n*v

Colgan, Bridget (pseud.). *See* James, Lydia
colic
  abdominal, 1:139, 141, 144, 231
  anxiety and, 1:183, 246, 266
  convulsions and fits, 1:306
  medical histories, taking, 1:175, 183
  mental hygiene of pre-school children and, 1:399, 400
  micturition disturbances and, 1:320
  temperature and medical charts, 1:201
colitis, 1:266, 271; 7:73–74
Collected papers: Through Paediatrics to Psychoanalysis (1958), 1:245; 2:3; 3:59, 117, 201, 245, 333, 447; 5:3, 12, 239, 345; 6:293, 401; 8:165*n*1, 165, 318; 9:92
  letter to Harvard-Watts on status of, 6:109
  preface to, 5:**301–302**
Collected Works of D. W. Winnicott (2017), 9:3
  arrangement of, 12:l–lii
  compilation of, 12:xlix–l, lv–lix
  online and in print, 12:lx
  selection of contents, 12:lii–lv
'A Collection of Children's Books' (reviewed 1967), 8:**203–204**
Collingwood, R. G., 10:5
Collinson, Michael P., letter to (1969), 9:**43–45**
Cologne, Germany, DWW on medical exhibition in, 1:**45–48**
Colonna, Alice B., 7:376
colostomy, 1:70
'Comforters' (1955), **5:12**, 77
comics, DWW recommending, 10:144, 154
'Commentary on *Play Therapy*' by Virginia Axline (book published 1947; comments recorded 1969), 9:**159–164**
'Comment on Obsessional Neurosis and "Frankie"' (1966), 7:**193–195**; 9:317*n*4
'Comments on Joseph Sandler's "On the Concept of the Superego"' (1960), 6:14–15, **127–133**
'Comments on My Paper "The Use of an Object"' (1968), 6:17; 8:15, 355, 390*n*iii, **393–395**; 9:33
'Comments on "Problems of Research in Psycho-Analysis" by Joseph Sandler' (1961), 6:**223–225**
'Comments on the Report of the Committee on Punishment in Prisons and Borstals' (1961), 6:17, **273–278**
common versus uncommon illnesses, 1:169–170
Commonwealth Fund, 9:63, 176
'Communal Feeding in Schools' (letter to *The British Medical Journal*; 1941), 2:**107–108**
communication
  between analyst and patient, 5:81; 10:32, 189
  antisocial behaviour cured through, 10:305
  'Breast-feeding as Communication' (1968), 8:**341–348**, 355
  'Communicating and Not Communicating Leading to a Study of Certain Opposites' (1963), 6:7, 10–11, **433–445**; 8:312*n*1; 11:15; 9:10
  'Communication Between Infant and Mother, and Mother and Infant, Compared and Contrasted' (1968), 8:6–7, 17, **227–237**, 249*n*i, 355
  between infant and mother, 8:86, 233–234
  'Interpretation in Psycho-analysis' (1968), 8:17, **253–255**
  'Interrelating Apart from Instinctual Drive and in Terms of Cross-identifications' (1971), 9:**319–336**
  mother-child mutuality and, 9:134–135
  noncommunication, distinguished from failure to communicate, 6:11
  objectively perceived object and, 6:437–442
  opposites of, 6:442
  physical movement as, 8:233
  string as symbol of, 6:138
  theory of, 6:436–437
compulsion
  in eating, 11:178
  in masturbation, 11:70
concentration, 6:441
  inability to concentrate, 6:394
conception, beginning of individual at, 7:449–450
'The Concept of a Healthy Individual' (1971), 8:11, **65–77**; 11:8, 9, 10
'The Concept of Clinical Regression Compared with that of Defence Organisation' (1967), 8:16; 8:30; 8:**183–189**
'The Concept of the False Self' (1964), 6:159; 7:**27–31**
'The Concept of Trauma in Relation to the Development of the Individual Within the Family' (1965), 7:**169–187**
concepts and conceptualisation, 6:15
concept-testing, 6:230
concern. *See* guilt; pre-concern; stage of; stage of concern
  capacity for, 11:15, 60, 93, 106
  transition from ruthlessness to, 11:36, 91, 151
confusion
  acute confusional state, 10:202, 204, 210, 212, 321
  'Fragments Concerning Varieties of Clinical Confusion' (1956), 5:**125–128**
congenital diseases. *See also* specific congenital conditions
  in children, 1:170–171, 214, 216–217, 290; 2:25
  heart disease, 7:384, 386*n*2
  psychological health and, 11:48–49

Congress of the International Housing and Town Planning, 1:31
Conran, Michael B., letter to (1969), 9:**53–56**
conscience, development of, 1:409
conscious, as term, 5:80
'Considerations in the Study of Homosexuality' (1963), 6:**407–408**
constipation
  anxiety and, 1:255
  central nervous system and, 1:281, 283
  convulsions and fits, 1:303
  eating disorders and, 1:414, 429
  masturbation and, 1:326
  in medical histories, 1:176–179, 182, 191–192
  in only children, 1:108
constructive activity and aggression, 7:132–133
consultations, therapeutic. *See* therapeutic consultations
'Contemporary Concepts of Adolescent Development and Their Implications for Higher Education' (1971), 8:269*n*iv; 9:57*n*i, 167*n*i, 169*n*ii, **337–348**
contented state of infant, mother's familiarity with, 2:223–224
continuity of being
  before and after birth, 11:144
  birth memories as break in, 3:212, 215–216, 217–218
  child development and, 3:404; 6:150; 10:15
  early infant agonies disrupting, 7:4–5, 46–47
  infant building, 6:155–156
  mind and its relationship to psyche-soma, 3:247, 248, 249, 250, 256
continuity of environment, importance of, 6:349
continuity of management, child's need for, 3:24
contraception. *See* birth control
'The Contribution of Psycho-Analysis to Midwifery' (1957), 5:**225–232**, 239*n*i; 8:34
'Contribution to a Discussion on Enuresis' (1936), 1:**391–395**
'Contribution to a Symposium on Envy and Jealousy' (1969), 9:**47–49**
'Contribution to the Final Number of *Case Conference*' (1970), 9:**179–180**
controlled projection test, 3:149
Controversial Discussions (1942–44), 1: lviii, lxiii–lxv, 17; 5:8, 261*n*ii; 6:217; 7:3, 377*n*i; 11:13. *See also* British Psychoanalytical Society; Klein, Melanie.
conversion hysteria, 1:135, 243, 277, 307, 321, 331, 334
conversion symptoms, 6:257
convulsions and fits
  anxiety and, 1:268, 306–307
  biting and, 1:309–312, 314*n*3

'Convulsions, Fits' in *Clinical Notes* (1931), 1:**303–314**; 8:285–287
  electrically induced. *See* shock therapy
  epilepsy, 1:146, 268, 301, 305–307, 308–314
  'Facial Nerve Paralysis, Associated with Fits' (1928), 1:**113**
  fainting attacks and, 1:307
  physical bases for, 1:303–308
  psychological basis for, 1:305–306
  pykenolepsy, 1:308
  'Treatment of Mental Disease by Induction of Fits', 2:207*n*i, **211–216**
  without physical basis, 1:308–314
Cooper, David, 9:55*n*ii
Cornell University Medical School, 1: xlvii–xlviii
corporal punishment
  of adolescents, 5:192–193
  hate in the countertransference and, 3:65
  in hostels, 2:18, 349–351, 374; 3:84, 93*n*3, 432
  'Memorandum on Corporal Punishment' (1945), 2:18, **349–351**
  progressive schools and, 7:158
  psychoanalytic research and, 7:154
  'Psychogenesis of a Beating Fantasy' (1958), 5:**313–315**
  'Psychological Aspects of Birching' (abstract; 1944), 2:**247–249**
  in school, 6:378*n*ii
  as substitute climax, 3:105
correspondents of DWW, biographies of, 12:193–210
cosmetic medical treatments, 1:70
Cottington, F., 3:356
cotton-reel game (S. Freud), 2:11, 136–137, 138*n*1, 138*n*6
couch, as symbol, 4:210, 211
'Counterfeit and Alone' (1955), 5:55
countertransference
  anticipation by DWW of later developments in understanding, 3:3–4
  in care-cure position, 9:195
  classification of phenomena of, 3:60
  'Counter-Transference' (1959), 5:**505–511**
  DWW avoiding use of technical language, 7:14
  S. Freud's introduction of term, 7:13
  hate in, 2:19
  'Hate in the Countertransference' (1947), 1: lxii; 2:230*n*i; 3:3–4, 7, 8–9, 15, **59–68**; 5:505; 9:4, 55, 355
  interpsychic processes, DWW's account of, 3:7–9
  reassurance and, 4:215; 5:107
  regression analysis and, 4:203
  split-off male and female elements in men and women and, 9:152

cousins, lack of, 4:255–256
couvade, 7:109, 371
Creak, E. Mildred, 1:463; 2:205, 205ni; 3:356; 4:35, 228, 239; 5:186
creativity. *See also* art
   artistic creation versus creative living, 9:216–217
   being and doing, 9:13–15, 215
   common to men and women, 7:318
   concept of creative living, 9:299–305
   as conceptualised by DWW, 1: lxvi–lxx; 2:16; 9:3–15
   'Creative Activity and the Search for the Self: An Added Observation on Psychotherapy in This Area' (lecture 1967), 8:169
   'Creativity and Its Origins' (1971), 8:169–170; 9:5, 6, 14, 15, 82n1, 298n3, **299–317**, 330; 10:10; 11:15–16
   defined, 9:213–215
   drives and, 9:11–13
   of everyday life, 9:5–6, 216–217
   in first year of life, 5:328
   and illusion, 11:120–121, 127, 130
   Klein on, 9:6, 11, 13, 303–304
   language as indicator of, 4:4
   'Living Creatively' (1970), 9:5, **213–224**
   maintaining, 9:215–216
   in marriage, 9:217–220
   mental illness and, 9:300–302
   and objective perception, 4:162, 169
   origins of, 9:215, 221–224
   of play, 8:274; 9:376, 377
   play and creativity, example of client in session, 8:172–179
   primary psychic creativity, 4:135, 162; 5:153, 415; 11:16, 126–128
   psychology of, 4:61
   Sargant, William, 'The Physiology of Faith' (1969), and, 9:60
   split-off male and female elements in men and women and, 9:13–15, 305–317
   subjective object and, 9:7–11
   thinking as part of, 7:144
   transitional object and, 5:410
A Criança Portuguesa (journal), 5:351; 10:165, 519
Crichton-Miller, Hugh, 3:327ni
crime. *See also* anti-social behaviour; delinquent children; punishment
   character disorder and, 6:455
   'The Child, the Family and the Offender' (1965), 7:**203–205**
   'The Child, the Family and the Young Offender' (UK Government Home Office White Paper), 7:203–205
   'Crime: A Challenge' (Oxford University group), 7:27

criminal versus lunatic, 4:97
   expiation and propitiation, value to criminal of, 3:241–242
   letter to *The Times* (1949) on punishment and crime, 3:**237–238**, 239, 241–242
   penal reform, 3:357–359
   as psychological illness, 3:44–45
   'Punishment and Crime: A Psychologist's View' (letter to *the Times*; 1949), 3:**237–238**, 241, 359, 359ni
   revenge as mitigating factor in criminal proceedings, 2:19
   WWII and increase in, 3:410
Crime, law and corrections (ed. Slovenko), 10:307
Criminal Justice Act (1948), 3:432
Cripplegate Institution, 1:59
Cromwell, Oliver, 8:366–368
cross-dressing, in *Holding and Interpretation*, 4:337
Crosse, Mary, 11:137n2
cross-identification
   case studies, 9:319–328, 330–334
   changes in patient capacity and, 9:335
   'La Interrelación en Terminos de Identificaciones Cruzadas' (1968), 9:**328–336**; 336n4
   'Interrelating Apart from Instinctual Drive and in Terms of Cross-identifications' (1971), 9:**319–336**; 10:16
   in medical profession, 9:195
   theoretical statement, 9:328–336
Crothers, B., 1:295, 297n4
cruelty
   of care-cure position, 9:195
   of children, 2:71
   enjoyment of, 2:97, 115
   in mental hospitals, 2:265
   in war, 2:90, 97–99
Cruse Clubs (later Cruse Bereavement Care), 7:99; 8:147, 149, 277
crying
   adopted child, crying to express sadness, 2:242–243
   anger, baby crying due to, 2:240–241, 244
   in *Holding and Interpretation*, 4:304, 409
   immaturity of mother and, 2:186
   pain, baby crying due to, 2:239–240, 244
   pleasure, baby crying for, 2:238; 9:302
   sadness, baby crying due to, 2:241–243, 244–245; 8:140–142
   patient not able to, 9:96–98
   'Why Do Babies Cry?' (published 1945; radio broadcast 1944), 1: lxvi; 2:21niii, **237–245**; 8:**137–142**
CSI (chronic staphylococcal infection), 1:69
Cubley, A., 1:127

Culpin, Millais, 2:29
cultural experience
　'Addendum to "The Location of Cultural
　　Experience"' (1967), 8:**207–209**
　beginning of individual and, 7:453
　concept of healthy individual and, 8:75–76
　importance of, 7:214
　letter to Renata Gaddini on (1967), 8:79–80
　'The Location of Cultural Experience' (1966),
　　7:**429–436**; 8:13, 79nii, 167, 205, 219, 300, 364
　'The Place Where We Live' (1968), 8:169,
　　221–226
　play and, 8:11
　'Playing and Culture' (1968), 8:**263–266**
　Strachey and, 8:125
'Cure' (1970), 9:**191–197**
Curtis, Myra, 2:369
Curtis Committee (Home Office Care of Children
　Committee), 2:5, 17, 18, 369; 3:162, 439
'Curtis Report on the Care of Children' (1946),
　2:**369–377**; 3:92n2, 149, 162, 350, 423; 5:72
Cuthbert, Martin, ' "Descriptive" Medicine in the
　Lay Press' (letter), 2:230
cyanosis, 1:81, 145, 212, 216–217, 305
cystitis, 1:146, 155–156, 231, 317–318, 416

Dahlberg, Charles Clay, 8:320nii
　letter to (1967), 8:**167**
Dale, Henry, 'A Prospect in Therapeutics'
　(lecture), 2:255
Danaides, 9:76
danger
　male seeking of, 7:110–111
　teaching children about, 6:31–42
Dartington Hall, Devon (progressive school),
　7:157, 163
Darwin, Charles, 1:xvi, 295; 4:62; 7:6; 8:40; 10:8
　Origin of the Species, 2:384; 7:17–18; 8:10
Darwinism, 4:62
Davidson, J. A., 1:77, 78, 82
Davidson, S. S.
　on Klein on envy, 6:316
　letter to (1952), 4:**49**
Davidson Clinic (Edinburgh), 6:523, 523n1
Davies, W. H., 'Infancy', 3:132
Davis, John, 1:7, 10; 5:438; 7:42
　letter to (1971), 9:**255**; 9:*256*
Davis, Madeleine, 1: xlviii, xlix; 9:255, 255ni; 11:3
　*Boundary and Space: An Introduction to the
　Work of D. W. Winnicott* (co-author David
　Wallbridge), 9:255ni
daydreaming
　The Daydreamer (undated short story),
　　9:**361–363**
　'Day Dreaming' (1970), 9:**247–248**
　dreaming versus, 7:10, 132

day nurseries
　initiative to close down, 4:231–232
　versus nursery school, 3:471; 4:256
deafness
　hysterical, 1:334–335, 336n4
　misdiagnosis of mental defect and, 1:302
　muteness and, 1:334–335
　in 'Speech Disorders', from *Clinical Notes*
　　(1931), 1:329
death. *See also* grief, mourning, sadness and loss
　of analyst, 8:360; 9:331
　annihilation, 6:150
　of baby under anaesthetic, 2:27
　certainty of, 8:272
　child's understanding of, 2:58–59
　coffins, actual and psychological weight
　　of, 7:150
　'Death and Murder in the Adolescent Process'
　　(1969), 9:337, **342–348**, 348n2
　of father, 9:35, 230–232
　fear of, 6:528–529
　hate and, 6:444
　lying on back equated with, 4:423–424
　of monarch, 9:181, 184, 186
　of mother, to infant, 9:285
　of parents and close family members, 1:405,
　　445–446; 11:170
　in *The Piggle*, 11:224, 232, 239–240, 247, 259, 266,
　　271–272, 307, 309–310, 315
　DWW and, 8:381, 383; 9:175, 351–353
　siblings, 1:394–395, 445–446
　in war, 2:83, 94, 97
　unconscious death wish of parents for
　　baby, 8:164
death instinct, 4:65, 66; 5:448, 501; 6:11, 17, 444;
　7:341, 413; 8:4, 45, 321, 330–331; 9:13, 34, 37,
　304; 11:17, 151
death of father. *See also* delayed reaction to death
　of father
　before child was born, 2:214–215
　found dead in road by child, 1:405
　inability to accept, 4:288–289, 339, 374–375
　Torrie, Margaret, *The Widow's Child* (foreword
　　by DWW; 1964), 7:**99**
　trauma of melancholic mother after, 7:174–176
Debré, 1:81, 83
'Deductions Drawn from a Psychotherapeutic
　Interview with an Adolescent' (1964),
　6:440nii; 7:6, **51–65**
defaecation. *See* excretion
defiance, 6:15, 118–119, 128, 132–133
　dependency and, 5:190, 270, 427
　group, 5:69, 191–192
defiance-dependency paradox, 5:190, 270, 427;
　6:189, 193, 429

deformity or difference. *See* physical deformity or difference
de Gaulle, Charles, 8:246–247
de-integration, 8:51
delayed reaction to death of father
 'A Child Psychiatry Case Illustrating Delayed Reaction to Loss' (1965), 7:11, **279–304**
'Delinquency: Continued' (ca. 1930s), 10:17
delinquent children
 Aichhorn, August, *Wayward Youth* (reviewed 1936), 1:**433–436**
 antisocial behaviour and, 3:46; 5:149; 6:158*n*16, 437i; 8:91–97; 10:17
 'The Antisocial Tendency' (1956), 1:12
 anxiety and, 1:277–278
 Auden, G. A., *The Difficult Child* (1929), discussion of (1934), 1:**353–355**
 in borstals, 6:276–278. *See also* punishment
 British Paediatric Association's interest in, 2:203
 'The Child, the Family and the Offender' (1965), 7:**203–205**
 'The Child, the Family and the Young Offender' (UK Government Home Office White Paper), 7:203–205
 child psychosis and, 3:353
 'Comments on the Report of the Committee on Punishment in Prisons and Borstals' (1961), 6:**273–278**
 confession by child, 8:95
 'Delinquency: Continued' (ca. 1930s), 2:**73–75**; 10:17
 'Delinquency as a Sign of Hope' (1968), 8:17*n*2, **91–97**
 delinquency as a symptom, 2:198
 'Delinquency Research' (1943), 2:**195–200**, 233, 234; 11:27
 'The Delinquent and Habitual Offender' (ca. 1939), 2:**31–33**
 deprivation, link to, 3:42–43, 45–47, 95; 5:151, 330, 368; 11:6
 dissociation and, 2:366
 DWW's experience of therapeutic community and, 2:8
 fear of madness in, 2:200
 A. Freud on, 7:222–225
 hostels and prevention of, 3:26, 47, 81–82
 Institute for the Scientific Treatment of Delinquency, 2:248, 291
 letter to *The Times* (1949) on punishment and crime, 3:**237–238**
 magistrate's role requiring knowledge of treatment methods, 2:233–236
 'manic defence' and, 1:366, 368, 369
 parents blamed for, 1:277
 placement of, 2:234–236, 372
 in Poor Law homes/workhouses, 1:409*n*iii
 pre-school children, mental hygiene of, 1:410–411
 probation officer, role of, 2:234–235
 psychoanalysis of, 2:32, 196, 233–235
 'Psychological Aspects of Juvenile Delinquency' (undated; ca. late 1940s), 3:**49–55**
 psychopaths and psychopathy, 5:152, 454–455
 management of, 4:279–280; 7:249*n*i
 separation from mother as cause of, 2:47–48
 'Some Psychological Aspects of Juvenile Delinquency' (1946), 3:**43–48**, 322*n*1
 stealing by. *See* stealing
 study of, 2:32, 382
 teachers, parents, and doctors, collaboration of, 1:382
 treatment of, 2:32, 203
delusional transference. *See* transference
democracy. *See also* freedom
 defined, 3:408
 developmental growth of child towards, 3:398; 5:49, 272
 education in, 3:419
 as exercise of freedom, 2:92
 gender, political leadership, and fear of women, 3:416–417, 421*n*4
 geographical boundaries, 3:418–419
 group formation and, 5:49
 immature identification with authority/society and, 3:410–411
 innate democratic tendency, 3:410–412, 421*n*2
 machinery of, 3:409–410
 ordinary good homes fostering, 3:412–414, 415, 421*n*3
 parent–child relationship in, 3:417–418
 proportional representation, 3:421*n*1
 psychiatric health and, 3:408–409
 social unrest and memory of dependence, 3:339*n*iii
 'Some Thoughts on the Meaning of the Word Democracy' (1950), 3:195*n*i, 197, 199, 405*n*1, **407–421**; 8:145*n*i
 voting and elections, 3:409, 414–415
 at war, 3:419–420
de Monchaux, C., 6:444
denial of inner reality, in manic defence, 1:363
Departmental Committee on Homosexual Offences and Prostitution (Wolfenden Report), 5:27
de Paul, St Vincent, 9:194, 195, 205
dependence, 4:194. *See also* defiance
 absolute dependence, 4:91, 185, 275, 297; 5:56, 62, 130, 294; 6:148, 471–473, 525; 8:287
 anaclitic, 5:184, 241, 446, 454
 'Dependence in Child Care' (1970), 9:247, **249–252**, 371*n*ii

dependence-independence transition, 4:38, 210, 275; 5:321; 6:40, 42, 118–119, 130, 149, 319, 351, 475–483
'Dependence in Infant-Care, in Child-Care and in the Psycho-Analytic Setting' (1962), 6:27, **333–342**; 7:176*n*ii; 8:184*n*i
'Dependence to Independence' (lecture; 1963), 6:469
double dependence, 4:197; 6:4, 414, 417; 5:321, 455, 457
DWW's focus on, 8:45
early, 11:55, 120, 149
emotional development as progression away from, 9:172
environment and, 9:304
extreme dependence, 4:276, 308; 5:252; 6:345
fear of woman and, 5:187, 294–295
infantile dependence, 4:134, 154, 252, 285, 295; 5:321; 6:145
'From Dependence Towards Independence in the Development of the Individual' (1963), 6:9, **469–477**; 8:184*n*i
healthy states of, 4:251
illness and, 9:194
inherited potential and, 6:146–147, 487–488
internal mother and, 7:411–412
memory of, 4:204
'The Mother-Infant Experience of Mutuality' (1969), 9:**131–139**
mother's death and stepmother's role, case study of, 6:474–476
mother's identification with infant and, 5:184
need satisfaction and, 7:373–374
personality growth, as part of, 7:305
pre-dependence, 11:17, 150–151
pre-dependent aloneness of newborn, 11:149–152
regression to, 4:154, 206, 207, 213, 262; 5:63, 133, 212, 448, 497; 6:7; 8:16, 186–187; 11:83, 85, 159, 174, 176
relative dependence, 6:148, 320, 473–474
reliability and, 9:192–197
risks of, 6:488–489
social unrest and memory of, 3:339*n*iii
subjective objects and, 9:133
transference and, 6:145, 334
transition to maturity, 11:10, 60, 65, 91, 136–137
trauma as failure relative to, 7:184–185
depersonalisation, 2:362–363; 4:57, 194; 6:415, 521; 9:225; 11:140–141
depression. *See also* manic defence; melancholia; stage of concern
adolescents, psychotherapeutic interviews with, 7:59, 60
anxiety and, 4:191–194
child psychosis and, 3:353; 4:276
in classification of psychiatric disorders, 5:368, 449–450; 6:254
clinical observations of parents with, 5:373–376
common occurrence of, 2:258; 259
'A Contribution to the Psychogenesis of Manic-Depressive States' (Klein, 1935), 1:14
control and, 9:116
creativity and, 9:216
definition of, 4:14; 6:461
delinquent children and, 1:434
depressed patients allowed to experience, 7:152–153
deprived children and, 3:370–371
destructive internal forces leading to, 2:69
different levels of, 5:372–373; 6:412–413, 465–466
disintegration and, 6:465
eating disorders and, 1:414, 418, 424
encephalitis and, 1:84
enuresis and, 1:392, 394
eye problems and, 2:316–317
'The Family Affected by Depressive Illness in One or Both Parents' (1958), 5:275*n*2, **367–377**
father's death before child was born leading to child's, 2:214–215
gender and, 6:464
in girls, 9:379
grief, mourning, sadness, and loss, and, 4:36; 5:127–128, 333–335; 6:413
guilt and, 5:140
health and, 4:198; 6:15, 259; 8:74
helping friends with, 3:424–425
Holding and Interpretation: Fragment of an Analysis (1955), 4:329–330
hope implied by, 5:126, 372–373
hostels for homeless children specialising in, 2:308
impurities of depression mood, 6:465–466
inner world of the child and, 11:104–105
integration of paediatrics and psychoanalysis by DWW and, 1:14, 15, 16
of Jung's mother, 7:119, 122
Kleinian terminology, Winnicott's doubts, 1: lxvi
Klein on children and, 11:105
lack of, in dictatorship, 9:118
management of, 5:371–372
medical histories, taking, 1:159, 175
mental defect and, 1:300
mother's depression affecting child, 2:156, 188–189; 6:20, 444–445; 10:138, 143–144, 153, 155, 339, 346, 365–366, 370, 399, 402*n*3, 420, 438, 518
nature of crisis, 6:464–465
as 'noble' illness, 2:259

depression (*Cont.*)
  normal emotional development and, 5:377, 452
  obsession and, 5:126
  origins of, 6:261
  of parents, 5:369–370, 373–376, 519–520
  persecution and, 5:368; 6:466
  physical examinations and, 1:188
  in *The Piggle*, 11:233, 239, 260, 277, 284, 285, 295
  post-partum, 7:180–181, 362
  pre-depressive stage, 1: lxxii
  pre-school children and, 1:399, 400, 403, 404, 406, 407, 408, 409, 411
  psyche-soma and, 1:159
  psychoanalysis of, 1: lxxii; 2:63*n*4, 252, 358–359; 6:413, 480–481, 489
  of psychoanalyst, 1: lxv
  psychology of, 5:376–377; 6:463–464
  psychoneurosis linked to, 6:463
  reactive, 5:211, 456; 6:413–414
  'Reparation in Respect of Mother's Organized Defence Against Depression' (1948), 3:12–13, 14–15, **117–122**; 5:126*n*ii
  Romeo in *Romeo and Juliet,* latent depressed mood of, 3:186, 190–191
  schizoid depression, 1: lxvii, lxxii; 6:413–414, 465, 466
  shock therapy for, 2:268; 3:73. *See also* shock therapy
  skin changes and, 1:449, 450, 453, 457, 458
  somatic effect of, 9:68–69
  spontaneous recovery from, 2:252, 258
  survival of subjective object and, 9:10*n*1
  teachers, parents, and doctors, collaboration of, 1:378, 382, 383, 386
  tendency to recover, 6:462
  therapeutic consultation, 10:397, 399, 444
  'The Value of Depression' (1963), 6:15, **4671–467**
  weaning and, 3:187–189; 4:36, 190; 6:13
  the west as a depressive society, 7:215
  WWII's effect on children, 2:98
depressive position in emotional development, 5:126
  beginnings of, 5:143, 252
  BPAS controversy over, 11:101*n*5
  'The Depressive Position' (from *Human Nature*; 1988), 11:**91–102**
  'The Depressive Position in Normal Emotional Development' (1954), 4:8, 11, 14–15, **189–204**; 5:152–153; 6:157*n*6, 233*n*i; 9:75
  diagrams of, 11:94, 96
  dramatisation of chaos after achievement of, 11:144
  grief, sadness, and, 5:127–128
  guilt in, 3:457; 11:91–93
  inner world of the child and, 11:95, 101, 104–105
  Klein on, 3:157–158, 335, 402, 457–458; 4:37, 189–204; 5:10, 11, 130, 152–153, 242, 252, 450, 499; 6:15–16, 17, 113–114, 329–330, 386, 511; 7:440; 9:75, 329; 11:15, 101*n*2
  managing bad forces and objects, 11:99–101
  preconditions for, 4:187
  recapitulation of, 11:97–99
  relationship concerns and, 11:91–93
  repression and, 11:99
  transitional objects and phenomena and, 3:457–458
deprivation
  adopted children, 5:72
  antisocial behaviour and, 5:151, 152; 6:255, 448; 7:306; 8:92; 10:304, 305, 333, 527–529
  assessment of deprivation, 3:368–371
  Bowlby on, 4:1162
  classification of broken homes, 3:368–369
  cultural experience and, 7:431, 435
  delinquency and, 3:43, 47–48; 11:6
  depression and, 3:158, 370
  'The Deprived Child and How He Can Be Compensated for Loss of Family Life' (1950), 3:**367–380**; 10:17
  diagnosis of, 7:160–161
  early history of child, importance of taking, 3:376–378
  effects on emotional development, 3:438–439; 4:133; 6:63–64, 417
  father's absence as cause of, 10:410, 418, 418*n*1
  foster parents, 3:373, 375
  hospital, visiting children in, 3:438, 441–445
  hostels, 3:373–374
  lack of time with mother before another child causing, 10:476, 492
  large institutions, 3:374, 375–376, 377–378
  love to offset, 8:317
  management of deprived child, 3:373–376, 444; 6:202–204
  non-interference with functioning households, 3:367–368
  physical care as psychological care, 3:98
  privation versus deprivation, 7:306
  resentment of deprived children, 6:81
  sexual development and, 5:28–29, 30
  symbolisation in drawings, 10:329
  therapeutic consultation, 10:399, 400, 420, 421, 438, 442, 443
  transitional objects and, 3:378–380; 10:17
  types of deprivation, 8:43
'The Deprived Mother'
  (radio broadcast; 1939), 2:5; 12:8
  (1940), 2:**35–41**
dermatology. *See* skin
de Saussure, Ferdinand, 7:407

Descuret, J. B. Felix, 3:157
desire versus need, 7:373
De Souza, Professor, 9:151
despair in clinical work, 6:72
Despert, J. L., 3:356
destruction adolescence and compulsive destructiveness, 6:103
   delinquency and, 2:71, 197–198
   loving and, 6:17
   morals and education, 6:385
   in normal children, 2:284; 6:11; 8:287
   obsessional tendency and, 6:257
   in *The Piggle*, 11:205, 213, 223, 233, 250, 253, 264, 269, 284, 286
   saying 'no' and, 6:41
   survival of breast and, 8:346–347, 361
   use of an object and, 8:394
determinism, 9:80–81
Deutsch, Helene, 3:490
development. *See* child development; emotional development; infant development
'The Development of a Child's Sense of Right and Wrong' (1962), 6:13, **295–298**
'The Development of the Capacity for Concern' (1962), 6:16–17, **351–356**
'Development of the Theme of the Inner World' (from *Human Nature*; 1988), 11:**103–106**
'Development of the Theme of the Mother's Unconscious as Discovered in Psycho-Analytic Practice' (1969), 9:**75–78**
Devine, H., 5:392
Devon and Exeter Association for Mental Health, 7:437
Devon Centre for Further Education, 7:139
devotion, 4:22, 36
diabetes, 1:66, 170, 184–185, 316; 9:193
'The Diagnosis of Chorea' (1929), 1:9, **133–140**
diagnosis of psychoses. *See* psychoanalysis
diarrhoea, 2:131
Diatkine, René, 9:130
Dibdin, Thomas, 9:187
Dick-Read, Grantly, 3:203–204; 5:239, 533
   Childbirth Without Fear: The Principles and Practice of Natural Childbirth (British Title *Revelation of Childbirth*; 1942), 5:12–13, 305
   letter to (1958), 5:**305**
   Natural Childbirth (1933), 5:12, 305
dictatorships, 2:92–93, 97; 9:118
'Didactic Statement on Child Development' (lecture; 1962), 6:325
difference, physical. *See* physical deformity or difference; race and ethnicity
'difficult child'. *See also* delinquent children
   concept of, 1:353–355

'Difficult Children' (Home Service BBC broadcast; 1945), 2:335, 343; 12:10
   foster parents, problems in placing with, 2:371
   teaching, 8:53
digitalis, 1:215, 217–218
diphtheria
   convulsions and fits, 1:305
   heart conditions and, 1:207, 213, 218
   'Hemiplegia Noticed after Diphtheria' (1929), 1:**127–128**
   measles and, 1:118
   physical examinations and, 1:188, 189
   rheumatic fever and, 1:222
   speech disorders and, 1:329
diplegia, 1:189, 292, 304; 6:66
disarmament agreements, 2:142
discipline, 4:233. *See also* corporal punishment; morality and ethics
   'Saying "No"' (1960), 6:**31–42**, 86
'Discussion of War Aims' (1940), 2:16–17, **87–94**
'Discussion on ocular psychoneuroses.'
   See 'Ocular Psychoneuroses of Childhood'
discussions (at societal meetings)
   Alger, Ian, *The Clinical Handling of the Analyst's Response* (1966), 7:**457–458**
   Auden, G. A., *The Difficult Child* (1929), discussion of (1934), 1:**353–355**
   on 'Consultation Technique' at BPAS (1946), 3:42*n*i
   'Contribution to a Discussion on Enuresis' (1936), 1:**391–395**
   Controversial Discussions (1942–44), 1: lviii, lxiii–lxv, 17; 5:8, 261*n*ii; 6:217; 7:3, 379*n*i; 11:13
   'Discussion of "Grief and Mourning in Infancy" by John Bowlby' (1959), 5:6, **495–500**; 10:18
   free discussions on specific themes or words, 5:171
   'Neurosis in the Child' (1936), 1:15
   'Notes on the Discussion Held on Dr Winnicott's Paper "The Birth Trauma"' (1949), 3:**225–228**
   'On "Separation Anxiety" by John Bowlby' (1958), 5:6, **379–381**
   of 'Skin Changes in Relation to Emotional Disorder' (1938), 1:460–462
'Disease of the Nervous System', from *Clinical Notes* (1931), 1:**281–290**
disillusionment, 2:280, 284; 6:78, 415, 472, 484
   babies as persons and, 3:99–100
   depressive position and, 4:200*n*8
   'Early Disillusion' (1939), 2:**43–45**
   family/mother providing, 7:184
   illusion-disillusionment, 4:168–171; 9:273–278; 9:276; 10:10

disillusionment (*Cont.*)
   James, Martin, on, 5:221
   process of, 8:134
   psychosis and, 4:37
   stealing impulse and, 3:322
   theory of illusion-disillusionment, development of, 4:171
   transitional objects and, 3:458; 5:413–418
   translation of term into French, 5:387
   weaning and, 3:306, 4:37, 170–171, 200n8
disintegration, 7:8–10, 8:70–71, 11:154. *See also* integration; unintegration,
   ACPP and use of term, 8:51
   anxiety associated with insecurity and, 4:57
   in artistic achievement, 8:77n1
   concern, capacity for, 6:355
   as defensive process, 11:136
   depression and, 6:465
   ego integration and, 6:394
   fear of, 2:197, 366
   in *Holding and Interpretation*, 4:313
   in letter to Masud Khan, 6:233–234
   opposed to unintegration, 2:14, 361–362, 366, 11:154
   primitive emotional development and, 2:14, 361–362, 366
   psycho-neurosis and, 6:253
   social worker's role to counteract, 6:418
   split-off elements in men and women and, 6:521
   squiggle game and, 10:119
   suffering, 8:77n1, 97, 237
'Disorders of Childhood' (1948), 3:**153–155**
displacement, and transitional objects, 3:456
Disraeli, Benjamin, 6:225
dissociation
   case studies, 7:246–247, 251–273; 10:328, 333, 334, 495
   defined, 7:247–248; 10:15; 11:154–155
   denial of antisocial behaviour, 7:245, 246, 247, 250–251, 267–269
   delinquency and, 2:366
   'Dissociation Revealed in a Therapeutic Consultation' (1966), 7:12, **245–273**; 10:307
   'Dreaming, Fantasying and Living: A Case-History Describing a Primary Dissociation' (1971), 9:**289–298**
   formlessness and, 9:295–298
   frequency of occurrence in case histories, 7:245, 246–247
   interest of DWW in, 7:8–10
   in letter to Masud Khan, 6:233–234
   lying versus, 7:247
   obsessional neurosis and, 7:198–200
   omnipotence experience distinguished, 9:298n4
   personality split distinguished, 7:247
   primitive emotional development and, 2:15–16, 363–364
   psychosomatic disorders and, 7:73–74
   simplified theoretical statement about, 7:249–250
   split-off male and female elements in men and women and, 7:321, 322, 328; 9:308–309
   stealing and, 7:245, 251–273; 10:333, 334
   symbolisation in drawings, 10:328
   theory underlying antisocial behaviour and, 7:248
   therapeutic consultation, 10:393, 402
   between true and false self, 7:305–3068
   unintegration and, 2:363; 6:233–234
distortion
   avoidable, 8:85
   classification by environmental distortion, 5:457
   'Ego Distortion in Terms of True and False Self' (1960), 3:4, 14
'Ditty on Enoch Powell' (undated, possibly 1968), 9:**395**
divorce and child development, 3:367
Dobinson, C. H., 3:472
Dockar-Drysdale, Barbara, *Therapy in Care* (foreword by DWW, 1968), 8:**409–410**
'A Doctor Looks at the Psychiatric Social Worker' (1943), 2:9, **177–193**
doctor-patient relationship, 2:17, 159–160, 266–267, 288–289, 390–391
doing and being. *See* being and doing
dolls
   DWW's childhood dolls, 3:331; 9:352; 12:300, 308
   overindulgent childhood and, 4:236
   punishment of, 12:253
   in *The Piggle* (baba; Galli-Galli; Frances), 11:204, 205, 210, 213, 217, 220–221, 225, 273, 275
   with sex organs, 3:183–184
   as transitional objects, 9:266
domination
   fear of, 5:294–295
   Holding and Interpretation: Fragment of an Analysis (1955), 4:318, 329, 336, 372
Donne, John, 9:261
Doppelgänger myth, 6:128
'Do Progressive Schools Give Too Much Freedom to the Child?' (1965), 7:**157–161**
Dostoyevsky, Fyodor, 1:308; 9:6
Dover Wilson, John, 8:397
   The Essential Shakespeare: A Biographical Adventure, 8:397ni
Dowling, R. S. W., letter to (1967), 8:**205–206**
Down's syndrome (Mongolism), 1:296n2, 301
Drake, Francis, 5:4; 6:218ni
drawings by patients. *See also* squiggle game

Complete Index of the Collected Works 383

autism and, 7:352, 353
by children with physical deformities, 9:226, 230, 231–232, 237–240, 243–244
delayed reaction to death of father, 7:281–292, 295, 296, 299, 300
dissociation case study, 7:251–273
hospitalised prepubertal child exposed to adult pervert, 7:172
Me and *Not-Me*, 11:90
in *The Piggle*, 11:310, 312–313
on suicide of sister, 9:356
trauma, the family, and therapeutic consultations, 7:172, 180–183
dreams
  aggression and, 7:132
  of anorexia patient, 7:71
  bed wetting and, 10:208
  of birth experience, 3:212–213
  of children the night before sessions, 10:30
  of children with physical deformities, 9:230–231, 238, 239
  daydreaming versus, 7:10, 132
  defence element of, 10:67
  delayed reaction to death of father and, 7:288–289, 294–297, 299
  destructive dreams, 6:55
  'Dreaming, Fantasying and Living: A Case-History Describing a Primary Dissociation' (1971), 8:171; 9:**289–298**
  dream screen (Lewin's concept), 8:418; 10:13
  'D. W. W.'s Dream Related to Reviewing Jung' (1963), 6:**501–503**; 8:355
  of DWW, 6:499; 8:208–209; 9:109
  Fairbairn on, 4:131
  in first years of life, 5:363–364; 6:148
  S. Freud on, 3:458, 461; 4:131; 9:317*n*3
  'Hallucination and Dehallucination' (1957), 5:171*n*i, **257–260**
  of hate, 4:250
  healing, 3:62–63
  horse dream in *The Piggle*, 11:273–274
  interpretation in analysis, in case study, 8:47, 101–103, 174–175, 256. *See also Holding and Interpretation: Fragment of an Analysis* (1955)
  Interrelating Apart from Instinctual Drive and in Terms of Cross-identifications' (1971), 9:322, 323; 10:16
  Jung's childhood dreams, 7:118
  reality and, 3:220*n*3, 262, 295, 296, 337
  on screaming, 9:97
  sexuality and, 3:105
  squiggle game and, 10:134
  suicidal, 6:334
  therapeutic consultation and, 10:47, 66–68, 162–163, 176–178, 199, 205, 208–210, 225–226, 229–230, 238, 244, 247, 268, 289–294, 320–324, 364, 371, 378–379, 396, 399, 434, 446–448, 451, 466–467, 469–472, 486–487, 491, 495, 512
  transitional objects and, 5:104–105
  trio of women in myths and dreams, 11:5, 74
  unconscious nature of, 10:13
dressing, in *Holding and Interpretation*
  cross-dressing, 4:337
  patient's choices, 4:424–425
drives
  creativity and, 9:11–13
  mother-child mutuality not related to, 9:136–137
  split-off male and female elements in men and women and, 9:314
  theory of, 6:17
dropping and throwing away, 3:287, 304–305; 4:186; 5:282
drugs. *See* medicines and drugs
Drysdale, Charles Robert, 2:256, 256*n*i
dummies, as transitional objects, 3:452
Dunnico, H. R., '"Pin-Up" Pictures at Approved School' (1954), 4:279–280
Durbin, Evan, 2:6
'D. W. W. on D. W. W.' (1967), 1: lxiv; 2:145; 4:137*n*i; 8:10, **35–47**, 333*n*i; 10:4, 5
'D. W. W.'s Dream Related to Reviewing Jung' (1963), 6:**501–503**; 9:33
'D. W. W.'s Notes for the Vienna Congress 1971' (Appendix I to 'The Use of an Object and Relating Through Identifications'), 8:**363–364**
'Dwelling of Psyche in Body' (from *Human Nature*, 1988), 11:**139–141**
'Dynamic Psychiatry and the G.P.' (1967), 8:129
Dynamische Psychiatrie, 8:283
dysentery, 9:107
dysuria, 1:144, 146, 316

eagerness, 8:394
earache and ear problems, 2:138–139*n*8, 186
'The Earliest States' (from *Human Nature*; 1988), 11:**143–148**
'Early Disillusion' (1939), 2:**43–45**
eating disorders
  adult cases, 1:424–425
  anorexia, 1:180–182, 413, 414; 2:189; 4:49*n*i; 6:343, 436; 7:31, 70–72, 373–374, 455; 9:244
  'Appetite and Emotional Disorder' (1936), 1:8, 14, 15, 16, **413–431**
  case studies, 1:417–424
  commonness and interrelatedness of different types of, 1:413–414
  greed and appetite, 1:413, 417, 424–425
  oral fantasy. about internal milieu and, 1:414–417
  out-patient clinic observations, 1:425–430

Ebdon, Stephanie, 1: lii, liii
Ecclesiastes 38:25, 8:271
ecology, 4:233
economics, 2:342
economics of child psychiatry, 10:526
ECT (electro-convulsive therapy). *See* shock therapy
eczema, 1:351, 357, 458, 461
Ede, Harold Stanley 'Jim', 1:**29–30**, 55*n*ii; 12:303
Ede family, 1:55
Edelston, Harry, 'Separation Anxiety in Young Children: A Study of Hospital Cases' (1943), 10:528
Eder, David, 1:11; 6:368
education. *See also* schools and teaching; training
careers in child development, 9:176–177
Chair of Child Psychiatry, need for, 5:161–163
as childhood stage, 4:233
'Contemporary Concepts of Adolescent Development and Their Implications for Higher Education' (1971), 8:269*n*iv; 9:57*n*i, 167*n*i, 169*n*ii, **337–348**
and democracy, 3:415, 419, 421
'Health Education Through Broadcasting' (1957), 5:**297–300**
moral education, 6:377–388
of parents, 3:399–401; 9:122–123
in psychoanalysis, 7:217–219
Education Act (1944), 2:5
'Educational Diagnosis' (1946), 3:**29–33**
EEGs (electroencephalograms), 9:298*n*7
'The Effect of Loss on the Young' (1968), 8:**277–278**
'The Effect of Psychosis on Family Life' (1960), 5:275*n*2; 6:12, 14, **65–72**
'The Effect of Psychotic Parents on the Emotional Development of the Child' (1959), 5:275*n*2, **513–522**; 6:135*n*i, 312*n*i
ego
body ego, 6:415, 472; 7:75
'Clinical Varieties of Transference' (1955) and, 5:61, 63, 65
communication and ego development, 6:441
depression and failures of ego organisation, 6:465
difference from American ego psychology, 6:9
ego distortion, 6:152, 159–171, 290
'Ego Distortion in Terms of True and False Self' (1960; 1965), 3:4, 14; 6:9–10, **159–171**; 7:27; 8:185*n*ii, 215, 309; 9:12–13, 278, 298*n*6, 302
ego-experience, 6:389
ego-ideal, 4:16
ego-integration, 8:112
'Ego Integration in Child Development' (1962), 6:11, **389–395**; 7:329; 8:13, 29, 184*n*iv, 186*n*vi, 305, 310*n*1, 364; 9:8, 298*n*4, 304, 316, 329; 10:6

ego mechanisms of defence, 6:145
ego nuclei, 4:43, 43*f*; 5:127
ego orgasm, 5:247
ego psychology, 9:3, 44
ego-regression, 6:342*n*3
ego-relatedness, 5:243, 245–247; 6:9, 434
ego repair, 8:280–281
ego-strength, 6:287, 336, 390, 462, 483, 489
ego structuring, 6:258, 352, 462
emergence of ego, 6:389; 7:305–306
Erikson on development of, 4:125
Fairbairn on development of, 4:134
good breast and, 5:123
Freudian theory and, 5:446; 11:79–80
infant's ego-needs, 6:160–161, 483
Kleinians and ego immaturity, 4:65; 5:181
'Mother's Madness Appearing in the Clinical Material as an Ego-Alien Factor' (1969), 9:**141–148**
naughtiness and ego development, 11:205
object-relating and, 6:392
observer ego, 4:212
premature ego development, 8:291
primary maternal preoccupation and, 5:186–188
psychoanalysis affecting, 6:287
regression and, 4:206
self versus, 7:122
Slavson on development of, 4:234
stages of development of, 6:392, 482; 8:112
use of term, 5:79; 6:389
ego support
mother giving to infant, 6:89–90, 142, 149, 230, 290, 391, 483; 7:90; 8:417
squiggle game and, 10:42
therapeutic consultation providing, 10:299, 528
Ehrenzweig, A., 9:6
Eigen, M., 8:7, 14, 16
Eissler, Kurt R., 7:408
'Ego-psychological Implications of the Psychoanalytic Treatment of Delinquents' (1950), 7:225
Eissler, Ruth S., 6:46*n*i. *See also The Psychoanalytic Study of the Child*
Ekstein, Rudolf, 8:280
Electra complex, 11:72–73
electric shock. *See* shock therapy
electroencephalograms (EEGs), 9:298*n*7
Eliot, T. S., 6:225; 8:157; 9:351; 12:307
Four Quartets, 11:20
'"Eliza" aet 7½ years' (1971), 8:413; 10:**83–112**
background, 10:83–84, 88
exploitation of the first hour, as example of, 10:111–112
hats, significance of and phobia about, 10:88, 110
pregnancy of mother as main theme, 10:110–111

Complete Index of the Collected Works

squiggle game and, 10:*84–108*, 84–109
Ellis, R. W. B., 4:228
emotional development.
  adolescent, 5:426–427
  adult, 5:426
  advice for persons seeking careers in, 9:176–177
  analysis and, 11:193
  autism as problem of, 7:351
  as basis for illness, 1:171–172
  'The Bearing of Emotional Development on Feeding Problems' (1996), 8:81
  'The Depressive Position in Normal Emotional Development', 4:**185–200**
  'The Earliest States' (from *Human Nature*, 1988), 11:**143–148**
  early infancy, emotional disturbances in, 5:73
  'The Effect of Psychotic Parents on the Emotional Development of the Child' (1959), 5:275*n*2, **513–522**; 6:135*n*1
  'Emotional Development Characteristic of Infancy' (introduction to Part III of *Human Nature*, 1988), 11:**89–90**
  'The Emotional Development of the Human Being' (Part II of *Human Nature*, 1988), 11:27, **59–86**
  environment and, 7:89–90, 180; 9:172–174; 10:31
  gender and, 7:103–105; 11:69–72
  guilt, morality, and ethics, 7:440–442
  health as emotional maturity, 5:426–428
  independence, as progression toward, 9:172
  of individuals, 5:46–48; 10:14
  of infants, 5:428
  innate tendency towards, 5:320
  instinct and, 11:65–72
  jealousy and. *See* jealousy
  Kanner and, 4:238
  in latency period, 5:427
  maturity. *See* maturity
  moral codes and, 6:383
  object relationships in, 9:328–220
  parental knowledge about, 9:123
  parental psychosis and, 5:522
  physiotherapy and, 9:69–73
  of pre-school children, 5:427–428
  'Primitive Emotional Development' (Introduction to Part IV of *Human Nature*, 1988), 11:**117**
  'Primitive Emotional Development' (lecture & published 1945), 1: lxii, lxv–lxvii, lxxi; 2:3, 12–16, 21*n*iii, **357–368**; 6:157*n*1; 9:7, 11; 11:7–8, 117*n*1
  stages of, 4:37–43, 202; 6:346–347; 8:70–72
  therapeutic consultation and, 10:155
  'Emotionally Disturbed Adolescents' (lecture; 1961). *See* 'Adolescence: Struggling through the Doldrums' (1962)

empathy, 6:359; 9:195
Empedocles, 9:34–37
emptiness, feeling of, 2:110; 6:529
empyaema, 1:190, 196, 289
encephalitis. *See also* 'Varicella Encephalitis and Vaccinia Encephalitis'
  anxiety due to, 1:272
  chorea, diagnosis of, 1:133, 250
  convulsions and fits, 1:304
  diagnosis and treatment, 1:285–288
  early experience of DWW with, 9:99–100
  'Encephalitis after Measles and Chicken-pox' (1928), 1:**115–116**
  'Measles Encephalitis' (1929), 1:**129–130**
  pathological sleeping, child with, 1:150
  post-encephalitis garrulity, 1:334
  psychosis as after-effect of, 6:66; 8:162
  Schilder's *encephalitis periaxialis diffusa*, 1:292
  'Symptoms Suggesting Post-Encephalitis' (1929), 1:**131–132**
  'Two Cases of Post-Encephalitic Hyperpnoea' (1926), 1:**95–97**
encopresis, 6:237
'The End of the Digestive Process' (1949), 3:**281–284**; 8:131
enemas, 1:178, 191, 325–326
England. *See* entries at Britain *and* British
enuresis
  Addis, Robina, paper of, 1:389–390
  anxiety and, 1:320–321
  'Contribution to a Discussion on Enuresis' (1936), 1:**391–395**
  dreams and, 10:208
  emotional diuresis and, 4:321–322
  'Enuresis' (abstract; 1929), 1:**141–142**
  'Enuresis: Notes for a Lecture to the Tavistock Children's Department' (ca. 1949), 3:**327–328**
  'History-Taking', from *Clinical Notes* (1931), 1:179–180
  in 'Micturition Disturbances', from *Clinical Notes* (1931), 1:319–322
  pathological sleeping, 1:149
  psychoanalysis and, 1:391, 393–394; 4:81–95
  'Short Communication on Enuresis' (1930), 1:**143–147**
  as symptom, not illness, 2:283; 4:831–95
  toilet training and, 1:393
environment
  for adolescents, 6:189
  African Americans, social subculture of, 7:33–34
  antisocial behaviour and, 5:150, 152
  'average expectable environment', 9:86, 137; 10:31
  birth memories and, 3:204, 210, 211–212

environment (*Cont.*)
  child's need for environmental stability, 3:24, 88, 128
  classification of environmental factors, 3:223, 381; 4:205–206, 237; 5:457
  communication between mother and child and, 5:85
  continuity of environment, importance of, 6:349
  delinquent children and, 2:234–236; 3:51–53
  dependence and, 9:304
  at different stages of development, 11:169–171
  dwelling of psyche in body and, *11:141*
  at earliest stages, 11:143–147; *11:144–146*
  emotional development and, 5:47; 7:89–90; 9:172–174; 10:31, 528
  'Environment' (from *Human Nature*; 1988), 11:**169–174**
  environmental failure, 5:46, 127, 156, 212, 455–458; 6:345, 417, 451; 10:130, 528–529
  'Environmental Health in Infancy', 8:**81–87**
  'Environmental Needs; the Early Stages; Total Dependence and Essential Independence' (1948), 3:**171–176**, 185; 10:8
  environment-individual set-up, 4:10, 37–43, 38–40*f*, 67
  environment mother versus object mother, 6:16, 353–355, 385, 436
  freedom and, 9:79–80, 85–87
  function of environment, 4:1988–191
  good-enough mothering/environment, 3:247–248, 369–370; 4:65; 5:48, 61, 244, 329; 6:11, 19, 89, 151–152, 164, 290, 320, 323, 346, 380, 390; 7:326; 8:66, 188, 314; 9:122, 134, 274, 340–342, 360
  growth and development resulting from, 3:397–398
  in hostels, 3:90–92
  importance of, 6:316–317; 7:6, 38, 306; 10:5
  infant development and, 1: lxv–lxix, 14–16, 172; 2:13; 6:150–151; 8:42–43; 9:133
  innate, inherited, or inborn tendencies and, 9:43–44
  'The Innate Morality of the Baby' (1949), 3:**299–302**
  integration into unit status and, 11:134
  Klein birthday book and, 3:223, 229, 381
  Kleinian psychology and envy theory, 9:48–49
  maladaption to, and intellectual development, 11:157
  maturational processes in context of. *See* maturity
  for mental health, 6:344
  mother-child relationship, 6:146–147; 11:171–173
  natural childbirth movement and, 5:13
  non-human, 6:505–507
  parental knowledge about, 9:123–124
  primary home experience, concept of, 3:80–81
  in psychoanalysis, 3:63–64; 4:9, 13; 7:13–14, 85–90
  psychosis and environmental deficiency, 5:455–456
  reliability of, 6:142, 151; 10:528
  schizophrenia as environmental deficiency disease, 7:233
  sense of responsibility for, 3:250
  shock treatment and, 2:265–266
  split-off male and female elements in men and women, 7:326–327
  stress as environmental issue, 9:126–127
envy, 2:17, 18
  'The Beginnings of a Formulation of an Appreciation and Criticism of Klein's Envy Statement' (1962), 1: lxviii; 5:11; 6:**315–324**; 9:47
  of breast, 9:314
  breast envy, 5:129; 6:16, 270–271, 361; 7:90
  case studies, 6:**269–271**, **403–405**
  communications between analysts, 5:85, 366
  contributing to libidinal desires, 2:134
  'Contribution to a Symposium on Envy and Jealousy' (1969), 9:**47–49**
  DWW's views on, 5:11; 6:18; 8:4
  'Envy: A Male Patient Near the End of His Analysis' (1961), 6:**269–271**, 315; 9:47
  jealousy and, 6:51
  Klein, Melanie, *Envy and Gratitude* (1957; reviewed 1959), 5:11, **433–436**
  Klein on, 5:87; 6:18, 231, 315–324, 361; 7:90, 190, 412–413; 8:45, 280, 330–332; 9:47–49
  mother's, of good care of children, 2:38
  'A Note on a Case Involving Envy' (1963), 6:**403–405**
  of opposite sex, 7:108
  oral sadism and, 5:11, 365, 433, 434, 436
  patient's envy of analyst, 6:404–405
  penis envy, 2:154; 5:122, 129, 185; 6:316
  Rosenfeld and, 5:365–366
  'A Study on Envy and Gratitude' (1956), 5:**131–132**; 9:47
epilepsy, 1:146, 268, 301, 305–307, 308–314. *See also* convulsions and fits
epiphysitis, 1:296
epistaxis, 1:183, 267
Eppel, E. M., and M. Eppel, *Adolescents and Morality* (1966; review by DWW), 7:**401–402**
Erb's paralysis, 1:295
Erb's Scapulo-Humeral Muscular Dystrophy, 1:294
Erikson, Erik, 6:388*n*2; 7:230, 326; 8:36, 47; 9:313
  Childhood and Society (1950/1951), 4:117; 7:236*n*1

Childhood and Society (1953, DWW's review of 1951 edition), 4:**125–126**
Childhood and Society (1965 paperback edition reviewed), 7:**213–214**
Young Man Luther (1958), 6:444; 7:213
Erikson, Milton, 9:150
Erleigh, Viscountess, *The mind of the growing child* (1928), 1:101
erotogenic zones, 8:67–69
errors, making use of, 9:25–26
Escalona, Sibylle, 4:117; 5:**317–318**
E.S.P. (extra sensory perception), 6:211*n*i, 211–212
Essen, Germany, 1:**31–33**
essential thrombocytopoenic purpura hæmorrhagica, 1:182
'Establishment of Relationship with External Reality' (from *Human Nature*; 1988), 11:**119–131**
ethics. *See* morality and ethics
'Ethics of Prefrontal Leucotomy' (letter to the *British Medical Journal*; 1951), 3:**467–468**
ethnic groups. *See* race and ethnicity
Europe, post-World War II
 hostels for homeless children in, 2:299–311
 refugees, 5:198, 536–537
European Congress of Child Psychiatry
 (1963), 6:447
 (Wiesbaden 1967), 8:99
euthanasia, 3:260
evacuation of children (World War II), 2:5–6, 35–41, 81–83
 antisocial behaviour of, 3:23–27, 79–81, 410
 British Paediatric Association and, 2:202
 Cambridge Evacuation Survey, 2:117–119
 'The Deprived Mother' (published 1940 & radio broadcast 1939), 2:5, **35–41**; 12:8
 development of hostels for, 3:77–78; 4:239
 'The Evacuated Child' (published & radio broadcast 1945), 2:**329–333**
 'Evacuation of Small Children' (*British Medical Journal* letter with Bowlby & Miller; 1939), 2:6, **47–48**; 10:17
 experiences of DWW with, 8:42; 9:100; 10:17
 'Home Again' (1945), 2:**353–356**
 Oxfordshire Evacuation Scheme, 1: lix; 2:8–9, 300–301; 8:42; 9:199; 12:306
 parents' relations with foster parents after return of child, 2:336
 problems with hostels for, 2:310–311
 psychological dangers of, 5:5–6
 'The Return of the Evacuated Child' (1945), 2:**335–339**
 transitional objects and separation anxiety, 9:281–283, 285–288

Evans, Philip, *Infant Feeding and Feeding Difficulties* (reviewed 1951), 3:**491–493**; 6:401*n*i
'Evidence Given to the Home Office Committee on Children's Homes' (1945), 2:349, **369–377**
evolution of human species, 6:379
examinations, physical. *See* physical examinations
excitability. *See* fidgetiness and excitability
excitement
 child management of excited state, 3:401–403
 defined and described, 5:290–291
 excited and quiet relationships, 11:119–123, *120*
 excited and quiet states, 11:77, 91, 198, 119
 'Excitement in the Aetiology of Coronary Thrombosis' (1957), 5:9, **287–291**
 experience of, 4:304, 307, 309–311, 313–314
 and first feed, 11:119–121
 instinct and, 11:66
 phases of, 9:67–68
 physiology of, 5:289–290
 primary excited impulse, 11:102*n*6
excretion. *See also* constipation; enuresis
 in '"Alfred" *aet* 10 Years', 10:180
 child's reactions to, 3:395
 control over, 6:383; 8:85–87
 depressive position and, 11:100
 disgust at, 3:395
 'The End of the Digestive Process' (1949), 3:**281–284**; 8:131
 enemas, 1:178, 191, 325–326
 flatus, manipulation of, 5:314
 incontinence of child, 2:187–188; 8:294–296
 in *The Piggle*, 11:219–221, 245–246, 257*n*IV, 274–275, 276
 psychological health and, 11:50
 relation to mother, 3:99. *See also* mother-child relationship
 toilet training, 1:393; 3:282–283; 8:293–294; 10:336
existentialism, 6:227
Exodus 3:14, 8:269*n*iv
expectancy, 10:10
experience
 concept of, 4:67
 of others, child living through, 6:56–58
 primary, 8:410
explanations, stage of, 6:37, 42
'The Exploitation of the First Interview with a Child: A Study of the Dangers and the Potential Value of Such Procedure' (lecture; 1968), 8:349
external reality. *See* reality
extra sensory perception (E. S. P.), 6:211*n*i, 211–212

eyes. *See also* blindness
  anxiety and, 1:269–270
  blinking, 1:136, 179, 246, 264, 270, 406–407
  depression and, 2:316–317
  eye-rubbing, 2:314–315
  glasses, attitude of children toward, 2:315
  interaction of infant with mother through, 8:259–260
  squinting, 2:318
  as symbol and as organ of excretion, 2:319
Ezriel, H.
  letter to (1952), 4:5, **51–52**
  'Notes on Personality Structure Suggested by the Analysis of a Schizophrenic' (1952), 4:51*n*i

Fabozzi, Paolo, 1:lxiv, lxvii, lxviii; 3:3, 9, 11
face, meaning of child putting hand to, 4:446, 457; 10:72
face masks, wearing while nursing infants, 2:227
'Facial Nerve Paralysis' (1928), 1:**111–112**
'Facial Nerve Paralysis, Associated with Fits' (1928), 1:**113**
Facio-Scapulo-Humeral Muscular Dystrophy, 1:294
faeces. *See* excretion
failure
  of adaptation, 8:44, 83, 233, 441
  of analyst/analysis, 5:64–65, 447, 482, 505; 8:357, 369, 443
  'The Aetiology of Infantile Schizophrenia in Terms of Adaptive Failure', 8:**161–165**
  creativity and, 8:77*n*1, 171, 226
  of environmental provision, 8:172, 185–188, 233, 236
  freezing of failure situation, 4:205, 224
  of reliability, 8:232
Fain, Michel, 3:341, 347*n*1
  'Importance du Rôle de la Motricité dans la Relation d'Objet' (with Pierre Marty; 1955), 5:197
fainting attacks, 1:267–268, 307; 7:120
Fairbairn, W. R. D., 1: lxvii, lxx; 4:67, 200*n*6; 5:419*n*1; 6:261; 7:434; 9:135, 373
  'Endopsychic Structure Considered in Terms of Object-relationships' (1944), 3:461
  S. Freud and, 4:129–130, 257–258, 261–263
  Guntrip in treatment with, 4:257*n*i; 6:261*n*i
  influence of, 8:4, 36, 45, 47
  Klein disagreement with, 4:264
  Psychoanalytic Studies of the Personality (1952; reviewed 1953), 4:**129–137**; 9:139*n*3
  'The Analysis of a Patient with a Genital Abnormality' (1931), 4:130
Fairfield, Letitia, 2:107–108
Fairhurst, William, 3:161

false self, 11:125–126, 131, 154. *See also* true and false self
family. *See also* death of father; father-child relationship; home; mother-child relationship; parents; siblings; trauma and the family
  breakup of, 11:170
  'The Child, the Family and the Offender' (1965), 7:**203–205**
  'The Child, the Family and the Young Offender' (UK Government Home Office White Paper), 7:203–205
  'The Child in the Family Group' (1966), 7:**387–396**
  'A Clinical Approach to Family Problems: The Family' (1959), 5:**543–545**
  Clyne, Max B., *Absent: School Refusal as an Expression of Disturbed Family Relationships* (1966; reviewed by DWW), 7:**405–406**
  dependence on. *See* dependence
  'The Effect of Psychosis on Family Life' (1960), 5:275*n*2; 6:12, 14, **65–72**
  'The Effect of Psychotic Parents on the Emotional Development of the Child' (1959), 5:275*n*2, **513–522**; 6:135*n*i
  'The Family Affected by Depressive Illness in One or Both Parents' (1958), 5:275*n*2, **367–377**
  'The Family and Emotional Maturity' (1960), 6:**117–123**
  The Family and Individual Development (1965), 9:92
  good-enough families, 7:170–171
  group in relation to individual, 7:389–390
  independence from. *See* independence
  'Integrative and Disruptive Factors in Family Life', 5:**265–275**
  interpersonal relationships and, 11:65
  at intersection of child and society, 7:309
  leaving and returning to, 7:392–393
  loyalty conflicts and, 7:393–396
  rehabilitation of, 10:19
  transitional objects and, 7:390–392
  value of, to growth, 11:73, 84
The Family and Individual Development (1965), 3:367, 397, 407; 6:423; 7:75, 75*n*iii; 8:34, 146*n*iii
  Gaddini translation to Italian, 8:8, 79, 145, 197
  letter of DWW to Italian translator (1966), 7:**399–400**
  Mazzantini translation to Italian, 8:197*n*i
  preface to English edition, 7:**309, 423**
  preface to Italian translation, 7:**419–422**, 424*n*i
family doctors, 7:155
Family Evangelism conference (1968), 8:313
Family Welfare Association, 8:58–59

Complete Index of the Collected Works 389

fantasies (phantasies)
  about the analyst, 2:155, 360
  of adoption, 5:22–23
  aggression and, 2:66, 68–69, 74, 96, 3:165, 311, 402; 7:132, 167, 190
  alimentary fantasy system, 8:437–438
  anxiety and, 1:259, 260, 268, 269, 270, 273n2, 277; 2:132, 152–153
  asphyxiation as masturbation fantasy, 3:215
  attack on mother in, 2:11, 392
  of being found, 6:433
  of birth, 3:216, 218, 251
  breastfeeding and, 2:13, 133, 392; 8:346
  breast, good and bad, 4:169, 221–222, 224
  capacity for, 7:391, 412
  of conflict against parents, 3:80, 103
  creativity and, 1: lviii, lxvi
  destruction and survival of breast, 8:346–347
  destruction and survival of cathected objects, 8:359, 362
  destructive elements of, 2:43–44, 134
  in difficult children, 1:354
  'Dreaming, Fantasying and Living: A Case-History Describing a Primary Dissociation' (1971), 9:**289-298**
  in DWW's integration of psychoanalysis and paediatrics, 1:13–16
  eating disorders and, 1:414–417, 415, 416, 417, 421, 427, 428, 429, 430
  eating fantasy of infant, 6:296–297
  emphasis of DWW on, 6:131, 133
  enuresis and, 1:141, 144–147, 390, 392–394
  environment and, 1: lxvi–lxvix; 2:70
  versus reality, 3:296, 337; 7:90, 107. *See also* reality
  fear of domination by fantasy women, 3:417
  in first year of life, 5:324; 6:354
  frustration and, 2:70
  gender and, 7:107
  hate and, 2:70
  heart disorders and, 1:208
  illusion and, 2:365; 4:161
  illusion-disillusionment, 4:168–171
  imagination and, 5:324, 386
  imaginative elaboration of function, 7:141, 166; 11:75–76
  inadequacy of idea of, 11:110
  of infants, 2:130, 132–133
  inner world and, 1:xxiii–xxiv
  instinct theory and, 11:81–82
  in Kanner's *Child Psychiatry*, 1:440
  'manic defence' and, 1:359–364, 366, 368, 369, 371–373, 373n1
  masturbation fantasies, 1:141, 144, 157, 320, 323–328; 2:44, 69–70, 169, 199; 4:282, 318, 353

  medical histories, taking, 1:182
  micturition disturbances and, 1:320, 321
  myth and, 4:196
  neurosis and, 5:165–166
  of only children, 1:104, 106
  oral fantasies and eating, 5:468
  oral hostility, 1:182
  orgiastic functioning and, 9:369–370, 390
  papular urticaria and, 1:344, 347–352
  pathological sleeping and, 1:150
  penis and, 2:133
  persecution fantasies, 1:14, 376, 377, 379–380, 382, 384–387, 434, 447, 457
  of personality and body, effect of the treatment on, 2:267–269
  phallic woman/woman with penis, 4:16, 327, 339
  physical examinations and, 1:188
  play and, 2:168–169
  of pre-school children, 1:400, 403, 404, 405, 407, 408, 409
  primitive fantasy, 6:64, 157n9
  of primitive love impulse, 3:314, 320
  psyche-soma and, 1:xxix, 159
  'Psychogenesis of a Beating Fantasy', 5:**313-15**
  in psychoanalysis, 3:121–122
  of re-entry into mother head-first, 3:214
  regression and, 4:55
  repressed fantasy, 6:257
  rheumatism and, 2:58–60, 63n4
  richness of concept, 7:412
  sex fantasies, 3:104–106; 5:267–268
  shock therapy and, 2:268
  shyness and, 1:448
  siblings and, 1:157
  skin and, 1:453, 454, 455, 456, 458, 459
  speech disorders and, 1:330, 336n4
  subjective object and creative illusion, 9:7–8
  term usage for, 6:260n2
  therapeutic consultation and, 10:377, 389, 399, 466, 471, 491–492
  thinking and, 7:143
  toys as means of expressing, 1:374n7
  transitional objects and, 3:458, 459; 5:387
  transitional objects and phenomena in analysis of adult patient, 9:284–288
  uses of, 1:359
  value of illusion and transitional states, 4:169–171; 11:123–126
  withdrawal and, 4:308, 309
  WWII's effect on children and, 2:83, 99
Farjeon, Eleanor, *The Wonderful Knight* (reviewed 1967), 8:203–204
Farrington, B., *Greek Science* (1953), 8:390, 390niii, 394nii, 401; 9:38n3
fat distribution, in children, 1:119; *1:121*

'The Fate of the Transitional Object' (1959), 5:12, **523–528**; 11:130nⅲ
father-child relationship. *See also* death of father; parents
  abusive fathers, 9:30
  adopted child, 4:152
  birth process and, 5:176, 226–227
  delayed reaction to loss of. *See* delayed reaction to death of father
  depressive position in emotional development and, 11:92
  discipline and, 6:42
  DWW's view of father's role, 6:6, 9
  family, role in, 7:389
  father-daughter relationship, 2:274
  father-son relationship, 2:275
  S. Freud on, 9:33–35
  guilt of child over death of father, 5:140–141
  loyalty conflicts and, 7:394
  new baby and father's role, 8:33
  paternal and maternal phalluses, 5:160
  preparation for, 7:331–332
  psychotic parents, children with, 5:517
  separateness, establishment of, 6:6–7
  sexual development in children and, 3:102–104, 105–106
  sibling rivalry, role of father in, 6:59
  Torrie, Margaret, *The Widow's Child* (foreword by DWW; 1964), 7:**99**
  true and false self and, 7:29
  'What About Father?' (published 1945 & radio broadcast 1944), 2:21nⅲ, **271–275**
  whole object, father as, 6:6
'fathers and mothers' (childhood game), 3:106, 307–308, 445; 4:251, 276
fear
  of being laughed at, 4:309, 401, 404
  of breakdown, 5:459; 6:466, 523–531, 531nⅱ
  chorea, as cause of, 2:50
  of death, 6:528–529
  of domination, 5:294–295
  'Fear of Breakdown' (ca. 1963), 5:458nⅱ; 6:**523–531**; 7:4–5, 6, 233nⅰ, 238; 8:269nⅳ
  of homosexuality, 4:324
  infant's fears upon coming independent, 6:295
  Ernest Jones on, 3:490
  leucotomy, associated with, 3:481
  of madness, 4:58, 6:275; 7:229, 233–238
  normal, 3:396; 6:208–209
  of nuclear war, 5:6; 7:152, 403
  psychology of, 11:85n2
  of women, 3:416–417; 5:187, 294–295; 7:126–127
Federn, Paul
  'Ego Psychology and the Psychoses' (1952), 3:179nⅰ
  letter to (1949), 3:**179–180**
feeding. *See also* breastfeeding; weaning
  advising parents about, 5:280–281; 8:119–120, 152–153
  'The Bearing of Emotional Development on Feeding Problems' (1996), 8:81
  belching, 3:278–279
  bottle versus breast, 2:391–393; 3:277–278, 304; 5:419–420n9; 8:342, 343; 9:288n2
  'Close-up of Mother Feeding Baby' (1949), 3:**289–292**
  digestive process, 3:278–280; 8:295–296
  disturbance in infancy, 2:124–125, 284–285
  'The End of the Digestive Process' (1949), 3:**281–284**; 8:131
  Evans, Philip, and Ronald MacKeith, *Infant Feeding and Feeding Difficulties* (reviewed 1951), 3:**491–493**; 6:401nⅰ
  as focus of newborn, 8:344
  'Infant Feeding' (published 1945 & radio broadcast 1943–44), 2:21nⅲ, **293–297**
  'Infant Feeding and Emotional Development' (1968), 8:81
  institutional versus maternal, 3:289–292
  maternal knowledge about, 3:388
  mother-child relationship and, 3:309
  paediatrics and psychiatry, interplay between, 3:125, 130–133
  psychological health and, 11:49–50
  reality, introduction of child to, 3:296–297
  refusal of food and finickiness, 2:283; 3:395; 6:132; 8:152–153
  spoon game (spatula game), 3:285–288, 304
  theoretical first feed, 4:38, 40f
  transitional objects and, 5:116–117, 118
  'Where the Food Goes' (1949), 3:**277–280**
'Feeling Guilty' (1961), 6:**205–210**
Fees, C., 2:8
female sexuality, 11:70
feminism. *See also* gender
  DWW's definition of, 7:106
  'This Feminism' (1986), 7:5, **103–111**, 126nⅰ
Fenichel, O., *The Theory of Neurosis* (1945), 6:447–448, 459n1
Ferenczi, Sandor, 1: lvii, lxii, lxxii; 5:392, 398n8, 446–447; 6:5; 7:14; 8:44
Ferrier, Camilla, 1:xliii
Ferro, A., 1: lxv
Ferruta, Anna, 1: lxxviii; 7:3
fertilised ovum/ova and creation of twins, 2:343–344
fertility symbols, numbers as, 10:330, *331*–332
fetishes and fetishism, 5:417–418, 419; 9:273
feverish attacks, 1:197–201, 227
fidgetiness and excitability

chorea and, 1:136–140, 247–253; 2:50
common fidgetiness due to anxiety, 1:245–246, 250, 266
crying by baby. See crying
differential diagnosis of, 1:249–253; 4:195
enuresis and, 1:144
'Fidgetiness', from *Clinical Notes* (1931), 1:**245–253**
micturition difficulties leading to, 1:192
mother's familiarity with excited state of infant, 2:223–224
tics or habit-spasms, 1:246–247, 250
Field, Joanna, 3:461
Fieldman (one of analysts of patient Q), 4:75, 77
fierceness, 8:367, 425, 428–429, 430, 437, 438–439
Fine, Bernard D., 8:12, 391, 393, 393*n*i; 9:36
finger-sucking, 2:367–368; 3:452, 454; 4:418; 5:101–102. See also thumb-sucking
Finland
  Finnish Psychoanalytic Society, 1: lix; 6:237, 241; 8:8, 18*n*6
  '"Iiro" case study. See '"Iiro" aet 9 Years 9 Months'
  '"Matti," aet 12 1/2 years: A Therapeutic Consultation' (1961), 6:**237–239**; 10:15
  'Sakari: A Therapeutic Consultation' (1961), 6:**241–253**; 10:15
'First Experiments in Independence' (1955), 5:12, **101–105**
'First Interview with Child May Start Resumption of Maturation' (1968) (report quoting DWW), 8:**349–354**; 10:253
First World War. See World War I
'The First Year of Life: Modern Views on the Emotional Development' (1958), 5:**319–331**; 7:43; 8:34
  Luria letter on, 6:105
Fisher, Dr, Archbishop of Canterbury, 7:449, 452
fits. See convulsions and fits
Fitzgerald, Otho W. S., letter to (1950), 3:**351–352**
FitzHerbert, Joan, letter to (1961), 6:**211–212**
'The Five-Year-Old' (1962), 6:135*n*i, **309–314**
fixation
  fixation points in emotional development, 4:205
  oral fixation, 4:131–132
  Wilson, Ambrose Cyril, 'The Rôle of Fixation in Perversion and Masturbation' (1947), 5:399
Flarsheim, Alfred, 1: lxxiii*n*iv; 8:388
flatus, 5:314
Fleming, G. W., 2:107–108, 207
flight to external reality from internal reality, in manic defence, 1:363
flight to sanity, 4:210; 8:73
Flügel, J. C., 2:19; 3:147*n*i; 5:392

The Moral Paradox of Peace and War (reviewed 1941), 2:115*n*i, **115–116**
foetus
  miscarriage and mother-foetus relationship, 9:390
  'A Note on the Mother-Foetus Relationship' (undated; first published 1989), 9:**389–390**
  quickening of, 7:450
  viability of, 7:451
Folger, 1:85
Follett, M. P., *Creative Experience* (1924), 3:483
food. See eating disorders; feeding
Foord, Alan, 4:117
Foote, Estelle J., *Six Children* (1956; reviewed 1957), 5:**223–224**
Fordham, Frieda, 7:192
Fordham, Michael
  'Counter-transference' (1960), 5:506, 508, 509, 510
  on de-integration, 8:51
  'The Empirical Foundation and Theories of the Self in Jung's Work' (1963), 7:122, 124*n*3
  An Evaluation of Jung's Work (1962), 7:122, 124*n*2
  influence of, 8:38
  on isolation, 6:443
  letters from DWW (1965) to, 7:17, **145, 189–190, 191–192**
  letter to (1954), 4:**245**
  letter to (1955), 5:**79–80**
  letter to (1970), 9:**169–170**
  letter to DWW (1965) from, 7:145*n*i
  letter to *The Times* (1966) with DWW and others, 7:365–366
  'Reflections on Training Analysis' (1970), 9:169
forewords by DWW
  Briance, Prunella, *Childbirth with Confidence*, 5:**533–534**
  The Case as the Patient Sees It: Psychoanalysis, National Association of Mental Health (1957), 5:**235–236**
  Dockar-Drysdale, Barbara, *Therapy in Care* (1968), 8:**409–410**
  Gardner, D. E. M. *Susan Isaacs: The First Biography* (1969), 8:**333–334**
  Graham, Joan (Malleson, J. Graham), *Any Wife, Any Husband* (1955), 5:**99**
  Milner, Marion, *The Hands of the Living God* (1969), 2:19; 8:**115–116**
  Tod, Robert, *Disturbed Children* (1968), 8:10, **261–262**
  Torrie, Margaret, *The Widow's Child* (1964), 7:**99**; 8:277
formlessness, 9:295–298
'For Stepparents' (1955), 5:**55–59**

Forster, E. M., *The Hill of Devi* (1953), 8:407
Forsyth, David, 1:11, 18; 5:392
 'The Psychology of the New Born Infant' (1919), 1:11
Fortes, Professor, 7:407
Fortnightly (Leys School magazine), 1:31, 39, 45
Forum (journal), 9:317n7
Foss, B. M., *Determinants of Infant Behavior, Vol. 2* (1962), 7:44
foster parents
 adoption compared, 5:70–72
 analogous situation to evacuated children homes, 2:332–333
 of child of psychotic parent, 5:513–516
 for children from broken homes, 3:373, 375
 difficult children, problems in placing with, 2:371
 psychiatric social workers and, 3:426
 social change and policy toward, 4:254
 Tod, Robert, *Disturbed Children*, 8:261–262
Foucault, Michel, *Les mots et les choses* (1966), 9:303
'The Foundation of Mental Health' (1951), 3:**437–439**
'Found Objects and Waifs' (undated; from 'Ideas' file), 9:**373–374**; 10:4, 10, 13
'Fragments Concerning Varieties of Clinical Confusion' (1956), 5:**125–128**
Francis, Sir Frank, 7:407
Frank, Klara
 'A Case of Over Indulgence', 4:234
 letter to (1954), 4:**234–236**
Frankl, Liselotte, 6:233, 399; 7:221
Franklin, Marjorie, 2:7–8, 103, 103nii, 291
 letter to (1944), 2:**291**
Fraser, Francis, 1:4, 5, 6, 167
 Surgery of childhood (1926), 1:335n1
Frazer, J. G., *The Golden Bough* (1911), 1:441; 9:107nii
free association
 Holding and Interpretation: Fragment of an Analysis (1955), 4:449
 Klein treating play as equivalent of, 5:7
 in latency period, 5:356
 relaxation and, 8:171
freedom. *See also* democracy
 in child psychiatry, 9:172
 determinism, resistance to concept of, 9:80–81
 environment and, 9:79–80, 85–87
 'Freedom' (1969), 9:**79–82**
 personality effects of, 2:91; 6:94
 psychiatric disorder and sense of loss of, 9:81–82, 84–85
 'Responsibility and Freedom' (letter to *British Medical Journal*; 1943), 2:217–219
 sharing of responsibility and, 2:93

 'The Threat to Freedom' (1969), 9:**83–87**
 willingness to fight to preserve, 2:89–90
Freeman, Tom, 7:227
freezing of the failure situation, 4:205, 224
Fremont-Smith, Frank, 3:487
French-British disagreement over psychoanalysis, 6:45–46
Freud, Anna. *See also The Psychoanalytic Study of the Child*
 on adaptation, 8:16
 on adolescents, 5:173
 on aggression, at Royal Society of Medicine symposium (1947), 3:148niii, 333, 473
 American psychiatry and, 4:239
 arrival in Britain, 5:7; 8:41
 background of, 4:219, 241
 basic principles of psychoanalysis and, 5:353
 'B' Group in BPAS and, 5:7, 261
 Bonnard and, 4:45
 Bowlby and, 5:496–497; 6:283
 'breast', wider meaning of, 5:420n9
 Burlingham as co-author with, 4:37, 101
 Casuso and, 5:159ni
 circle of influence, 3:474
 classification of psychiatric conditions and, 5:446, 447
 Controversial Discussions (1940s), 1: lviii, lxxiii–lxxv; 5:8, 261nii
 developmental model of, 1:xvi
 discussion groups with, 2:80
 DWW compared, 1:xv
 DWW influenced by, 4:203n7; 11:6, 32
 DWW relationship with, 5:8; 6:8; 8:4, 336; 10:18
 ego-regression and, 6:342n3
 Hampstead Clinic. *See* Hampstead Child Therapy Course and Clinic (now Anna Freud Centre)
 Hampstead War Nurseries, 9:94
 Harms, Ernest, ed. *Handbook of Child Guidance* (1947; reviewed 1949), 3:235
 Hoffer and, 8:9, 110
 on identification with the aggressor, 3:347n6
 on importance of technique in caring for infants, 11:128
 influence of, 6:325; 8:4, 39, 279
 Klein-Freud controversy, 2:5, 9; 4:64, 174n11; 5:6–8, 10–11, 12, 19–20, 33, 87, 261nii, 366; 6:325, 331
 latency period, psychoanalysis in, 5:354, 355
 letter to (1948), 3:**147–148**
 letter to (1955), 5:**87–88**
 letters to (1958), 5:**337, 347, 383**
 letter from (1968), 9:7
 letter to (1969), 8:15, 18n8; 9:**41–42**
 letter to *The Times* (1966) with DWW and others, 7:365–366

on losing and being lost, 8:279
on masturbation and antisocial behaviour, 2:70
Mead, Margaret, and, 5:204
on mother-child relationship, 3:126; 4:75
Nagera, Humberto, and, 7:147
on need satisfaction, 7:373
on onset of separation anxiety, 2:359
on oral instinct and fantasy, 1:429
on parent-infant relationship, 6:4
photograph of, *4:17*
primary maternal preoccupation and, 5:183–184
'Psycho-Analysis and Education', 5:87
publication of *Standard Edition of the Psychological Works of Sigmund Freud* (1966) and, 7:408, 410
reparation, DWW's concept of, 3:13
review of JamesRobertson's *Going to Hospital with Mother* (film), 5:531*n*1
Ries, Hertha, and, 4:123
Riviere, Joan, and, 5:255
Rosenfeld, Eva, and, 6:211*n*ii
seventieth birthday of, 7:243
Sigmund Freud's principles carried on by, 9:93–94
Spitz, René and, 5:255*n*i
transitional objects and, 8:11, 301
Young-Breuehl's work on, 1: liii
Freud, Anna, works of
'Aggression in Relation to Emotional Development: Normal and Pathological' (1947), 3:147*n*i, 148*n*iii
'Contributions of Direct Child Observation to Psychoanalysis', 5:261*n*iii
The Ego and the Mechanisms of Defence (1937), 3:460–461; 6:157*n*5, 255, 263, 331; 8:393; 11:85*n*1
Indications for Child Analysis and Other Papers (1968/1969; reviewed 1969), 9:**93–94**
Menninger Bulletin paper on ego-regression (1963), 6:342*n*3
Normality and Pathology in Childhood (1965; reviewed by DWW), 7:14, 16, **217–225**, 227, 377
'Problems of Infantile Neurosis' in *Psychoanalytic Study of the Child*, 5:183
The Psycho-Analytical Treatment of Children (1946), 5:355
The Psychoanalytic Study of the Child, Volume 20 (multiple editors; 1966; reviewed by DWW), 7:**375–376**
'The Widening Scope of Indications for Psycho-Analysis' (1954), 5:62
Young Children in Wartime: A Year's Work in a Residential War Nursery (with Dorothy Burlingham; 1942), 5:497; 10:18
Freud, Ernst, 7:407; 9:41
Freud, Mrs. Ernst, 7:407

Freud, Sigmund
accomplishments of, 3:397
adult findings applied to children by, 2:131
on aggression, 3:339; 8:331
on anaclitic dependence, 5:184, 241, 446, 454
on analyst's voluntary state of attentiveness, 6:155
Angst defined by, 3:208
Anna Freud and, 6:325; 7:217, 219; 9:93–94
on antisocial behaviour, 5:147, 149, 153; 11:6
on anxiety, 2:129; 5:383; 6:157*n*15
arrival in Britain, 5:7, 203
Balint on, 6:43–44
basic principles of psychoanalysis and, 4:115
Beyond the Pleasure Principle, 3:208
Bion and, 7:96
on birth trauma and anxiety, 3:201–202, 207, 208, 209, 217, 228; 11:162, 165, 167*n*1
on bisexuality, 9:14
Bowlby and, 4:113; 5:379
Bund and, 6:368
censor, use of, 1:341
Centenary celebrations, 5:395–396
on character and analysis, 6:448
on childhood roots of adult psychoneurosis, 3:123
on child psycho-neuroses, 5:251–252, 352
on children and childhood, 5:130
choice of cases by, 4:207
classical interpretative techniques of, 11:13
classification of psychiatric conditions and, 5:445–446, 449, 451, 454
commemorative statue, committee for, 8:381, 381*n*i; 9:*18*; 12:3–4
comparing psychoanalysis to archaeology, 8:280
cotton-reel game, 2:11, 138*n*1; 6:142; 136–137
countertransference, introduction of term by, 7:13
on creativity, 9:6, 11–12, 13, 304
cultural experience and, 7:429, 433
cure as secondary aim of psychoanalysis, 2:146
on death instinct, 4:65, 68; 5:180, 501; 6:17, 330; 7:413; 8:321, 330–331; 9:304; 11:17, 150
on denial, 3:14
on dream formation, 9:317*n*3
on drives, 6:17
DWW compared, 1: lvii; 2:136–137; 4:15; 9:3; 11:18, 19
DWW criticism of, 6:7, 18, 330
DWW influenced by, 1: lvix, lx, lxii–lxiii, lxxviii, 53, 54, 167; 2:19, 109, 147–148, 358; 4:7; 6:3, 330; 8:4, 10, 35, 38, 42, 65, 170, 187; 11:10, 32
DWW's loyalty to, 9:60
DWW's theoretical writings and, 7:4, 229
on the ego, 5:79; 6:415; 7:75; 9:359

Freud, Sigmund (*Cont.*)
  on emotional development after age five, 9:207–208
  English translations of, 1:11
  on epilepsy, 1:308
  on evolution of humans, 6:379
  Fairbairn and, 4:129–130, 257–258, 261–263
  on father-child relationship, 9:33–35
  on fusion, 6:352
  on guilt, 5:136–137, 138, 145, 329; 7:440
  Guthrie and, 1:5–6
  on hallucinatory wish-fulfilment, 6:5, 152
  in Harms, Ernest (ed.), *Handbook of Child Guidance* (1947; reviewed 1949), 3:235
  Human Nature (DWW) and, 11:4, 6, 63
  on hypnosis, 4:459, 461
  on id-establishment, 8:67
  on infancy, 6:4, 142–145, 150, 152, 352–353; 7:305
  on infantile sexuality, 3:102, 103, 397, 490; 5:326, 428; 6:156; 11:80–81
  on inorganic state, 11:150, 151
  instinct theory of, 11:18, 79–80, 81
  International Psycho-Analytical Library and, 6:235
  on interpersonal relationships, 11:63, 89
  Isaacs, Susan, and, 3:161
  as Jew, 6:368
  Jones, Ernest, and, 3:489, 490; 4:53; 5:203, 309, 310, 311, 389–397
  Jung and, 7:15, 115, 116–117, 119–121; 8:62
  Klein, Melanie and, 6:113, 145
  Moses and, 9:303
  on knowledge, 9:391
  language use and terminology of, 4:6–7
  life of, 5:7; 6:367–370
  Little Hans analysis, 6:142–143
  'love' as used by, 1:438; 6:213
  manic defence and, 1:362
  marriage of, 6:369
  on maternal care's importance, 6:143
  Margaret Mead and, 5:203
  on melancholia, 2:252; 5:10, 153, 333, 449
  methodological approach of DWW and, 3:6; 4:207–208
  modification of theory of, 9:133, 356
  on mother-child relationship, 3:66
  narcissism and, 6:44
  Nemon's statue of, *9:18*; 12:3–4
  neurosis and, 4:124; 11:59–60, 63
  obsessional neurosis, theory of, 3:257n1
  Oedipal complex and, 3:102–103; 6:15, 129, 479; 11:72–73, 78, 83
  other analysts' view of, 4:472
  paediatrics and child psychiatry, 5:424
  on phallic phase, 7:105–106
  poetry and mental illness, 7:315
  on pregenital versus genital sexuality, 6:160
  on pre-school children, 5:130
  psychoanalysis, development and theories of, 2:146–147, 216, 384–386; 4:207–209; 6:217–220, 481; 8:11, 14, 42, 222
  psychoanalysis, influence on, 9:26, 60, 80, 135, 330, 391
  psychoanalytic setting of, 6:203
  psychological paediatrics and, 5:170
  on reaction to loss, 4:198
  on regression, 4:201, 207–208, 217n1; 7:85
  reparation, DWW's concept of, 3:13
  on repetition-compulsion, 4:131
  on repression, 5:180, 363; 6:142
  Rickman, J., personal communication to (1905), 11:167n1
  Riviere, Joan, as translator of, 3:221
  Rosenfeld, Eva, and, 6:211nii
  Sargant, William, 'The Physiology of Faith' (1969) on, 9:59–60
  scientific psychology and, 3:70
  on self-preservation, 6:17
  on sexual trauma in childhood, 6:335
  society and culture permeated by ideas of, 7:156, 425
  on stages of emotional development, 5:61
  Strachey, James, and, 3:435; 4:53; 8:124–126
  on superego, 6:15, 127–133; 7:439; 11:79
  on transference and countertransference, 5:506, 507
  on transitional objects, 3:458–459, 460, 461
  on 'tripartite division of mind', 4:130
  on the unconscious, 3:43, 54; 4:107; 6:438, 526–527
  Zetzel on, 6:335
Freud, Sigmund, works of
  'Analysis of a Phobia in a Five-Year-Old Boy' (1909), 11:191, 192n4
  Analysis Terminable and Interminable (1937), 9:33, 34, 38n4
  Beyond the Pleasure Principle (1920), 5:501
  'Case of Dora', 4:173n2
  'A Child Is Being Beaten', 5:313
  '"Civilized" Sexual Morality and Modern Nervous Illness' (1908), 9:12
  'Collected Papers' Vol. 3, 3:459
  'Creative Writers and Day-dreaming' (1908), 9:11–12
  'Dostoevsky and Parricide' (1905), 1:314n1
  The Ego and the Id (1923), 3:460; 4:168; 9:274
  Female Sexuality (1931), 11:4, 74
  Fliess Letters (1895), 3:461
  Formulations on the Two Principles of Mental Functioning (1911), 6:4, 143–144
  Group Psychology and the Analysis of the Ego (1921), 3:202, 460; 4:173n9; 5:419n7
  'Inhibitions, Symptoms and Anxiety' (1926), 5:380; 6:8
  Instincts and their Vicissitudes (1915), 3:65

International Psychoanalytical Library, works included in, 6:235*n*i
The Interpretation of Dreams (1900), 1:10; 2:385; 3:458; 4:131; 6:220; 7:409; 9:60, 317*n*3
'Introductory Lectures on Psychoanalysis' (1916–1917), 2:384; 3:459
Letters of Sigmund Freud, 1873–1939 (E. Jones, ed.; 1961; reviewed 1962), 6:**367–370**
Moses and Monotheism (1939), 5:397; 9:33–38, 303
'Mourning and Melancholia' (1917), 4:37; 5:449; 6:328; 11:101*n*3
The origins of psycho-analysis (1950), 4:418*n*8
Project for a Scientific Psychology, 3:461*n*i
The Psychopathology of Everyday Life, 2:385
Standard Edition of the Complete Psychological Works of Sigmund Freud (Strachey, ed. 1966), 1: lxxviii; 7:15, 18, **407–410**, 431; 8:123, 126; 9:12
'Three Essays on the Theory of Sexuality' (1915), 3:459; 9:12
Totem and Taboo, 4:472–473; 6:6
Freud, Sophie, 6:370
Freud, W. Ernest, 8:281
Freudenberg, R., 2:261
Friedlander, Kate, 1: lxiv; 2:195, 233, 234; 3:126–127
letter to, 2:**79–80**
Friedmann, Manna, 5:536–537
Friedmann, Oscar, 5:173
obituary, 5:**535–537**
Friedreich's ataxia, 1:293
friendship
adolescent's friendship, 2:190
desire for, in *Holding and Interpretation: Fragment of an Analysis* (1955), 4:321, 361, 449
psychotherapy resembling, 6:203
fright. *See* fear
'From Dependence Towards Independence in the Development of the Individual' (1963), 6:9, **469–477**; 8:184*n*i
'From Instinct Theory to Ego Theory' (Part IV of *Human Nature*, 1988), 11:27, **117–178**
Fromm, Erich, 8:320*n*ii
From Paediatrics to Psychoanalysis (1958), 1: lxix
Frontiers of Clinical Psychiatry, 8:349
frozen (affectionless) child, 8:409
frozen failure situation, 4:205, 224
frustration
aggression and, 6:214
failure situation and, 4:224
fantasy and, 2:70
of mothers and what irks them, 6:73–86
newborn and, 4:23, 168; 6:290
tolerance/intolerance of, 4:63, 154, 168
weaning and, 4:170
Fry, Margery, *Child Care and the Growth of Love* (1953), 3:405*n*2
'Funeral Address for Ernest Jones' (1958), 5:**309–311**, 349

'Further Clinical Illustration of "The Use of an Object"' (1968), 8:**369–377**
'Further Clinical Material on the Theme of a Male Patient's Exploitation of His Female Self' (1963), 6:**519–522**
'Further Thoughts on Babies as Persons' (1947), 3:**95–100**
fusion, 6:148, 352, 435
futility, 4:67; 6:10, 100–101, 192, 527–528

Gabrielle. *See The Piggle*
Gaddini, Eugenio, 7:16; 8:401; 9:39, 111, 189
'On Imitation' (1969), 9:112
Gaddini, Renata
letter to (1969), 9:**39–40**
letter to Renata and family (1969), 9:**111–113**
letter to (1970), 9:**189**
background of, 8:8, 79, 145, 197, 401
on DWW as both paediatrician and psychologist, 8:8
The Family and Individual Development (Preface to Italian translation by), 7:419–422
letter to (1964), 7:**83–84**
letters to (1966), 7:16, **399–400**, **423**
letter to (September 1966), 8:197*n*i
letter to (November 1966), 8:197*n*i
letter to (March 1967), 8:**79–80**, 197*n*i
letter to (September 1967), 8:**145–146**
letter to (November 1967), 8:**197–198**
letter to (October 1968), 8:325, **337**
letter to (December 1968), 8:**401**
letter to (1969), 8:18*n*8
on paper of E. Gaddini, 9:112*n*ii
on transitional objects and phenomena, 9:263
Gaddini, Sylvia, 9:112
Galeerd, Elizabeth, 3:157
Galli, P., 1:79, 88
Gallup Polls, 7:426
Galsworthy, John, *Forsyte Saga* (1922), 8:209
games. *See also* play; squiggle game
cotton-reel game (S. Freud), 2:11, 136–137, 138*n*1, 138*n*6
'doctors and nurses' (childhood game), 4:251
'fathers and mothers' (childhood game), 2:273; 3:106, 307–308, 445; 4:251, 276
Jason playing game with DWW, 10:*488–490*, 488–491
King of the Castle game, 7:75, 80; 9:343; 11:243, 244, 245
noughts and crosses, playing with DWW, 10:276, *277*, 288, 288–289, 408
Patty-cake (game and song), 11:280–281
pencil game, 4:277–278
spatula game, 1: lxiii, 5, 8, 138, 188, 190, 273, 310, **425–431**; 2:10–11, 16, 122–126, 132–138; 3:285–288, 304; 8:309–310

Gardner, Dorothy E. M.
  letter to (1959), 5:**473-474**
  Susan Isaacs: The First Biography (foreword by DWW; 1969), 8:**333-334**
Garma, Angel, 6:4
Garrod, Archibald, 1:4-5, 6
  introductory chapter to *Diseases of Children* (1913), 1:5, 296*n*1
gastric ulcer, 11:177-178
Gay (encephalitis researcher), 1:83
gaze, 8:5, 259-260
Geigy Bequest Lecture, Sussex Postgraduate Federation (1968), 8:221
gender. *See also* split-off male and female elements in men and women
  adopter preference for female babies, 7:312
  aggression and, 8:93-94
  birth of male sibling and girl's desire to be a boy, 9:231
  'Case Notes for a Psychoanalytic Seminar: Withdrawal, Regression, Male Identification' (1965), 7:**239-242**
  character disorders at adolescence, 6:455-456
  'Clinical Material on the Theme of a Male Patient's Exploitation of His Female Self' (1959), 5:**539-541**
  cross-identification of, 7:104
  danger, male seeking of, 7:110-111
  depression and, 6:464
  differences between sexes, 7:103, 109-110
  emotional development and, 7:103-105; 11:69-72
  envy of the opposite sex, 7:108-110
  false self, disclosure of, 6:69
  fantasy and, 7:107
  female imaginative identification with male, 11:69-70
  feminism and, 7:106, 110-111
  goat as symbol of male instinct, 8:435
  in letter to a Confidant ('M') (1966), 7:**371-372**
  masculinity, in *Holding and Interpretation: Fragment of an Analysis* (1955), 4:325, 339, 342
  mother's depression, reaction to, 9:76
  narcissism and, 6:425
  not-me possession, no gender difference in use of, 4:163
  phallic phase and, 7:105-107
  pre-school children and gender identity, 7:104-105
  'The Split-Off Male and Female Elements to Be Found in Men and Women', 6:519
  therapeutic consultation and gender identity, 10:260, 269, 284, 344, 530
  'This Feminism' (1986), 7:5, **103-111**, 126*n*1
  transitional objects and phenomena, 9:269
  trio of women in myths and dreams, 11:5, 74
  true and false self and, 7:29
  woman, birth of all men and women out of, 7:108-110
  woman patient's acute sense of women as third-class citizens, 9:330, 333-334
general paralysis of the insane, 7:232
Genesis 1:2, 11:16
genetics and heredity, 5:69, 457; 8:44-45, 70
  adoption and, 5:76
  environment and, 8:66, 184, 236*n*1
  as external factors, 8:66, 236*n*1
  inherited tendency towards growth, 8:184, 227-228, 232, 235, 272, 314-315, 324, 350; 9:43-44
  integration activity and, 4:44
  Klein on inheritance, 8:332
  psychological health and, 11:47
  schizophrenia and, 4:439
genital dominance, stage of, 4:205, 206; 11:1, 67, 68, 69-71, 74
geographical boundaries of democracies, 3:418-419
'"George" aet 13 Years', 10:**495-514**
  acting in plays and acting as way of getting real feelings, 10:512
  admitting to delinquencies, 10:512
  annihilation of self and, 10:508
  crying as a baby and, 10:510
  delinquent behaviour, 10:495, 509-510
  difficulty of case and treatment required, 10:512-513
  dissociation and, 10:495
  dreams and, 10:495, 512
  forgetfulness and, 10:512
  gender identity and, 10:509
  hoarding and, 10:510, 513
  lack of sense of humour and, 10:497, 503
  noise, desirability of, 10:512
  sleep issues and, 10:511
  spoiling George as family's way of dealing with him, 10:511
  squiggle game and, 10:496-508, *497-508*
  stealing as issue, 10:496, 509
  transitional phenomena and, 10:511-512
  unwanted pregnancy producing George, effect of, 10:511
George III (king of England), mental illness of, 7:315
Gerber Baby Council, 8:81
Germany
  allied occupation of, 5:6
  British versus German behaviour, 2:88-89
  Essen, Germany, DWW on, 1:**31-33**
  post-World War I, 8:145
Gesell, Arnold, 3:461; 4:104; 6:371
gestalt psychology, 4:52
'Getting to Know Your Baby' paper (1944), 9:134*n*1

paper (1945), 2:**221–225**, 287*n*i, 293
radio broadcast (1943–44), 2:21*n*iii, 221; 8:117
radio broadcast (1945), 12:10–11, **245–249**
pamphlet (1945), 12:lvi, 9, 11, 20
Giannakoulas, Andreas, 3:11; 4:107
Gibbs, Edith, 1:59
Gibbs, Nancy, 1:75
Gilbert and Sullivan, 'The Yeoman of the Guard', 5:125*n*i
Gillespie, R. D., 11:101*n*4
Gillespie, William H., 1: lxix*n*iii, 9, 353; 3:225; 5:365
  The Edge of Objectivity: An Essay in the History of Scientific Ideas (1960), 9:317*n*2
  letter to (1966), 7:**403–404**
gingivitis, 1:296
Giovacchini, Peter, letter to (1970), 9:**167**
Gisburne House, Watford
  letter to Miss Maw on (1959), 5:439
  'Memorandum on Gisburne House' (1959), 5:**441–443**
Glover, Edward, 1:10; 2:5; 3:121, 167; 4:30, 64; 5:127, 392, 394, 399, 400; 7:14, 221, 409*n*7; 11:101*n*5, 137*n*1. *See also The Psychoanalytic Study of the Child*
  On the Early Development of Mind (1956), 5:456
  letter to (1951), 3:**475**
  'The Position of Psycho-Analysis in Great Britain' (1949), 5:456–457
  Psycho-Analysis and Child Psychiatry (reviewed 1953), 4:**115**
Glover, James, 5:392, 399, 400
goat, symbolism of, 10:105
God. *See also* religion
  child presenting himself at analysis as, 11:108–109
  as the 'Great I AM', 7:75
  Jones, Ernest, 'The God Complex', 5:397
  '"Milton" *aet* 8 Years' and, 10:294–295
  one-ness with God/Universe, 6:530–531
  of seventeenth century compared with God of present day, 8:366–367
  theological paradox of existence of God, 8:265
'going concern', family as, 8:94
Goldfarb, William, 4:113
  Childhood Schizophrenia (1961; reviewed 1963), 6:**509–510**
Goldman, Dodi, 1: lxxi
Goldsmith, W. N., 1:454
Gombrich, Professor, 7:407
gonorrhoea, 1:4, 68
Goodacre, Iris, *Adoption Policy and Practice* (1966; reviewed by DWW), 7:**427–428**
Goodall, E. W., 1:115, 132
'good' as cliché, 8:332*n*1
good breast, 6:16, 270, 320–324; 7:96; 8:340; 11:95–96

Goodenough, Sir William, and Goodenough Report, 3:243
good-enough analyst, 6:322–323, 335; 8:6; 10:8
good-enough families, 7:170–171
good-enough mothering/environment, 3:247–248, 343, 369–370; 4:65; 5:48, 61, 244, 329; 6:11, 19, 89, 151–152, 164, 290, 320, 323, 346, 380, 390; 7:326; 8:66, 188, 314; 9:122, 134, 274, 340–342, 360
'good-enough' versus good, DWW's use of, 9:91
Goodhart, J. F., 2:49, 51; 7:380
good internal object, 5:244
Good King Wenceslaus (Christmas carol), 11:310
'good mother', 4:63–64
goodness, 2:88; 6:378
Gordon, M. B., 1:79
Gordon, R. G., *A Survey of Child Psychiatry* (1939), 1:18
Gorer, G., 5:198
  The People of Great Russia: A Psychological Study (with J. Rickman; 1949), 11:141*n*1
Gorky, Maxim, 4:126; 7:214
gossip, 4:365
Gough, Donald, 8:212
  letter to (1968), 8:9, 212*n*i, 234*n*iv, **259–260**
Gould, Stephen J., 7:18
Government Paper on Children in Hospital (1959), 5:544
Graham, Joan. *See* Malleson, Joan Graham
grandparent-child relationship, 2:186
Grant, Duncan, 7:409
Grassi, Aldo, 7:18
gratitude
  Klein's envy statement and, 6:319
  of patients for medical professionals, 9:195–196
  residential therapy and, 9:204–205
  'A Study on Envy and Gratitude' (1956), 5:**131–132**
Graves, Robert, 7:315; 9:59
  Graves & Podro, *Nazarene Gospel Restored*, 8:158
  letter to *The Times* (1966), 7:315–316*n*i
  Mammon, 8:105–106
gravity, effects of, 11:147–148
Great Britain. *See entries at* Britain *and* British
greed, 1:392, 413; 2:135; 5:154–155, 198, 330; 6:486–487
  aggression and, 68, 89
  appetite and, 1:422
  economics and, 2:342
  feeding and, 2:44, 225, 239
  healthy, 2:285
  inhibition of, 1:418–419, 423, 424
  love, hate and, 1:14, 362, 372, 377
  as primitive form of love, 2:68, 89, 134, 342
  normal greediness, 1:15, 425
  in war, 2:142

Greek mythology, 6:517; 9:76, 311, 381. *See also* Oedipal complex
Green, André, 1: lvii, lxv; 11:10, 13, 14, 19
 'The Dead Mother' (1980), 3:15*n*vi
Green, F. H. K., 1:61, 290*n*2
Greenacre, Phyllis, 3:201, 202–203, 207, 217, 220*n*1, 222, 226, 227; 5:184; 6:4, 9, 160; 8:391; 9:39; 10:17
 'Awe in Childhood', 5:318
 'The Childhood of the Artist', 5:363
 'Considerations Regarding the Parent-Infant Relationship' (1960), 8:272*n*v
 influence on DWW, 8:12, 36, 44, 363*n*1
 on parent-infant relationship, 6:4, 115, 359, 363
 in *The Psychoanalytic Study of the Child,* Vol. 15 (1961), 6:284
Greenfield, J. G., 1:132
Greenson, Ralph R., 7:199; 8:29
grief, mourning, sadness, and loss. *See also* death
 baby crying due to sadness, 2:241–243, 244–245; 8:140–142
 Bowlby's 'Separation Anxiety' on, 5:496–500
 depression and, 5:127–128; 6:413
 'The Effect of Loss on the Young' (1968), 8:**277–278**
 A. Freud on, 8:279–280
 love associated with sadness, 4:312
 psychology of mourning and separation anxiety, 5:334–335
 reaction to loss, 4:198; 6:133
 'A Tendency in Therapeutics' (1944), 2:258–259
 tendency to recover, 6:462
Griffith, Dr, 1:461, 462
Griffith, George, *Valdar the Oft-born,* 8:228, 228*n*i
Grinstein, Alexander, 5:390
 The Index of Psychoanalytic Writings (1957), 5:398*n*2
Groarke, Steven, 1:xlii, lxxiv; 11:3
Grolnick, S. A., 8:17
Grosskurth, P., 1:12
groups
 adolescence as group management issue, 5:190–193, 427
 classification of cases and, 5:52–54
 formation of, 5:48–50
 group defiance, 5:69, 192
 'Group Influences and the Maladjusted Child: The School Aspect' (1955), 5:**45–54**; 8:79*n*i
 group therapy, 9:201–202
growing pains
 anxiety and, 1:266
 chorea and, 1:9, 138, 171
 fidgetiness and, 1:251, 252
 'Growing Pains', in *Clinical Notes* (1931), 1:**235–238**

rheumatic fever and rheumatic carditis, 1:171, 216, 219, 227
tonsillectomies and, 1:205
'Growth and Development in Immaturity' (1950), 3:**397–405**
Grunhut, Max, 7:27
Guerin, Carroll, 9:111
guilt
 absence of sense of, 5:144–145; 7:442–446
 'The Absence of a Sense of Guilt' (1966), 7:**437–452**
 'Aggression, Guilt and Reparation' (1960), 6:**97–104**
 antisocial behaviour and, 2:198, 200, 248; 3:241–242
 autistic children, guilt feelings of parents of, 7:347, 349, 354, 360–362
 child's symptoms as cause of parental guilt, 2:150; 6:69
 creative artists and, 5:145
 depressive position and, 3:457; 11:91–97; 11:94, 96
 destructiveness as cause of, 2:43, 134, 197, 359
 development of sense of, 4:154, 193; 5:136–141, 377, 449; 6:17, 303, 383, 391
 emotional development process and, 7:440–444
 expiated, as defence, 11:85
 'Feeling Guilty' (1961), 6:**205–210**
 in first year of life, 5:329
 gang membership and, 2:200
 intention, residing in, 5:135, 136
 Ernest Jones on, 3:490
 Klein on, 4:75, 193
 loss and recovery of sense of, 5:145–147
 masturbation and, 2:199; 8:432
 origin of sense of, 2:391, 5:141
 parents and, 5:298; 6:13
 'Psycho-Analysis and the Sense of Guilt' (1956), 5:**135–147**; 6:157*n*6, 473*n*2
 psychopathology of guilt sense, 5:139–141
 punishment and, 2:350
 relief from, 2:70, 244
 reparation and, 3:117; 5:56, 131
 sexual, 10:54
 shock therapy and, 2:267
 sickness a bodily form of, 2:198
 stage of concern and, 3:335–336, 402–403; 4:14; 5:329; 6:351
 superego and, 5:136, 138–139
 war as cause of, 2:94, 142
Gull, William, 1:127
Guntrip, Harry, 1: lxxii; 4:261; 6; 6:235
 letter to (1961), 4:137*n*i; 6:**261**
 'My Experience of Analysis with Fairbairn and Winnicott' (1975), 6:261*n*i
Guthrie, Leonard, 1:5–6

Functional Nervous Disorders in Childhood
  (1907), 1:5; 11:38*n*1
'Functional Nervous Disorders' in *Diseases of*
  Children (1913), 1:5
'The Gwrw Tree' (1948), 3:**143–145**

habit-spasms or tics, 1:136, 246–247, 250
haematuria, 1:79, 183, 318, 347
'Hæmoptysis: Case for Diagnosis' (1931),
  1:**151–152**; *1:152*
hæmorrhagic nephritis, 1:79, 183, 318, 203221
hair-pulling by infant, 8:327–328, 337, 3357*n*i
Haldane Report, 1:4
Hall, Maida, 7:191
hallucinations
  auditory, 9:145–147
  creation and, 11:123
  as dream phenomena, 9:300
  'hallucinated satisfaction', 6:150
  'Hallucination and Dehallucination' (1957),
    5:171*n*i, **257–260**; 7:151*n*i
  'hallucinatory magic omnipotence', 6:5
  persecutory, 7:290–291, 292, 301
  and transitional object, 5:409, 523–524
  wish-fulfilment, hallucinatory, 6:5, 152
Halmos, Paul, 7:37–39
  letter to (1959), 5:**467–468**
Hambling, John, 5:288
  'Emotions and Symptoms in Essential
    Hypertension' (1951), 5:291*n*1
  'Psychosomatic Aspects of Arterial
    Hypertension' (1952), 5:291*n*1
Hampstead Child Therapy Course and Clinic
  (now Anna Freud Centre), 5:87, 337*n*ii, 536;
    6:306; 7:147, 217, 220–221, 375; 9:41
Hampstead War Nurseries, 5:8, 87, 337*n*ii, 497; 8:9,
    110; 9:94; 10:18
handling
  inducing psychosomatic partnership in
    infant, 6:91
  as maternal function, 7:43
hands, child's reluctance to draw, 7:257–260,
  257–261, 265, 266, 267. *See also* Ada
happiness
  patient's refusal to acknowledge, 4:235
Hardcastle, D. N., 2:268, 269*n*2
Hardenberg, Janet, 7:127
Harding, D. W.
  'Donne's Anticipation of Experience' (1963),
    7:144*n*1
  'The Hinterland of Thought' (1963),
    7:141*n*ii, 144*n*1
Hardy, Thomas, 'The Self-Unseeing', 7:144*n*1
Harms, Ernest (ed.), *Handbook of Child Guidance*
  (1947; reviewed 1949), 3:**235**
Harrington squares, 5:102; 11:124
Harris, Armstrong, 8:17*n*1

Harris, W., 1:118*n*1
Hart, Bernard, 1:9, 11
Hartmann, Heinz, 3:341; 4:219; 5:256, 318, 364, 447;
  6:450, 506; 8:12, 36, 38, 44, 391; 9:86, 93, 137.
    See also The Psychoanalytic Study of the Child
  Ego Psychology and the Problem of Adaptation
    (1939), 7:391*n*i; 9:87*n*1, 304
  Ego Psychology and the Problem of Adaptation
    (1958), 8:162*n*ii
  libidinal theory of
    Hartmann-Kris-Loewenstein, 8:393
Harvard-Watts, John, letter to (1960), 6:**109–110**
Haskell, Arnold, 3:119
hate and hatred. *See also* love
  within aggressive impulse, 2:16, 65, 68
  in analysis, 2:359; 9:55, 194
  of analyst, 5:506
  of babies, 9:107–108
  capacity for feeling, 2:17; 3:80, 148, 369; 11:170
  in care-cure position, 9:194–195
  child's, for foster parents, 3:375
  death and, 6:444
  dependence and, 9:325–326
  dreams of, 4:250
  DWW recognising within himself, 2:19;
    3:38; 4:259
  fantasy and, 2:70
  for father, 3:103; 5:137; 9:30; 11:73, 77–78, 84
  feelings of, in baby or child, 8:134, 141
  frustration and, 2:70, 197; 3:311
  'Hate in the Counter-transference' (1947),
    2:230*n*i; 3:3–4, 7, 8–9, 15, **59–68**; 5:505; 6:86*n*i;
    9:4, 55, 355
  Jones, Ernest, on, 3:490
  love and, 2: 65, 134, 197, 215, 347, 367; 3:61, 64;
    4:22, 153–154, 178, 186, 193, 202, 208, 251;
    5:137–140, 166–167, 427; 6:214, 383; 9:127, 346;
    11:36, 97, 155, 176, 178
  manifested as envy, 2:17
  masturbation and, 5:243
  in mother-child relationship, 3:66–67; 5:56–57;
    6:17; 9:77–78, 293
  mother's hate of baby or child, 5:58, 447
  mourning and, 5:334
  for new baby, 2:325; 4:22
  for parents, 2:213–214, 243, 248, 273–274,
    356; 5:269
  play as release for, 2:167
  projection of, 2:268; 4:66, 133
  repressed, 3:44, 370
  for rivals, 4:464, 468, 470, 473
  sentimentalism as denial of, 9:4–5
  in transference, 3:**59–68**, 70
  'Trips into Partisanship', 8:**191–193**
  in wartime, 2:97, 99
hats, child's phobia of women with, 8:293,
  438; 10:110

Hazlehurst, R. S., letter to (1949), 3:**239**
headaches, migraines, in anxious children, 1:139, 198, 237, 267
head-banging, 4:294
healing, social worker's role in, 6:419
healing dreams, 3:62–63
health. *See also* mental health
   of adolescents, 6:193–194
   'The Concept of a Healthy Individual' 8:11, **65–77**
   'The Concept of Health Using Instinct Theory' (from *Human Nature*, 1988), 11:**75–86**
   as continuity of being, 11:144, 149–150
   depression and healthy individual, 6:259
   development and living fully, 6:12–18, 347
   DWW's concept of, 11:11–14, 17–18, 36–38
   as emotional maturity, 3:95, 408–409; 5:426–428; 6:10, 13, 121–123, 344, 410, 414
   'Hypochondriacal Anxiety' (from *Human Nature*; 1988), 11:**113–114**
   'Ill-Health' (from *Human Nature*; 1988), 11:**43–46**
   intellect and, 11:40–41
   life's purpose and, 8:74–75
   psyche health, 11:40
   psyche ill-health, 11:44–45
   social health, 8:65, 69–70
   somatic health, 11:39–40
   somatic ill-health, 11:43–44
   three lives of healthy people, 8:11, 75–76
   types of people divided into classes by psychological health, 8:72–73
Health Act, 5:438
'Health Education Through Broadcasting' (1957), 5:**297–300**
'Health Magazine' (Home Service BBC broadcast; 1945), 2:353
health visitors
   training of, 5:339–344
   weaning and, 3:303
Heaney, Seamus, 1: lix
heart and heart disease. *See also* cardiac neurosis; chorea; pre-systolic murmur; rheumatic fever; thrill
   'Active Heart Disease', from *Clinical Notes* (1931), 1:**229–233**
   auscultation, 1:212–213
   congenital conditions, 1:214, 216–217; 7:384, 388*n*2
   examination of the heart, 1:208–209, 212–213, 231–232
   'Excitement in the Aetiology of Coronary Thrombosis' (1957), 5:9, **287–291**
   'The Heart, with Special Reference to Rheumatic Carditis', from *Clinical Notes* (1931), 1:**207–218**, 232

heart failure, 1:217–218
   hypertrophy, 1:135, 208, 209, 210–211, 232, 251–252
   mitral stenosis, 1:153–154, 211, 212, 215–216, 232
   'On Cardiac Neurosis in Children' (1966), 7:**379–386**
   percussion, 1:211–212
   position of the apex beat, 1:209–214
   'Pre-systolic Murmur, Possibly Not Due to Mitral Stenosis' (1931), 1:**153–154**
   systolic murmur, 1:214, 231–232
   systolic thrills, 1:209
Heimann, Paula, 1: lxv; 3:226, 229, 233; 4:30, 52, 61, 123; 5:307, 349; 6:330; 7:377*n*i; 11:101*n*2
   'A Contribution to the Re-evaluation of the Oedipus Complex: The Early Stages' (1951), 7:230, 238*n*2
   letter to (1959), 5:**501**
   'On Counter-transference' (1950), 3:3*n*ii
Hellman, Ilse, 6:115
   letter to (1960), 6:**107**
Hellmann, Miss, 5:173
hemiplagia
   'Case for Diagnosis (? Infantile Hemiplegia)' (1926), 1:**93–94**
   chorea, diagnosis of, 1:134
   convulsions and fits associated with, 1:304
   'Hemiplegia Noticed after Diphtheria' (1929), 1:**127–128**
   mental defect and, 1:299
   walking disorders and, 1:295
Henderson, David K., 1:439*n*1, 11:101*n*4
   letter to (10 May 1954), 4:**227–229**
   letter to (20 May 1954), 4:**227–239**
Hendrick, Harry
   Children, Childhood and English Society, 1880–1990 (1994), 1:17*n*viii
   Child Welfare: England: 1872–1989 (1997), 1:17*n*viii
Hendrick, Ives, 4:117
Henoch, E., 2:49; 7:380
   Lectures on children's diseases (1889), 1:253*n*1, 308, 314*n*2; 8:284*n*i, 282–284, 296*nn*1–2, 321, 323*n*1, 335
Henriques, Basil, 3:431
Henry, Hannah 'Queen'
   DWW staying with, after separation from first wife, 3:197, 383
   letter to (1950), 3:**383–384**
Henry Ittleson Centre (New York City), 6:509–510
heredity. *See* genetics and heredity
Hermann, I., 4:56
hermeneutics of suspicion, 11:13
Hernandez, M., 3:11
hernia operation, 10:453, 474, 476
Heseltine, Philip, 9:117

hesitancy, 2:10–11
'"Hesta" aet 16 Years', 8:351*n*i; 10:**253–274**
  background, 10:253–254
  dreams and, 10:268
  gender identity and, 10:260, 269
  manic-depressive disease and, 10:254, 272
  patient's acceptance of mental illness as diagnosis, 10:253
  penis envy and, 10:261–262, 265
  squiggle game and, 10:254–264, 254–272, 269–272
hidden antisocials, 3:410–411, 420
hierarchies, in psychoanalysis, 9:193–194
Hill, Adrian, *Art Versus Illness* (1948; reviewed 1949), 3:**265–267**
Hill, Sir Dennis, 7:339, 407
Hill, Geoffrey, 11:20
Hill, T. R., 1:142
Hillary, Sir Edmund, 7:262
Hiller, Eric, 5:392
Hilton, Annie, 1:43
Hilton Hotel (London), 8:192, 192*n*ii
Hippocrates, 5:507; 7:417; 11:83
Hirschberg, J. Cotter, 8:349, 352–355
history-taking. *See* medical histories, taking
Hjulmand, Knud, 12:5
Hitler, Adolf, 2:88; 4:126; 7:214
HMS *Lucifer*, DWW's service on, 1:3–4
Hoares, Sir Frederick, 7:4079
Hobhouse, Neill, 1:91, 94
Hodge, S. H., letter to (1949), 3:**241–242**
Hoffer, Willi, 5:198, 261, 408; 7:436*n*2; 9:202, 202*n*i. *See also The Psychoanalytic Study of the Child*
  'Development of the Body Ego' (1950), 8:9, 110, 112–113
  'Infant Observation and Concepts Relating to Infancy' (1966), 8:110
  letter to (1952), 4:**47–48**
  on mothering in infant care, 6:157*n*5
  'Mouth, Hand, and Ego-Integration' (1949), 8:9, 110*n*i, 110–112
  'The Mutual Influences in the Development of Ego and Id: Earliest Stages', 6:467*n*1
  The Psychoanalytic Study of the Child, 4:173*n*2
  on transitional objects, 3:461
  tribute to (1967), 8:9, **107–113**
Hogarth Press, 6:235*n*i
Holder, Carole, 9:63, 64, 65
holding (concept of)
  as authority function, 7:80
  babies as persons and, 3:96–97
  birth memories and, 3:209
  care-cure position of medical professionals and, 9:196–197
  in casework, 5:486, 490, 491; 6:158*n*19, 489
  communication and, 8:231–232
  failures in, 6:9–10; 7:42–43; 8:7; 10:136
  elevator phobia and, 7:194
  gravity, effects of, 11:148
  healthy being and, 8:70
  infant development during holding phase, 6:147–148; 8:83–84
  insecurity first associated with, 4:56
  knowing/learning and, 3:388–391
  mother-child mutuality and, 9:137–139
  mother's holding, 4:155, 187, 191, 194, 197–199, 251–253; 6:4–5, 90–91, 201; 8:315
  primary introduction to reality and, 3:168
  psychotherapeutic consultation as type of, 8:414
  residential therapy as form of, 9:203–204
  satisfactory parental care and, 6:146–147
Holding and Interpretation: Fragment of an Analysis (1955), 1: lxi, lxxiii; 4:**303–474**
  abstraction becoming reality, 4:446
  analyst's role, 4:349–350
  anger, 4:433–434, 450, 452
  antisocial behaviour, 4:336–337, 400–401, 425–426
  anxiety, perfection to counter, 4:328
  boredom, 4:446
  break in between sessions, patient's reaction to, 4:286–288, 332, 373–374, 379, 390
  breast-feeding, reliving of, 4:351
  cannibalism, 4:308, 309, 311, 315, 349, 350
  career management, 4:315–316, 348, 376–378, 386–387, 393, 394, 416, 442, 461–465, 464, 468–469
  castration anxiety, 4:310, 323, 384, 396, 398
  child putting hand to face, meaning of, 4:446, 457
  cigarette smoking, 4:418–419, 420
  conditional love versus love, 4:402
  crying, 4:409
  death, lying on back equated with, 4:423–424
  depression, 4:329–330
  domination, 4:318, 336, 374
  dream of girls with penis, 4:326, 329, 372
  dreams, 4:319–320, 324, 326, 329, 331–332, 363–364, 400, 407, 409, 423, 425, 445, 450, 453–456, 461, 464–465
  dressing, patient's choices, 4:337, 424–425
  excitement, experience of, 4:304, 307, 309–311, 313–314, 369
  father-daughter relationship, 4:319–320, 336, 351, 371
  father's death, 4:339, 374–375, 390, 425, 427
  father's role and failure, 4:353, 362, 357
  father-substitute, psychoanalyst as, 4:366, 405, 414, 473
  fear of being laughed at, 4:309, 401, 404
  finger-sucking, 4:418
  free association, 4:449

Holding and Interpretation: Fragment of an Analysis (1955) (*Cont.*)
  friendship, desire for, 4:321, 361, 449
  gender equality, 4:325–326
  general practitioners (GPs), 4:441
  gossip, 4:365
  guilt, 4:306, 422
  hatred for analyst, 4:370
  hatred for rivals, 4:464, 468, 470
  homosexuality, 4:304, 322–323, 324, 409, 424
  hopelessness, expression of, 4:434–435, 445, 458, 460
  impotence, 4:339–340, 344, 346, 347, 382, 390
  incest, 4:319, 323–324, 338, 368
  latency period, 4:427
  masculinity, 4:326, 339, 342
  masturbation, 4:318, 319, 321, 353, 358, 398
  Montessori principle, 4:376
  mother-father relationship, 4:380–382, 404
  mother-in-law, relationship with, 4:409, 410, 451
  mother's analysis, 4:396
  mother's attitude toward son and his analysis, 4:337, 352, 361, 377, 380, 403, 405, 413, 426, 429, 435, 443, 448, 451, 453, 457
  mother-substitute, psychoanalyst as, 4:414, 427, 456, 473
  penis, dream of girls with, 4:326, 329, 372
  perfection, attainment of, 4:328, 380–381, 383, 431–432, 453
  play, 4:316–317
  prattling, 4:310, 312, 401, 403, 405, 410, 429, 454
  premature ejaculation, 4:319
  progress in analysis, assessment of, 4:309, 321, 340–342, 343, 349–350, 357, 358–359, 411, 416, 428, 447, 450, 455, 471
  promiscuity as option for future, 4:357
  psychosis versus neurosis, 4:438
  punctuality of patient, 4:324, 334, 415–416
  punishment, 4:351
  reality, 4:328–3340, 369
  schizophrenia as diagnosis, 4:439, 440
  separation, acceptance of, 4:468
  sexual intercourse, 4:286, 304, 319, 334, 361, 371
  showing off to mother, 4:340, 342
  silence during sessions, 4:388, 427–429, 431
  sisters, relationship with, 4:336, 396, 426, 437–439, 463
  sleepiness or sleeping during analysis, 4:323, 332–333, 344, 345–346, 349, 389, 396, 407, 422, 423, 426–427, 428, 430, 432–433, 435, 444, 446, 450, 451–452, 455, 467, 468
  smoking by patient, 4:418–419, 420
  son, patient having daughters instead of, 4:336, 381
  speaking freely, 4:365
  temper of patient, 4:423
  termination of analysis, 4:375, 378–379, 382, 392, 412, 417, 419, 433, 470–471
  thumb-sucking, 4:307, 337
  tiredness of patient, 4:324
  triangular relationship, 4:320, 323, 354, 360, 400, 453
  true and false self, 4:337, 411, 415, 418
  wet dream, 4:340
Holloway Gaol, 3:237
Hollowood, Jane, *Maggie* books, 8:203–204
Holmes, Oliver Wendell, *The Autocrat at the Breakfast Table* (1898), 7:190
home
  'A Case Managed at Home' (1955), 5:**89–97**
  'Home Again' (1945), 2:**353–356**
  hospital versus home birth, 5:175–178
  school attendance, effects on home life of, 1:443–444
  sexuality and home life, 5:28–29
  stability despite child's dreams of hate, 4:250
  value of stays away from, 3:444; 5:96
homelessness
  'Homeless Children and Childless Homes' (1955), 5:**21–23**
  'The Problem of Homeless Children' (with Clare Britton; 1944), 2:291*n*i, **299–311**; 3:27*n*1
Home Office Care of Children Committee (Curtis Committee), 2:5, 17, 18, 369; 3:162, 439
  'Evidence Given to the Home Office Committee on Children's Homes' (1945), 2:349, **369–377**
homeopathy, 3:141
Homer, 1:40
homosexuality
  absence of, 5:314
  adolescents, psychotherapeutic interviews with, 7:57, 60, 61–63
  anal pruritis and, 1:456, 457
  assault, homosexual, 5:28
  birth memories and, 3:214
  child's bed-wetting and mother's represses homosexuality, 5:357
  child sexual development and, 3:104
  Commission on, 4:267
  compromise with parents, in development of child, 11:70, 78, 81, 170
  compromise with rival, 11:84
  'Considerations in the Study of Homosexuality' (1963), 6:**407–408**
  decriminalisation of, 5:27
  early development and, 5:28–30, 53
  of father, 2:159
  father-deprivation and, 7:276

of father-son relationship, 10:492
female self and, 5:539
friendship among boys as healthy sublimation of, 10:153
'Further Clinical Material on the Theme of a Male Patient's Exploitation of His Female Self' (1963), 6:**519–522**
gender and, 7:104
Greek myth and, 7:323; 9:311
Holding and Interpretation: Fragment of an Analysis (1955), 4:304, 322–323, 324, 409, 424
'Homosexuality and the Law' (1955), 5:25, **27–30**
interpretation, in *Holding and Interpretation*, 4:304, 322–323, 324, 409, 424
of Leonardo da Vinci, 9:303
male ability to identify with women distinguished, 7:371–372
maternal identification of boy to develop into, 6:138, 407–408
normal versus manifest, 11:74n6
psychiatric illness and, 5:27, 29–30
reinforcement of, 6:408
in relation to mother, 9:238, 282
reparation and, 3:119
repression of, 1:456, 457; 5:30; 6:405, 407
split-off male and female elements in men and women and, 7:318, 323; 9:151, 306, 310–311
transference and, 4:285–286
unconscious, 5:30
value of, to society, 11:72
Wilson, Ambrose Cyril, 'Homosexuality' (1946), 5:399
honesty, 2:45–46
Hood, Catriona, 1: xlviii
Hooker, Miss, 5:439
hope, antisocial behaviour implying, 5:152; 10:17, 304, 529
hopelessness, expression of, 4:434–435, 445, 458, 460; 6:202; 8:201; 10:529
Hopkins, Gerard Manley
'Carrion Comfort', 8:175, 177, 179n4
correspondence of, 11:5
'Spring and Fall', 8:178, 179n5
'The Wreck of the *Deutschland*' (1918), 9:333, 333n1
Horace, 8:269, 269niv; 9:343
Horder, Thomas, 1:4, 5; 8:284; 12:305
Horne, Ann, 1:xlii; 8:3
Horney, Karen, 3:490
horse dream, in *The Piggle*, 11:273–274
Hoskyns, Katharine, and Jenny Joseph, *Water and Wind* (reviewed 1967), 8:203
'Hospital Care Supplementing Intensive Psychotherapy in Adolescence' (1963), 6:18, **491–497**

Hospital for Sick Children, Great Ormond Street, London, 1:149
hospitals. *See also* mental hospitals; visiting children in hospital
child exposed to adult pervert in, 7:171–174
child psychiatry and, 4:2439
child's need for acceptance and cooperation with, 9:226–227
home birth versus hospital birth, 5:175–178
'The Niffle' (probably before 1961; published 1996), 9:**383–387**
Robertson, James, *Going to Hospital with Mother* (film, 1958; reviewed 1959), 5:**529–531**
Robertson, James, *A Two-year-old Goes to Hospital* (film, 1953), 5:317, 419n2, 497, 529, 531n1
Robertson, James, *Young Children in Hospital* (1958), 5:531, 531n3
hostels
administrative development of, 3:82–83
adolescents with mental disorders, lack of provision for, 7:339–340
antisocial behaviour and, 3:23–27
central therapeutic idea of, 3:88–92
'Children's Hostels in War and Peace' (1948), 3:**23–27**; 4:239n1
corporal punishment in, 2:349–351, 374–376
delinquency, preventing, 3:26, 47, 81–82
for delinquent children, 2:235–236
deprived children, providing care for, 3:373–374
development of wartime hostels scheme for evacuated children, 3:77–78
environment of, 3:90–92
for evacuated children. *See* evacuation of children
group work in, 5:50–52
for homeless children as result of WWII, 2:300–301
incorporating features from, into existing local authority homes, 2:369
location of, 2:370
'Maladjusted Children: Damaging Effect of Delay' (letter to the *Times*, 1950), 3:**361–362**
nature of, 2:304–306
number of children for best results, 2:372–373
placement of children in, 3:25–26, 85–88
post-war status of, 2:376
as primary home experience, 3:80–81
provision of, 3:25
psychiatric social worker's role in, 2:302–303
psychiatric teams in, 3:83–85
psychiatrist's role in, 2:301–302
purpose and effectiveness of, 3:81–82

hostels (*Cont.*)
   'Residential Management as Treatment for Difficult Children' (with Clare Britton; 1947), 3:27*n*1, **77–93**
   self-government, problem of, 3:93*n*5
   staffing, adequate, 2:373
   teaching of children in, 2:370
   training of staff, 2:376–377; 3:89–90
   transfer of child to different type of hostel, 2:309–310, 373–374
   types of, 2:307–309, 371–372
   warden's selection and role in, 2:303–304
Housman, A. E., *A Shropshire Lad* (1896), 1:57
Howard League for Penal Reform, 2:247
Howell, B. Whitchurch, 1:92, 93
Howells, J. G. (ed.), *Modern perspectives in child psychiatry*, 10:525
hubris, 6:461
Human Nature (1954/1967/1988), 1: xlvii, lxi, 6; 4:247*n*i; 7:12; 8:14; 9:8; 10:6, 12
   central dialectic of, 11:14–18
   circumstances of composition of, 11:3–4, 5
   publication history, 11:3
   unfinished at DWW's death, 11:3, 7
human nature
   developmental approach to, 11:41–42
   health as conceived by DWW and, 11:11–14, 17–18, 42–44
Human Relations, 3:27*n*1, 195, 407
humour, 6:259; 10:65, 109, 394
Humphreys, Robert, 7:339
Humpty Dumpty, 11:134, 298, 299
Hungarian Uprising (1956), 5:6
Hunter, D. D., 5:352*n*i
Hunter, V., 'John Bowlby: An Interview' (1971), 10:18
husband-wife relationship. *See* marital problems; parents
Hussey, B. J., 3:181
Hutchinson, Ann, 7:307
Hutchison, Robert, 7:380
   Lectures on diseases of children (1904), 1:236; 7:380*n*ii
Hutton, Dr, 2:207
hyperaemia, 1:204, 269, 270, 296
hyperaesthesia, 1:82, 264, 269, 320
hypermotility, 5:198
hyperpnoea, post-encephalitic: 'Two Cases of Post-Encephalitic Hyperpnoea' (1926), 1:**95–97**
hypertrophy, cardiac, 1:135, 208, 209, 210–211, 232, 251–252
hypnosis, 1:53–54, 268, 275, 319, 321, 394; 4:459, 461; 10:30
'Hypochondriacal Anxiety' (from *Human Nature*; 1988), 11:**113–114**

hypochondriacal anxiety. *See* anxiety
hypochondriacs, 2:132, 219, 316; 3:117–122; 5:365; 6:257, 404, 461, 466
hypo-manic patients, 3:60; 6:461, 466
hysteria, request to share clinical responsibility in case of, 7:403–404
hysteria in children
   anxiety hysteria, 1:138, 231, 263, 273*n*5, 326, 331
   Bowlby, John, 'Hysteria in Children' (1939), 1:465
   conversion hysteria, 1:135, 243, 277, 307, 321, 331, 334
   epilepsy and, 1:308
   S. Freud on, 1:5–6
   mental defect and, 1:301
   post-encephalitic hyperpnoea and, 1:96
   skin disorders and, 1:357
hysterical blindness, 1:269
hysterical deafness, 1:334–335, 336*n*4
hysterical mutism, 1:270, 334, 335
hysterical vomiting, 1:281, 418

IACAPAP (International Association for Child and Adolescent Psychiatry and Allied Professions), 8:49, 49*n*i
I AM state, 4:274–281; 5:47, 48; 6:12; 7:75, 3386–337, 440; 8:267–269; 9:329; 10:15, 78–79
id
   erotogenic zones and, 8:67
   id-functioning, 6:389; 8:69
   infant's id-needs, 6:11, 160–161
   restatement of Freud's instinct theory and, 11:79–80
   satisfaction of id-drives, 6:490; 8:68
idealisation, 4:16; 10:8
idealism, of adolescents, 9:347
'Ideals in Education' (conference, Lady Margaret Hall, University of Oxford; 1936), 1:375
'Ideas and Definitions' (undated, possibly early 1950s; published 1989), 1: lxxv; 6:159; 9:**359–360**
'Ideas' file of DWW, 6:519; 9:359, 373, 375
identification
   infant's identification with the mother, 6:89–90
   maternal identification, 6:138, 155, 349–350
   primary identification, 4:134
   secondary identification, 4:134
   superego and, 6:15
identity
   establishment of personal identity, 6:9, 121
   gender identity, 7:104–105; 10:260, 269, 284, 344, 509, 530
   problems of, 4:16; 7:213–214
'"Iiro" aet 9 Years 9 Months', 8:7–8; 9:226; 10:13, 15, 31–32, **37–55**, **515**

background in selecting child for case
presentation, 10:37
dreams and, 10:47
interview with mother, 10:53–55
squiggle game and, 10:38–53, 39–53
surgery to remedy disabilities, 10:48, 49, 515
Ilg, Frances, 3:461
illegitimacy, 3:325, 369; 5:74–75
'Illegitimacy and the Broken Home'
(1959), 7:27n1
Illingworth, R. S., 5:408
'Sleep Disturbances in Young Children' (1951),
3:461; 4:173n6
illness
affecting mental attitudes, 6:410
concept of, 9:194
'Ill-Health' (from *Human Nature*, 1988),
11:**43–46**
psyche ill-health, 11:44–45
somatic ill-health, 11:43–44
illusion. *See also* disillusion
fantasy and, *See* fantasies (phantasies)
capacity for, 4:40, 170
of contact with external reality, 11:130, 154, 171
creativity and, 11:119–120, 122, 124
illusion-disillusionment, 4:168–171; 11:120
in normal cultural life, 6:62
of omnipotence, 6:3, 163
as overlap of hallucination and external
reality, 2:364
positive value of, 4:173, 175n10
reality and, 6:229, 484
religion and the arts and, 11:127
transition to disillusion, 2:280, 284
and transitional states, 11:123–124
imagination
adulthood and staying open to, 6:440
children in world of, 2:285–286
existence from start of life, 4:26; 5:116
feeding as imaginative experience,
5:116–117, 118
in first year of life, 5:324
body functioning, imaginative elaboration of,
5:386; 11:75–76
psyche as location of, 6:15
as relief from need for destructive action, 6:55
squiggle game and. *See* squiggle game
Imago group, 8:263n1
imitation, 6:15
immaturity
of adolescents, 9:338, 344–345
as mental ill health, 6:344
immorality. *See* morality and ethics
immunisation. *See* vaccination
impetigo, 1:348, 452–453
impingement, need for freedom from, 2:17–18

'The Importance of the Setting in Meeting
Regression in Psychoanalysis' (1989), 7:6–7,
13, **85–90**
impotence, 4:339–340, 344–347, 382, 390; 7:133, 312,
323; 8:69; 9:310
'The Impulse to Steal' (1949), 3:**319–322**
I'm the King of the Castle/ You're the Dirty Rascal!
See King of the Castle game
inability to concentrate, 6:400
incontinence of child, 2:187–188; 8:294–296.
See also enuresis
independence. *See also* dependence
dependence-independence transition, 4:38, 275;
6:40, 42, 118–119, 130, 149, 313, 469–477
'Environmental Needs; the Early Stages; Total
Dependence and Essential Independence'
(1948), 3:**171–176**, 185
'First Experiments in Independence' (1955),
5:12, **101–105**
striving toward, 6:118–119
Independents, 8:12, 16. *See also* 'Middle Group';
1952 Club
Indian tribes, Erikson's study of, 4:125
individuals
'The Beginning of the Individual' (1966),
7:**449–454**
benign and persecutory elements, containment
of, 9:116–118
'Berlin Walls' (1969), 9:**115–119**
family group in relation to, 7:389–390
'The Individual and the Community: Current
Perspectives in Rehabilitation' (clinical
symposium 1963), 6:491
'Individuation' (1970), 9:**207–211**
as modern concept, 9:115–116
necessity of understanding child as, 7:387–389
political divisions and, 9:117–119
'The Infancy of Juliet' (1949), 3:174n1, **185–193**
infant development. *See also* 'The First Year
of Life'
changing attitudes toward, 5:227
communication between infant and
mother, 8:86
devotion to child in early months of life, 7:5, 42,
91–93, 333–334
DWW's theory of, 1: lxv–lxix; 2:357–368; 7:4–8
'The Earliest States' (from *Human Nature*;
1988), 11:**143–148**
early abnormalities, 6:361
'Emotional Development Characteristic of
Infancy' (introduction to Part III of *Human
Nature;* 1988), 11:**89–90**
environment, importance of, 9:133
'Environmental Health in Infancy', 8:**81–87**
'Further Thoughts on Babies as Persons' (1947),
3:**95–100**

infant development (*Cont.*)
  going-on-being, 6:123, 142, 149, 334, 339, 381, 393, 417, 472; 10:15
  'Growth and Development in Immaturity' (1950), 3:**397–405**
  during holding phase, 6:147–148; 8:83–84. See also holding
  'How a Baby Begins to Feel Sorry and to Make Amends' (1967), 8:**131–136**
  infant care and, 4:57–68, 265
  love and, 6:213–215
  meaning of 'infant', 6:144–146
  mental health of infant, 4:25
  mother's role in, 2:223–224; 8:66–67, 119–120. See also mother-child relationship
  'The Neonate and His Mother' (1964), 7:4, 5, **41–50**, 84*n*i
  no madness phase in, 7:231–232
  normal emotional development patterns, 5:428
  'The Observation of Infants in a Set Situation' (1941), 1: lxii, 8, 310*n*ii, 431*n*5; 2:3, 10, 16, **121–139**; 6:467*n*2; 8:285*n*ii, 310
  omnipotence and. *See* omnipotence
  paediatrics and psychiatry, interaction of, 3:124, 128–136
  parental psychosis and, 5:522
  parents and. *See* father-child relationship; mother-child relationship; parents
  physiotherapy and, 9:69–73
  'Primitive Emotional Development' (lecture, published 1945), 1: lxii, lxvi–lxviii, lxxii; 2:3, 12–16, 21*n*iii, **357–368**; 9:11
  psychoanalytical evolution in thinking about, 6:359
  psychoanalytical re-enactment of, 3:132–136
  psychosis and, 1: lxvi–lxviii; 2:357–358, 387
  social anthropology and, 9:43–45
  stage of concern, 6:352
  training infants, 2:296
  unintegration, state of, in early infancy, 7:4
'Infant Feeding'
  paper (1945), 2:**293–297**; 7:148*n*i
  radio broadcast (1943–44), 2:21*n*iii; 8:117
'Infant Feeding and Emotional Development' (1968), 8:81
infantile behaviour
  primitive infantile behaviour, 4:74
  regression and, 4:208
  sexuality, 6:156
  in transference, 4:71
infantile schizophrenia, 1:439*n*i; 6:391; 8:161–163; 10:122, 138, 139, 518
infantile sexuality, 5:326, 428; 11:80–81
infection
  streptococcal, 1:120, 220–221, 288

treatment methods, 2:255–259, 294
'The Wearing of Masks in the Nursing of Premature and Older Infants' (abstract; 1943), 2:**227**
infestation, phobia of, 1:458–459, 461
'On Influencing and Being Influenced', 2:**109–113**
Ingram, John T., 'The Personality of the Skin' (1933), 1:344, 352*n*3, 454
inherited traits. *See* genetics and heredity
inhibitions
  in adolescence, 6:14
  civilization and, 11:162
  as defence, 11:84
  feeding, 6:132
  ill-health and, 11:73
  reparation and, 11:93
  repression and, 11:51, 54
innate, inherited, or inborn tendencies, 9:43–44
'The Innate Morality of the Baby' (1949), 3:**299–302**; 8:151
inner world of the child
  aggression and, 3:336–339
  cultural experience and, 7:431, 436
  depressive position and, 4:195–196; 11:95, 100, 104–105
  'Development of the Theme of the Inner World' (from *Human Nature*; 1988), 11:**103–106**
  environmental needs and, 3:173
  in first year of life, 5:324–325
  importance in DWW's work, 1: lxiv; 8:4
  manic defence and, 1:363; 11:105–106
  material presented by patients in analysis from, 11:109–111
  pre-school children and, 1:407–411
  transitional objects and, 4:161
  Wickes' *Inner World of Man* and, 3:463
'insane', use of word, 3:92*n*3
instinct, 2:368*n*6; 3:6, 14; 6:9. *See also* death instinct
  aggression and, 3:335, 340 345; 6:17
  of aggressiveness and love, 2:68
  antedated experiences of baby and, 4:56
  baby as instinct-driven, 2:14
  chart of psychology of small boy in terms of, 11:84–85
  'The Concept of Health Using Instinct Theory' (from *Human Nature*; 1988), 11:**75–86**
  conscience and, 2:387
  control of, 4:158
  death instinct, 4:65. *See also* death instinct
  defined, 11:66
  development of instinct quality, 4:153, 205–206, 225; 6:346
  DWW's restatement of, 11:80–81
  of the ego, 3:9, 340

emotional development and, 11:65–72
excited and unexcited states, 11:77–78
in first year of life, 5:325–326; 6:35460
of four-year-old, 4:250
S. Freud on, 5:352; 11:18, 79–80, 81
imaginative elaboration of function, 11:75–76
inner reality and, 2:70, 131, 269, 358
instinct-gratification 439, 4:206
'Instincts and Normal Difficulties' (1950), 3:**393–396**; 8:151
instinctual love, 4:188, 191–193
instinctual tension, 4:135, 169, 188–190, 200*n*5; 10:10
Jungian archetypes and, 2:368*n*6
maternal instinct, 2:185, 287–289, 296, 337; 4:21–22; 6:88; 8:153
as maturational process, 3:15–17, 128, 167–168, 403
non-integration and, 3:14
Oedipus complex and, 11:78–79
origin of, 2:62, 292
pent up, 2:66
of the personality, 3:70, 167, 334–335
pregenital instinctual functions, 6:15, 117, 130–131, 188, 326, 469
progression from alimentary instinctual life to genital instinctual life, 6:347
psyche, development of, 11:76
reality and fantasy, distinguishing, 2:44; 11:81–82
the soul and, 11:76–77
transitional objects and instinct tensions, 3:457; 4:200*n*5
techniques of infant care and, 4:56
the unconscious, 11:82–83
Institute for Psycho-Analysis, 9:100
Institute for the Scientific Treatment of Delinquency, 2:234, 248, 291
Institute for the Study and Treatment of Delinquency, 5:400
Institute of Child Health, University of Manchester, Catherine Chisholm Memorial Lecture (1968), 8:283
Institute of Child Psychology, 3:183
Institute of Education, University of London, 1:18; 2:6; 3:171; 5:9, 400; 6:377; 8:43, 333; 11:3, 25
Institute of Human Relations, 5:479
Institute of Psycho-Analysis, London, 1:11; 4:227; 5:169, 234, 236; 6:305–306; 11:63. *See also* British Psychoanalytical Society
Child Department, 2:3, 6, 7, 149–163; 6:182
DWW training at, 2:179; 6:180; 8:333; 11:32
Paddington Green Children's Hospital working with, 6:182
setting for regression, third-year students discussing, 7:13, 85

Institute of Psychology, 1:15
Institute of Public Health and Hygiene, 3:153
Institute of the Pennsylvania Hospital (Philadelphia), 6:479
insult, infant experiencing, 8:83–84
integration, 2:14–15, 168–169, 227, 318, 361–363; 3:6, 14; 6:415. *See also* disintegration; unintegration
as achievement, 4:65; 11:116, 126
aggression and, 3:335, 340 345
character and, 6:448
development of self and, 4:106
disintegration and, 11:133–136, 153
ego-integration, 3:9, 340; 8:112, 273
'Ego Integration in Child Development' (1962), 6:11, **389–395**; 10:6
in first year of life, 5:321–322; 6:483
guilt, capacity for, 5:145
hate and, 3:65–66
in *Holding and Interpretation: Fragment of an Analysis* (1955), 4:320
importance in childhood, 3:128, 167–168, 403; 6:346; 10:6
individual emotional development and, 5:47–48; 8:271–272
'Integration' (from *Human Nature*; 1988), 11:**133–137**
'Integrative and Disruptive Factors in Family Life', 5:**265–275**
and management of the body, 11:139–140, 141
as maturational process, 3:15–17, 128, 167–168, 403; 4:43–44, 44*f*; 6:98; 8:70–71
as natural tendency, 6:227, 233
non-integration and, 3:14
'ordinary devoted mother' factor in, 7:7, 336
personal omnipotence as essential step in, 7:6
of the personality, 3:70, 167, 334–335
psychosomatic disorders and, 7:75–77
psychotic anxiety and, 8:188
in *Romeo and Juliet*, 3:186, 192
social worker's role to counteract disintegration, 6:418
in time, 6:355, 415
trauma and, 7:186
unintegration, state of, in early infancy, 7:4
intellect and intellectual development. *See also* mind
health and intellect, 11:40–41
'The Intellectual Function' (from *Human Nature*; 1988), 11:**157–158**
Isaacs, Susan, *Intellectual Growth in Young Children* (1930), 1:279, 280*n*5; 3:161
mind and health, 8:77*n*2
of pre-school children, 1:398–399; 8:270
psyche-soma and intellectual life, 7:198–199

intelligence testing and intelligence quotient (IQ)
  academic psychology and, 5:421
  administration of tests, 2:180
  autism and, 7:351, 358, 359
  Axline, Virginia A., *Dibs: In Search of Self* (reviewed 1966), 7:367
  educational diagnosis and, 3:30
  obsessional neurosis and IQ, 7:198
  in private practice, 5:36
  of psychologists as a group, 9:156
  therapeutic consultations and, 7:274, 278*n*1; 10:522
Interdepartmental Committee on Medical Schools, 3:243*n*i
interference
  doctors and nurses' need to avoid, 8:85–87, 344
  mother alternating between neglect and, 6:290
  mother viewing pregnancy in terms of interference in her life, 8:117
intermediate area, 3:6–7, 16; 4:66, 171; 6:202, 318, 436, 443
intermediate object, 6:291–292
intermediate state, 11:172–173
internal mother, 7:411–412
internal object, Kleinian concept of, 4:167–168; 5:244, 413; 7:412; 9:273
'internal', use of, 5:209–210
International Association for Child and Adolescent Psychiatry and Allied Professions (IACAPAP), 8:49, 49*n*i
International Conference on Mental Health (11–21 August 1948), 3:147*n*i
International Congress for Analytical Psychology, 5:307*n*i
International Congress of Child Psychiatry, 5:351
International Congress of Paediatrics, 5:165, 217
International Congress of Psychotherapy, 5:345*n*i
International Journal of Child Psychotherapy, 9:225
International Journal of Offender Therapy, 2:195*n*i
International Journal of Psychoanalysis, 1:11, 357, 439; 2:115*n*i, 357; 3:59, 223, 447, 460; 4:129, 159, 201; 5:12, 61, 241, 309, 389, 392, 394, 399, 401, 405, 529, 535; 6:141, 333, 359, 363, 505; 7:67, 115, 193, 429; 8:12, 18*n*10, 121, 123, 299, 355; 9:75, 265; 10:37, 113, 515, 517
International Psychoanalytical Association (IPA)
  accreditation of Finnish Psychoanalytic Society, 6:237, 241; 8:8, 18*n*6
  Amsterdam Conference (1965), 7:193, 197
  Amsterdam Congress (1951), DWW at, 3:20
  'Clinical Varieties of Transference' (1955) read before, 5:16; 5:61
  Copenhagen Congress (1959), 5:465*n*i
  Copenhagen Congress (1967), 8:7–8; 10:37, 515
  DWW and, 1: lix
  DWW on European committee investigating Lacanian group, 6:46*n*i
  Edinburgh Congress (1961), 6:3–4, 46*n*i, 141, 359, 363; 10:17
  Geneva Congress (1955), DWW at, 5:*16*; 9:48
  Geneva Congress (1955), Melanie Klein at, 6:315
  'Notes for the Vienna Congress' (1971), 9:15, **355–356**
  Paris Congress (1957), 5:249; 9:371
  publication of Standard Edition of Freud's works and, 7:407, 410
  Rome Congress (1969), 8:18*n*6; 9:75, 109; 11:190
  Statute III, 2:145; 147
  Stockholm Congress (1963), DWW at, 6:24–26
  Vienna Congress (1971), 9:15, 355–356
International Psycho-Analytical Library, 5:395; 6:233, 235–236; 8:363*n*1; 9:29, 93, 94
International Psycho-Analytical Press, 5:392
International Review of Psychoanalysis, 6:523
interpersonal relationships
  depressive position and, 11:91–97; 11:*94*, 96
  DWW's thinking in terms of, 4:9–10; 8:33–34
  the family and, 11:64
  instinct and, 11:65–72
  'Interpersonal Relationships' (from *Human Nature*; 1988), 11:**63–74**
  love relationships, 11:72–74
  neurosis, understanding of healthy child through study of, 11:63–64
  'The Relationship of a Mother to Her Baby at the Beginning' (1960), 6:12, **87–92**; 8:34
'Interpretation in Psycho-analysis' (1968), 8:17, **253–257**
interpreter, use of, 6:237, 241; 10:32, 37, 53
'La Interrelación en Terminos de Identificaciones Cruzadas' (1968), 9:**328–336**; 336*n*4
'Interrelating Apart from Instinctual Drive and in Terms of Cross-identifications' (1971), 9:**319–336**; 10:16
'Inter-Relationship of Body Disease and Psychological Disorder' (from *Human Nature*; 1988), 11:**47–52**
interruptions
  to mother's routine, 6:85
  to satisfactory maternal care, 6:154
intimacy between therapist and child, 10:12–13, 29
intracranial disease. *See* brain disease
introductions (by DWW)
  The Child, the Family, and the Outside World (1964), 7:**125–127**
  Human Nature (1988), 11:5, **31–32**, **41–44**, **65–67**, **95–96**, **123**
  The Maturational Processes and the Facilitating Environment (1965), 7:**305–307**

The Piggle (1977), 11:3, 5, **193–195**
Playing and Reality (1971), 9:**261–263**
'Introduction to a Symposium on the Psycho-Analytic Contribution to the Theory of Shock Therapy' (1944), 2:**261–264**
introjection
  depression and, 6:462
  infantile maturational processes and, 6:481–482
  introjected mothering, 7:179
  introjective and projective identifications, 9:135, 319–320, 328–336, 330–331
  Kleinian contribution and, 6:328
  superego and, 6:15, 132
  transitional objects and, 3:456
introversion
  childhood psychoses and, 4:35
  hostels for homeless children specialising in, 2:308
  shock therapy for, 2:268
IPA. *See* International Psychoanalytical Association
IQ. *See* intelligence testing and intelligence quotient (IQ)
'I Qant Stand It' (letter to *The Times* 1957), 5:**219**
Irish Adoption Act, 5:75
Isaacs, Nathan, 3:163; 8:334
Isaacs, Susan, 1:11, 18, 398; 2:11, 63n4, 119ni; 3:169, 472; 4:104, 124, 260; 5:473; 7:16, 154, 217; 8:43; 11:3, 25, 101n2
  Childhood and After, 3:162, 460
  'Children in Institutions' in *Childhood and After*, 3:162
  The Children We Teach, 3:162
  Gardner, D. E. M. *Susan Isaacs: The First Biography* (1969, foreword by DWW), 8:**333–334**
  'Habit', in *On the Bringing Up of Children* (1936), 1:437, 438
  Intellectual Growth in Young Children (1930), 1:279, 280n5; 3:161
  Melanie Klein and, 3:162, 163; 6:114, 330
  'The Nursery as a Community', in *On the bringing up of children* (1936), 1:437, 438
  The Nursery Years (1929), 3:162
  obituary, 3:**161–163**; 8:333
  Mr Q. and, 4:75, 77
  Social Development in Young Children (1933), 3:161
isolation, 4:38, 39f; 6:11
  of individual, 4:38, 40, 44, 445–447; 6:149, 189, 425–426, 440–441, 443–445
  primary isolation, 4:44
Issroff, Judith, 11:29
  Donald Winnicott and John Bowlby: Personal and Professional Perspectives (2005), 10:18
Itard, Jean, 10:5

Jackson, Lydia, *Aggression and Its Interpretation* (1954; reviewed 1954), 4:**247–248**; 5:345; 11:137
Jacobsen (New York Psychoanalytic Society discussant), 9:36
Jacobson, Edith, 6:399; 8:12
James, Henry, 6:514–515; 12:304
James, Lydia, 7:227
  letter to (1961), 6:**175**
James, Martin, 1: xlviii; 5:447; 6:175, 360–361
  letter to (1957), 5:**221**
  letter to (1965), 7:217, **227**
  'The Mothers Children Need', 7:91, 93
James Spence Gold Medal for Paediatrics, 1:xvii
Janet, Pierre, 1:142
Jaques, Elliot, 5:347
  'Disturbances in the Capacity to Work' (1959), 5:493ni
  letter to (1959), 5:**493–494**
'"Jason" aet 8 Years 9 Months', 10:**453–493**
  aggressiveness and, 10:473–474, 478
  appendicitis and hernia operation and, 10:453, 469–471, 474, 476
  background, 10:453–454
  blinking and, 10:454, 476
  car hitting Jason, Jason's part in causing, 10:478, 492
  deprivation due to lack of time with mother before another child, 10:476, 492
  desire of parents to have a girl instead of boys, 10:476
  drawings and, 10:467–470
  dreams and, 10:466–467, 469–472, 486–487, 491
  fantasying and, 10:466, 471, 491–492
  father's role and, 10:473–475, 478–479, 491, 493
  homosexuality of father-son relationship, 10:492
  mother's childhood, 10:476–477
  mother's subsequent pregnancy, effect on Jason, 10:473
  parents viewing Jason as a pest, 10:474–475
  playing game with DWW, 10:488–490, 488–491
  preference for father over mother, 10:471, 474
  punishment techniques used by parents, 10:475
  siblings of Jason, 10:476, 492
  squiggle game and, 10:455–465, 455–469, 479–488, 479–492
  stealing as issue, 10:454, 478, 486
  teasing and, 10:475
  transitional phenomena and, 10:475–476
jaw, sarcoma of, 1:70

jealousy
  of child for father, 2:285
  'Contribution to a Symposium on Envy and Jealousy' (1969), 9:**47–49**
  of friends, 10:443
  of infant as part of normal development, 6:13, 49
  of infant when deprived of breast or mother's attention, 2:134–135
  'Jealousy' (BBC talk; 1960), 6:13, **47–61**
  Ernest Jones on, 3:490
  of mother for father-daughter relationship, 2:274
  of mother for temporary family's mother of evacuated children, 2:39
  of older sibling for younger sibling, 2:84, 127, 158; 6:13, 47–61; 8:297–298; 10:142, 153. *See also* sibling rivalry
  relationship to mother as basis for, 6:51
  Ziman, Edmund, *Jealousy in Children* (reviewed 1951), 3:**469**
Jemstedt, Arne, 1:xlv; 9:3
Jews
  amaurotic family idiocy primarily affecting, 1:292
  S. Freud as, 6:368
  A. Freud's clinical study of German-Jewish orphans whose parents died under Hitler, 9:94
  Friedmann, Oscar and Manna, and Jewish refugee children, 5:536–537
  hidden identity of, 2:154
  Jewish Refugees Boys' Hostels, 5:536
  Jones, Ernest, Jewish analysts helped out of Germany by, 1: lxiii
  letter to Mrs. Neville (Ann) Chamberlain (1938) on views of prime minister regarding, 1:463
  Nazi treatment of, 1: lxiv, 17, 408, 463
J. N. (DWW's patient), 8:385, 387, 389, 399*n*i, 403, 405*n*iv, 405–406
Johns, Jennifer, 1: lxv, lvii*n*1; 5:3
Johns, Marcus, 1:lv; 5:3
Johns Hopkins Hospital, 10:6
Jokl, Katherine (later Jones), 5:311, 393, 394, 395, 398
Jolly, T., 5:437
Jones, Ernest
  'Address Introducing Margaret Mead, VIIIth Ernest Jones Lecture' (1957), by DWW, 5:**203–204**
  'Alcoholic Cirrhosis of the Liver in Children', 5:390
  analysands of, 2:115*n*i; 7:95
  on aphanisis, 5:391; 8:443; 11:18
  children referred to DWW by, 1:18
  on delinquent children, 1:369, 373*n*6
  DWW referred for analysis by, 11:11–12, 189
  'The Early Development of Female Sexuality' (1927), 8:443*n*ii; 11:4, 74
  editor, *Letters of Sigmund Freud, 1873–1939* (1961; reviewed 1962), 6:**367–370**
  Essays in Applied Psycho-Analysis (1951), 5:398*n*6, 398*n*17
  establishment of psychoanalysis in Britain and, 1:11; 3:475; 8:124
  Free Association: Memories of a Psycho-Analyst (1959), 5:398*n*1
  S. Freud and, 5:203, 309, 310, 311, 389–395
  'Funeral Address for Ernest Jones' (DWW, 1958), 5:**309–311**, 349
  'The God Complex', 5:397
  on 'Homosexuality and the Law' (1955), 5:25
  influence of, 6:326
  International Psycho-Analytical Library and, 6:235, 235*n*i; 9:93
  Jewish analysts helped out of Germany by, 1: lxiii
  Klein and, 1: lxiii, 16; 5:7; 6:327
  letter to (1952), 4:**53–54**
  on mind, 3:245
  'The Nature of Genius' (1956), 5:395
  On the Nightmare, 5:390
  obituary (1958), 5:**389–398**
  'On Symbolism' (1916), 1: lxxv–lxxvii
  'Our Attitude towards Greatness' (1956), 5:395
  Papers on Psycho-Analysis (1948; reviewed 1951), 3:**489–490**
  'Psychiatry before and after Freud' (1956), 5:395
  'The Question of the Side Affected in Hemiplegia in Arterial Lesions of the Brain', 5:390
  Riviere and, 5:349, 350
  Sigmund Freud: Four Centenary Addresses (1956), 5:398*n*14
  Sigmund Freud: Life and Work, Vol. 3 (1957), 5:398*n*9
  'Sigmund Freud: The Man and His Achievements', 5:395
  'The Significance of the Phrictopathic Sensation', 5:390–391
  on Strachey's translation of Freud, 7:409
  'The Symbolic Significance of Salt', 5:390
  'Treatment of the Neuroses' (1920), 1:328*n*2
  'A Valedictory Address' (1946), 5:398*n*9
  Wilson, Ambrose Cyril, and, 5:399
  on writings of DWW, 4:225
Jones, Gwenith, 5:393, 398*n*11
Jones, Katherine Jokl, 5:311, 393, 394, 395, 398; 8:263*n*i

Jones, Lewis, 5:393
Jones, Mervyn, 5:393
Jones, Morfydd Owen, 5:393, 398*n*10
Jones, Nesta, 5:393
Jones, Robert, 2:178
Joseph, Betty, 7:411; 11:13
   letter to (1954), 4:**221–222**
   on wishes, 4:224
Joseph, Jenny
   Judy and Jasmin and *Tim and Terry*, 8:2013–204
   Water and Wind (with Katharine Hoskyns; reviewed 1967), 8:203
Josiah H. Macy, Jr. Foundation, 3:487; 4:117
Journal of Abnormal Psychology, 5:391
Journal of Child Psychology and Psychiatry, 6:373
Journal of Child Psychotherapy, 10:419, 527
Journal of Nervous and Mental Diseases, 5:398*n*7
Journal of the Royal Institute of Public Health and Hygiene, 3:153
Journal of State Medicine, 1:353
'Journées d'Etudes sur les Psychoses chez l'Enfant' (Paris conference, 1967), 8:161
Joyce, Angela, 1:ix; 6:1; 8:11
Judge Baker Guidance Center (Boston), 10:419
Jung, Carl, and Jungian analysis
   analytical psychology and, 2:368*n*6; 3:54, 122, 352
   anima/animus, 9:14, 169
   childhood psychosis and emotional development of, 7:116–120
   conceptualisation styles, 7:142
   on continuous development throughout life, 9:207
   depressive position and, 4:196
   'D. W. W.'s Dream Related to Reviewing Jung' (1963), 6:**501–503**; 8:355; 9:33
   expressions used by DWW, 3:202
   Fordham, Michael, and, 4:241; 5; 5:79–80, 506, 509; 508
   S. Freud and, 7:15, 115, 116–117, 119–121
   in Harms' *Handbook*, 3:235
   Jones, Ernest, and, 5:392
   Jungian training, 6:305
   Lowenfeld and, 10:5
   Memories, Dreams, and Reflections (1963; reviewed 1964), 7:15–16, **115–124**
   on poetry and mental illness, 7:315
   psychotherapy and, 8:62
   Sargant, William, 'The Physiology of Faith' (1969), 9:60
   'self', use of, 7:122–123
   shadow mother, 4:60
   society and culture permeated by ideas of, 7:425
   on the unconscious, 7:120–122
   Wickes' *Inner World of Man* and, 3:463

Juvenile Courts
   asking for analytic treatment, 2:196
   'The Child, the Family and the Young Offender' (UK Government Home Office White Paper), 7:204
   hostel committees and, 3:47
   magistrates', 2:233–236
   private practice and, 5:36
   psychological methods, use of, 3:44
   Watson, J. A. F., *The Child and the Magistrate* (1950; reviewed 1951), 3:**431–432**
juvenile delinquency. *See* delinquent children

Kabesh, Amal Treacher, 1:li; 12:xlix
Kahne, Merton J., letter to (1960), 6:**63–64**
Kahr, Brett, 1: lvii*n*1; 8:13
   D. W. Winnicott. A Biographical Portrait (1996), 1: lvii*n*i, 3*n*ii; 5:8
Kalff, Dora, 10:5
Kalmanovitch, Jeannine, letters to (1971), 9:**257, 259–260**
Kanner, Leo, 3:354; 4:228, 238–239; 5:186; 7:397; 8:161–162; 10:5–6
   Child Psychiatry (1935/1937) (reviewed by DWW), 1:**439–440**; 2:9; 8:159*n*i
Kanter, Joel, 5:9; 6:6
Karnac, Harry, 1:ix, 12:5
Karpf, Anne, 1: lxxviii; 2:221, 12:9, 15*n*14, 15*n*19, 15*n*21, 15*n*23, 15*n*26, 239
Keate, John, 6: 384, 385
Keats, John, 5:369; 6:433, 433*n*i, 528; 9:172
   'On First Looking into Chapman's Homer', 2:384; 8:405*n*iii
Keene, Mr., 1:61
Kendrick, W., and P. Meisel (eds.), *Letters of James and Alix Strachey*, 8:124*n*i
Kennedy, H., 8:16
Kennel, Professor, 7:407
Ker, C. B., 1:115, 132
Kernig's sign, 1:80, 192, 283, 288
Keynes, Geoffrey, 7:409
Keynes, John Maynard, 7:409, 426; 9:84
Khan, Masud
   acknowledged in DWW texts, 2:388; 5:302; 7:307, 309; 9:263
   on auto-erotism, 8:300
   Balint on aggression and, 8:77*n*1, 171
   bibliography of DWW's works, 12:5
   'The Concept of Cumulative Trauma', 8:189*n*vii
   as discussant, 1: lxix*n*iii; 6:4; 8:xxiii*n*3, 17*n*1
   on dreaming ego, 3:12
   DWW using as critical and editorial commentator, 1: xlvii; 12:157
   editorial role of, 10:3, 23

Khan, Masud (*Cont.*)
  as editor of *International Psycho-Analytical Library*, 9:93
  'Ego Distortion, Cumulative Trauma, and the Role of Reconstruction in the Analytic Situation' (1964), 9:139n7
  'The Function of Intimacy and Acting Out in Perversions' (1964), 8:312
  Gaddini, Eugenio, 'On Imitation', comments on, 9:112nii
  introductions and forewords to DWW's works by, 1: lxxiiinv; 5:3; 8:xxviin4; 11:190
  letter to (1961), 6:**233–234**
  Playing and Reality (1971), editing of, 10:3
  The Privacy of the Self (1974), 8:189nvii
  Psychoanalytic Studies of the Personality (Fairbairn 1952; review co-author with DWW 1953), 4:**129–137**
  Rapaport, David, recommended to, 4:121
  Smirnoff, Victor, and, 5:385
  on split-off male and female elements, 9:149–150
A Kid for Two Farthings (novel, 1953 and film, 1958), 9:381ni
killing of children, 9:106–108
'Kinds of Psychological Effect of Shock Therapy' (1944), 2:207ni, 261, **265–269**
King, Allan, 8:167ni
King, Pearl, 2:9, 14; 5:263; 8:8, 17n1
  The Freud-Klein Controversies, 1941–45 (1991), 5:7; 7:377–378ni
  letter to (1961), 6:**235–236**
King, Truby, 9:341
King of the Castle game, 7:75, 80; 9:343; 11:243, 244, 245
Kinnear, J., 'Urticaria Papulosa' (1933), 1:343, 352n2
Kirk, H. David, *Shared Fate* (reviewed 1965), 7:**311–312**
Klein, Eric/Erik, 1:12; 2:7; 4:62, 62ni; 6:114
Klein, Judy, 4:642, 62ni
Klein, Melanie
  on aggression, 3:335, 338, 347n6; 4:247; 6:97, 145, 321, 324; 8:280, 331
  'A' Group in BPAS and, 5:7, 261nii
  analysis of two-year-old children, 2:130
  on anxiety drive, 6:450, 511
  background of, 4:59, 247; 6:113
  on 'bad mother', 4:63–64, 65–66, 127–128
  Baumann, Marianne, and, 5:307, 345
  'The Beginnings of a Formulation of an Appreciation and Criticism of Klein's Envy Statement' (DWW, 1962), 1: lxviii; 5:11; 6:**315–324**; 10:47
  Bion and, 5:83, 84; 6:279; 7:17, 96; 8:157
  on Bonnard, 4:48
  Bowlby's 'Separation Anxiety' and, 5:496, 499
  'breast', wider meaning of, 5:420n9
  children of, 1:18; 2:195ni
  classification of psychiatric conditions and, 5:447, 449–450
  on conflict between love and hate, 6:17
  Controversial Discussions (Freud-Klein controversy), 1: lxiv; 2:5; 4:174n11; 5:6–8, 10–11, 12, 19–20, 33, 87, 261nii, 366; 6:325, 331
  on creativity, 9:6, 11, 13, 303–304
  on death instinct, 6:17; 8:45
  death of, 6:18, 113
  on dependence, 6:145
  on depression, 2:63n4; 4:37; 6:15–16; 11:105
  on depressive position in emotional development, 3:157–158, 335, 457; 4:134, 185–200, 276; 5:10, 11, 130, 152–153, 242, 252, 353, 450, 498, 499; 6:17, 113–114, 321, 329–330, 386, 511; 7:440; 9:75, 329; 11:15, 101n2
  on drives, 9:11, 13
  DWW, children referred to, 1:18
  DWW compared, 1: lvii
  DWW estranged from, 1: lxviii–lxix, 16; 2:10
  DWW moving away from conceptualisations of, 2:13–14, 19; 4:30, 183; 6:11, 16, 18, 3371–332; 8:4, 45, 265
  DWW not considered Kleinian by, 6:18, 310
  DWW's paper on transitional objects, discussant of, 1:lxviiiniii; 2:12
  DWW studying under and influenced by, 1: lxii, 11–15, 431n2; 2:4, 10, 12; 4:7, 123; 5:7, 8; 6:18, 327–330; 8:4, 35, 37, 41–42, 46, 334; 9:60; 10:5; 11:6, 10, 15, 32, 101n2
  DWW's theory of infant development and, 1: lxvi–lxvii; 6:7, 361
  DWW's works, editing and publication of, 1:viii
  environment and, 3:223, 381, 385; 4:189
  on envy, 5:87, **433–436**; 6:18, 231, 315–324, 361; 7:90, 190, 412–413; 8:45, 280, 330–332; 9:47–49. *See also* her writings on envy listed below
  on envy of the good breast, 6:16, 270–271, 316, 318, 361; 7:90
  on internal factors, 2:192
  Fairbairn and, 4:133–135, 261–262, 263
  on fear of loss of mother, 2:137
  A. Freud and, 2:5, 9; 7:218, 219 (*see also* Controversial Discussions)
  S. Freud and, 4:202; 6:113, 129, 145
  Glover's critique of, 3:121, 475
  on good internal object, 5:244
  on good mother, 4:63–64
  on guilt, 4:75, 193; 5:141, 143–144, 329
  Harms, Ernest (ed.), *Handbook of Child Guidance* (1947; reviewed 1949), 3:235
  IJPA birthday festschrift (1952), 1: lxix, lxx; 3:223, 229, 231, 365ni, 381, 385

on inner and outer reality of young
   children, 2:131
internal objects and, 4:167–168; 5:244, 413;
   7:412; 9:273
International Journal of Psychoanalysis issue
   devoted to, 4:47
Isaacs, Susan, and, 3:162, 163; 6:114, 330
Jacques, Elliot, and, 5:347
Jones and, 5:396
latency period, psychoanalysis in, 5:354, 355
letter of DWW to Joan Riviere on, 5:121–124
letter to (1952), 4:4, 5, 7; 5:123*n*iii; 7:14; 9:4
letter to (1954), 4:**241–243**
letter to (1957), 5:**209–210**
Lowenfeld and, 10:5
loyalties of followers to, 5:20; 9:60
on the manic defence, 1:359, 373*n*3, 374*n*7
on maternal care, 6:4, 152
'Melanie Klein: On Her Concept of Envy'
   (1989), 6:269, 315
Meltzer, Donald, and, 5:463; 7:411–413
Money-Kyrle, Roger, as follower of, 1:441; 4:63
on mother affected by child's neurosis, 1:278
'Mourning and Its Relation to Manic-
   depressive States' (1940), 9:277
Nagera, Humberto, and, 7:147
normal child behaviour compared to psychosis,
   by, 3:13
'Notes on Some Schizoid Mechanisms'
   (1946), 1:xxv
obituary for (1960), 6:**113–114**
Oedipus complex and, 9:38*n*1
oral fantasies of two-year-old children
   and, 2:130
on paranoid anxiety, 3:217
on paranoid position, 4:37, 43*n*2, 110, 134; 5:252;
   6:330; 9:37
'A Personal View of the Kleinian Contribution'
   (DWW, 1962), 6:16, 18, **325–332**
on play, 5:7; 6:438–439; 8:301
potential space, DWW's concept of, 3:12
on pregenital instinctual life, 6:15
on pre-Oedipal development, 6:4
on primary aggression, 5:180–181
on primitive fantasy, 6:157*n*9
on projective and introjective identifications,
   9:135, 330
propaganda and followers of, 4:74; 5:20
on psychic reality, 6:129
psychoanalysis approach of, 2:145; 6:481; 8:14
psychoanalysis of children in London and, 1:11
on psycho-neurosis of children, 6:259
reparation and, 3:13, 14, 121, 402; 7:166; 9:37;
   11:286*n*2
Riviere, Joan, and, 4:61, 242; 5:121–124
Rodrigue, Emilio, and, 5:31–32

Rosenfeld, Herbert and, 4:73, 79
Rosenfeld, Eva, and, 6:211*n*ii
on schizoid position, 4:130, 134
scientific psychology and, 3:70
Segal, Hannah, and, 4:71; 5:209*n*i
on sexual development in girls, 3:490
Stokes and, 5:33*n*i
superego and, 6:129–132; 7:439
theories of, 1: lviii; 2:137, 216, 368*n*1; 3:5, 12–13
toys used in diagnosing and treating children,
   1:374*n*7
transitional objects and, 3:460, 461; 4:171; 5:12,
   413, 416, 420*n*9, 527
understanding of psychotic people, 4:74
Wilson, Ambrose Cyril, and, 5:399
Zetzel on, 5:318
Klein, Melanie, works of
   Contributions to Psycho-Analysis (1948),
      6:114, 260*n*3
   'A Contribution to the Psychogenesis of Manic-
      Depressive States' (1934), 1:14; 9:273, 329;
      11:101*n*4
   'The Depressive Position in Emotional
      Development', 6:97; 7:440
   Developments in Psycho-Analysis (1952), 6:114
   'Early Anxiety Situations and Ego
      Development' in *The Psychoanalysis of
      Children* (1931), 1:13
   'Envy' (1955), 1: lxviii; 6:231; 8:280
   Envy and Gratitude (1957; reviewed 1959), 5:11,
      433–436; 6:315; 7:190; 9:330
   'The Importance of Symbol Formation in
      Development of Ego' (1930), 1: lxii, 301, 302*n*2
   Love, Hate and Reparation (with Joan Riviere;
      1937), 1:413
   Narrative of a Child Analysis (1961), 6:374
   'Notes on Some Schizoid Mechanisms' (1946),
      3:4–5, 256*n*12; 5:7
   'The Oedipus Complex in the Light of Early
      Anxieties' (1945), 6:260*n*3
   'On the Sense of Loneliness' (1963), 1: lxvii
   The Psycho-Analysis of Children (1932), 1:14,
      273*n*1; 3:460; 5:354, 496; 6:114; 9:139*n*2, 330;
      11:101*n*4
   'The Psychogenesis of the Manic-Depressive
      States' (1935), 1:16; 3:461
   'The Significance of Early Anxiety-Situations in
      the Development of the Ego', 2:21*n*i
   'Some Theoretical Conclusions Regarding the
      Emotional Life of the Infant' (1944), 2:13
   'A Study of Envy and Gratitude' (1956), 5:7, 11,
      121–122, **129–132**; 6:270*n*i, 315*n*i
   'Weaning', in *On the bringing up of children*
      (1936), 1:18, 437, 438
Klumke's paralysis, 1:295
Knight, Desmond, 8:203–204

Knight, Mrs, 6:379
Knights, L. C., 7:328
   Explorations (1946), 9:316
Knopf, Mrs. B. J., letter to (1964), 7:17, **113**
knowledge
   'Knowing and Learning' (broadcast 1950, published 1957), 3:**387–391**, 7:187n1
   'Knowing and Not Knowing' (undated; first published 1989), 9:**367–368**
   'Outline for a Study in the Sociology of Knowledge' (incomplete and undated), 9:**391–394**
Knox, Ronald, 5:524; 8:265; 11:136niii
Koplik, H., 1:78, 88
Korean War, 5:6
Kornitzer, Margaret, 7:312
Krabbe, K. H., 1:82, 83, 88
Kris, Ernst, 2:79; 4:117, 219; 5:249, 364, 447; 8:39, 195, 300; 9:93. See also *The Psychoanalytic Study of the Child*
   libidinal theory of Hartmann-Kris-Loewenstein, 8:393
   'Opening Remarks on Psychoanalytic Child Psychology' (1951), 5:251, 252
   'Recovery of Childhood Memories in Psycho-analysis', 5:318
Kris, Marian[ne], 8:195
   The Psychoanalytic Study of the Child, Volume 20 (multiple editors; 1966; reviewed by DWW), 7:**375–376**
Kristeva, J., 1: lxix–lxx
Krupp foundry (Essen, Germany), 1:31
Kulka, Anna M.
   'Kinesthetic Needs and Motility in Earliest Infancy' (1957), 5:197

letter to (1957), 5:**197–198**
Lacan, Jacques, 1:xvii; 4:4; 6:6–7, 45, 46ni
   The Four Fundamental Concepts of Psychoanalysis, 6:6
   International Psychoanalytical Association's European committee investigating, 6:46ni
   Le nom du Père, 6:6
   letter to (1960), 6:**45–46**
   'Le Stade du Miroir' (1949), 8:211, 217
Lagache, Daniel, 6:4; 7:408
Laing, Adrian, *R. D. Laing: A Life* (1997), 5:361ni
Laing, Ronald D., 6:443, 445; 7:233, 237; 8:36
   'The Divided Self', 5:361–362; 6:109
   letter to (1958), 5:**361–362**
Lamb, Charles, *Essays of Elia* (1905), 7:449
Lampl-de-Groot, Jeanne, 6:284; 8:280
The Lancet
   'Frontal Lobes of the Human Brain' (letter; 1943), 4:**33**
   'Leucotomy in Psychosomatic Disorders' (letter; 1951), 3:**465–466**
   'Prefrontal Leucotomy' (letter; 1943), 2:207ni, **207–208**
   'Prefrontal Leucotomy' (unpublished letter; 1943), 2:**209**
   review in, 3:463
   William Sargant on leucotomy for obsessional neurosis in, 3:467
Langdon-Browne, Walter, 'On Getting the Rash Out' (1937), 1:455
Langs, Robert, 8:13
language of psychoanalysis, 4:4–5, 14; 6:360
   Balint on, 6:360
   S. Freud's language use and terminology, 4:6–7
Lantos, Barbara, 1: lxviii
   letter to (1956), 5:**179–181**
   'On the Problem of Aggression', 5:179ni
Lartigue/Lartigout, 1:81, 88
Lasix, DWW taking, 9:189
Lask, Aaron, *Asthma: Attitude and Milieu* (1966; reviewed by DWW), 7:**417–418**
latency period, 11:78, 80, 83
   defined and described, 5:354–357; 8:67
   ending treatment in, 5:358–359
   environment in, 11:169
   normal emotional development in, 5:427
   psychoanalysis in, 5:351–359
   WWII's effect on children in, 2:95–96
latent neurosis or psychosis, 4:42; 5:436
lay analysis, 4:237–238
laziness, 10:13
lead poisoning (Pink's disease), 11:105, 106n3
Lear, Edward, 12:307
Lebovici, Serge, 6:4, 115, 359
   Un Cas de Psychose Infantile (with Joyce McDougall, 1960; reviewed 1962), 6:**379–381**
   Dialogue with Sammy (with Joyce McDougall, 1969), preface by DWW, 9:**129–130**
   letter to (1960), 6:**115–116**
   'The Narcissistic Foundation of Object Relation', 6:115ni
lectures given by DWW, list of, 12:213–232
Lees, Kenneth, 1:115
Lehmann, Liza, 1:60
Lemma, Alessandra, 6:235ni
Lenox Hill Cardiac Care Unit, New York, 8:379, 390; 9:23, 24, 38
Leonardo da Vinci, 9:6, 302–303
LeShan, Eda J., *How to Survive Parenthood* (1965; reviewed 1967), 8:**181–182**°°°
letters, lists of, 12:171–192
leucorrhoea, 8:240–241, 243
leucotomy
   'Battle Neurosis Treated With Leucotomy' (*British Medical Journal* letter; 1947), 3:**113**

benefits of, 3:259, 260
DWW's critique of, 2:18, 379; 3:59, 72, 259–263; 4:210; 6:304, 12:12
'Ethics of Prefrontal Leucotomy' (*British Medical Journal* letter; 1951), 3:**467–468**
'Frontal Lobes of the Human Brain' (*The Lancet* letter; 1943), 4:**33**
'Leucotomy' (1949), 3:59, **259–263**
'Leucotomy in Psychosomatic Disorders' (*The Lancet* letter; 1951), 3:**465–466**
'Notes on the General Implications of Leucotomy' (1951), 2:207*n*i; 3:**477–481**
'Prefrontal Leucotomy' (*British Medical Journal* letter; 1956), 5:10, **119–120**
'Prefrontal Leucotomy' (*The Lancet* letter; 1943), 2:207*n*i, **207–208**
'Prefrontal Leucotomy' (*The Lancet* unpublished letter; 1943), 2:**209**
soul, DWW on, 11:76–77
Lévy-Solal, 1:81
Lewin, Bertram D., 6:405; 8:416; 10:13. *See also* dream screen
'Inferences from the Dream Screen' (1948), 8:416*n*ii
Lewis, Sir Aubrey
letter to (January 1961), 6:**177–178**
letter to (October 1961), 6:**267**
Lewis, Gwen, 1:11
Lewis, J. B. S., 2:209
Leys School, Cambridge, 1:xvi; 1:22; 1:31, 35*n*i, 37, 39–41, 45, 49, 55; 12:301
Leyton School Medical Service, 1:131
Lezany, 1:83
The Liberal Magazine, 2:341
Liberal Party, 2:341
libido, 4:132
life
meaning of life, cultural experience, and psychiatric treatment, 7:432, 433
origins of individual, 7:455–460
life instinct, 6:444; 9:37
Lightwood, Reginald, letter to (1959), 5:**437–438**
Likierman, Meira, 1: lxvii
Lilith, mythology of, 2:368*n*4
'"Lily" aet 5 Years', 10:17, 19, **451–452**
rehabilitation of the family as important aspect of case, 10:452
stealing as issue, 10:452
Limentani, Adam, letter to (1968), 8:3, **335–336**
Lindner, S., 5:419*n*5
Ling, T. M., 1:150
'A Link Between Paediatrics and Child Psychology: Clinical Observations' (1968), 1:310*n*ii; 2:125*n*ii; 8:**283–298**; 10:6
lip-sucking, compulsive, 1:450
Literary Editors of DWW's work, 1: xlviii

literature of medicine, 1:70
lithaemia, 1:237
Little, H. M., 3:356
Little, Margaret, 1: lxix*n*iii, lxxii; 3:218; 5:258, 511; 6:341; 8:4, 36, 46, 390; 11:7
'On Delusional Transference (Transference Psychosis)' (1958), 5:260*n*1; 7:173, 176*n*ii, 234, 238*n*4
'"R" - The analyst's total response to his patient's needs', 5:511*n*ii
Little's disease, 1:295; 6:391
'Living Creatively' (1970), 9:5, **213–224**. *See also* creativity
Lloyd George, David, 2:93
'The Location of Cultural Experience' (1966), 7:**429–436**; 8:13, 79*n*ii, 167, 205, 219, 300, 364; 9:12, 330
Loewenstein, Rudolph
libidinal theory of Hartmann-Kris-Loewenstein, 8:393
'Theory and Practice of Psychoanalysis', 5:363
London, changing architecture of, 8:191–193
London Child Guidance Clinic, 1:17; 2:47
London Clinic of Psychoanalysis, 1:xvii; 5:9
London County Council Children's Department, 6:423
London County Council Rheumatism Clinic, 9:99
London Hospital, 5:437–438
London Psycho-Analytical Society, 1:11
London School of Economics (LSE), 5:9, 473, 543; 9:57, 179*n*iii, 262
'Notes on the General Implications of Leucotomy', 2:207*n*i; 3:477
'Yes, but How Do We Know It's True?' (1950) given to students at, 3:423
London Society for Psycho-Analysts, 5:392
loneliness
'Loneliness in Infancy' (letter to *The British Medical Journal*; 1942), 2:**165**
'Loneliness in Infants' (Bakwin 1942), 4:265
Longchampt, 1:81
Loos, Anita: *Gentlemen Prefer Blondes*, 8:77*n*3
Lorenz, Konrad, 8:321
Lorenz, William F., 5:204
Los Angeles Psychoanalytical Society, 6:325; 333
loss. *See* grief, mourning, sadness, and loss
love. *See also* hate and hatred; primitive love
aggression and, 2:16, 65; 7:132, 133–134
appetite-love, 2:68
capacity to love, 10:385, 400
in care-cure position, 9:194–195
conditional love versus, 4:402
definition of, 6:383
deprived child's need for, 8:317
of DWW for wife Clare, 3:331
for environment mother, 6:16

love (*Cont.*)
  fathers and, 9:30
  in first year of life, 4:22; 5:330
  hate, coincidence with, 3:61, 64; 6:214, 383
  holding, as form of loving, 6:151
  influence in relationship and, 2:111
  love relationships, 11:72–74
  jealousy and, 6:47
  'The Meaning of Mother Love', 8:**117–120**
  moral education not a substitute for, 6:381
  in mother-child relationship, 3:270–271, 274; 6:16, 213–215, 350, 364
  as physical care, 11:36, 83, 120, 134, 147, 149, 172
  primal or primary repression and, 5:181
  primary love, 6:320
  primitive love impulse, 3:340, 394, 457; 4:65, 251; 5:155; 9:5, 183–184
  in psychoanalysis (letter to *New Society*, 1964), 7:**37–39**
  psychoanalysts disagreeing over topic of, 6:213–214
  religion and, 6:213
  sadness associated with, 4:311
  of son for mother, 11:73, 78, 84, 95
  transitional objects and, 5:117, 385
love and hate. *See also* hate. 1:110, 280, 320, 360, 377–378, 401, 413
  'love plus hate', 1:279*n*4, 312, 313
  enuresis and, 1:392
  mother's love and hate for child, 8:164, 308
Lovelace, Richard, 6:93
  'To Althea, From Prison' (1642), 9:79i
Low, Barbara, 1:17; 2:147; 5:392; 6:368
Lowenfeld, Margaret, 1:9, 15, 17, 404; 8:35, 41, 300; 9:176; 10:5
  'The World Technique', 10:5
Lowry, Oliver H., letter to (1956), 5:**161–163**
loyalty conflicts and the family, 7:393–396
LSE. *See* London School of Economics
Lucifer (Royal Navy vessel), DWW's service on, 1:3–4
Lucksch, F., 1:85, 86, 87, 88
Lundgren, Ester Ringner, *Little Trulsa's Secret* (reviewed 1967), 8:203
Lundholm, Helge, 'Repression and Rationalisation' (abstract; 1933), 1:**341**
Luria, Alexander, letter to (1960), 6:**105**
lying
  as antisocial behaviour, 10:370, 401, 438, 532
  dissociation versus, 7:247
  'Stealing and Telling Lies' (1949), 3:**313–317**

Maberley, Alan, 2:205, 205*n*i
MacAlpine, I., 3:246
MacCarthy, Dermod, 5:530

MacCormac, H., 1:462
Mackay, Helen, 1:145, 290*n*5
MacKeith, Ronald, 7:365–366
  The Child and His Symptoms: A Psychosomatic Approach (with J. Apley as co-author; 1962), 6:401*n*i
  Infant Feeding and Feeding Difficulties (with Philip Evans as co-author; reviewed 1951), 3:**491–493**; 6:401*n*i
  letter to (1963), 6:**401–402**
madness, psychology of
  aetiology of schizophrenia, 7:233
  borderline cases, based on, 7:232
  defining madness for purposes of, 7:229
  fear of madness, 7:229, 233–238
  infant development, no madness phase in, 7:231–232
  physiological problems and, 7:232–233
  polymorpho-perverse symptomatology of childhood and, 7:229–230
  'The Psychology of Madness' (1965), 7:4, 5, **229–238**
  therapy of psychosis linked with psychoanalytic practice, 7:230–231
magic
  in child's inner world, 2:285, 363
  illusion and magical control , 4:169
  infantile, 7:134
  projection/introjection and, 4:195, 197–199, 261
  magical destruction, 2:66; 7:10, 134–135
  magical control, 2:79–80, 284
  magical control of transitional object, 4:168
  medicine as, 2:54, 219, 256, 383
Mahler, Margaret S., 5:183, 186; 6:399; 9:329
maiming, 6:150
Main, Thomas
  'The Ailment', 5:201*n*i
  letters to (1957), 5:**201, 207–208**
  'Psychoanalysis as a Cross-Bearing' (1967), 8:149*n*i, 149–150
maladjusted children
  antisocial behaviour and, 5:151
  in Foote's *Six Children* (1956), 5:223
  'Group Influences and the Maladjusted Child: The School Aspect' (1955), 5:**45–54**
  'Maladjusted Children: Damaging Effect of Delay' (letter to the *Times*, 1950), 3:**361–362**
  transitional object, lack of, 3:379
  use of word", 3:92
Malan, David, 5:477–478
Malan Triangles, 5:477*n*i
Malev, Milton, 8:12, 387, 391
Malleson, Joan Graham, 3:181–182
  Any Wife, Any Husband (writing as Joan Graham; foreword by DWW; 1955), 5:**99**

Malthus, Thomas, 9:106
Maltings House School, 5:473
Manheimer, Marcel, 10:5
mania, 5:126
    meaning of 'manic', 8:438n2; 10:112n1
    omnipotence of, 4:136
manic defence, 1:14, 15,
    ascensive defence and, 1:364–365
    characteristics of, 1:362–366; 4:194–195
    clinical examples of, 1:366–372; 4:276; 5:470
    as defence against depression, 4:194, 210, 276
    denial of inner reality, 1:363
    depression and, 6:461, 466
    excitement versus, 5:290
    fantasy and, 1:359, 360, 362, 373n1
    flight to external reality from internal reality, 1:363
    hospitalisation of mother and, 7:291, 293, 302
    hypomania as clinical expression of, 5:450
    inner world of the child and, 11:105–106
    mania versus, 5:126
    'The Manic Defence' (1935), **359–374**; 3:14; 5:126nii, 498; 9:298n1
    as opposite in reassurance, 1:364
    play affected by, 5:247
    stages of grief leading to, 5:496
    suspended animation, 1:363–364
    symbolism and, 1:365–366
manic-depressive disease, 2:32; 3:137; 4:199–200; 6:65, 466; 10:254, 272
manic restlessness, 4:195
'A Man Looks at Motherhood' (1949), 3:**269–271**; 8:117
Mannheim, Hermann, 3:49, 49n1
    Young Offenders (1942), 2:196, 200n1
The Man Who Came to Dinner (play, 1939; movie, 1942), 7:332
Marfan, A. B., 1:78, 88
marital problems
    adolescents, psychotherapeutic interviews with, 7:54–55
    envy of the opposite sex and, 7:108
    incontinence of child as result of, 2:187–188
    of Jung's parents, 7:117–119
    quarrelling between parents, 3:338
    resentment of mother against child and, 2:186–187
'"Mark" aet 12 Years', 10:**369–402**, **525–526**
    capacity to love and, 10:385, 400
    depression and, 10:397, 399
    deprivation and, 10:399, 400
    dissociation and, 10:393, 402
    dreams and, 10:371, 378–379, 396, 399
    fantasy, expression of, 10:377, 389, 399
    lying as issue, 10:370, 401

    mother's depression and, 10:370, 399, 402n3
    parents doing bulk of management, 10:402
    sea-fixation, 10:380, 385, 399–402, 402n3
    sense of humour and, 10:394
    separation from mother and, 10:397–398
    sleep routine and, 10:371, 377
    squiggle game and, 10:372–378, *372–379*, 380–387, *381–387*, 388–398, *388–398*
    stealing as issue, 10:370, 393, 399–401
    weaning difficulties and fixation on mother and, 10:370, 399–400
Market End House (Bicester). *See* Q-Camps
married life
    creativity in, 9:217–220
    social work training on, 5:342–343
Marty, Pierre, 3:341, 347n1
    'Importance du Rôle de la Motricité dans la Relation d'Objet' (with Michel Fain; 1955), 5:197
Marx, Harpo, 10:269
masculinity, in *Holding and Interpretation: Fragment of an Analysis* (1955), 4:325, 339, 342
masochism, 2:70, 267
mastectomy, 8:147
masturbation, 3:108–110
    in adolescence, 6:425; 9:378
    aggressiveness and, 2:69
    antisocial behaviour resulting from giving up, 2:69–70
    anxiety and, 1:13, 156–157, 266, 268–269, 320, 328; 2:199
    asphyxiation as fantasy of, 3:215
    compulsive, 3:109–110, 459; 7:358
    daydreaming and, 9:248
    deprivation and, 11:70
    eating disorders and, 1:427–428
    enuresis and, 1:392
    excitement and, 5:290–291
    fantasy and. *See* fantasies
    guilt and, *see also* guilt. 1:141, 144; 8:432; 10:103
    Holding and Interpretation: Fragment of an Analysis (1955), 4:318, 319, 321, 353, 358, 398
    instincts and, 11:77
    masturbation fantasies, 1:141, 144, 157, 320, 323, 324; 4:318, 353
    'Masturbation', from *Clinical Notes* (1931), 1:**323–328**, 343n1
    papular urticaria and, 1:155–157, 324–325, 327, 344, 345–351
    penis, child complaining of pain in, 1:155
    in *The Piggle*, 11:212, 222, 232, 243nIV, 273nIII
    play as alternative to, 2:169; 8:300–301
    primal scene and, 5:243–244
    sex education in schools and, 3:324

masturbation (*Cont.*)
　sexual development in children and, 3:108–111
　spider symbolising in dream, 10:324
　squiggle game and, 10:103
　skin excitement and, 1:347, 348, 352, 455
　treatment of, 1:326–328
　stealing and, 7:257, 260, 265; 10:313
　therapeutic consultation and, 10:442
　Wilson, Ambrose Cyril, 'The Rôle of Fixation in Perversion and Masturbation' (1947), 5:399
materialism, 9:80
material presented by patients in analysis, 11:107–111
'Maternal Care and the Welfare State' (with Alice Stewart; 1959), 5:467*n*i
Maternity and Child Welfare, 1:101
mathematics, 8:14, 267–274
Mathematics Teaching, 8:267
Matthew, Gospel of
　7:5, 9:192*n*ii
　13:9, 8:259*n*ii
'"Matti," *aet* 12 1/2 years: A Therapeutic Consultation' (1961), 6:**237–239**; 10:15
maturity
　defined, 5:543–544
　democracy and, 3:408
　as development process, 3:397; 7:89
　DWW's criterion for, 11:19, 155
　environment in, 11:169
　'The Family and Emotional Maturity' (1960), 6:**117–123**
　health as emotional maturity, 3:95, 408–409; 5:426–428; 6:10, 344, 410, 414; 8:66
　integration and. *See* integration
The Maturational Processes and the Facilitating Environment (1965), 7:75*n*iii, **305–307**, 374; 8:167, 363*n*1; 9:29, 36, 43, 92, 300; 11:190, 192*n*2, 206*n*3
　maturational processes in context of environmental provision, 3:397–398; 6:9, 91, 117–123, 3460, 363–364, 380, 393, 434, 450, 462, 471, 5495; 8:44, 67
　'Psychiatric Disorder in Terms of Infantile Maturational Processes' (1963), 6:13, **479–490**
　socialisation and, 6:470
　war resulting in, 2:94
Maudsley Hospital, 3:266, 357; 4:239; 6:299
Maw, Miss, letter to (1959), 5:**439**
McAlpine, D., 1:290*n*3
McCarthy, Desmond, 3:174
McDougall, Joyce, and Serge Lebovici
　Un Cas de Psychose Infantile (with Joyce McDougall, 1960; reviewed 1962), 6:**379–381**
　Dialogue with Sammy (with Joyce McDougall, 1969), DWW's preface to, 9:**129–130**

Un Cas de Psychose Infantile (with Joyce McDougall, 1960; reviewed 1962), 6:**379–381**
McDougall, Kay, 9:179, 179*n*iii
McKissock, W., 2:207, 209
McLean Hospital (Belmont, Massachusetts), 6:491; *8*:30; 8:183
McMillan, Margaret, 3:472; 4:256; 7:154
McWhinnie, A. M., *Adopted Children*, 8:275
Mead, Margaret, 3:147*n*i; 7:326; 9:150, 151, 313
　'Address Introducing Margaret Mead, VIIIth Ernest Jones Lecture' (1957), by DWW, 5:**203–204**
　'Changing patterns of parent-child relations in an urban world' (1957), 5:204
　'Discussions on Child Development', 5:204
　letter to (1957), 5:**205**
meal planning, 6:84
Me and *Not-Me*, 11:149
　aggression and, 3:344–347
　beginning of individual and, 7:452–453
　concern, development of capacity for, 6:17, 353
　ego integration and, 6:393–394; 8:273
　envy and, 9:48–49
　failures in holding and, 6:9
　first not-me possession, 4:160–161, 167, 177*n*1; 5:406–410
　in *Holding and Interpretation*, 4:159
　not-me objects, 4:275–276
　object relating and, 9:329
　omnipotence, experience of, 9:298*n*4
　in *The Piggle*, 11:230*n*XV, 251*n*V, 252
　repudiated *Not-Me*, 4:274
　Spock, Benjamin, and, 6:291
　subjective objects and, 9:133
　transitional objects and, 3:447, 456; 5:406–410, 527; 9:265, 266
　unit status, establishment of, 11:90
meaning of life, cultural experience, and psychiatric treatment, 7:432, 433
measles
　'Encephalitis after Measles and Chicken-pox' (1928), 1:**115–116**
　'Measles Encephalitis' (1929), 1:**129–130**
　measles encephalitis in 'Varicella Encephalitis and Vaccinia Encephalitis' (with Nancy Gibbs; 1926), 1:88–89
　'Muscle Weakness, Altered Gait and Absent Deep Reflexes after Measles' (1928), 1:**117–118**
medical charts, 1:195–201
medical histories,
　adolescent patient, taking history from, 7:52
　birth process, 11:165–166
　cardiac neurosis, 7:381–382
　central nervous system diseases, 1:281–282
　deprived children, 3:376–378

examples and case studies, 1:176–185
excreta, parental reticence about, 1:315
family history, 1:173
'History-Taking', from *Clinical Notes* (1931), 1:9, **173–185**
interviews with child, 7:52, 280; 10:528
onset of condition, 1:175–176
paediatrics and psychiatry, interplay between, 3:124–125, 136–137
parental testimony, importance of, 1:155, 156, 381
past history of child, 1:174–175
'The Snag' (1921), 1:**65–66**
social worker taking, 2:180, 182
taking child's history from mother in front of the child, 2:182
teachers and, 1:381–382, 445–446
therapeutic consultation, 10:111, 183, 184, 233, 305, 308, 371, 403, 410, 442, 519, 528
transitional objects, use of, 4:297–298; 9:268
value of, 4:37, 166; 6:19
Medical News Magazine, 7:415; 8:323
Medical Press, 3:323; 4:291; 5:319
medical profession. *See also* nurses; paediatrics and paediatricians
  advisers, doctors as, 5:422–423
  'Advising Parents' (1957), 5:**277–284**
  Balint, Michael, *The Doctor, His Patients, and the Illness* (1957; reviewed 1958), 5:213ni, 215ni, 261ni, **401–404**
  Chair of Child Psychiatry, need for, 5:161–163
  'Cure' (1970), 9:**191–197**
  disorders of childhood, lessons learned from, 3:153–155
  DWW continuing to work in, 11:5–6
  DWW on, 1:67–71, 169–170, 451–452
  DWW's early interest in, 1:29–30
  family doctors, 7:155
  as friends to child, 1:275, 276
  interference of, 8:85–87, 344
  inter-speciality discussion, 3:351–352, 487
  mother, doctor, and nurse, relationship between, 5:228–229
  mother-child relationship and, 3:291–292, 310–311
  multidisciplinary teams, benefits of, 6:19–20
  nationalisation of, 3:37–38, 39, 141
  personal versus public doctor, 2:217–219
  psychoanalytic research and, 7:153–154, 155
  psychology, as professional field, 5:421–425
  psychosomatics and, 5:423; 11:53
  science in medical practice, 3:69–70
  training for, 5:403
medicines and drugs
  attitude of child toward, 9:53–54
  bromide, 1:268, 276, 305, 306, 308, 310
  calamine lotion, 1:327, 344
  DWW on use of, 1:279n3
  eating disorders in infants and, 1:431n1
  Lasix, DWW taking, 9:189
  magical action of, 2:54, 219, 256, 383
  'The Pill' (1969), 9:**101–110**
  sulphanilamide, 2:255–256
  'A Tendency in Therapeutics' (1944), 2:207ni, **255–259**
  tincture of stramonium, 1:287–288
  treatment of mental illness with, 7:315, 316ni
Medico-Psychological Clinic, Brunswick Square, London, 1:11
'Meeting the Challenge of the Case in Child Psychiatry' (1968), 8:438n1
'Meet to Be Stolen From' (ca. 1939–1945), 2:16–17, **141–142**
Megson, Barbara, and Clegg, Alec, *Children in Distress* (reviewed 1968), 8:**339**
Meisel, P., and W. Kendrick, eds., *Letters of James and Alix Strachey*, 8:124ni
melancholia, 3:137; 6:463, 464. *See also* depression
  Abraham on, 5:153, 449
  Burton, Robert, *Anatomy of Melancholy*, 5:137, 142
  defined, 5:140
  S. Freud on, 2:252; 5:10, 153, 333, 449
  Klein's depressive position and, 5:153
  as psychosis, 6:65
  trauma of melancholic mother after death of father, 7:174–176
'Melanie Klein: On her Concept of Envy' (1989), 6:269
Meltzer, Donald, 6:316, 322
  letter to (1959), 5:**463–464**
  letter to (1966), 7:**411–414**; 9:47
  'Notes on a Transient Inhibition of Chewing', 5:463ni
  'Sexuality' (1966), 7:411ni
memoranda
  'Memorandum from Paddington Green Children's Hospital Psychology Department on Homosexuality and the Law' (1955), 4:267
  'Memorandum on Corporal Punishment' (1945), 2:18, **349–351**
  'Memorandum on Gisburne House' (1959), 5:**441–443**
  'Memorandum on Organisational Aspects of Child Care at Paddington Green Children's Hospital (Psychology Department)' (1961), 6:19, **179–185**
  'Memorandum on "The Relation Between Clinical Paediatrics and Child Psychology"' (1943), 2:7, **201–205**

memory. *See also* birth memories
  accumulation of good memories in the child, 6:56
  Bion on 'memory and desire', 8:157
  five-year-old's ability to have memories, 6:310
  infancy and childhood, adult memory of, 3:101
  repressed memories, regaining, 3:101–102
meningitis, tuberculous, 1:119, 192, 282–284
meningococcal meningitis, 1:288–289, 290n5
meningo-encephalitis, 1:288
Menko, M. L. H. S., 1:78–79, 88
Menninger, K., 5:452
Menninger Clinic Bulletin, 6:342n3, 351
Menninger School of Psychiatry Forums Committee, 6:357
menopause, 6:409
menorrhagia, 1:192–193
menstruation
  anxieties regarding, 1:453
  onset of, 10:447
mental breakdown. *See* breakdown
mental disability
  attainment of child and, 1:299–301
  classification of, 1:299; 7:450
  definition of mental illness, 2:257; 6:410
  educational diagnosis of, 3:30
  'Mental Defect', in *Clinical Notes* (1931), 1:**299–302**
  'The Mentally Ill in Your Caseload' (1963), 6:13, **409–420**
  Mongolism (Down's syndrome), 1:296n2, 301
  parental point of view and, 1:301
  patient's acceptance of mental illness as diagnosis, 10:253
  psychological point of view on, 1:301–302; 2:160–161
  psychosis confused with, 3:134, 204, 353
  speech disorders and, 1:330
mental health. *See also* health
  aetiology of, 6:13
  development of, 3:126–127, 274
  distinguishing mental from physiological illness, 7:7, 232–233, 315–316, 456
  'The Foundation of Mental Health' (1951), 3:**437–439**
  as maturity, 3:95
  'The Psychotherapy of Character Disorders' (1963), 6:13, **447–459**
  society in terms of its mental illness or health, 9:338–340
  theory of, 3:71–72
  of therapists, 6:19
mental hospitals
  adolescents, lack of provision for, 7:339–340
  cruelty in, 2:265

  effect of therapy on staff and atmosphere of, 2:265–266
Mental Hygiene, 1:339
'Mental Hygiene of the Pre-School Child' (1936), 1:**397–411**. *See also* pre-school children
mental illness
  Mental Illness Association: Social and Medical Aspects (MIASMA), 6:197
  'The Mentally Ill in Your Caseload' (1963), 7:75, 75ni
  poetry and, 7:315
merging, 6:152, 507; 8:259–260
metaphysical poets, 9:261
'Metapsychological and Clinical Aspects of Regression within the Psychoanalytical Set-up' (1954), 7:124n1; 9:371nii
metapsychology, 4:5
  S. Freud on, 6:218–219
  'Metapsychological and Clinical Aspects of Regression within the Psychoanalytical Set-up' (1954), 1:373n6; 3:257n2; 4:8, 11–12, **205–221**, 225ni, 227ni, 261ni; 6:157n2, 159; 8:187nv, 218n2
  terminology of, 4:219
Metcalfe, Arthur J., letter to (1959), 5:**475–476**
Methodism, DWW influenced by, 5:4; 8:313–314; 12:301
Meyer, Adolf, 10:5
  preface to Kanner's *Child psychiatry* (1935), 1:439
Meyer, C. G. S., 8:1224
MIASMA (Mental Illness Association: Social and Medical Aspects), 6:197
micro-cephalia, 1:301
micturition. *See also* enuresis
  anxiety and urgency of, 1:156–157, 246, 250, 266, 315–316
  circumcision and, 2:26
  diabetes and, 1:316
  dreams and, 10:132
  dysuria, 1:144, 146, 316
  examination and testing of urine, 1:316–319
  girl's delusion of having a penis and diffidence about, 9:149
  haematuria, 1:79, 183, 318, 347
  'Micturition Disturbances', from *Clinical Notes* (1931), 1:**315–322**
  narrow meatal opening, 1:192
mid-diastolic murmur, 1:232
'Middle Group' (later the Independents), 3:41; 5:7–8, 501; 6:175, 211nii, 235
Middlemore, Merell P., 5:496, 524; 7:436n2; 8:41
  on nurses' efforts to assist mother's feeding of child, 2:296
  The Nursing Couple (1941), 5:528n2

paediatrics and psychiatry, interaction of, 3:124, 130
on presentation of feeding situation, 11:123
review (1941), 1: lxiv–lxv, 18; 2:12, **171–174**
'The Uses of Sensuality', in *On the Bringing up of Children* (1936), 1:437
midwifery, 1:68
  'Advising Parents' (1957), 5:**277–284**
  'The Contribution of Psycho-Analysis to Midwifery' (1957), 5:**225–232**, 239*n*i
Meitner-Graf, Lotte, photographs of DWW, 8:21–30
migraines, 1:267; 10:416
Miller, Arthur, 8:301
  Jane's Blanket (1963), 8:195*n*ii, 312*n*2
  letter to (1967), 8:**195**, 301*n*i
Miller, Emanuel, 1:9, 17, 18; 2:6; 5:5; 7:365–366; 9:176
  'Evacuation of Small Children' (*British Medical Journal* letter with DWW; 1939), 2:6, 47–48; 10:17
Miller, Jacques Alain, 6:46*n*i
Miller, Reginald, 1:77, 78, 82, 88, 91, 167, 237, 243*n*1; 2:55–58, 61
Mill Hill (former location of Maudsley Hospital), 3:266
Milne, A. A., 8:301
Milner, Dennis, 2:7, 10
Milner, Marion, 1: xlvii, lxv, lxix, lxix*n*nii–iii, lxxv, lxxvi; 2:7, 10, 19; 4:63, 178*n*10, 273–274; 5:43, 361*n*i, 419*n*8; 6:20; 7:96, 431; 8:171, 299–300; 9:5, 6, 329, 340; 11:13
  'Aspects of Symbolism in Comprehension of the Not-Self', 1: lxxv; 6:467*n*1
  in 'Cleopatra Anamnesis Imphiccough', 9:381
  The Hands of the Living God (preface by DWW; 1969), 2:19; 8:**115–116**
  On Not Being Able to Paint (1950; reviewed 1951), 1: lxxvi–lxxvii; 3:461, **483–485**
  'The Role of Illusion in Symbol Formation' (1952), 1: lxxv
  The Suppressed Madness of Sane Men: Forty-four Years of Exploring Psychoanalysis (1987), 9:6
Milton, John, 1:40
'"Milton" *aet* 8 Years', 10:**275–299, 521–523**
  bragging and, 10:294, 297–298
  breasts, sadistic attack on, 10:296
  bullying and, 10:276, 293, 294
  deeper level work, 10:289–297
  drawings of dreams and, 10:290–292, 290–292
  dreams and, 10:289–293, 294
  gender identity and, 10:284
  God and religion and, 10:294–295
  mother's later pregnancy and, 10:296
  noughts and crosses, DWW playing with, 10:276, *277*, 288, *288–289*
  oral sadism and, 10:298
  period of reassessment, 10:287–289
  primitive love impulse and, 10:298
  psychotherapeutic interview and, 10:276
  repression and, 10:293
  sado-masochism and, 10:276, 293, 295–296
  sibling rivalry and, 10:275
  squiggles game and, 10:277–287, *278–287*
  stealing and, 10:293–294
  transitional phenomena and, 10:280
mind
  brain and, 3:260
  'division into compartments, 10:196, 202
  as entity, 3:245
  false self and, 6:15, 163
  in first year of life, 5:323–324
  as function of psyche-soma, 3:246–247
  intellect and health, 8:77*n*2
  location of, 3:254–256; 8:169, 295
  Mind and Its Relation to the Psyche-Soma' (1949), 1: lxxi; 3:17, 220*nn*5–6, **245–257**; 4:203*n*i; 6:128, 163; 8:6, 185*n*iii, 447, 448; 9:329; 11:39*n*i
  'Mind and Its Relation to the Psyche-Soma' (1954), 7:69; 8:443
  as mother-substitute, 11:157–158
  'The Psyche-Soma and the Mind' (*Human Nature*; 1988), 11:**39–41**
  psyche versus, 6:15, 148
  reliving birth experience and, 3:250–254
  theory of, 3:247–250
Mind (organisation). *See* National Association for Mental Health
Ministry of Health
  complaints of, 5:488
  Goodenough Report, 3:243*n*i
  Government Paper on Children in Hospital (1959), 5:544*n*i
  hostels, establishment of, 3:26, 47, 78, 79, 82, 92*n*1
  Q Camps Report, 2:104–105
Ministry of Information, 2:5
mirroring, 8:5–7
  'Mirror-Role of Mother and Family' (1971), 7:329*n*1
  'Mirror-Role of Mother and Family in Child Development' (1967), 6:7, 11; 8:5, 13–14, **211–218**, 234*n*iv, 259*n*i, 304; 9:317*n*8
miscarriage and mother-foetus relationship, 9:390
mistakes, making use of, 9:25–26
Mitchell, Guy, 7:339
Mitchison, Naomi, *The Big Surprise* (reviewed 1967), 8:203–204

mitral regurgitation, 1:214
mitral stenosis, 1:153–154, 211, 212, 215–216, 232
Modern perspectives in child psychiatry (Howells, ed.), 10:525
modified analysis, 11:9
Molière, *Les Fourberies de Scapin* (1671), 8:62*n*iii
monarchy, 7:315; 8:367–368; 9:181–187
Moncrieff, A., 1:92; 3:181; 6:177
Money-Kyrle, Helen 'Minora' (née Fox), 1:442
Money-Kyrle, Roger
  background of, 4:63, 269
  democracy defined by, 3:408
  as discussant of DWW's paper on transitional objects, 1: lxxvi*n*iii
  letter to (1937), 1:**441–442**
  letters to (1949), 3:**195**, **197**, **199**, 223, 229, 231
  letters to (1950), 3:**365**, **381**, **385**
  letters to (1952), 1: lxviii; 3:10; 4:**63–67**
  letter to (1954), 4:**269–270**
  letters to (1955), 5:11, **19–20**, 33
  Mead, Margaret, and, 5:204
  Meltzer, Donald, and, 7:411
  Psychoanalysis and Politics (1951), 3:365; 11:86*n*4
  'Some Aspects of State and Character in Germany' (1951), 3:408*n*i
  Wisdom, John, writing on dissolution of Imago group, 8:263*n*i
Mongolism (Down's syndrome), 1:296*n*2, 301
Montefiore, Mr. (placing Jewish refugee children in England), 5:536
Montessori principle, 4:376
mood and psychosomatic disorders, 9:68–69
Moody, Robert, 5:258
moon landing
  letter to Renata Gaddini on (1969), 9:39–40
  'Moon Landing' (poem; 1969), 9:**89–90**, 109–110
Moore, Henry, 7:281
Moore, N., 1:60
Moore, Sheila, 1:61
morality and ethics. *See also* guilt
  'The Absence of a Sense of Guilt' (1966), 7:**437–452**
  attitude in psychotherapy, 8:231, 254
  in child emotional development, 3:171, 299–302; 6:13, 42, 6:297; 7:440–442, 453; 8:312, 316
  'The Development of the Child's Sense of Right and Wrong' (1962), 6:13, **301–304**
  Eppel, E. M., and M. Eppel, *Adolescents and Morality* (1966; review by DWW), 7:**401–402**
  'Ethics of Prefrontal Leucotomy' (*British Medical Journal* letter 1951), 3:**467–468**
  imposition of, 3:312, 325
  innate, inherited, or inborn tendencies, 7:437–438, 9:44

'The Innate Morality of the Baby' (1949), 3:**299–302**
  lack of moral sense, 5:144–145
  of leucotomy and shock therapy, 3:465, 467, 478
  'Morals and Education' (1962), 6:13, **377–388**; 7:187*n*5; 8:17; 9:300
  residential therapy and, 9:204
  sense of values, 6:383–386
Morley, Robert, 7:332
Morley, Mrs. Royston, *see* Benzie, Isa
Moro Response (Moro Reflex), 7:4, 46–48, 8:83
Morris, Professor, 7:407
Morrison, N. R. McLeod, 1:60
Morton, J. M., *Box and Cox* (1848), 7:77
'Mother, Teacher, and the Child's Needs' (1953), 4:**151–158**
Mother and Child (U.S. title of *The Child and the Family*), 5:297; 6:109, 293
mother-child relationship. *See also* ordinary devoted mother; parents; primary maternal preoccupation
  adaptation of mother to infant, 4:22, 36, 38–44, 168–170, 252–253; 6:5, 165, 214, 230, 381, 415, 472; 8:45, 66, 272, 315
  aggression and, 3:5, 165–166, 311–312
  anthropological study of, 7:389
  anxiety in, 9:243, 244
  'The Baby as a Going Concern' (1949), 3:**273–276**
  'The Baby as a Person' (1949), 3:**285–288**
  baby equated to mother-infant relationship, 2:14
  'bad mother', 4:63–64, 65–66, 127–128
  birth memories and, 3:215, 227–228
  'blood-tie child' case, harm to child from delay in placement, 7:365–366, 369
  books about child care, DWW on mothers reading, 7:83, 113, 125–126
  breastfeeding. *See* breastfeeding
  capacity to be alone and, 5:242–243
  career of mother, 6:75; 7:16–17, 92, 93, 332, 358–359
  caretaker, mother described as, 7:221, 222
  cathected internal mother imago, 6:132–133, 165, 3655
  chaotic mothers, 5:518–519
  'Children and Their Mothers' (1940), 2:**81–86**
  cleverness of mother versus devotion of mother, 7:16–17, 91–93
  communication between mother and child, 5:84–85
  cultural experience, location of, 7:429–430
  'dead mother', Greene's concept of, 3:15*n*vi
  deformity of mother passed down to child and, 10:54

depression of mother. *See* depression
depressive position in emotional development
    and, 11:91–93
development of, 3:126–127
'Development of the Theme of the Mother's
    Unconscious as Discovered in Psycho-
    Analytic Practice' (1969), 9:**75–78**
early separation, 2:31–32, 47–48
easing tension by management of triangular
    relationship, 2:187
ego of infant, mother providing support for.
    See ego
'ego relatedness' between infant and
    mother, 6:9
enjoyment and pleasure in, 3:274–275
evacuation during WWII. *See* evacuation of
    children; World War II
excited relationships, setting for,
    11:119–121; *11:120*
excretion, maternal management of, 3:282–284
failure and blame, 1:172, 277, 7:331–332, 334–335
father, existing within structure provided by,
    3:6*n*iii, 273–274
feeding. *See* breastfeeding; feeding
'Feeling Guilty' (1961), 6:**205–210**
A. Freud on, 3:126; 4:75
'Getting to Know Your Baby' (1945), 2:**221–225**
good-enough mothering/environment,
    3:247–248, 369–370; 4:65; 5:48, 61, 244, 329;
    6:11, 19, 89, 151–152, 164, 290, 320, 323, 346,
    380, 390; 7:326; 8:66, 188, 314; 9:122, 134, 274,
    340–342, 360
hate and, 3:66–67; 9:78
holding and, 3:96–97, 168, 209, 388–391; 4:11,
    252–253; 6:4–5. *See also* holding (concept of)
hypochondria in mothers, 3:117–122
illness of the mother, 10:419–420, 441, 449
illness versus normal behaviour, 3:393–396
individual emotional development and,
    5:46–47, 48
individuation and, 9:208–209
infant development, DWW's theory of, 1:
    lxv–lxvi; 6:150–156, 338–341
infant's identification with the mother, 6:89–90
influence of, 2:110; 7:126–127; 8:112; 112
'The Innate Morality of the Baby' (1949),
    3:**299–302**
'Instincts and Normal Difficulties' (1950),
    3:**393–396**
instinctual experience of infant and, 4:56
intellectual understanding of infant's needs,
    6:348; 7:16–17, 91–93
internal mother, 2:11
interpsychic processes, DWW's awareness
    of, 3:7–9

introducing infant to external world, 11:171–173
intuitive actions of, 1:101
'Knowing and Learning' (1950), 3:**387–391**
love-hate relationship with children, 1:277,
    278–279*n*4
love in, 3:270–271, 274; 8:117–120
loyalty conflicts and, 7:394
'A Man Looks at Motherhood' (1949),
    3:**269–271**
Maternal Care and Mental Health (Bowlby 1951;
    reviewed 1953), 4:**111–114**
maternal care function, 6:90–91, 150–156, 157*n*3;
    7:43, 194–195
maternal instinct, 4:21–22; 8:153, 236
Mead, Margaret, on, 5:204
medical professionals and, 2:288–289; 3:291–292,
    310–311
medicines and drugs, attitude of child
    toward, 9:53
mental health and, 3:126–128
methodological approach of DWW to child
    development and, 3:6–7
mind as mother-substitute, 11:157–158
mirror role of mother, 6:5–6. *See also* mirroring
Mother and Child (U.S. version of *The Child
    and the Family*), 9:92
'The Mother-Infant Experience of Mutuality'
    (1969), 9:**131–139**
'The Mother's Contribution to Society' (1957),
    5:13, **293–296**
'Mother's Madness Appearing in the Clinical
    Material as an Ego-Alien Factor' (1969),
    9:**141–148**
'The Neonate and His Mother' (1964), 7:4, 5,
    41–50, 84*n*i
'A Note on the Mother-Foetus Relationship'
    (undated; first published 1989), 9:**389–390**
object-mother versus environment-mother,
    6:16, 353–355, 385, 436
'ordinary devoted mother' factor in
    integration, 7:7
overidentification of mother with child, 9:139*n*6
overindulgenge, 4:235–236
personhood of baby and, 3:96–100, 285–288,
    308–310
phallus, maternal, 5:160, 418
physical care as psychological care, 3:98–99
preparation for, 7:331–332
primary maternal preoccupation. *See also*
    primary maternal preoccupation, 8:230
primary narcissism in, 3:10–11
privacy of mother sacrificed, 6:8, 78–79
psychoanalytic research and, 7:154–155
psychotic parents, children with, 5:517
reality, relationship with, 3:130–132, 11:128–129

mother-child relationship (*Cont.*)
  'The Relationship of a Mother to Her Baby at the Beginning' (1960), 6:12, **87–92**
  reparation and, 3:12–15
  result of psychotherapeutic interview in improved relationship, 10:333–334
  Rickman (ed.), *On the bringing up of children* (1936), review on maternal reading of, 1:437–438
  role in treatment of anxiety in children, 1:277–278
  'Saying "No"' (1960) 6:**31–42**, 86
  self-confidence of mother, 2:159
  sense of security, 6:36, 93–96
  sexual development in children and, 3:102–104, 105–106, 107
  social worker's assistance to mother, 2:183
  stealing as looking for mother, 3:46, 314–315, 320, 336*n*ii, 371; 5:150–151, 153–154
  surrender of mother at beginning, 6:81
  talking to mothers about, 3:425; 6:31–42, 73–86
  thinking, as mother-substitute, 7:142–144
  tiredness of mothers, 6:74
  toilet training and, 1:393
  transient total devotion to child in early months of life, 7:5, 42, 91–93, 333–334, 335–337
  transitional object, mother as, 9:360
  transitional objects, DWW's theory of, 1: lxix
  transitivity of experience in, 2:15
  twins and, 2:344–345
  unawareness of satisfactory maternal care, 6:154
  unit, mother and baby as, 5:7, 8, 11, 12, 13–14, 31–32, 181; 6:6–7
  untidiness as irksome in, 6:73–77
  'What Irks?' (1960), 6:**73–86**
  'The World in Small Doses' (1949), 3:**293–297**
'The Mother's Contribution to Society', 3:421*n*4; 7:126*n*i
motility, 5:197–198, 328–329; 7:130–131
Mount Everest, 7:260
mourning, 11:93. *See* grief, mourning, sadness, and loss
mouth. *See also* finger-sucking; thumb-sucking
  causing anxiety and fear in infants, 2:227
mouthing, 5:386
Moynihan, Rodrigo, 5:394
'"Mrs X" *aet* 30 Years', 10:19, **441–450**
  anger and, 10:444–445
  depression and, 10:444
  deprived childhood of mother, 10:442–443
  dreams and, 10:446–447, 448
  jealousy of friends and, 10:443
  masturbation and, 10:442
  mother consulting on behalf of her daughter when illness really mother's, 10:441, 449
  mother insisting upon her being a bad person, 10:442–443
  onset of menstruation and, 10:447
  orphanage experience of, 10:443–444, 446–449
  religion and, 10:445
  searching for her mother who abandoned her to orphanage, 10:446
  sexual excitement from holding children, 10:445
  stealing as issue, 10:445, 446
Mulberry Bush school (residential special school), 8:409*n*i
Müller-Braunsweig, Ada, 5:536
multidisciplinary teams, benefits of, 6:19–20
multiple personalities, 4:130
Munro, Dr, 4:270
Murray, Gilbert, 5:543; 7:408; 9:340
muscle erotism, 6:17
'Muscle Weakness, Altered Gait and Absent Deep Reflexes after Measles' (1928), 1:**117–118**
muscular atrophy, 1:293
muscular dystrophies, 1:293–294
music
  in dream, 8:101
  as occupation therapy, 3:266–267
Mussolini, Benito, 2:89
muteness
  deafness, due to, 1:334–335
  hysterical mutism, 1:270, 334, 335
mutuality
  in basic care and holding, 9:137–133
  communication and, 9:134–135
  drives, not related to, 9:136–137
  'The Mother-Infant Experience of Mutuality' (1969), 9:**131–139**
  subjective object and, 9:132–134
M'Uzan, Michel de, 4:13
Myers, F. W. H., 8:124*n*i
mysticism, 6:439
myths and dreams, trio of women in, 11:5, 74
myxoedema, 6:409

Nagera, Humberto, 8:281
  'Early Childhood' (1964), 7:147
  letter to (1965), 7:**147–148**
  in *The Psychoanalytic Study of the Child*, Volume 20 (1966; reviewed by DWW), 7:376
nail-biting, 2:367; 5:104
naiveté and dwelling of psyche in body, 11:141
NAMH. *See* National Association for Mental Health
narcissism, 4:16, 206; 5:242, 448; 6:44, 425; 7:6
narcolepsy, 1:150

nasal problems. *See* nose and throat
National Association for Mental Health (NAMH; later Mind), 3:147*n*i; 7:14, 149, 243, 429
The Case as the Patient Sees It: Psychoanalysis (foreword by DWW; 1957), 5:233–234, **235–236**
National Childbirth Conference (London 1968), 8:341
National Childbirth Trust (formerly Natural Childbirth Association), 5:13, 239, 305; 10:138
National Children's Home, Simey's Convocation Lecture (1960), 6:213
National Froebel Foundation Bulletin, 3:29
National Health Service (NHS), 2:18, 217–219; 3:37–38, 39, 141; 5:8–9, 233
National Health Service Act (1947), 2:5
National Institute of Industrial Psychology, 2:163*n*2
nationalism, 6:123*n*2
National Marriage Guidance Council Journal, 8:411
National service (military) in Britain, 5:6
National Society for the Prevention of Cruelty to Children, 3:349
National Society of Day Nurseries, 1:17, 101
Natural Childbirth Association (later National Childbirth Trust), 5:13, 239, 305
natural childbirth movement, 5:12–13; 10:138
natural cure, 6:450
Nature, obituary for Susan Isaacs in, 3:161; 8:333
Nazis and Nazism, 1: lxiv, 17, 408, 463; 2:89–90, 93; 3:35; 5:7, 394–395, 535–536; 9:94. *See also* World War II
need satisfaction, 6:15, 132; 7:373–374; 9:139*n*4
'Needs of the Under-Fives' (1954), 4:**249–256**
negative mother transference, 3:233
neglect
  mother alternating between interference and, 6:290
  'Neglected Children' (letter to the *Times*; 1950), 3:**349–350**
Nelson, Gillian, letter to (1967), 8:**159–160**
Nemon, Oscar
  bust of D. W. Winnicott (1971), 1:*ii, and front matter of each volume*
  DWW in studio of, 9:18
  S. Freud, statue of, *9:19*; 12:3–4
'The Neonate and His Mother' (1964), 7:4, 5, **41–50**, 84*n*i
nephritis
  albuminuria and, 1:317
  hæmorrhagic, 1:79, 183, 318, 203221
  pyelo-nephritis or pyelitis, 1:317
  red corpuscles in urine and active forms of, 1:318
nervousness. *See* anxiety

nervous system. *See* central nervous system
Netter, H., 1:81
neurosis. *See also* obsessional neurosis; psychoneurosis; transference
  analyst, neurotic patient's view of, 3:60
  Bion on, 5:86
  'A Case Managed at Home' (1955), 5:89, 92, 96–97
  classification of psychiatric disorders, 5:367–368, 450–452
  defined and described, 5:165–167; 6:199; 11:44
  developmental stage linked to, 6:13–14
  DWW on neurotic children, 1:15–16*n*vii, 16
  English inhibited pattern of, 9:175
  hysteria and, 4:58
  infantile, 7:148
  Jones, Ernest: 'Treatment of the Neuroses' (1920), 1:328*n*2
  latent neurosis in children, 5:426
  manifest neurosis in children, 5:425
  mother affected by child's neurosis, 1:278
  'Neurosis in the Child' (discussion, 1936), 1:15
  obsessional neurosis, 11:154
  'Ocular Psychoneuroses of Childhood' (1944), 2:3, **313–319**
  'On Cardiac Neurosis in Children' (1966), 1:123*n*i; 7:**379–386**; 10:6
  origins of, 4:36, 1106; 11:60, 64–65, 72, 74
  'Paediatrics and Childhood Neurosis' (1956), 5:**165–170**
  of parents, 1:172, 275
  psychoanalytical environment and, 3:64
  psycho-neurosis versus, 6:253; 11:82, 140
  psychosis versus, 4:71–72, 128, 441
  relation to emotional development, 2:257, 387
  transference neurosis, 4:73, 196, 205, 234, 304, 307; 5:62, 64, 133*n*i, 446, 482, 506–510; 6:412
  treatment of, 5:168; 6:201, 203
  understanding of healthy child through study of, 11:63–64
  war-neurosis, treatment of, 4:136
  in women or girls, 11:70, 71
neurosurgery and psychology, 3:261, 466
Neville, L. Crofts, 1:60, 61
newborn. *See also* infant development
  development of acceptance of psychology of, 1:432*n*2
  devotion to, 4:22
  'The New Baby' (1945), 2:21*n*iii
  social change and policy toward mother-infant relationship, 4:254
New Directions in Psychoanalysis, 3:223
New Education Fellowship Monograph, 2:299
New Era in Home and School, 3:43, 95, 441; 4:103; 6:423; 9:179; 11:27

New Library of Psychoanalysis, 6:235*n*i
'New Light on Children's Thinking' (1965), 1: lxxi; 7:7, **139–144**
New Society, 6:423; 7:79; 9:93, 101
    letter to (1964), 7:16, **37–39**
    reviews published in, 7:33, 213, 311, 367, 401, 417, 427; 8:89, 105, 129, 181, 203, 275, 279, 339
New Statesman, 8:124, 321; 9:84
New York Herald-Tribune, 5:109
New York Psychoanalytic Society and Institute, 8:3, 12, 355, 363, 365; 9:3, 26, 36; 12:4
New York State serum, 1:290*n*5
NHS, *see* National Health Service
Niblett, W. R., 6:378, 387
Niederland, William, 5:363–364
'The Niffle' (probably before 1961; published 1996), 9:**383–387**
Nigeria, paranoia in, 7:215
'The Night Attack' (1914), 1:**39–41**
nightmare, 11:101
    in *The Piggle*, 11:201, 203, 204, 212
night terrors
    active heart disease and, 1:230, 235, 237
    anxiety and, 1:261, 263, 265, 268
    arthritis and, 1:240, 241, 242
    chorea and, 1:134, 136, 137, 138
    convulsions and fits, 1:308, 312
    fidgetiness and, 1:246, 251
    medical histories, taking, 1:174, 177, 180
    in only children, 1:108
    pathological sleeping and, 1:149, 150
    post-encephalitic hyperpnoea and, 1:95–96
    pre-school children and, 1:405
    rheumatic fever and, 1:225, 227
    sexual climax and, 3:105
    speech disorders and, 1:332
1952 Club, 8:3–4, 12–13, 17*n*1, 35, 335
nocturnal epilepsy, 1:146
noncommunication, distinguished from failure to communicate, 6:11
non-directive play therapy, 9:159–164
non-existence, 6:530–531
'The Non-Pharmacological Treatment of Psychosis in Childhood' (1968), 8:**99–104**
nonverbal approach, 8:16, 117–118
normal and pathological, continuity between, 7:6, 31
normal children
    defining normality, 7:158–160
    A. Freud on, 7:220
    normal psychology, 4:153–155
    'What Do We Mean by a Normal Child?' (published 1946 & radio broadcast), 2:21*n*iii, **281–286**
normal difficulties of life, children dealing with, 5:425

normal shyness, 1:447
Norman, Lady, 7:407
North, Roger (Lord), 2:19, 195, 233*n*i
    letter from (reprint of), 2:234
    letter to (1944), 2:195, **233–236**
Northern Ireland, Catholic-Protestant divide in, 9:118
nose and throat
    adenoids, 1:203–204, 329
    nasal congestion due to anxiety, 1:267, 270
    'The Nose and Throat', from *Clinical Notes* (1931), 1:**203–205**
    obsessive nose-picking, 1:270, 455
    throat issues due to anxiety, 1:270–271
    tonsils, tonsilitis, and tonsillectomies, 1:204–205
'A Note on a Case Involving Envy' (1963), 6:**403–405**
'Note on Infant Observation' (undated; written after Paris IPA Congress of 1957), 9:**371–372**
'A Note on Normality and Anxiety', from *Clinical Notes* (1931), 1:**255–273**; 7:148*n*i. *See also* anxiety
'A Note on Regression and Reassurance' (1955), 5:**107–108**
'A Note on Temperature and the Importance of Charts', from *Clinical Notes* (1931), 1:**195–201**
'A Note on the Mother-Foetus Relationship'(undated; first published 1989), 9:**389–390**
'Notes for a Discussion on Technique in Analysis of Psychotics' (undated), 9:**365–366**
'Notes for the Vienna Congress' (1971), 9:15, **355–356**
'Notes Made in the Train' (1965), 7:**163–167**; 8:18*n*7, 355; 9:33
'Notes on Adolescence' (1956), 5:**189–193**
'Notes on a Little Boy' (1938), 1:376*n*1, **443–444**
'Notes on Play' (undated, before late 1960s; in 'Ideas' file), 9:**375–379**
'Notes on the Discussion Held on Dr Winnicott's Paper "The Birth Trauma"' (1949), 3:**225–228**
'Notes on the General Implications of Leucotomy' (1951), 2:207*n*i; 3:**477–481**
'Notes on the Time Factor in Treatment' (1961), 6:**225–227**; 8:269*n*iv
'Notes on Withdrawal and Regression' (1989), 7:6
'Nothing at the Centre' (1959), 5:**469–471**
'Not Less than Everything', 8:245; 9:**351–353**; 10:3
Nouvelle Revue de Psychanalyse, 9:79, 225, 259
nuclear war, fear of, 5:6; 7:152, 403
numbers as fertility symbols, 10:330, *331*–332
Nursery Journal, 4:249
nursery rhymes, 8:269*n*iv, 270
nursery schools, 4:154, 231
    adopted children and, 4:151–152

day nurseries versus, 3:471; 4:235–236, 260
education of teachers for, 4:256
five-year-old at, 6:310–311
individual emotional development and, 5:46
letter to *The Times* on importance of
(1959), 5:**461**
mental hygiene of pre-school children and,
1:402–404
'Nursery Schools: A Definition of Functions'
(letter to *the Times*; 1951), 3:**471–472**
in *The Piggle*, 11:213, 247, 276, 285
play in, 6:3171
psychoanalytic research and, 7:154
as substitute for family support, 4:255
teacher's role in, 4:155–158
Nursery Schools Association, 1:397; 7:14, 331, 387
nurses
breastfeeding and, 2:390–391; 3:291–292;
5:230–232; 11:122–123
depression in parents, dealing with, 5:372–373
DWW opinion while in NYC hospital, 8:385
as maternal aides, disadvantages of use of, 2:224
mother, doctor, and nurse, relationship
between, 5:228–229
mother-child relationship and, 3:291–292,
310–311
visiting children in hospital and, 3:438, 441–445
Nurses' Home Fund, 1:59
nursing baby. *See* breastfeeding
nursing couple, neonate and mother referred to
as, 7:41, 436*n*2
Nursing Mirror, 5:225, 239
nurture, 4:233

obituaries
Oscar Friedmann (1959), 5:**535–537**
Susan Isaacs (1948), 3:**161–163**; 8:333
Ernest Jones (1958), 5:**389–398**
Melanie Klein (1960), 6:**113–114**
James Strachey (1969), 8:**123–127**; 10:9
Ambrose Cyril Wilson (1958), 5:**399–400**
object relationships. *See also* entries at 'The Use of
an Object...'
aggression and, 6:435
capacity to communicate and, 6:434–436
'Clinical Illustration of "The Use of an Object"'
(1968), 8:**365–368**
'Comments on My Paper "The Use of an
Object"' (1968), 6:17; 8:15, 355, 390*n*iii,
393–395
definition and description, 6:328; 8:71, 357–358
destruction and survival, 8:346–347, 359, 363,
394–395
ego initiating, 6:392, 395
in emotional development of individual,
9:328–220

faulty, 6:91
in first year of life, 4:134; 5:327; 6:148, 4839;
8:84–85
five-year-olds and, 6:3193–314
'Found Objects and Waifs' (undated; from
'Ideas' file), 9:**373–374**
maternal adaptation facilitating, 6:415
mother-child communication and
object-relating, 9:135
objectively perceived object, 6:437–442
object-presenting, 6:525; 7:43
object-seeking, 8:47
primitive aspects of, 6:482
sequence of, 8:362, 363
split-off male and female elements in men and
women and, 7:324–326; 9:311–313
state of affairs preceding, 4:57
two-body relationship and, 4:57; 8:358
observations, clinical. *See* clinical observations
The Observer, 4:308, 315; 6:175, 461
letters to (1964), 7:17, **91–93**, **101**, 113, 345*n*i
obsessional neurosis
in adolescence, 6:14
analyst, obsessional neurotic's view of, 3:60
'Comment on Obsessional Neurosis and
"Frankie"' (1966), 7:**193–195**; 9:317*n*4
depression and, 5:126
destructive impulse and, 6:257
'Fragments Concerning Varieties of Clinical
Confusion' (1956), 5:**125–128**
S. Freud's theory of, 3:257*n*1
guilt in, 5:139–140
intelligence quotient and, 7:198
obsessive compulsive disorder, 10:16
'Spoken Comments on Obsessional Neurosis
and Frankie' (1965), 7:**197–201**
occupation therapy
Adrian Hill on, 3:266–267
use of term, 2:252
'Ocular Psychoneuroses of Childhood' (1944), 2:3,
313–319
O'Donovan, W. J., 1:451, 462
Oedipus complex
aetiology of illness and, 6:188
aggression and, 3:339
anxiety and, 11:78–79
as achievement of health, 11:73
Balint on, 4:276
basic principles of psychoanalysis and,
5:352–353
capacity to be alone and, 5:244
changing views of, 5:449
death wish and, 11:74
direct childhood observation and, 5:251
DWW's paediatric training and, 1:13–14
in DWW's psychoanalytical training, 8:35, 41

Oedipus complex (*Cont.*)
  DWW versus Freud and other analysts on,
    1: lxxiv, 431*n*2; 4:15
  envy and, 6:269
  S. Freud on, 3:102–103; 6:15, 129, 479;
    11:72–73, 78, 83
  gender and emotional development, 7:104–105
  good-enough provision and, 6:346
  guilt and, 5:137, 138, 141, 145
  in *Holding and Interpretation*, 4:16
  homosexuality and, 6:407
  impatience of parents and teachers with,
    11:60–61
  infant development and, 2:134
  instinct theory and, 11:78–79
  inverted Oedipus Complex, 11:78, 89
  Jung and, 7:121
  Klein on, 5:7; 9:38*n*1
  love relationships and, 11:72–74
  need to separate from mother and, 6:317
  neurosis and, 5:167, 450, 452
  normal development and, 4:185–200, 205; 6:255
  passing of, 6:129–133, 144
  persons never reaching, 9:34
  The Piggle, Oedipal fantasies in, 11:212
  play as means of working through, 2:156
  psychoanalytic preoccupation with,
    6:326–330; 9:131
  in psychoanalytic technique, 5:211; 6:8, 220,
    258; 8:41
  psychology of madness and, 7:230
  psychosis and, 6:411, 9:38
  re-situated by DWW, 11:14, 18
  stage of concern and, 6:352
  superego and, 5:446
  twins and, 4:106
O'Flynn, Elizabeth, 1:99, 111, 152, 167
  'Abscess in Frontal Lobe: Post-Mortem
    Findings' (with DWW; 1928), 1:**119–121**;
    1:120, 121
Ogden, Thomas, 1:xlix, lxi, lxv, lxvii; 3:4; 6:523
Old Sir Simon the King (nursery rhyme),
  11:264, 269*n*1
omnipotence, 4:136–1437, 169
  of analyst, 6:486; 8:17
  dissociation versus experience of, 9:298*n*4
  of ego, 6:527
  illusion and, 6:5; 9:7
  of infant, 6:141–142, 149, 164–165, 167, 271, 341,
    364, 365, 390, 394, 395, 434, 503, 517; 7:6; 8:67,
    71–72, 234
  of patient, 8:375
  shock of loss of, 9:9
  trauma and the family, 7:184, 185
'On Acting Out and Its Role in the Psychoanalytic
  Process' (IPA congress 1967), 8:7

'On Adoption' (1957), 5:**21–23**
'On Cardiac Neurosis in Children' (1966), 1:123*n*i;
  7:**379–386**; 10:6
'On Child Analysis and Paediatrics' (IPA
  congress; 1967), 8:7–8
'On the Contribution of Direct Child Observation
  to Psycho-Analysis' (1957), 5:**249–254**, 457
'On Influencing and Being Influenced' (1941),
  2:**109–113**
'On In-Patient Treatment for Rheumatic Fever
  and Chorea' (ca. 1923–1931), 1:**161–163**
only child
  advantages of being, 2:324
  from age five in father-mother-child triad,
    1:103–107
  care and treatment of, 1:109–110; 4:255
  care of ageing parents and, 2:326
  disadvantages of being, 2:324–327
  as family member, 1:107–108
  as an infant, 1:101–103
  letting each new infant have 'only child'
    experience, 7:17, 93
  medical problems of, 1:102, 108
  'The Only Child' (1927), 1:15, 17, **101–110**
  'The Only Child' (published & radio broadcast;
    1945), 2:21*n*iii, **323–327**
  play groups, value of, 7:395
  reasons parents may choose to have only one
    child, 2:323–324
'On Scientific Aims in Psychoanalysis' (British
  Psychoanalytical Society; 1942), 2:10
'On Security' (1960), 6:**93–96**
'On "Separation Anxiety" by John Bowlby' (1958),
  5:6, **379–381**
'On the Nature of Mental Breakdown' (1963),
  6:523, 537*n*ii
'On the Occasion of the Publication of the
  *Standard Edition of the Psychological Works
  of Sigmund Freud*', 7:15, 18, **407–410**, 429
'On the Origins of Violence' (1964; now
  lost), 7:129
Operation Pied Piper. *See* evacuation of children
Ophuijsen, J. H. W., 'On the Origin of the Feeling
  of Persecution' (1920), 11:102*n*7
Opie, I, and P. Opie, *The Oxford Dictionary of
  Nursery Rhymes* (1951), 9:343
Oppenheim's disease, 1:293
opportunity, provision of, 6:386–388
oral erotism, 3:214, 334; 4:203
oral fixation, 4:131–132
oral sadism, 6:239; 8:286
  anger and, 6:336
  confusion and, 5:125
  eating and fantasy of eating, 5:470
  envy and, 5:11, 365, 433, 434, 436
  instinct-drive episodes and, 6:354

Klein on, 4:196; 5:142
in latency period, 5:357
mistaken for compulsive greed, 6:487
psychiatric classification and, 5:448
therapeutic consultation, 10:229, 298
in transference, 4:203
the ordinary devoted mother
  autism and, 7:331–332, 352–354, 355, 356, 360–363
  definition of devoted, 7:332
  failure and blame, 7:331–332, 334–335, 360–261
  integration made possible by, 7:7, 336–337
  intense early period of infant care, 7:333–334, 335–337
  'The Ordinary Devoted Mother' (1966), 2:13, 221; 6:514; 7:7, **331–337**; 12:12
  The Ordinary Devoted Mother and Her Baby (BBC series and publication; 1949), 3:269, 273, 277, 281, 285, 289, 293, 299, 303; 6:171*n*1; 12:12–14
  The Ordinary Devoted Mother and Her Children (BBC series; 1960), 6:31, 47, 73, 299; 7:331; 12:10
  origin of term, 12:12–13
  preparation for arrival of child, 7:332–333
orgiastic functioning and fantasies, 9:369–370, 390
original sin, 4:472–473; 6:378
orphanage experience, 10:443–444, 446–449
Osler, William (with Ernest Jones in Canada), 5:391
osteopathy, 2:218–219; 3:29, 39, 141, 167
'Other Sex Identifications' (1970), 9:169*n*ii
'Outline for a Study in the Sociology of Knowledge' (incomplete and undated), 9:**391–394**
out-patient department, 2:181–185
Owen, Morfydd, 5:393, 398*n*10
The Owl and the Pussycat (Edward Lear), 12:307
The Oxford Dictionary of Nursery Rhymes (Iona and Peter Opie, Eds., 1951), 8:269*n*iv
Oxfordshire Evacuation Scheme, 1: lix, 18; 2:8–9, 300–301; 6:17, 181; 8:42; 9:199; 12:306
Oxford University Scientific Society, 6:217

Paddington Green Children's Hospital, London
  DWW as physician-in-charge of, 6:181
  DWW, retirement from, 6:3, 19, 182–183, 264–265
  DWW, work at, 1: lviii, lxii, 5–8, 18, 75, 161, 167, 353; 2:3, 6, 179, 183; 3:24, 227; 5:9, 27, 35, 307, 438, 475, 482, 488; 6:180–181; 8:150; 9:99; 10:4, 7–8, 451; 11:5, 189; 12:305–306
  educational psychologist, employment of, 6:181
  future of, DWW advice for, 6:183–185
  Guthrie, Leonard, at, 11:38*n*1
  Institute of Psycho-Analysis working with, 6:182
  'Memorandum from Paddington Green Children's Hospital Psychology Department on Homosexuality and the Law' (1955), 4:267
  'Memorandum on Organisational Aspects of Child Care at Paddington Green Children's Hospital (Psychology Department)' (1961), 6:19; **6:179–185**
  merger of St Mary's Hospital, 6:181, 307. See also St Mary's Hospital Paddington Green
  organisation of, 6:181–182
  'Paddington Green Children's Hospital' (letter to the *British Medical Journal* 1949), 3:**243–244**
  post–World War II, 6:181
  senior registrar, appointment of, 6:181, 185
  social workers, appointment of, 6:180–181, 184–185
  in 'String', 9:279
  submission to the Committee on Homosexuality (1954), 4:267*n*ii
  threat to close, 3:221–222, 243–244
paediatrics and paediatricians
  childhood psychosis, awareness of, 3:353; 4:36
  child psychiatry and, 2:10; 4:78, 117, 228; 5:423–424; 6:20, 177, 269–271, 310–311; 9:174, 176; 10:5; 11:37
  childhood sexuality and, 3:108–109
  as field of study, 8:54–55
  'A Link Between Paediatrics and Child Psychology: Clinical Observations' (1968), 1:310*n*ii; 2:125*n*ii; 8:**283–298**; 10:6
  'The Paediatric Department of Psychology' (1961), 6:**263–265**, 273; 10:6
  'Paediatrics and Childhood Neurosis' (1956), 5:**165–170**
  'Paediatrics and Psychiatry' (1948), 1: lxii; 3:13–14, **123–139**; 4:43; 6:467*n*1; 9:304; 10:8; 11:129*n*II
  preventive medicine, importance for, 2:202
  psychiatrists, psychologists and, shortage of, 2:185, 202
  psychiatry and, 3:126, 136, 487
  psychoanalysis and, 1:12–17; 6:183–184, 304–305, 484; 8:81, 283–298; 11:5, 37
  psychology and, 2:201; 4:80–81, 269
  rareness of physical disease in, 2:202
  'Relationship between Clinical Paediatrics and Child Psychology', 2:**201–205**
  social change and, 4:254
  specialties of, 2:201
  'Taking Children's Temperatures' (letter to *British Medical Journal*; 1949), 3:**181–182**
  University Chair in Paediatrics, need for two professors in, 6:265

pain
  baby crying due to, 2:239–240, 244
  as lesson of learning what is dangerous, 6:31–42
  transitional objects and pleasure-pain principle, 3:455–456
panic attacks, 3:12
papular urticaria
  calamine lotion as treatment for, 1:327, 344
  case studies, 1:345–351
  in *Clinical Notes* (1931), 1:324–325, 327
  defined, 1:343
  differential diagnosis, 1:345
  masturbation and skin excitation, 1:155–157, 324–325, 327, 344, 345–351
  'Papular Urticaria and the Dynamics of Skin Sensation' (1934), 1: lxii, **343–352**, 429*n*1
  skin involvement with feelings and mental states, 1:455–456, 461
paracentesis, 1:70, 184
paradox, acceptance of, 9:4, 182, 185–186, 208, 262, 304, 349
paranoia
  congenital versus constitutional, 11:166
  birth memories and, 3:217, 225–227
  cultural manifestations of, 7:215
  defensive pathological introversion and, 4:44
  delayed reaction to death of father and, 7:281, 292, 296–297
  dwelling of psyche in body and, 11:141
  expectation of persecution and, 11:50, 104, 141
  home management of case of psychosis and, 5:92, 94
  homosexuality and, 5:29
  inner world of the child and, 11:103–104
  integration and, 11:136
  Klein on paranoid position, 4:43*n*2, 114, 138; 5:252; 6:330; 9:37
  Laing on, 5:361–362
  physiological causes for, 7:232–233
  as regression from Oedipal complex, 9:38
  shock therapy for, 2:268
paranoid-schizoid position, 1: lxvii, 16; 6:330
parasitophobia, 1:458–459, 461
parents. *See also* death; father-child relationship; foster parents; hate and hatred; love; mother-child relationship; stepparents
  adolescents as, 5:269
  'Advising Parents' (1957), 5:**277–284**; 8:34
  authority over children, 2:71; 4:254–255
  'The Building Up of Trust' (1969), 9:**121–128**
  bulk of management of disturbed child falling on, 10:402, 403
  care of ageing parents by only child, 2:326
  'A Case Managed at Home' (1955), 5:**89–97**

children as integrative and disruptive factors for, 5:266–269
and childrens' psychopathologies, 9:281–283
Child Study Association of America, *Parents' Questions* (reviewed 1947), 3:**151**
complaints from, 5:488
continued existence, infant's awareness of, 1: lxxvi
deaths of, 1:446
democracy, ordinary good homes fostering, 3:412–414, 415, 421*n*3
democracy, parent-child relationship in, 3:417–418
desire of parents to have a girl instead of boys, 10:476
disillusionment as job of, 3:99–100, 306, 322
disruptive factors coming from, 5:269–271
education of, 3:399–401
'The Effect of Psychotic Parents on the Emotional Development of the Child' (1959), 5:275*n*2, **513–522**; 6:135*n*i, 312*n*i
enuresis and, 1:146–147
evacuation of children during WWII. *See* evacuation of children
excreta, modesty about, 1:315
'The Family Affected by Depressive Illness in One or Both Parents' (1958), 5:275*n*2, **367–377**
fantasy and reality of child, ability to distinguish between, 11:81–82
foster parents, 3:373, 375, 380
of four-year-old, 4:250
guilt of, 8:162, 275
homosexuality and, 5:29
illness of parental figure, 6:287; 10:33
importance of psychoanalyst working with, 11:188
interaction between parents and children, 9:124
LeShan, Eda J., *How to Survive Parenthood* (1965; reviewed 1967), 8:**181–182**
medical histories and, taking of, 1:155, 156, 381
and medical issues, 8:82, 86, 240
medical professionals, what parents need from, 3:154
mental defect, view of, 1:301
mental nursing role of, 6:368
morality and standards, role of, 3:299–302
mother-child relationship existing within structure provided by father, 3:6*n*iii, 273–274
neurosis in, 1:172, 275
nursing couple, 6:87–89
Oedipal complex, impatience with concept of, 11:60–61
parental attitude, 6:40, 58, 152–153
parental care, evolution into family, 6:118, 146

perplexity of, 6:510
physical deformity or difference, response to, 9:390
of the Piggle. *See under The Piggle*
preparation for parenthood, 7:331–333
psyche–soma, DWW on, 1:lxix–lxxi
psychosis of parent, effect on children, 6:70–71
quarreling between, 3:338
relationship between, 2:272, 275; 6:76, 86
role in childhood, 9:122–128
satisfactory parental care, 6:146–147
school refusal, dealing with, 10:81–82
sense of their job in child development, 4:253–254
sexual relationship of, 5:266–268
standards of, 8:155
stress, dealing with, 9:124–127
style of childraising, difference between two parents, 2:158
superego support from, 6:130–131, 142. *See also* ego
'Support for Normal Parents' (published 1945 & radio broadcast 1943–44), 2:21*n*iii, **287–289**
'The Teacher, the Parent and the Doctor' (1936), 1:17, **375–387**. *See also* school and teaching
and teaching of children, 8:53, 63
'The Theory of the Parent-Infant Relationship' (1960), 6:3–9, 115, **141–158**; 8:232*n*ii; 9:303, 306; 10:518
'The Theory of the Parent-Infant Relationship: Contributions to Discussion', 6:**363–365**
'The Theory of the Parent-Infant Relationship: Further Remarks', 6:**369–361**
therapists for their own children, 5:520–522
of timid children, 2:155
Parents' Magazine, 3:162; 8:117, 131, 151
Parfitt, D. N., 5:441
  letter to (1966), 7:**455–456**
Park, Edwards A., preface to Kanner's *Child Psychiatry* (1935), 1:439
Parkinsonian syndrome/Parkinsonism, 1:287
Parrishes Food, 9:53–54
Parsons, Marianne, 1: lii
Parsons, Michael, 1: lxxvii; 11:11
parthenogenesis, 7:450
part objects, transitional objects as, 3:456
Paterson, Mark, 1: lii
Paterson, R., 1:273*n*3
pathology
  A. Freud on, 7:220–226
  normal and pathological, continuity between, 7:6, 31
  ''Pathies in a State Service' (letter to the *British Medical Journal*; 1948), 3:**141**

'Pathological Sleeping' (1930), 1:13, **149–150**
pattern-making, 4:52; 6:258, 424; 8:214
Patty-cake (game and song), 11:280–281
Payne, M. A., *Oliver Untwisted* (1929), 1:409, 409*n*iii
Payne, Sylvia, 1: lxiv, 11; 2:79; 4:241, 243; 5:392, 394; 7:377*n*i, 410
  letter to (1953), 4:**119–120**
  letter to (1966), 7:**377–378**
Peanuts cartoon strip (Charles Schulz), 5:109; 9:261
Pearn, Clay, 1:li; 12:xlix, 5, 15
Pearson, W. J., 1:172*n*1
Pedder, Jonathan, 1: xlviii
Pediatrics (journal), 9:337, 348*n*2
Peller, Lili E., letter to (1966), 7:**373–374**
penal reform, 3:357–359
pencil game, 4:277–278
penis. *See also* castration; castration anxiety
  Casuso, 'Anxiety Related to the "Discovery" of the Penis' (1957), 5:159*n*i
  circumcision, 2:25–27
  clitoris and, 1:323
  dream of girl with, 4:326, 329, 372
  fantasies and, 2:133
  female imaginative identification with male, 11:69–70
  girl's delusion of having a penis, 9:149
  identification of whole body with, 3:214
  maternal phallus, 5:160, 418
  pain in, as symptom, 1:155–156
  paternal phallus, 5:160
  penis envy, 2:154; 3:110, 490; 5:122, 129, 185; 6:316
  in *The Piggle*, 11:282–283, 284, 290–292
  possession of, 4:326–336
  protecting, gesture for, 10:129
  skin excitement and, 1:268–269, 327, 343
  snake interpreted as penis symbol, 10:35, 68
  squiggle game and, 10:129, 133, 152, 201
penis envy, 7:105, 318, 322; 9:231; 10:261–262, 265; 11:70, 73
Pennington, Lady Sarah, 'Letter to Miss Louisa ******, on the Management and Education of Infant Children' (1824), 1:402*n*i; 3:227
Penrose, Professor, 7:407
PEP (Psychoanalytic Electronic Publishing), 9:3
perception's relation to apperception, 6:230–231; 8:5
percussion, examination of heart, 1:211–212
perfection, attainment of, in *Holding and Interpretation*, 4:328, 380–381, 383, 432
pericardial adhesion, 1:135, 208
pericardial effusion, 1:211, 212, 232
pericardial rub, 1:135, 216
pericarditis, 1:196, 208, 211, 216, 229, 232, 233

periodic group defiance, *see* defiance
peritonitis, tuberculous, 1:191
Perkins, H., 1:167
Perrotti, Professor, 8:146
persecution, 4:44, 196–198, 274
  depression and, 6:466
  fantasies of, 1:14, 376, 379–380, 384–387, 447, 457
  'The persecution that wasn't' (1984), 8:105
  persecutory and depressive position, 4:65
  persecutory expectation, 6:254, 394
  persecutory hallucinations, in case study, 7:290–291, 292, 303*n*1
  regress to, 4:110
personalisation, 2:361, 362–363; 5:322–323; 6:392, 415, 483; 9:225–226
personality development, theory of, 6:303–304, 344; 9:69–73
personality, silent core at centre of, 9:10–11
personality split, 4:41, 42*f*
  dissociation distinguished, 7:247
  'Knowing and Not Knowing' (undated; first published 1989), 9:**367–368**
personal management, child's need for, 3:24
personal omnipotence, infant experience of, 7:6
personal pattern, development of, 4:161–164
'A Personal Statement on Child Psychiatry' (1971), 9:**175–178**
'A Personal View of the Kleinian Contribution' (1962), 6:16, 18, **325–332**; 11:189, 192*n*1
personhood
  of baby, 3:96–100, 285–288, 308–310
  'The Baby as a Person' (1949), 3:**285–288**
  'The Baby as a Person' (BBC radio broadcast), 2:14
  of child, 7:415
perversion
  'Perversions and Pregenital Fantasy' (1963), 6:**511–512**
  therapeutic consultation, 10:276
'"Peter" *aet* 13 Years', 10:**403–418**
  deprivation caused by father's absence, 10:410, 418, 418*n*1
  desire to live at home as opposed to boarding school, 10:408
  home used as mental hospital for Peter, 10:408, 412, 418
  illness at school and, 10:415–416
  leaving school due to mental illness and living at home, 10:411–412
  migraines and, 10:416, 417
  noughts and crosses, playing with DWW, 10:408
  parents doing bulk of management, 10:403
  sheet-slashing and opening mail addressed to others, 10:403–404
  sibling rivalry and, 10:406–407, 415

  sleep routine and, 10:406, 411, 412
  squiggle game and, 10:406, 407
  stealing as issue, 10:403–404, 406, 407, 412
Pfister, Oskar, *The Psychoanalytic Method* (1915), 1:10
phallic phase, 7:105–107; 11:1, 67, 68, 69, 74
phallic woman fantasy, 4:16
phantasies. *See* fantasies
Phelps, Cecily, 1:75, 76
Philadelphia Psychiatric Society, Dorothy Head Memorial Lecture (1963), 6:479
Phillips, Adam, 1: lvii*n*1; 6:20; 8:14
philosophy of reality, 11:130
phobias. *See also specific common types (e.g. agoraphobia)*
  in adolescence, 6:14
  as defence, 6:257; 7:200
  of elevators, 7:194
  and hallucination, in case study, 7:290
  infestation, phobia of, 1:458–459, 461
  parasitophobia, 1:458–459, 461
  skin conditions and, 1:458–459, 461
  syphilophobia, 1:461
  vomiting, fear of, 1:265, 380
  of women with hats, 8:293, 438
phrictopathic sensation, 5:390–391
phthisis, 1:69, 119; 6:414
phylogenesis, 6:214
'Physical and Emotional Disturbances in an Adolescent Girl' (1968), 8:**239–241**3
physical care as psychological care, 3:98–99
physical deformity or difference
  'Basis for Self in Body' (1970), 9:**225–234**
  children's need for acceptance as they are, 9:226–227, 233–234, 243
  drawings by children with deformities, 9:226, 230, 231–232, 237–240, 243–244
  dreams of children with deformities, 9:230–231, 238, 239
  Hannah, age 18 (girl with spina bifida), 9:235–243
  Iiro, age 9 (child with syndactele), 9:226–228, 233
  Jill, age 18 (girl with one leg shorter than the other), 9:228–233
  Mollie, age 8 (child with very dark skin in fair-skinned adoptive family), 9:243–245
  mother's deformity passed down to child, 10:54
  parental response to, 9:390
  'Two Further Clinical Examples' (undated, probably 1970), 9:225, **235–245**
physical examinations
  anxiety preventing, 1:273
  cardiac neurosis, 7:383–384
  central nervous system diseases, 1:281–282
  heart, examination of, 1:208–209, 231–232

Complete Index of the Collected Works

'Physical Examination', from *Clinical Notes* (1931), 1:**187–194**
posture and movement, 1:294–296
physical therapy. *See also* leucotomies; shock therapy
'Physical Therapy in Mental Disorder' (letter to *The British Medical Journal*; 1945), 2:**379–380**
'Physical Therapy of Mental Disorder' (1946), 2:207*n*i
'Physical Therapy of Mental Disorder' (1947), 3:59, **69–75**
Physiotherapy (1969), 9:67
'Physiotherapy and Human Relations' (1969), 9:**67–73**
Piaget, Jean, 4:104; 6:371; 7:140
Picasso, Pablo, 7:287; 9:223
picking up and holding babies, 3:96–97, 168, 209, 388–391
The Piggle. An Account of the Psychoanalytic Treatment of a Little Girl (1964–1966/1977), 1: li, lxv; 5:171*n*i; 6:351*n*i; 7:12, 151*n*i, 207; 8:269*n*iv; 10:3, 4; 11:**185–318**
 aggression, naughtiness, and destructive behaviour, 11:205, 213, 223, 233, 250, 253, 264, 269, 284, 286
 anxiety in, 11:209, 214, 219, 220, 221, 229, 236, 252*n*IX, 266, 267, 274, 288
 artificial voice in, 11:201, 204, 214, 223
 attitude of child toward DWW and sessions, 11:199, 204, 213, 214, 218, 222, 224, 227–228, 232, 239, 259, 260, 261, 265, 266, 268–269, 276, 284–286, 294–295, 302, 310–314, 316, 318
 attitude of child toward parents, 11:197, 200–203, 212, 231–232, 242
 babacar, 11:8, 198, 200, 201, 202, 205, 206, 207, 218, 220–221, 222, 224, 228, 232, 237
 baby, desire of child to have, 11:237–238, 243
 birthing play, 11:210–211, 219, 229, 307–308
 black mummy and concern with blackness in, 11:8, 198, 200–203, 205, 212–214, 218, 220–224, 228–231, 238, 245, 246, 249, 253, 257, 259, 260, 264, 265–266, 268, 289, 316
 breasts (yams), 11:8, 198, 214, 224–225, 232, 238, 276, 282, 290, 291
 calling child Gabrielle versus Piggle, 11:216, 230*n*XV, 241, 244, 247*n*2
 church, Gabrielle's inquiries about going to, 11:306–307
 comments by DWW, 11:202–203, 211, 221–222, 231–232, 238, 245, 252–253, 258, 267–268, 275–276, 283–284, 293, 303, 308, 314
 comments of mother on transcript of, 11:195*n*2, 239–240
 daddy's little girl, mummy wanting to be, 11:230–231, 232
 dead things and death in, 11:224, 232, 239–240, 247, 259, 266, 271–272, 307, 309–310, 315
 death of DWW, child's response to, 11:318
 depression in, 11:233, 239, 260, 277, 284, 285, 295
 dolls (baba; Galli-Galli; Frances), 11:204, 205, 210, 213, 217, 220–221, 225, 273, 275
 excretion (bryyyyyh and wee), 11:219–221, 245–246, 257*n*IV, 274–275, 276
 'greedy Winnicott baby' play in, 11:10, 208–210, 212, 213, 219–220
 horse dream (of parental intercourse), 11:273–274
 identity establishment in, 11:197, 203, 211*n*XIII, 242–245, 251, 260–261
 involvement of parents in composition of story, 11:193, 194
 letters from DWW to parents, 11:239, 246, 284
 letters from father to DWW, 11:203–205, 206, 213–214, 258–259
 letters from Gabrielle to DWW (dictated), 11:285, 294
 letters from mother to DWW, 11:197–198, 205–206, 211–213, 222–225, 232–233, 238–239, 245–246, 259, 261, 268–269, 276–277, 284–286, 293–295
 letters from parents to DWW, 11:203–205, 245–247, 253, 259, 260, 268, 303–304
 lullaby, child's ambivalence about, 11:201, 206*n*2
 masturbation in, 11:212, 222, 232, 243*n*IV, 273*n*III
 mending in, 11:297–299, 304*n*2
 Mrs. Winnicott in, 11:237, 238, 253*n*2
 nursery school, 11:213, 247, 276, 285
 Oedipal fantasies in, 11:212
 'on demand' method used for, 11:194, 240*n*3, 317
 penises (wee-wees) in, 11:282–283, 284, 290–292
 plan of DWW's working space at 87 Chester Square, London, *11:186*
 play as condition for analytic treatment in, 11:10–11, 19, 187, 231, 302
 publication history, 11:3
 regression in, 11:203, 210, 258
 Renata (au pair), 11:220
 roller game in, 11:307, 309–310, 315
 sessions with DWW, 11:199–201, 207–211, 217–221, 227–231, 235–238, 241–244, 249–252, 255–258, 263–267, 271–275, 279–283, 287–293, 297–303, 305–308, 309–314, 315–316
 shyness, 11:199, 202, 203, 206, 210, 316
 sibling of Gabrielle in (Sush Baby/Susan), 11:197, 198*n*2, 199–200, 203, 204, 205, 213, 214, 222, 223, 238, 242, 245, 256–258, 259, 263–265, 267, 268, 272, 279–281, 284, 285, 292, 295, 297–298, 301, 303–304
 sibling of mother in, 11:198*n*2, 294

The Piggle. An Account of the Psychoanalytic Treatment of a Little Girl (*Cont.*)
  sickness, child's preoccupation with, 11:207–209, 211, 218, 220, 235, 236nIII, 243
  telephone calls from mother to DWW, 11:239
  termination of sessions, 11:310–316
  thumb of father, sucking, 11:227, 230, 231
  tidying and washing, child's interest in, 11:200–201, 205, 215, 220, 229, 233, 239–240, 244, 245, 252, 258, 259, 286, 301
  toilet training, 11:201
  transference in, 11:310–314
  transitional objects and phenomena, 11:209
  unfinished at DWW's death, 11:3
  verbalisation in analytical process, importance of, 11:9
  the Wattie (family domestic help), 11:214, 253, 285
Pilgrim's Progress (John Bunyan), 5:139
'The Pill' (1969), 9:**101–110**
Pink's disease (lead poisoning), 11:111, 112n3
'Pitfalls in Adoption' (1954), 4:**291–296**
pituitary tumours and abnormalities, 1:119, 257, 290
'The Place of the Monarchy' (1970), 8:355; 9:**181–187**
'The Place Where We Live' (1968), 8:169, **221–226**; 9:11
Planned Environment Therapy Trust (PETT), 2:291
Platt, Harry, 5:544nii
Plaut, Fred, 7:435
  'Reflections About Not Being Able to Imagine' (1966), 8:77n4
  on trust, 8:76
play. *See also* games
  as achievement, 9:375–376
  adolescence and, 9:378–379
  of adopted child, 4:294–295
  in adult analysis, 4:282
  aggression and, 7:132–133
  beginning of individual and, 7:453
  breastfeeding and, 2:224, 227, 238, 392–393
  case study, 8:172–179
  '"Cecil" aet 21 Months at First Consultation' on play capacity, 10:340, 344
  child inventing during therapy, 6:475
  'Commentary on *Play Therapy*' by Virginia Axline (book published 1947; comments recorded 1969), 9:**159–164**
  as communication between mother and infant, 8:233–234
  as condition for analytic treatment, 11:10–11, 19, 187
  as creative activity, 8:274; 9:376, 377
  cultural experience and, 7:429–436
  daydreaming and, 9:247–248
  developmental advantages of, 9:377
  dolls with sex organs, letter to manufacturer of, 3:183–184
  in dreams, 4:330
  drives and, 9:13
  DWW's focus on, 8:3, 11–12
  emotional health and, 5:104
  expression of aggressiveness and destructive urges in, 2:183, 366
  in genital phase, 11:71
  hide-and-seek, 6:439
  hospital experience and, 3:445
  imagination and, 3:286, 288, 290; 9:376
  importance for children, 2:285–286, 324–325, 354; 4:281
  and inner world, 11:92, 109–110, 181
  instincts and, 5:117, 247
  Jung on, 7:121–122
  Klein on, 5:7; 6:438–439
  masturbation and, 2:169; 8:300–301
  material presented by patients in analysis during, 11:107–111
  Me and *Not-Me*, distinguishing, 5:117
  mother-child mutuality and development of, 9:134
  'Notes on Play' (undated, before late 1960s; in 'Ideas' file), 9:**375–379**
  noughts and crosses, DWW playing with Milton, 10:276, *277*, 288
  in nursery school, 4:154
  parents and infant trust in, 1:15
  in *The Piggle*, 11:10–11, 19, 187, 231, 302
  'Playing: A theoretical statement' (1968), 1:310nii; 2:125nii; 8:11–12, 167, 283nii, 287niii, **297–310**; 9:11, 12, 13; 10:267
  'Playing: Creative Activity and the Search for the Self' (1967), 8:**169–179**, 414ni
  'Playing: Its Theoretical Status in the Clinical Situation' (1968), 8:12, 13, 298, 364
  'Playing and Culture' (1968), 8:**263–266**; 9:11
  Playing and Reality (1971), 1: lxix, lxxv, lxxvii; 3:447; 5:12; 8:3, 11, 15; 9:4, 112ni, 167ni, **261–263** (introduction), 265, 337, **349** (tailpiece); 10:3; 11:206n3
  'Play in the Analytic Situation' (1954), 4:**281–282**
  pleasure as characteristic of, 9:375
  psychiatric social worker engaging child in, 2:182–183
  psychopathology of, 9:378
  psychotherapy and, 8:299, 310–311
  psychotic children and, 4:453
  reparation in, 2:138

search for self and, 8:170–172
sexuality and, 3:104–106
spoon (spatula) game, 3:285–288, 304
symbols and 7:132; 9:375, 376
theory of, 8:307–310
in time and space, 8:302–307
transitional objects and, 5:104
transitional phenomena and, 8:301–302
in triangular relationship, 4:251
'Why Children Play' (1942), 1: lxxvii; **2:167–170**
work and, 7:413–414
pleasure
baby crying for, 2:238
play, as characteristic of, 9:375
'pleasure principle', 4:105; 6:133, 143–144, 146, 201
transitional objects and pleasure-pain principle, 3:455–456; 9:274
Pliny, 8:394
Plowden, Victoria, 9:247, 249
pneumococcal meningitis, 1:289
pneumonia
anxiety and, 1:257, 268, 272
central nervous system disease and, 1:288
chemotherapy for, 2:255–256
convulsions and fits, 1:303, 304
haemoptysis and, 1:152
heart problems and rheumatic fever, 1:207, 212, 218, 222
temperature and charts, 1:196
walking problems and, 1:296
Podro, Joshua, & Graves, Robert, *Nazarene Gospel Restored*, 8:158
poetry and poems. *See also* Hopkins, Gerard Manley; Keats, John; Wordsworth, William
Blake, William, 'I fear'd the fury of my wind', 8:366–367
Calverley, Charles Stuart, *Humorous Poems III. Parodies: Imitations*, 8:267ni
'Ditty on Enoch Powell' (undated, possibly 1968), 9:**395**
Housman, A. E., *A Shropshire Lad* (1896), 1:57
imaginative life and being a poet, 6:440
mental illness and, 7:315
metaphysical poets, 9:261
'Moon Landing' (poem by DWW; 1969), 9:**89–90**, 109–110
Penguin Book of English Verse, 8:407
Reeves, *Georgian Poetry*, 8:407
Rosetti, Christina, 'Passing Away', 8:174
'A Shropshire Surgeon' (poem by DWW; 1920), 1:**57**
'The Silent Kill' (poem by DWW; 1969), 9:102, 108
'The Tree' (poem by DWW; 1963), 6:20, **499–500**

'A Point in Technique' (undated; originally published 1989), 9:**369–370**
polioencephalitis, 1:76, 304
poliomyelitis, 1:87, 91–92, 139, 284–285, 286, 288, 296; 9:99–100
politics and politicians, 2:341; 9:117–119, 395
polymorpho-perverse symptomatology of childhood, 7:229–230
polyneuritis, 1:118
Pond, Desmond, 7:407
Pontalis, Jean-Bertrand, 9:225
Poor Law homes, 1:409*n*iii
population explosion and psychoanalytic research, 7:152
porphyria, of King George III, 7:315–316*n*i
Portman Clinic (formerly Psychopathic Clinic), 5:400
possessing, 2:141–142; 6:53–54
'The Possible Significance of the Nurse Scene in *Romeo and Juliet* (1966), 3:185
post-encephalitis. *See under* encephalitis
Postgraduate Medical Journal, 1:133
post-partum depression, 7:180–181, 362
potential space, 3: 6–7, 11–12; 8:224–226, 265, 302; 9:5–6, 8–9
Powell, Enoch
'Ditty on Enoch Powell' (undated, possibly 1968), 9:**395**
'Rivers of Blood' speech, 9:395
Poynton, F. J., 1:139, 253*n*2; 2:49, 51, 59; 7:380
The Practitioner, 3:101
prattling (chattering), in *Holding and Interpretation*, 4:309–314, 316, 404, 406, 408, 432, 456
pre-birth personal life of infant, 5:116
pre-concern, stage of. *See also* pre-ruth, 2:366, 368*n*5
predictability, 8:213
prefaces (by DWW). *See also* forewords by DWW
Collected papers: Through Paediatrics to Psychoanalysis (1958), 5:**301–302**
The Family and Individual Development (1965), preface to English edition, 7:**309**, 423
The Family and Individual Development (1965), preface to Italian translation, 7:**419–422**, 422*n*i
Lebovici, S. and J. McDougall, *Dialogue with Sammy* (1969), 9:**129–130**
Milner, Marion, *The Hands of the Living God* (1969), 2:19
Stevenson, Olive, *The First Treasured Possession* (1954), 4:**297–299**
Tod, Robert, *Disturbed Children* (1968), 8:10, **261–262**; 9:99
prefrontal leucotomy. *See* leucotomy

pregenital stage, 4:205–207; 11:67, 68, 69
  instinctual functions, pregenital, 6:15, 117, 130–131, 188, 326, 469
  'Perversions and Pregenital Fantasy' (1963), 6:**517–518**
  sexuality, pregenital, 6:145, 160, 411
pregnancy
  attitude of woman toward, 2:221–223; 6:12, 80, 154, 208
  child's anxiety brought on by mother's subsequent pregnancy, 2:152–153; 10:110–111, 296, 336–337, 338, 362, 473
  late pregnancy as illness, 6:12
prelatency period, 4:202, 207
premature infants
  emotional needs of, 11:129
  movement and mobility, 5:197
  'The Wearing of Masks in the Nursing of Premature and Older Infants' (1943), 2:**227**
pre-rheumatic children, 1:125, 171, 219, 225, 266
'pre-ruth', 2:15; 3:5, 335, 340; 5:153; 6:17
pre-school children. *See also* nursery schools
  conscience, development of, 1:409
  delinquency in, 1:410
  emotional development of, 1:399–403, 404–411; 5:427–428
  environment and, 11:169–171
  S. Freud on, 5:130
  frustrations experienced by, 1:403
  gender identification in, 7:104–105
  hospital treatment affecting, 1:405–406
  inner and outer world, establishing control of, 1:407–411
  intellectual development of, 1:398–399
  intensity of feeling in, 3:294
  'Mental Hygiene of the Pre-School Child' (1936), 1:**397–411**
  physical development of, 1:398
  reality, introduction of child to, 3:294–296
  'The Toddler, the Second Adoption, Telling Children About Adoption' (mid 1950s), 5:**111–112**
  Wolff, Werner, *The Personality of the Preschool Child: The Child's Search for His Self* (1947; reviewed 1948), 3:**159–160**
prescription drugs. *See* medicines and drugs
pre-systolic murmur
  'Active Heart Disease', from *Clinical Notes* (1931), 1:232–233
  'The Heart, with Special Reference to Rheumatic Carditis', from *Clinical Notes* (1931), 1:215, 216
  'Pre-systolic Murmur, Possibly Not Due to Mitral Stenosis' (1931), 1:**153–154**
pre-systolic thrill, 1:209, 232

pre-tubercular children, 1:171, 266
preventive medicine in paediatric practice, 2:202
'The Price of Disregarding Psychoanalytic Research' (1965), 5:171*n*i; 7:**149–156**, 207
'The Price of Mental Health' (1965), 7:149
primal or primary repression, 5:179, 180–181
primal scene, 5:243–244; 11:81
primary creativity, 11:16, 132–134
primary excited impulse, 11:102*n*6
primary home experience, 3:80–81, 86, 92
primary identification, 5:62
'Primary Introduction to External Reality: The Early Stages (1948)', 3:**165–170**, 185; 10:8
primary maternal preoccupation
  as ancient process, 9:173
  autism and, 7:346
  communication and, 6:434
  creativity and drives, 9:12
  definition of, 6:5; 7:42
  dependence and, 6:339–340, 471
  DWW's concept of, 6:12; 8:44
  good breast and, 5:123, 131; 6:270
  in letter to a Confidant ('M') (1966), 7:371
  object relationship and, 8:364
  in paediatrics and child psychology, 8:287
  'Primary Maternal Preoccupation' (1956), 1:439*n*1; 3:220*n*4; 5:13, **183–188**, 241, 256; 6:158*n*17, 166, 339–340; 7:346; 8:226*n*1, 230; 9:15, 128, 134, 209
  as transient total devotion of mother to child in early months of life, 7:5, 42, 91–93, 335–336
primary narcissism, 4:16, 206, 209, 273; 7:6; 11:147, 160, 172–173
primary schools, 6:311–313; 7:154, 395
'A Primary State of Being: Pre-Primitive Stages' (from *Human Nature*; 1988), 11:**149–152**
primary walking, 7:42
primitive behaviour
  aggression as primitive or magical destruction, 7:134–135
  DWW's word choice, versus Klein's, 2:13
  in *Human Nature*, 11:15–16
  primary excited impulse, 11:102*n*6
primitive agonies, 6:526
primitive anxiety, 10:130
'Primitive Emotional Development' (1945), 1: lxii, lxv–lxvii, lxxi; 2:3, 12–16, 21*n*iii, **357–368**; 3:4, 6, 9, 17, 139*n*3, 246; 5:3–4; 6:11, 12, 157*n*1; 8:232*n*iii; 9:7, 11, 304; 11:7–8, 117*n*1
'Primitive Emotional Development' (introduction to Part IV of *Human Nature*; 1988), 11:**117**
primitive love and destructiveness, 11:95, 96

primitive love impulse, 3:340, 394, 457; 5:155;
　　9:5, 183–184; 10:111, 298; 11:92, 151
primitive retaliation, 2:367–368
　　ruthlessness of, 11:98
　　Thomas, William, 'Primitive behaviour'
　　　　(1937), 1:441
primitive peoples and adolescent passage to
　　adulthood, 6:190, 426
Prince, Morton, 5:391
Princess Louise Hospital for Children, 3:243
'Principles of Direct Therapy in Child Psychiatry'
　　(lecture; 1967), 10:419
prisoners of war, 3:226
prisons
　　asylums versus, 4:98
　　'Comments on the Report of the Committee on
　　　　Punishment in Prisons and Borstals' (1961),
　　　　6:17, **273–278**
　　penal reform, 3:357–359
　　smoking by prisoners, 6:274–276
Prison Service Journal, 8:91
privacy of mother sacrificed, 6:8, 78–79
'Private Practice' (1955), 5:**35–42**
privation, 6:417
probation officers, 5:339–344
　　Association for Child Psychology and
　　　　Psychiatry and, 8:58
　　'The Child, the Family and the Young Offender'
　　　　(UK Government Home Office White
　　　　Paper), 7:203–204
　　role with delinquent children, 2:234–235
　　talk on 'Psychological Aspects of Juvenile
　　　　Delinquency' (undated; ca. late 1940s) given
　　　　to, 3:**49–55**
'The Problem of Homeless Children' (with Clare
　　Britton, 1944), 2:291*n*i, **299–311**; 3:27*n*1
problem solving, 8:351
Proceedings of the British Student Health
　　Association, 9:337
Proceedings of the Royal Society of Medicine, 1:91,
　　93, 95, 99, 111, 113, 115, 117, 119, 127, 129, 131, 141,
　　149, 151, 153, 391; 4:79
Progressive League, 6:97; 7:14, 129; 9:101, 213
progressive schools
　　control in, 7:166–167
　　defining, 7:157–158
　　'Do Progressive Schools Give Too Much
　　　　Freedom to the Child?' (1965), 7:**157–161**
　　'Notes Made in the Train' (1965), 7:**163–167**
　　positive and negative aspects of, 7:164–165
　　problems faced by, 7:165
projection
　　analyst's acceptance of patient's, 7:343–344
　　depression and, 6:462
　　DWW's use of concept, 6:5
　　identifications, projective and introjective, 3:5;
　　　　5:85, 121–122; 6:154, 373; 7:325, 356, 413; 9:135,
　　　　319–320, 328–336, 330–331
　　Kleinian contribution and, 6:326
　　parent-infant relationship and, 6:157*n*11
　　play and, 8:265
　　primary projection, 4:10–11
　　psychiatric disorder and infant development,
　　　　6:481–482
　　transitional objects and, 3:456
prophylaxis in medicine, 1:68–69
proportional representation, 3:421*n*1
prostitution
　　character disorders of adolescent girls and,
　　　　6:455–456
　　fear of venereal disease, 6:196*n*1
Protestant-Catholic divide in Northern
　　Ireland, 9:118
'Providing for the Child in Health and Crisis'
　　(1962), 6:**343–350**
pruritus, 1:350, 449, 456–458, 461, 462
　　anal, 1:456–458; 2:29
　　'Pruritus and Psychology' (letter to *The British*
　　　　Medical Journal; 1939), 2:**29**
pseudo-hypertrophic muscular dystrophy,
　　1:293–294
pseudologia fantastica, 5:419; 10:363
PSWs. *See* psychiatric social workers
psyche
　　development, or growth of, 11:36, 55, 51, 76, 158
　　'Dwelling of Psyche in Body' (from *Human*
　　　　Nature; 1988), 11:**139–141**
　　as imaginative elaboration of body functioning,
　　　　11:36, 37, 54–55, 66, 76, 140,
　　'Psyche Health' (from *Human Nature*;
　　　　1988), 11:**40**
　　'Psyche Ill-Health' (from *Human Nature*; 1988),
　　　　11:**44–46**
　　somatic basis in brain, 11:39, 55, 76, 140
Psyche (journal), 8:107
psyche-soma
　　'Dwelling of Psyche in Body' (from *Human*
　　　　Nature; 1988), 11:**139–141**
　　DWW's concept of, 1: lxx–lxxi, 9–10, 159–160,
　　　　357, 459; 6:5; 11:15
　　fantasies and, 1: lxxi, 159
　　in first year of life, 5:322–324
　　head, localisation of mind in, 3:254–256
　　'Hypochondriacal Anxiety' (from *Human*
　　　　Nature; 1988), 11:**113–114**
　　intellectual life and, 7:198–199
　　'Inter-Relationship of Body Disease and
　　　　Psychological Disorder' (from *Human*
　　　　Nature; 1988), 11:**47–52**
　　linkage of, 6:415

psyche-soma (*Cont.*)
   'Mind and Its Relation to the Psyche-Soma'
     (1949/1954), 1: lxxi; 3:17, 220*nn*5–6, **245–257**;
     4:203*n*i; 6:128, 163; 7:69; 8:6; 11:39*n*i
   mind as function of, 3:246–247; 8:270
   mind versus psyche, 6:15
   'The Psyche-Soma and the Mind' (from
     Human Nature; 1988), 11:**39–41**
   reliving birth experience and, 3:250–254
   theory of mind and, 3:247–250
psychiatric social workers (PSWs). *See also*
   casework
   antisocial children in hostels, arranging
     psychotherapy for, 3:25
   Association for Child Psychology and
     Psychiatry (ACPP) and, 8:61
   depression, management of patients with,
     5:371–373
   deprived children, taking histories of, 3:377–378
   'A Doctor Looks at the Psychiatric Social
     Worker' (1943), 2:9, **177–193**
   'The Family Affected by Depressive Illness in
     One or Both Parents' (1958), 5:275*n*2, **367–377**
   generic training and, 5:339–344
   in hostels for homeless children, 2:302–303
   infant-care, role in, 6:418–419
   love versus skill in work of, 7:37–39
   'The Mentally Ill in Your Caseload' (1963), 6:13,
     409–420
   Paddington Green Children's Hospital,
     6:180–181
   profession of, 2:193*n*1; 5:341–342; 6:19, 418–420
   psychosis versus psycho-neurosis, allowing for
     social work, 6:411–412
psychiatrist and psychiatry, 4:78, 185, 203, 11:37. *See*
   also child psychiatry
   antisocial children in hostels, arranging
     psychotherapy for, 3:24–25, 27*n*2
   'Child Psychiatry, Social Work, and Alternative
     Care' (1970), 9:**171–174**
   as field of study for Association for Child
     Psychology and Psychiatry, 8:56
   hate in the countertransference and, 3:59–68
   hostels for homeless children, role in, 2:301–302
   infant care and, 4:43
   inter-speciality discussion, 3:351–352, 487
   nature of psychiatric disorder, 6:483
   not symptom-curers, 4:80
   paediatrics and, 4:36, 117, 228
   patients dangerous to, 5:208
   personality development, theory of, 6:309–310
   psyche-somatic research and, 11:113
   'Psychiatric Disorder in Terms of Infantile
     Maturational Processes' (1963), 6:13,
     479–490

   'A Psychiatrist's Choice' (letter to *The Spectator*;
     1954), 4:**181–182**
   psychoanalytic research and, 7:152–153
   regression of patient, importance of adapting
     to, 3:234
   relationship of adult psychiatry to child
     psychiatry, 6:302–303
   reparation and, 3:121–122
psychoanalysis. *See also Holding and*
   Interpretation: Fragment of an Analysis
   (1955); therapeutic consultations
   Aichhorn, August, *Wayward Youth* (reviewed
     1936), 1:434–436
   aims and goals of, 6:198; 7:223
   'The Aims of Psycho-Analytical Treatment'
     (1962), 6:19, **285–288**
   Alexander, Franz, 'Psychoanalysis and
     Medicine' (abstract; 1932), 1:**339**
   Alger, Ian, 'The Clinical Handling of the
     Analyst's Responses' (1966), discussion of,
     7:13, **463–464**
   as an art, 3:41; 4:214
   antisocial behaviour and, 5:150, 157–158
   of anxiety, 1:275–276. *See also* anxiety
   of artist, 4:62
   Association for Child Psychology and
     Psychiatry (ACPP) and, 8:61–62
   basic principles, 4:212–214; 5:352–353
   of borderline patients, 4:13, 193, 238; 6:7. *See also*
     borderline cases
   of BPAS candidates, 3:233–234
   break in between sessions, patient's reaction to,
     in *Holding and Interpretation*, 4:286–288, 332,
     373–374, 379, 390
   case history, taking of, serving therapeutic
     purpose in, 6:198
   case studies. *See* case studies
   character disorders, 6:452–455
   child psychiatry and, 5: 351–352; 6:305–306,
     357–358; 10:27; 11:37
   children, orientation to, 5:424–425
   choice of analyst, 4:269–270
   choice of case, 4:124, 202
   comparison of British and American
     approaches, 8:13
   'The Contribution of Psycho-Analysis to
     Midwifery' (1957), 5:**225–232**, 239*n*i
   cultural and social acceptance of, 7:425–426
   'Cure' (1970), 9:**191–197**
   definition and description, 2:381–388; 3:54;
     4:2051–202; 6:217
   of delinquents. *See* delinquent children
   of depression, 1: lxxii; 2:63*n*4, 252, 358–359;
     6:480–481. *See also* depression
   depressive position in, 4:186–187, 193, 199, 202

development of, 7:218
diagnosis and, 5:353
diagnostic interviews with child, 3:125
different types of patients and, 5:207–208
education in, 7:217–219
as emotional experience shared by analyst, 7:9
enuresis and, 1:391, 393–394
environment for, 3:63–64
failure in, 4:60, 64, 238; 6:341, 418; 8:357, 369
first hours of treating children, 6:439
S. Freud's work in. *See* Freud, Sigmund
friendship, resemblance to, 6:203
gossip and, 4:365
'honeymoon period' of, 6:439
how little need be done, as guiding principle, 6:198; 7:277; 8:350; 10: 298, 519, 525; 11:192
illusion in, 4:174
infant care and, 4:58, 192
infant development, re-enactment of, 3:132–136
interpretation in, 6:286, 480–481; 10:9–10, 34; 11:83, 113–114
'Interpretation in Psycho-analysis' (1968), 8:17, **253–257**
Jones, Ernest, and use of term, 5:393–394
Klein's contribution to, 4:30, 193, 242
language of, 4:4–5, 219
in latency period, 5:351–359
lay practice of, 4:237–238
love versus skill in, 7:37–39
medicines and drugs believed to be superseding, 7:315, 316*n*i
modifications of technique, 6:488; 8:16
multidisciplinary teams, benefits of, 6:19–20
neurosis, treatment of. *See* neurosis
nonverbal approach, 8:16, 117–118
'Nothing at the Centre' (1959), 5:**469–471**
'on demand' method of, 11:191, 194, 240*n*3, 317
'On the Contribution of Direct Child Observation to Psycho-Analysis' (1957), 5:**249–254**, 457
openness of patient to, 6:199
opposition to, 1:408; 4:228; 5:170
paediatrics and, 1:12–17; 4:228; 6:183–184, 304–305, 484; 8:81; 11:5, 43
patient's view of, 5:233–234, 235–236
personal experience of DWW with, 9:175–176
'Play in the Analytic Situation', 4:**281–283**
potential space in, 3:12
'The Price of Disregarding Psychoanalytic Research' (1965), 7:**149–156**, 207
professional standards of psychoanalysts, 6:19
progress in, 4:204, 212; 8:256–257
'Psychoanalysis and Science: Friends or Relations' (1961), 6:**217–221**

'Psycho-Analysis and the Sense of Guilt' (1956), 5:**135–147**; 6:157*n*6, 467*n*2
'The Psycho-analyst and Child Psychiatry: A Matter of Economics' (1962), 6:**363–364**
Psychoanalytic Explorations (1989), 8:413; 10:3, 83
'The Psychology of Madness' (1965) as contribution from, 7:**229–238**
of psychotics, 4:731–72, 73–74. *See also* psychosis
public clinic compared to psychoanalytic consulting room, 6:19
punctuality, 4:211, 3106, 324, 334, 415–416; 6:19, 203
questionnaire on the analyst's practice and range of beliefs, 5:503*n*i
quick versus long treatments, 2:200*n*2
reflecting back principle, 8:257
regression in, 4:202, 213, 215–217, **283–289**, 11:147
relationship between child and adult analysis, 7:218–219, 223–224
'Remarks on a Discussion of Balint's Paper on Technique' (1957), 5:**211–212**
repressed memories, regaining, 3:101–102
research, dangers of disregarding, 7:149–156
'Resolution K: On Scientific Aims in Psychoanalysis' (1942), 1: lxiv; 2:**145–147**
science and, 6:217–221, 229–231
shyness, treating, 1:447
silence during, 4:213, 388, 427–429, 431
'Some Principles of Child Analysis' (1969), 9:**51**
speaking freely and, 4:365
termination of, in *Holding and Interpretation*, 4:332, 375, 378–379, 382, 392, 412, 417, 419, 433, 470–471, 474
therapeutic consultations distinguished, 7:273–274, 277; 8:413; 10:518
'Towards an Objective Study of Human Nature' (1945), 2:**381–388**
training of child analysts, need for, 2:162–163
training, 4:119–120, 215, 209–228, 238; 5:7–8; 6:177–178; 10:27, 369, 521–522
transference neurosis in, 11:82–83
transference, use of, 5:353–354; 6:198. *See also* transference
truth, as scientific aim of, 2:145–146
types of, 2:358; 6:19, 197–203, 489; 8:16, 18*n*9, 181–182; 11:107–111, 1985
'The Use of the Word "Use"' (1968), 8:**249–251**
'Varieties of Psychotherapy' (1961), 6:19, **197–204**
waiting-list and delay in children receiving, 2:161–162
'What Is Psychoanalysis?', 4:53

Psychoanalytic Forum, 7:457; 9:149
The Psychoanalytic Study of the Child
  Bowlby's 'Separation Anxiety' included in Vol. 15, 5:495
  Casuso's 'Anxiety Related to the "Discovery" of the Penis' in Vol. 12, 5:159*n*i
  Kulka and, 5:198
  on neurosis, in Vol. IX, 5:13, 183
  preface to *The First Treasured Possession* (DWW preface to Stevenson book), 4:**297–299**
  Sandler's 'On the Concept of the Superego', in Vol. 15 (1960), 6:127
  Spock's 'Observations on the Striving for Autonomy and some Regressive Object Relationships after six months of age' in Vol. 18, 8:295
  Volume 2 (eds. Anna Freud, W. Hoffer, and E. Glover, 1946; reviewed by DWW 1948), 3:**157–158**, 461, 475*n*i
  Volumes 3–4 and 5 (eds. Anna Freud, W. Hoffer, and E. Glover, 1949; reviewed by DWW 1951), 3:461, **473–474**; 8:110*n*ii
  Volume 11 (eds. Ruth S. Eissler, Anna Freud, Heinz Hartman, and Ernst Kris, 1957; reviewed by DWW 1958), 5:**317–318**, 531*n*2
  Volume 12 (eds. Ruth S. Eissler, Anna Freud, Heinz Hartman, and Ernst Kris, 1958; reviewed by DWW), 5:**363–364**
  Volume 15 (eds. R. S. Eissler, A. Freud, H. Hartmann, M. Kris, 1961; reviewed by DWW 1962), 6:**283–284**
  Volume 16 (eds. R. S. Eissler, A. Freud, H. Hartmann, M. Kris, 1962; reviewed by DWW 1963), 6:**399**
  Volume 20 (eds. Ruth S. Eissler, Heinz Hartman, and Ernst Kris, 1966; reviewed by DWW), 7:**375–376**; 8:337
  Volume 22 (eds. Ruth S. Eissler, Anna Freud, Heinz Hartman, and Ernst Kris, 1967; reviewed by DWW 1968), 8:**279–281**
'Psychogenesis of a Beating Fantasy' (1958), 5:**313–315**
Psychological Wednesday Society, 5:310
psychology
  classification and, 9:174
  of convulsions and fits, 1:305–306
  of depression, 5:376–377; 6:463–464
  as field of study for Association for Child Psychology and Psychiatry, 8:53–54
  as field of study for British Paediatric Association, 2:201–205
  as gradual extension from physiology, 7:42
  mental disability, psychological point of view on, 1:301–302; 6:409
  paediatrics, relationship with, 4:80–81
  as professional field, 5:421–425
  'Psychological Aspects of Birching' (abstract; 1944), 2:**247–249**
  'Psychological Aspects of Juvenile Delinquency' (undated; ca. late 1940s), 3:**49–55**
  'Psychologists as a Group' (1969), 8:49; 9:**155–158**
  'Psychology in the Child's Education' (letter to *British Medical Journal* 1946), 3:**35–36**
  'The Psychology of Juvenile Rheumatism' (1939), 1:14; 2:**49–63**; 7:386
  'The Psychology of Madness' (1965), 6:523; 7:4, 5, **229–238**
  'The Psychology of Separation' (1958), 5:**333–335**
  Sandström, Carl Ivar, *The Psychology of Childhood and Adolescence* (reviewed 1968), 8:10, **411–412**
  as science, 2:29, 382–386; 3:70
  stage of development at which psychology becomes meaningful, 7:451–452
  study of, 3:423–427
  'Theoretical Statement of the Field of Child Psychiatry' (1958), 5:**421–429**
  'Towards an Objective Study of Human Nature' (1945), 2:**381–388**
  of unwellness, 1:171–172
psychoneurosis. See also neurosis
  aetiology of, 8:186
  borderline cases. See borderline cases
  character disorders, 6:450
  definition and description of, 6: 254, 257, 417; 8:228–229
  depression linked to, 6:463
  DWW's reaction to, 6:14
  guilt, ethics, and morality, 7:445
  health as absence of psychoneurotic disorders, 8:69
  instinctual life and, 6:14
  psychoanalysis of, 6:489; 8:356
  'Psycho-Neurosis in Childhood' (1961), 6:13, 14, **253–260**
  psychosis versus, 4:207; 6:253, 410
  repression and, 6:410–411
  roots in young childhood, 7:44
psychopathology
  differential environmental impacts, 2:13
  of guilt sense, 5:139–141
  of play, 9:378
  transitional objects and, 9:279–284
psychopaths and psychopathy, 5:152, 454–455; 6:254–255, 416
psychosis
  analyst, psychotic patient's view of, 3:60
  Bion on, 5:85

'A Case Managed at Home' (1955), 5:**89-97**
changing views of, 4:271-272; 5:449
character disorders, 6:450-451, 457-459
   in childhood, 1:439*n*1; 4:8, 35, 38, 125,
   271-272; 7:116
'Childhood Psychosis' (1950), 3:**353-356**
classification of psychiatric disorders and,
   5:367-368, 450-452, 455-456, 517; 6:199
communication difficulties due to, 5:81
countertransference, DWW's understanding
   of, and, 3:4
definition and description of, 5:459*n*2; 6:65-66,
   253; 7:6; 11:44
developmental stage linked to, 6:13
diagnosis of, 4:203, 210
'The Effect of Psychosis on Family Life' (1960),
   5:275*n*2; 6:12, 14, **65-72**
'The Effect of Psychotic Parents on the
   Emotional Development of the Child' (1959),
   5:275*n*2, **513-522**; 6:135*n*i, 312*n*i
environmental causes of, 5:455-456; 6:14, 417
external factor at root of, 9:38
hate in the countertransference and, 3:59-68
health and, 4:207
infant development and, 1: lxv-lxvii; 2:357-358,
   387; 6:152; 8:161; 11:65, 166
infantile state in transference, 4:71
latent psychosis in children, 5:426
manifest psychosis in children, 5:425
mental disability confused with, 3:134, 204, 353
methodological approach of DWW to, 3:6-7
mother-infant mutuality and, 9:132
need satisfaction and, 7:374
neurosis versus, 4:71-72, 124, 185, 207, 439;
   6:253, 410
'The Non-Pharmacological Treatment of
   Psychosis in Childhood' (1968), 8:**99-104**
normal child behaviour compared, 3:13-14,
   125-126
'Notes for a Discussion on Technique in
   Analysis of Psychotics' (undated), 9:**365-366**
Oedipal complex and, 6:411
parent with psychosis, effect on children,
   6:70-71
psychoanalytical environment and, 3:64
psychoanalytic practice, therapy of psychosis
   linked with, 7:230-231
'Psychoses and Child Care' (1952), 3:248; 4:8,
   9, **35-43**; 6:157*n*4; 7:233; 8:184*n*i, 185; 9:7,
   38*n*8, 304
regressions, psychotic, 3:125
Segal's view on treatment of, 4:71
theories of DWW regarding, 11:7-8
treatment by psychoanalysis, 4:58, 203, 210, 216
psychosomatic disorders

'Additional Note on Psycho-Somatic Disorder'
   (1969), 9:**95-98**
allergy, 11:51
anorexia as, 7:70-72
asthma, 11:175-177
birth memories and, 3:217
classification, 7:75-77
clinical examples of, 7:70-74
complicating factors, 7:68-69
definition, 7:67-68
depression and psyche-soma, 1:159
excitement and, 9:67-68
'Excitement in the Aetiology of Coronary
   Thrombosis' (1957), 5:9, **287-291**
gastric ulcer, 11:177-178
heart condition of DWW and, 5:9
infant care and, 8:71
integration, as problem of, 7:75-77
of Jung, 7:117, 119
'Leucotomy in Psychosomatic Disorders' (letter
   to *The Lancet*; 1951), 3:**465-466**
medical profession and, 5:423
mood and, 9:68-69
in paediatrics, 3:139
personality disturbances and, 9:68
'Physiotherapy and Human Relations' (1969),
   9:**67-73**
positive aspects of, 7:75
'Psycho-somatic Disorder Reconsidered' (from
   Human Nature; 1988), 11:**175-178**
'The Psycho-Somatic Field' (from *Human
   Nature*; 1988), 11:**53-56**
'Psycho-somatic Illness in Its Positive and
   Negative Aspects' (1966), 11:247*n*1
'Psycho-Somatic Illness in Its Positive and
   Negative Aspects' (1966), 7:8, **67-77**; 8:54*n*ii,
   269*n*iv; 9:95
purpose of, 3:255-256
responsible agents, scattering of, 7:72-74
sexual development in children and, 3:108
skin and, 1:449-454; 9:95
as subject, 7:69-70
the unconscious and, 1: lxxi
'A Psychotherapeutic Interview in Child
   Psychiatry' (1963), 6:24-26
psychotherapy. *See also* psychoanalysis,
   psychology
for antisocial children in hostels, 3:24-25, 27*n*2
casework and, 5:481-482
friendship resembling, 6:203
'Hospital Care Supplementing Intensive
   Psychotherapy in Adolescence' (1963), 6:18,
   491-497
morality, ethics and, 8:231, 254
playing and, 8:299, 3010-311

psychotherapy (*Cont.*)
  'A Psychotherapeutic Consultation: A Case of Stammering', 10:165
  'A Psychotherapeutic Consultation in Child Psychiatry: A Comparative Study of the Dynamic Processes', 10:275
  'A Psychotherapeutic Interview in Child Psychiatry' (1963), 6:24–26
  'Psychotherapy of Character Disorders' (1963), 6:13, **447–459**
  suffering and, 6:449
  'Varieties of Psychotherapy' (1961), 6:19, **197–204**
puberty, 11:83, 84
  adolescence versus, 7:51
  new orientation to world required by, 5:68–69
  as stage in child development, 6:347; 8:67–68
  WWII's effect on children in, 2:96–97
public clinics, 6:19–20
public health, 1:31–33, 68. *See also* National Health Service
pulmonary stenosis, 1:217
punishment. *See also* corporal punishment
  'Comments on the Report of the Committee on Punishment in Prisons and Borstals' (1961), 6:17, **273–278**
  docking child, 2:350
  expiation and propitiation, value to criminal of, 3:241–242
  Holding and Interpretation: Fragment of an Analysis (1955), 4:351
  letter to *The Times* (1949) on punishment and crime, 3:**237–238**, 239, 241–242
  of naughtiness versus delinquency, 7:205
  penal reform, 3:357–359
  'Psychological Aspects of Birching' (1944), 2:**247–249**
  'Punishment and Crime: A Psychologist's View' (letter to *the Times*; 1949), 3:**237–238**, 241, 359, 359*n*i
  as substitute climax, 3:105
  techniques, 10:475
Putnam, M. C., 1:295, 297*n*4
pyelo-nephritis or pyelitis, 1:317
pykenolepsy, 1:308

Mr Q (American correspondent of DWW), letter to, 9:**29–31**
Qantas (airlines), DWW on spelling of, 5:219
Q Camps (Bicester Poor Law Institution), 2:7–8, 17–18, 291; 9:200–201
  'Report on Q Camps' (1941), 2:**103–105**, 349
Q principle, and antisocial behaviour, 2:105
Queen's Hospital for Children, Bethnal Green, London, 1: lviii, 6, 75, 95, 111, 117, 119, 123, 131, 149, 290*n*5; 2:6, 63*n*2, 178; 9:99; 10:4
questionnaires', 5:503*n*i; 6: 109–110; 7, 364, 400; 9:341
quickening of foetus, in development of individual, 7:450
quiet states and transitional objects, 3:457
Quigley, Janet, 2:221, 237, 271, 277, 281, 323, 329, 335, 343; 9:179, 12:8–11, 13–14

race and ethnicity
  African Americans, 7:33–34
  Australian Aborigines, eating of children by, 9:107
  black, idea of, 7:151
  breastfeeding in black versus white populations, 9:341
  dark-skinned child in fair-skinned adoptive family, 9:243–245
racial unconsciousness, 11:165
radio. *See also* BBC broadcasts
  DWW on value of radio broadcasting, 7:83–84
  'Health Education Through Broadcasting' (1957), 5:**297–300**
  as occupation therapy, 3:267
rage, in infants and young children, 3:394, 396. *See also* anger
Raison, Timothy, letter to (1963), 6:**421–422**
Ramzy, Ishak, 6:351*n*i; 10:4
  Editor's Foreword to *The Piggle* (1977), 11:**189–192**
  manuscript of *The Piggle* (1977) prepared by, 11:3
Rank, O., 7:14
  Trauma of Birth (1929), 3:212, 213; 7:49
Rapaport, David, letter to (1953), 4:**121–122**
Rapaport, J., 3:356
rationalisation, Helge Lundholm on, 1:341
Raum and *Welt* (Rilke), 8:395
Raven, John C., controlled projection test, 3:149
Rayner, Claire, 6:205–210
Rayner, Eric, *The Independent Mind in British Psychoanalysis* (1991), 2:6*n*i
'Reactions of Patients to the New Institute' (symposium), 4:29*n*i
reactive depression, 5:211, 456; 6:413–414
Read, Grantly Dick. *See* Dick-Read, Grantly
Read, Major Stanford, 5:392
reality
  abstraction becoming, 4:446
  beginning of individual and, 7:453–454
  child development and, 3:403–404; 6:41–42, 415–416
  creative illusion and, 9:7–8
  delinquency as defence against loss of objects and reality, 5:364
  denial of inner reality, in manic defence, 1:363, 372

environmental needs and, 3:172
'Establishment of Relationship with External Reality' (from *Human Nature*; 1988), 11:**119–131**
excited and quiet relationships with, 11:119–123; 11:*120*; 11:129
failure in initial contact with, 11:125–126, 131*n*3
fantasy versus, 2:36, 44, 99, 240, 365; 4:64, 164, 189–191, 213
flight to external reality from internal reality, in manic defence, 1:363
happiness/unhappiness, and acceptance of, 1:156–157, 158*n*1
Holding and Interpretation: Fragment of an Analysis (1955), 4:328–330, 369
individual babies and, 11:129
infant's appreciation of, 2:361, 364–366; 4:66
infant's clash of inner world with, 2:284–285
inner versus outer, 1:24, 359
instinct theory and, 11:81–82
Klein on psychic reality, 6:129
mother's importance in relationship with, 11:128–129
omnipotence, shock of loss of, 9:9–10
paediatrics and psychiatry, interaction of, 3:128–132, 135–136, 137–139
philosophy of, 11:130
Playing and Reality, 8:3
'Primary Introduction to External Reality: The Early Stages' (1948), 3:**165–170**, 185; 10:8
reality principle, 5:318; 6:41, 133, 146, 200, 201, 214, 279; 7:184, 185, 390–392; 8:71, 328, 358, 360; 9:7–10, 37, 49, 153, 208–209, 214
reality-testing, 4:161; 6:230
in *Romeo and Juliet*, 3:192
subjectivity of, 9:300
schizophrenia and, 3:172–173; 6:415–416
Searl, Nina, 'The Flight to Reality' (1929), 1:360
transitional objects and, 4:40; 5:407; 9:267, 273, 274
trauma and the family, 7:184, 185
value of illusion and transitional states, 11:123–126
'The World in Small Doses' (1949), 3:**293–297**
reassurance, 4:215
countertransference and, 4:215; 5:107
between DWW and child patient, 8:352
regression and, 4:215; 5:107–108
Recherches, 8:161
recidivism, 5:152
red blood corpuscles in urine, 1:318
Rees, J. R., 1:9
Reeves, C., 1: lv, lxiii; 2:3, 12; 8:13, 14; 11:18
 'Singing the Same Tune? Bowlby and Winnicott on Deprivation and Delinquency', 10:18
Reeves, James, *Georgian Poetry*, 8:407

refugees
 Friedmann, Oscar and Manna, and Jewish refugee children, 5:536–537
 Jewish Refugees Boys' Hostels, 5:536
 Russian, 5:198
 in WWII, 3:226
regression
 addiction and, 4:173
 advantage of, 4:293
 analyst needing to adapt to, 3:234; 4:123, 285; 6:7, 360
 anxiety, lack of, during, 4:58
 beating fantasy and, 5:314
 'Case Notes for a Psychoanalytic Seminar: Withdrawal, Regression, Male Identification' (1965), 7:**239–242**
 changing meaning of, 5:448
 in childhood schizophrenia, 3:134
 'The Concept of Clinical Regression Compared with that of Defence Organisation' (1967), 8:16; 8:*30*; 8:**183–189**
 defined, 4:98, 202–209; 9:360
 in delayed reaction to death of father, in case study, 7:294, 299
 to dependence, 1: lxxii; 4:206, 207, 210, 213; 5:133; 8:16, 184–185; 11:83, 174, 176
 environment and, 6:507; 7:13–14
 fantasies and, 4:55
 S. Freud on, 5:363
 'The Importance of the Setting in Meeting Regression in Psychoanalysis' (1989), 7:6–7, 13, **85–90**
 'Metapsychological and Clinical Aspects of Regression within the Psychoanalytical Set-up' (1954), 1:373*n*6; 4:**201–217**, 225*n*i; 6:159
 need versus wish in, 4:99
 'Notes on Withdrawal and Regression' (1989), 7:6
 omnipotence and, 4:136
 in *The Piggle*, 11:203, 210, 258
 professional attitude of therapist and, 5:510
 psychotic, 3:125
 reassurance and, 4:215; 5:107–108
 regressive object, 6:292
 schizophrenia and, 7:44–50; 8:183
 Scott on, 4:221–222, 223–225
 theory of mind and, 3:247, 251
 therapeutic consultation, 10:336, 360, 361, 364, 366, 367*n*6
 unintegration, progress from/regression into, 11:133–136
 'Withdrawal and Regression' (from *Human Nature*; 1988), 11:**159–160**
 'Withdrawal and Regression' (published 1955), 1: lxxiii; 4:**283–289**; 5:253*n*i; 6:170
 withdrawal distinguished, 7:6–7, 240

rehabilitation, 4:136; 10:19, 452
Reich, W., 7:14
Reichenhaimsche Waisenhaus, 5:536
relationships. *See* interpersonal relationships
relaxation and creativity, 8:171–172
reliability, 6:349, 381, 437, 448; 8:6–7, 314–315
  dependence and, 9:192–197
  failure of, 8:232; 10:124
  residential therapy providing, 9:202–203
religion. *See also* Jews; scriptural references
  blasphemy, 8:365–366
  Blessed Sacrament, for Catholics versus Protestants, 9:270
  child's thinking about, 9:386
  Christianity and the ascensive, 1:365
  Christian religion, characterisation of, 8:375
  conscience, development of, 1:409
  'Cure' (1970), 9:**191–197**
  environmental abnormalities and, 6:444
  existence of God, 8:265
  God, child presenting himself at analysis as, 11:108–109
  God as the 'Great I AM', 7:75
  God of seventeenth century compared with God of present day, 8:366–367
  goodness and, 6:378
  Graves & Podro, *Nazarene Gospel Restored*, 8:158
  Jung and, 7:121
  love and, 6:213
  Methodism, DWW influenced by, 5:4; 8:313–314; 12:301
  monotheism, 8:268–269
  Northern Ireland, Catholic-Protestant divide in, 9:118
  one-ness with God/Universe, 6:530–531
  original sin, 6:378
  The Piggle, inquiries about going to church in, 11:306–307
  Sargant, William, 'The Physiology of Faith' (1969), 9:59–61
  science compared to, 6:218
  the soul, DWW on, 11:76–77
  therapeutic consultation and, 10:445
remand homes, 3:51, 52
'Remarks on a Discussion of Balint's Paper on Technique' (1957), 1: lxxii; 3:215*n*i; 5:**211–212**
'A Reminder to the Binder' (1921), 1:**63**
removal of child from parents, cases requiring, 5:518
reparation, 11:92–94, 172
  adolescents and, 9:347
  'Aggression, Guilt and Reparation' (1960), 6:**97–104**
  in child development, 3:402; 4:194; 6:329–330
  DWW's understanding of, 3:12–15
  Klein's concept of, 9:37

'Reparation in Respect of Mother's Organized Defence Against Depression' (1948), 3:12–13, 14–15, **117–122**; 5:126*n*ii; 6:158*n*18; 9:75
repetition
  allowing child to sleep, 6:82–83
  symbolised in psychotherapy, 4:131; 7:189–190, 191–192
'Report on Child Department Consultations' (lecture, June 1942), 2:149
Report on Q Camps (1941), 2:8, 17, **103–105**, 349
repressed unconscious, 3:101–102, 208; 9:355; 11:82, 155
repression
  of anal erotism, 1:348, 350, 457
  defined, 11:155
  depressive position and, 11:99
  enuresis and, 1:320
  of genital erotism, 1:157, 347
  of homosexuality, 1:456, 457; 5:30; 6:405, 407
  Lundholm, Helge, 'Repression and rationalisation' (abstract; 1933), 1:**341**
  as management of antisocial behaviour, 6:387
  primal or primary, 5:179, 180–181; 6:142
  psycho-neurosis and, 6:410–411
  sense of guilt and, 1:320, 350
  therapeutic consultation and, 10:293
  toddler age and, 6:257
research, psychoanalytic, dangers of disregarding, 7:149–156
resentment
  of mother against child, 2:186–187; 6:79
  toward adolescents, 6:195, 423
'Residential Care as Therapy' (1970), 2:7, 103, 291; 9:**199–206**
residential child care, 8:60–61
'Residential Management as Treatment for Difficult Children' (with Clare Britton; 1947), 3:27*n*1, **77–93**. *See also* hostels
resilience of children, 6:309
'Resolution K: On Scientific Aims in Psychoanalysis' (1942), 1: lxiv; 2:**145–147**; 6:217
responsibility
  child growth and development and, 3:398–399; 6:35, 40; 8:155
  'Responsibility and Freedom' (letter to *The British Medical Journal*; 1943), 2:**217–219**
restlessness, 6:237, 394
retaliation
  on analyst, 8:360
  anxiety about, 10:129
  primitive, 2:367–368
return of evacuated children. *See* evacuation of children
revenge, 2:19; 6:18, 274, 427, 449

Complete Index of the Collected Works   445

of public, in punishment and legal procedures, 2:233, 235, 247, 375
reverie, 7:17, 96. *See also* daydreaming; fantasies
reviews. *See also The Psychoanalytic Study of the Child*
  Aichhorn, August, *Wayward Youth* (1936), 1:**433–436**
  Axline, Virginia, *Play Therapy* (book published 1947; comments recorded by DWW 1969), 9:**159–164**
  Axline, Virginia A., *Dibs: In Search of Self* (reviewed 1966), 7:**367–368**
  Bakwin, Harry and Bakwin, Ruth Morris, *Clinical Management of Behavior Disorders in Children* (1953; reviewed 1954), 4:**265–256**
  Balint, Michael, *The Doctor, His Patients, and the Illness* (1957; reviewed 1958), 5:**401–404**; 7:68n1
  Bergeron, Marcel, *Psychologie du Premier Age* (1961; reviewed 1962), 6:**371**
  Bowlby, John, *Maternal Care and Mental Health* (1951; reviewed 1953), 4:**111–114**
  Bowley, Agatha H., *The Psychology of the Unwanted Child* (1947; reviewed 1948), 3:**149–150**
  Burton, Lindy, *Vulnerable Children: Three Studies of Children in Conflict* (reviewed 1968), 8:**275–276**
  The Cambridge Evacuation Survey: A Wartime Study in Social Welfare and Education (1941), 2:**117–119**
  character and personality of DWW revealed in, 7:15–16
  Chess, S. et al, *Your Child Is a Person* (1960; reviewed 1966), 7:**415**
  Child Study Association of America, *Parents' Questions* (1947; reviewed 1948), 3:**151**
  Clegg, Alec and Megson, Barbara, *Children in Distress* (reviewed 1968), 8:**339**
  Clyne, Max B., *Absent: School Refusal as an Expression of Disturbed Family Relationships* (1966), 7:**405–406**
  Clyne, Max B., *Absent: School Refusal as an Expression of Disturbed Family Relationships* (1966; reviewed 1967), 8:**129–130**
  'A Collection of Children's Books' (1967), 8:**203–204**
  Direct Analysis. Selected Papers (Rosen 1953, reviewed 1953), 4:**127–128**
  Eissler, Ruth S., et al.,*The Psychoanalytic Study of the Child, Volume 20* (1966), 7:**377–378**
  Eppel, E. M., and M. Eppel, *Adolescents and Morality* (1966), 7:**403–404**
  Erikson, Erik, *Childhood and Society* (1951; reviewed 1953), 4:**125–126**
  Erikson, Erik, *Childhood and Society* (paperback edition, 1965), 7:**213–214**
  Evans, Philip, and Ronald MacKeith, *Infant Feeding and Feeding Difficulties* (1951), 3:**491–493**; 6:401n1
  Fairbairn, W. R. D., *Psychoanalytic Studies of the Personality* (1952; reviewed 1953), 4:**1329–137**
  Flügel, J. C., *The Moral Paradox of Peace and War* (1941), 2:**115–116**
  Foote, Estelle J., *Six Children* (1956; reviewed 1957), 5:**223–224**
  Freud, Anna, *Indications for Child Analysis and Other Papers* (1968/69; reviewed 1969), 9:**93–94**
  Freud, Anna, *Normality and Pathology in Childhood* (1965), 7:14, 16, **217–225**, 227, 375
  Glover, Edward, *Psycho-Analysis and Child Psychiatry* (1953), 4:**115**
  Goldfarb, William, *Childhood Schizophrenia* (1961; reviewed 1963), 6:**509–510**
  Goodacre, Iris, *Adoption Policy and Practice* (1966), 7:**427–428**
  Harms, Ernest, ed. *Handbook of Child Guidance* (1947; reviewed 1949), 3:**235**
  Hill, Adrian, *Art Versus Illness* (1948; reviewed 1949), 3:**265–267**
  Jackson, Lydia, *Aggression and Its Interpretation* (1954), 4:**247–248**
  Jones, Ernest, ed., *Letters of Sigmund Freud, 1873–1939* (1961; reviewed 1962), 6:**367–370**
  Jones, Ernest, *Papers on Psycho-Analysis* (1948, reviewed 1951), 3:**489–490**
  Jung, C. G., *Memories, Dreams, and Reflections* (1963; reviewed 1964), 7:15–16, **115–124**
  Kanner, Leo, *Child Psychiatry* (1935; reviewed 1937, 1938), 1:**439–440**, 2:9
  Kirk, H. David, *Shared Fate* (reviewed 1965), 7:**311–312**
  Klein, Melanie, *Envy and Gratitude* (1957; reviewed 1959), 5:11, **433–436**
  Lask, Aaron, *Asthma: Attitude and Milieu* (1966), 7:**417–418**
  Lebovici, S., and J. McDougall, *Un Cas de Psychose Infantile* (1960; reviewed 1962), 6:**373–375**
  LeShan, Eda J., *How to Survive Parenthood* (1965; reviewed 1967), 8:**181–182**
  Letters of Sigmund Freud, 1873–1939 (E. Jones, ed.; 1961; reviewed 1962), 6:**367–370**
  Middlemore, Merell P., *The Nursing Couple* (1942), 1: lxiv–lxv, 18; 2:12, **171–174**, 296, 297n1
  Milner, Marion, *On Not Being Able to Paint* (1950; reviewed 1951), 3:**483–485**
  Rickman, J., ed., *On the bringing up of children* (1936), 1:18, **437–438**

reviews (*Cont.*)
  Riese, Hertha, *Heal the Hurt Child* (1963; reviewed 1964), 7:**33–35**
  Rimland, Bernard, *Infantile Autism* (1964; reviewed 1966), 7:**397–398**
  Robertson, James, *Going to Hospital with Mother* (film, 1958; reviewed 1959), 5:**529–531**
  Rosen, John N., *Direct Analysis. Selected Papers* (1953), 4:**127–128**
  Sandström, Carl Ivar, *The Psychology of Childhood and Adolescence* (reviewed 1968), 8:10, **411–412**
  Searles, Harold F., *The Non-Human Environment in Normal Development and in Schizophrenia* (1960; reviewed 1963), 6:**505–507**
  Senn, M. J. (ed.), *Problems of Infancy and Childhood. Transactions of the Third Conference* (1949; reviewed 1951), 3:**487**; 4:**117**
  Simey, T. S., *The Concept of Love in Child Care* (1961), 6:**213–215**
  Slavson, S. R., *Child Psychotherapy* (1953), 4:**233–234**
  Soddy, Kenneth, *Clinical Child Psychiatry* (1960; reviewed 1961), 6:**223**
  Stein, Leopold, *The Infancy of Speech and the Speech of Infancy* (1949; reviewed 1950), 3:**363–364**
  Stewart, Sheila, *A Home from Home* (1967; reviewed 1967), 8:**105–106**
  Storr, Anthony, *Human Aggression* (reviewed 1968), 8:**321–322**, 329*n*i
  Thomson, Helen, *The Successful Step-Parent* (1966; reviewed 1967), 8:**89–90**
  Watson, J. A. F., *The Child and the Magistrate* (1950; reviewed 1951), 3:**431–432**
  Wickes, Frances G., *The Inner World of Man: With Psychological Drawings and Paintings* (1950; reviewed 1951), 3:**463**
  Wolff, Werner, *The Personality of the Preschool Child: The Child's Search for His Self* (1947; reviewed 1948), 3:**159–160**
  Ziman, Edmund, *Jealousy in Children* (1951), 3:**469**
Revista de Psicoanálisis, 9:336*n*4
Revue Française de Psychanalyse, 4:283; 5:249
rheumatic clinics
  cardiac neurosis, DWW's experience of, 7:3879, 380, 383
  London County Council Rheumatism Clinic, DWW at, 9:99
  Queen's Hospital, London, 1:123–125, 161
  'The Rheumatic Clinic', from *Clinical Notes* (1931), 1:**225–228**
rheumatic fever (rheumatism)
  acute, 1:196–198, 220–223; 2:54–62
  anxiety and, 1:272
  arthritis, rheumatic, 1:200
  chorea and rheumatic heart disease, 1:133, 161–163; 2:50
  diagnosis of, 1:226–228; 2:50–54
  DWW's experience of treating, 8:43
  fantasy and, 2:58–60
  frequency of occurrence in 1920s and virtual disappearance in 1930s and 1940s, 7:380–381, 384
  growing pains and, 1:235–238
  heart disease as result of, 2:49
  pre-rheumatic children, 1:125, 171, 219, 225, 266; 2:50–54
  psychological states and, 2:50–54, 54–62; 6:414; 11:50
  smouldering, 1:196, 220–223, 226
  subacute, 1:205, 226, 230; 2:54–62, 63*n*1
  systolic murmur and active rheumatism, 1:214
  terminology, 2:49
  tonsils, tonsilitis, and tonsillectomies, 1:124, 205, 221, 240
  'The Heart, with Special Reference to Rheumatic Carditis', from *Clinical Notes* (1931), 1:**207–218**
  'On In-Patient Treatment for Rheumatic Fever and Chorea' (ca. 1923–1931), 1:**161–163**
  'Rheumatic Fever', from *Clinical Notes* (1931), 1:**219–223**
  'Rheumatism in Children' (1928), 1:**123–125**
  'Rheumatism in Children' (1931), 7:379*n*i
Rhodes, E. C., *Young Offenders* (1942), 2:196, 200*n*1
Ribble, Margaret, 6:434; 8:35
  The Rights of Infants (1943), 7:415
rickets, 1:296, 297*n*5; 2:294
Rickman, John, 1: lxix*n*iii; 2:15; 3:147*n*i; 4:37; 5:211, 242, 392, 456; 6:203
  critiquing papers read at BPAS by Associate Members, 4:48
  definition of 'mental illness' by, 6:410
  editor, *On the bringing up of children* (reviewed 1936), 1:18, **437–438**
  'The Factor of Number in Individual-and Group-Dynamics' (1950), 5:211*n*i
  S. Freud's personal communication to (1905), 11:167*n*1
  The People of Great Russia: A Psychological Study (with G. Gorer, 1949), 11:141*n*1
Ricoeur, P., 11:13
riddance, 2:10–12, 137
Ries, Hannah, letter to (1953), 4:15*n*ii, **123–124**
Riese, Hertha, *Heal the Hurt Child* (1963; reviewed 1963), 7:**33–35**

Riggall, R. M., 5:392
Rilke, Rainer Maria, 8:395, 401
Rimland, Bernard, *Infantile Autism* (1964; reviewed by DWW 1964), 7:**397–398**
Ritvo, Samuel, 8:12
 'Correlation of a Childhood and Adult Neurosis: Based on the Adult Analysis of a Reported Childhood Case', 7:198
 as New York Psychoanalytic Society discussant, 9:36
rivalry. *See also* jealousy
 with foster parents, 2:38
 between mother and daughter, 2:214, 274
 over mother, 2:275
 sibling, *see* jealousy; sibling rivalry
Rivers, W. H. R., 5:392
Riviere, Joan
 birthday of, 5:349–350
 on depression and elation, 2:63n4
 Developments in Psychoanalysis (1952), 5:123niii; 8:331
 DWW acknowledging influence of, 8:364
 DWW in analysis with, 1: lviii, 12; 2:13; 4:60–61; 8:10, 42, 44; 9:356; 11:6
 on female sexual development, 3:490
 as founding member of BPAS, 1:11; 5:394
 on frustration in infants, 3:341
 Jones, Ernest, and, 5:392, 394–395, 396
 Klein and, 4:61, 242; 5:121–124; 6:330; 8:331
 letters to (1949), 3:**221–222, 233–234**
 letter to (1956), 5:11, **121–124**
 letter to (1957), 5:**237**; 329nii
 letter to (1958), 5:**349–350**
 letter to (1956), 9:47
 Love, Hate and Reparation (with Melanie Klein; 1937), 1:413
 on manic defence, 1:371
 on objectivity, 3:460
 'On the Genesis of Psychical Conflict in Earliest Infancy' (1936), 7:187n2; 9:277
 on reality-acceptance, 5:417
 during WWII, 2:6
'"Robert" aet 9 Years', 10:**141–156**
 mother's depression, effect on child, 10:143–144, 153, 155
 objective statement of home situation, 10:153–154
 squiggle game and, 10:*144–152, 144–153*
Robertson, James, 3:400; 4:114ni; 5:6, 255ni; 6:175; 7:156; 8:339; 9:127, 204; 10:528
 Going to Hospital with Mother (film, 1958; review 1959), 3:405n2; 5:**529–531**
 A Two-year-old Goes to Hospital (film, 1953), 9:127
 A Two-year-old Goes to Hospital (film, 1953), 3:405n2; 5:317, 419n2, 497, 529, 531n1; 10:18

Young Children in Hospital (film, 1958), 3:405n2; 5:531; 10:18
Robertson, Joyce, 4:114ni; 5:6; 7:156; 9:127, 204; 10:18, 528
 'A Mother's Observations on the Tonsillectomy of Her Four-year-old Daughter', 5:317, 531
'"Robin" aet 5 Years', 10:**57–82**
 dreams and, 10:66–68
 humour coming out in therapy session, 10:65
 regressive behaviour to get mother's attention, 10:57–58
 school refusal, 10:57, 81–82
 squiggle game and, 10:*58–67, 58–81, 69–81*
Robinson, Clive, 1:xii
Robinson, Helen Taylor, 1:xlix, lv; 12:xlix
Robinson, Ken, 1:3, 11niv, 479–480
 'Remembering, Repeating and Working Through' (2015), 7:378ni
Rocaz (encephalitis researcher), 1:81, 88
'Rockabye Baby', 3:67
rocking movement, 2:152; 3:171, 343; 6:372, 435; 7:190; 8:233; 9:137, 263, 360
'Rock of Ages, Cleft for Me' (Wesleyan hymn), 9:191ni
Rodman, F. Robert, 1: lviin1, lx; 2:21nii; 3:234nii; 5:9, 10; 6:20, 46ni
 'Accidental Technical Lapses as Therapy', 9:25
 letter to (1969), 8:15; 9:**25–27**
 Nemon, Oscar, DWW in studio of, 9:18
 providing footnote for 'The Use of an Object and Relating Through Identifications' (1968), 8:364
 Winnicott: Life and work (2003), 1:3nii, 35, 43, 49, 51; 2:6ni, 11, 21nii; 8:195
Rodrigue, Emilio, letter to (1955), 5:**31–32**
Rogerson, C. H., 2:252, 252ni
Rolleston, J. D., 1:78, 88, 115, 127, 132
 'Acute Infectious Diseases' (1929), 1:335n2
Romeo and Juliet (Shakespeare), 3:174, 185–193
Romulus and Remus, 7:335; 9:208
Roosevelt, Franklin D., 2:93
'Roots of Aggression' (1964), 7:9–10, **129–135**; 9:36
'Roots of Aggression' (1968), 8:10, **329–332**; 9:47
Rorschach test, 8:320
rosacea, 1:461–462
'"Rosemary" aet 10 Years', 10:**157–163**
 death-wish toward mother, 10:163
 dreams and, 10:162–163
 squiggle game and, 10:*157–163, 158–163*
Rosen, John N., 7:84; 11:166
 Direct Analysis. Selected Papers (reviewed 1953), 4:**127–128**
Rosenberg, Dr, 3:228
Rosenblut, D., 5:307
Rosenbluth, Michael, letter to (1969), 9:**23–24**

Rosenfeld, Eva, 6:211, 211*n*ii
Rosenfeld, Herbert, 1: lxviii; 9:112*n*ii, 151
  background of, 4:73, 77
  letter to (1958), 5:**365–366**
  letter to (1966), 7:**343–344**
  'Psychopathology of Hypochondriacal States',
    5:365*n*i
  'Some Observations on the Psychopathology of
    Hypochondriacal States', 5:365*n*i
Rosenheim, Professor, 7:407
Rosenthal, Arthur, 6:109, 109*n*i
Rosetti, Christina, 'Passing Away', 8:174
Ross, Helen, 5:337*n*i
Rothenstein, John, 8:218*n*3
Rowley, J. L., 4:64; 6:107
  'Rehearsal and Collusion' (1952), 4:61, 63*n*iv
Royal College of Midwives, 5:277, 390
Royal College of Physicians, 5:310; 7:407; 10:4
Royal Medico-Psychological Association (later
  Royal College of Psychiatrists), 7:407; 8:65,
  149*n*i; 11:12
Royal Society of Medicine, 1: l, 9, 143; 3:148, 333;
  4:79; 5:9, 337; 8:81; 10:7
Ruben, Margarete, 5:364
Rubinstein, L. H. (nominated as Scientific
  Secretary of BPAS by DWW), 5:347
Rudnytsky, P., 8:13
Runyan, Damon, 7:401
Rushdie, Salman, 'Is nothing sacred?' (1990), 9:5
Russell, H. B., 1:75, 83, 84, 86, 87, 88
Russia, communist disruption of family life in,
  2:32–33
'"Ruth" aet 8 Years', 7:180*n*iii; 10:**419–439, 527–533**
  deprivation and, 10:420, 421, 438, 527–528,
    530, 532
  dreams and, 10:434
  gender identity and, 10:530
  identification of Ruth with her mother, 10:424,
    436, 438
  illness of the mother and, 10:419–420
  lying as issue, 10:438, 532
  mother's depression, effect of, 10:420, 438
  squiggle game and, 10:421–439, *422–437*,
    530–531
  stealing as issue, 10:419, 421, 436, 438, 530, 532
ruthlessness
  change to concern, 11:36, 60, 67, 91, 151
  'pre-ruth', 2:15; 3:5, 335, 340; 5:153; 6:17
  primitive, 2:15, 366; 3:311, 457
  ruthless love, 3:66; 11:44, 91, 92
  as stage, 3:335, 339, 402
Rycroft, Charles, 1: lxviii, lxxvii; 4:276; 5:201, 361*n*i;
  8:17*n*1; 11:13
  'An Enquiry into the Function of Words in the
  Psycho-Analytical Situation', 5:199*n*i

letter to (1954), 4:**179–180**
letter to (1955), 5:**43**
letters to (1956), 5:**171, 173,** 258*n*i
letter to (1957), 5:**199**
letter to (1956), 7:151*n*i
'Some Observations on a Case of Vertigo'
  (1953), 4:55–56, 58

Sackett, H. L., 1:60
sadism. *See also* oral sadism
  cannibalism and, 4:313
  reparation phenomenon and, 4:313
  sadistic superego, 6:128
sadness. *See* grief, mourning, sadness, and loss
sado-masochism
  corporal punishment and, 2:247; 5:193
  'Psychogenesis of a Beating Fantasy' (1958),
    5:**313–315**
  therapeutic consultation, 10:276, 293, 295–296
St Ann's Road Hospital, Tottenham, London, 1:129
St Bartholomew's Hospital, London
  DWW's medical education at, 1:xvi, 3–5, 18,
    65–66, 67, 69; 2:256; 12:304–305
  'St Bartholomew's Hospital Amateur Dramatic
    Club' (1920), 1:**59–61**
  St Bartholomew's Hospital Journal, 1:57, 59, 63,
    65, 143
  *St John's Hospital Dermatological Society
    Report*, 1:449
St Luke's Church, Hatfield, 9:191
St Mary's Hospital Gazette, 6:263; 10:157
St Mary's Hospital Paddington Green, 2:177; 3:222,
  243–244; 5:438, 475, 488; 6:181, 183, 264,
  301. *See also* Paddington Green Children's
  Hospital
St Mary of Bethlehem (Bedlam) Hospital, 7:316*n*i
St Paul's School (London), 2:381
St Vincent de Paul, 9:194, 195, 205
St Vitus' Dance, 1:108, 332, 333, 383
'Sakari: A Therapeutic Consultation' (1961),
  6:**241–255**; 10:15
salt in water treatment for adenoids, 1:203–204
Salzburger, Miss, 5:307
Sandler, Joseph J., 7:377*n*i, 407; 8:16, 227
  'Comments on Joseph Sandler's "On the
    Concept of the Superego" (1960), 6:14–15,
    127–133
  'Comments on "Problems of Research
    in Psycho-Analysis"' (1961), 6:**229–231**
  FitzHerbert letter to (1961), 6:211
  From safety to superego, 6:127
Sandström, Carl Ivar, *The Psychology of Childhood
  and Adolescence* (reviewed 1968), 8:10,
  411–412
Sandy, J. R., 3:141

San Francisco Psychoanalytic Society, 6:343, 433
sanity, flight to, 4:210; 8:73
Sargant, William, 3:113, 465; 7:455
  letter to (1969), 9:**59–61**
  'The Mechanism of Conversion', 3:467
  'The Physiology of Faith' (1969), 9:59–61
Sargant-Florence, Mary, 8:126
satisfaction of infants, 2:365, 368n3; 6:150, 152, 290, 435
Sauget, Dr, 7:407
savants, autistic, 7:351, 352, 354
'Saying "No"' (1960), 6:**31–42**, 86
scalp condition, compulsive scalp excitement, and phobia of infestation, 1:458–459
Scandinavian Orthopsychiatric Congress, 6:253
Scarfone, Dominique, 1:liii; 4:3, 10
Schilder, P., 1:292; 4:56
Schindelha (encephalitis researcher), 1:85
schizoid states. *See also* schizophrenia
  in *Holding and Interpretation*, 4:308, 441
  child psychosis and, 3:353
  children of psychotic parents, 5:517–518
  concept of, 1: lxvii; 4:44f, 131
  countertransference, DWW's understanding of, and, 3:4
  creativity and, 9:300–301
  depression and, 6:465, 466
  Fairbairn on schizoid personality, 4:133–135
  guilt, morality, and ethics for, 7:442, 445
  gullibility of schizoid patients, 6:486
  hiding of schizoid disorder, 6:392
  Holding and Interpretation: Fragment of an Analysis (1955), 4:304, 441
  Klein, 'Notes on Some Schizoid Mechanisms' (1946), 1: lxvii
  Klein on schizoid position, 4:130, 134
  management of, 3:137
  mother-infant mutuality and, 9:132
  need satisfaction and, 7:373–374
  paranoid-schizoid position, 1:xxv, 16; 6:330
  psychoanalytic research and, 7:152, 153
  psychoanalytic technique and, 4:129–130; 5:212
  schizoid depression, 1: lxvii, lxxii; 6:4193–414
  schizoid position, 4:130, 134
  therapeutic consultation, 10:213–214, 231
  transitional objects and, 9:284
  trauma and the family, 7:183–184
schizophrenia
  'The Aetiology of Infantile Schizophrenia in Terms of Adaptive Failure' (1967), 1:439ni; 8:**161–165**; 9:91, 301, 302
  anxiety and, 6:391
  autism and, 7:345–346, 356, 359, 397
  basic fault and, 1: lxxii
  birth memories and, 3:212–213

borderline cases, 7:44, 247, 275. *See also* borderline cases
  in childhood, 2:153, 252; 3:353, 354; 7:116, 345–346, 356
  creativity and, 9:300–302
  as defence organisation, 8:183
  delinquency and, 2:212
  description of, 8:71
  diagnosis of, 6: 414, 496–497
  early development and, 3:125, 128, 134, 135, 137; 4:37–38, 74
  environmental deficiency and, 5:455; 7:233
  as genetic condition, 4:440
  Goldfarb, William, *Childhood Schizophrenia* (1961; reviewed 1963), 6:**509–510**
  infantile schizophrenia, 1:439ni; 6:391; 8:161–164; 10:122, 138, 139, 518
  latent, 6:392
  Milner on, 8:115–116
  as negative of maturational processes, 7:305
  as normal state of individual growing up in environment dominated by persons with schizophrenic traits, 7:233
  'Notes on Personality Structure Suggested by the Analysis of a Schizophrenic' (Ezriel, 1952), 4:51ni
  physical basis for, 2:207
  prophylaxis against, 11:128
  psychoanalytic research and, 7:153
  psychoanalytic technique and, 4:439; 5:212
  as psychological condition, 7:231
  as psychosis, 6:65
  reality, relationship to, 3:172–173; 5:517; 6:415–416
  regression and, 7:44–50; 8:183, 186; 9:38
  roots in neonatal period, 7:44
  Rosenfeld on, 4:73n1
  social work and, 2:190
  splitting of personality and, 4:109
  therapeutic consultation, 10:213
Schlesinger, Bernard E., 1:152, 154, 223n1, 253n2
Schmideberg, Melitta, 1:12, 369; 2:195, 195ni, 196, 198; 3:179; 6:114
Schmidt, Dr, of Essen, 1:31–33
schools and teaching. *See also* nursery schools; progressive schools
  adopted children and relationship with teachers, 4:152
  age for starting school, 7:395
  antisocial and delinquent children, 4:279–280
  approved schools, 4:279–280; 5:151
  child's adaptation to, 1:382–383; 4:154
  Clyne, Max B., *Absent: School Refusal as an Expression of Disturbed Family Relationships* (1966; reviewed by DWW), 7:**405–406**

schools and teaching (*Cont.*)
   'Communal Feeding in Schools' (letter to the *British Medical Journal*; 1941), 2:**107–108**
   continuity of teachers at a school, 3:175
   difficult children, 8:53
   distrust between parents and teachers, overcoming, 1:376–381
   'Educational Diagnosis' (1946), 3:**29–33**
   evacuated children in wartime and, 2:95–99, 330
   'Group Influences and the Maladjusted Child: The School Aspect' (1955), 5:**45–54**
   home life versus, 1:443–444; 7:393
   hostel, children in, 2:370
   influencing and being influenced in, 2:110; 111–112
   loyalty conflicts and, 7:395
   management of children in, 3:169
   medical history of child, usefulness of, 1:381–382
   Oedipal complex, teachers' impatience with concept of, 11:60–61
   persecution fantasies, 1:376, 379–380, 384–387
   'Primary Introduction to External Reality: The Early Stages' (1948), 3:**165–170**, 185
   primary schools, 6:311–313
   psychoanalytic research and, 7:154
   'Psychology in the Child's Education' (letter to the *British Medical Journal*, 1946), 3:**35–36**
   psychosomatic disorders and, 7:71, 73
   reality, introduction of child to, 3:295
   refusal of child to attend school, 2:151–152; 6:312; 8:129–130; 10:57, 81–82, 143
   relationship between teachers and children, 3:176; 8:52–53
   in H. Riese's educational therapy centre, 7:34–35
   'Sex Education in Schools' (1949), 3:**323–326**
   'Shyness and Nervous Disorders in Children' (1938), 1:17, **445–448**
   social worker, role of, 2:183, 189–190
   'The Teacher, the Parent and the Doctor' (1936), 1:17, **375–387**
   teachers' understanding of psychotherapy, 8:273
   treatment of children with emotional problems and, 1:383–384
   true and false self and, 7:28–30
Schorstein, Joseph, 3:467
Schulz, Charles M., 8:301; 9:261
   letter to (1955), 5:**109**; 8:195*n*i, 301*n*i
Schur, Max, 6:283
Schweitzer, Albert, 9:386
science
   human nature, scientific inquiry into, 3:404
   in medical practice, 3:69–70
   psychoanalysis and, 6:217–221, 229–231

'Psychoanalysis and Science: Friends or Relations' (1961), 6:**217–221**
psychology and, 3:70; 8:50–51
religion compared to, 6:218
'Resolution K: On Scientific Aims in Psychoanalysis' (1942), 1: lxvi; 2:**145–147**; 6:217
'The Scientific Foundations of Obstetrics and Gynaecology' (not published), 8:243
Scientific Bulletin (internal newsletter of British Psychoanalytic Society), 7:377
Scotland and England, border between, 9:119
Scott, P. D., letter to (1950), 3:**357–359**; 9:4
Scott, W. Clifford M., 1: lxix*n*iii, 11; 2:216; 3:245, 253, 255; 4:43*n*1; 5:419*n*4; 7:408
   'Blathering', 4:173*n*5
   on environmental factors, 3:228
   influence on DWW, 8:363*n*2
   letter to (1953), 4:**97–99**
   on pregnant mothers, 3:227
   on regression, 4:225–226, 227–229
screaming, *see* crying
scriptural references
   Ecclesiastes 38:25, 8:271
   Exodus 3:14, 8:269*n*iv
   Genesis 1:2, 11:16
   Matthew 7:5, 9:192*n*ii
   Matthew 13:9, 8:259*n*ii
scurvy, 1:169, 191, 295–296, 297*n*5, 318
sea-fixation, 10:380, 385, 399–402, 402*n*3
search for self, 8:170–172
Searl, Nina, 1:11, 12
   'The Flight to Reality' (1929), 1:360
   'Questions and Answers', in *On the Bringing up of Children* (1936), 1:437
Searles, Harold, 7:239
   The Non-Human Environment in Normal Development and in Schizophrenia (1960; reviewed 1963), 6:356*n*1, **505–507**
seborrhoea, 1:458
Sechehaye, Marguerite A., 3:347*n*2; 5:523; 6:164, 231, 348–349, 393; 7:96
   Symbolic Realization (1951), 5:63, 528*n*1; 6:350*n*1; 9:139*n*1
Second World War. *See* World War II
secret self, 6:439
security
   'Anxiety Associated with Insecurity' (1952), 4:**55–58**, 61*n*i
   child testing limits, 6:95–96
   'On Security' (1960), 6:36, **93–96**
Seebohm Report, 8:49
Segal, Hanna, 1: lxviii; 5:209–210, 262; 9:13; 11:13, 101*n*2
   letter to (1952), 1: lxviii; 4:**29–31**

letter to (1953), 4:**71–72**
letter to (1955), 5:11, **81**
'A Psychoanalytic Approach to Aesthetics' (1952/1955), 1: lxxvi
'Report on the Analysis of a Man of Seventy-Four', 5:209*n*i
self. *See also* true and false self
   'Basis for Self in Body' (1970), 9:**225–234**
   definition of, 9:259–260
   ego versus, 7:122
   French translation of, 9:260
   Jung's use of, 7:122–123
self-care (introjected mothering), 7:179
self-confidence of mother, 2:159
self-cure, 6:416, 419; 8:292, 307
self-expression, 4:153
self-preservation, 6:17
Senn, M. J., 2:47*n*i
   editor, *Problems of Infancy and Childhood. Transactions of the Third Conference* (1949; reviewed 1951), 3:**487**; 4:**117**
sentimentalism
   British monarchy and, 9:182
   concepts of DWW and, 9:4–5
separation. *See also* evacuation of children
   Bowlby on, 4:254
   Bowlby, John, 'Separation Anxiety' (1958), 5:379–381, 383*n*i
   'The Capacity to Be Alone' (1958), 5:13–14, **241–248**
   of child from mother, effects of, 2:47–48, 84–86, 189, 336–338, 359; 4:88, 136; 5:515, 520, 529; 6:137, 291, 369, 364; 9:96, 98, 280–284. *See also* evacuation of children; World War II
   Fairbairn on, 4:136
   'On "Separation Anxiety" by John Bowlby' (DWW, 1958), 5:6, **379–381**
   of parents, 9:161
   'The Psychology of Separation (1958), 5:**333–335**
   Robertson, James, *Going to Hospital with Mother* (film, 1958; reviewed 1959), 5:529
   string signifying denial of, 6:138–139
   transitional objects and, 5:103; 9:281–283, 285–288
'A 70th Birthday Present', 7:**243**
sexual assault of child, in Burton, Lindy, *Vulnerable Children: Three Studies of Children in Conflict* (reviewed 1968), 8:**275–276**
sexual climax
   ability to experience achievement and, 10:320
   night terrors and, 3:105
sexual excitement and erection, 10:133, 151–152, 210
sexual intercourse. *See also* birth control
   adolescents engaging in prior to readiness for sex, 6:189–190
   breathing and, 4:11.
   capacity to be alone after, 5:243
   creativity in married life and, 9:218–220
   dream of, 4:276
   Holding and Interpretation: Fragment of an Analysis (1955), 4:286, 304, 319, 334, 361, 371
   horse dream in *The Piggle*, 11:273–274
   men who prefer to initiate girls into sexual experience, 7:323–324; 9:310
   physical illness after, 7:320, 329*n*2
   primal scene, 5:243–244
   World War II interest of child linked to, 2:83
sexuality. *See also* bisexuality; gender; homosexuality; masturbation; split-off male and female elements in men and women; sexual intercourse
   adolescence and, 5:189; 8:241
   adopted children learning about, 5:68–69
   adult sexual disorders and childhood development, 3:104, 106–107, 111
   aggression and eroticism, 3:344–347; 6:148
   anal erotism, 3:108, 110, 181
   anxiety and, 1:262, 268–269, 277–278
   in boys, 3:102–103, 109–110
   'The Child and Sex' (1947), 3:**101–111**
   contact with reality and, 3:137
   creativity and drives, 9:12
   dolls with sex organs, letter to manufacturer of, 3:183–184
   enuresis and, 1:392
   fantasy of sex, 5:267–268
   'fathers and mothers' (childhood game), 3:106, 307
   S. Freud on childhood sexuality, 3:102, 103, 397, 490; 6:156
   genital excitement, onset of, 3:110; 6:160
   in girls, 3:103–104, 107, 110, 490
   Graham, Joan (Malleson, J. Graham), *Any Wife, Any Husband* (foreword by DDW; 1955), 5:**99**
   home life and, 5:28–29, 30
   illegitimacy and, 5:74–75
   infantile sexuality, 5:326, 428; 11:80–81
   Juliet's falling over in presence of nurse's husband in *Romeo and Juliet*, 3:187, 189, 193
   male genitalia, value placed on, 3:109–111
   masculine side of a female patient, 8:241–242
   maternal knowledge and handling of, 3:395
   menstruation anxieties, 1:453
   oral erotism, 3:214, 334
   parents, sexual relationship of, 5:266–268
   play and, 3:104–106
   precocity, sexual, 1:119

sexuality (*Cont.*)
    pregenital, 6:145, 160, 411
    psychosomatic disorders and, 3:108
    setting of patterns and trends by age 5, 5:28
    'Sex Education in Schools' (1949), 3:**323–326**
    sexual development, 6:121
    transitional objects, auto-erotism, and allo-erotism, 3:448, 455, 456, 459, 461
    urinary erotism, 3:110
Sexual Offences Act 1967, 5:27
sexual perverts
    assault by, 7:171–174, 276
    rehabilitation of, 4:136
Shakespeare, William
    Coriolanus, 8:397, 401
    DWW reading while recuperating in NYC, 8:401, 403, 407
    feuds, external and internal, 3:185–187
    Hamlet, 3:174, 426; 6:361; 7:28, 328; 9:315–316
    'The Infancy of Juliet' (1949), 3:174*n*i, **185–193**
    inner world of, 3:173
    Macbeth, 5:139–140
    Measure for Measure, 7:81
    plays of, 8:397*n*i, 401
    psychoanalytical knowledge of, 4:54
    Romeo and Juliet, 3:174, 185–193
    on seven ages of man, 1:397
    sonnet form used by, 9:172
    The Winter's Tale, 7:79, 80
Sharpe, Ella Freeman, 1:11, 12; 5:392
    letter to (1946), 3:**41**
    'Planning for Stability', in *On the bringing up of children* (1936), 1:437
Shaw, Bernard, 8:149
Sheldon, W., 1:223*n*1
Shelley, Percy Bysshe, 3:492
shell shock, 1:53; 3:113, 327*n*i; 5:391–392
Shenley Psychiatric Hospital, St Albans, 3:351; 9:53, 55
Shepherd, Ray, 1: liii
    editorial note to *Human Nature*, 11:3
    preface to *The Piggle*, 11:**187–188**
shock therapy, 2:18; 3:59, 70–71, 72–75; 4:210; 6:465, 12:12. *See also* leucotomy
    introduction into Nigeria, 7:215
    'Introduction to a Symposium on the Psycho-Analytic Contribution to the Theory of Shock Therapy' (1944), 2:**261–264**
    'Kinds of Psychological Effect of Shock Therapy' (1944), 2:207*n*i, 261, **265–269**
    'Physical Therapy in Mental Disorder' (letter to the *British Medical Journal*; 1945), 2:**379–380**
    'Shock Therapy' (letter to the *British Medical Journal*; 1944), 2:**251–253**
    'Shock Treatment of Mental Disorder (letter to the *British Medical Journal*; 1943), 2:207*n*i, **229–230**
    Wilson, Cyril: 'An Individual Point of View on Shock Therapy' (1943), 2:261
shopping, compulsive, 5:156
'Short Communication on Enuresis' (1930), 1:**143–147**
short oesophagus, 11:49
'A Shropshire Surgeon' (poem; 1920), 1:**57**
'Shyness and Nervous Disorders in Children' (1938), 1:17, **445–448**
sibling rivalry
    adolescents, psychotherapeutic interviews with, 7:52–65
    breastfeeding of new infant and, 8:109
    'Jealousy' (BBC talk; 1960), 6:**47–61**
    jealousy of younger sibling, 2:84, 158; 6:13, 47–61; 8:297–298; 10:142, 153
    regression and birth memories as means of dealing with, 7:45–46
    therapeutic consultation, 10:240–241, 251–252, 275, 344, 362, 406–407, 415
siblings. *See also* only child
    adopted children and, 5:111–112, 514
    anxiety at birth of, 1:255–256, 354; 4:253
    attention of older sibling transferred to younger sibling, 7:272
    birth of male sibling and girl's desire to be a boy, 9:231
    'A Clinical Example of Symptomatology Following the Birth of a Sibling' (ca. 1931), 1:**155–158**, 343*n*1
    deaths of, 1:394–395, 445–446
    differences between, 3:313
    of Gabrielle, in *The Piggle*, 11:197, 199–200, 203, 204, 205, 213, 214, 222, 223, 238, 242, 245, 256–258, 259, 263–265, 267, 268, 272, 279–281, 284, 285, 292, 295, 297–298, 301, 303–304
    guilt over death of, 5:138
    holding younger siblings, 3:388–389
    home management of case of psychosis and, 5:90–91, 92, 93, 95–96
    lack of, 4:255–256
    letting each new infant have 'only child' experience, 7:17, 93
    loyalty conflicts and, 7:394–395
    maternal role taken on by, 3:398
    of mother, in *The Piggle*, 11:198*n*2, 294
    quarrelling between, effect on parents, 6:82
    rivalry. *See* jealousy; sibling rivalry
    significance in child's emotional development, 9:133
    sisters, relationship with, in *Holding and Interpretation*, 4:336, 426, 437–438, 463

transitional objects, different uses of, 3:451–455
traumatic reaction to birth of, 7:178–182, 180–182
younger child persecuted by adopted child, 9:243
youngest child's fantasy of killing off other children, 9:108
sight. *See* blindness; eyes
Silcock, Dr, 1:461
silence during sessions, 8:46, 253–254, 369. *See also* psychoanalysis
'Two Notes on the Use of Silence' (1963), 6:**513–517**
silent hidden illness, 10:522
'The Silent Kill' (poem; 1969), 9:102, 108
Simey, T. S., *The Concept of Love in Child Care* (review, 1961), 6:**213–215**
Simmel, *Zur Psychoanalyse der Kriegsneurosen* (1919), 5:398*n*8
skin. *See also* popular urticaria; *other specific skin conditions*
 emotional development and skin erotism, 1:392; 11:68
 involvement in feelings and mental states, 1:454–459; 8:152
 lip-sucking, compulsive, 1:450
 phobias and skin conditions, 1:458–459, 461
 psyche-soma relationship and, 1:449–454; 9:95; 11:139–140
 self-roasting (in front of a fire), 1:450
 'Skin Changes in Relation to Emotional Disorder' (1938), 1:14, **449–462**
slavery, 2:90
Slavson, S. R., *Child Psychotherapy* (1953; reviewed 1954), 4:**233–234**
sleep,
 anxiety and, 4:43, 165
 child in same bed with parents, 2:83; 10:338–339, 344–345
 dissociation and, 4:177–178
 infant and, 4:23, 160, 162, 165, 190
 Illingworth, R. S., 'Sleep Disturbances in Young Children' (1951), 3:461
 narcolepsy, 1:150
 'Pathological Sleeping' (1930), 1:13, **149–150**
 pyknolepsy, 1:308
 REM and NREM sleep, 8:172
 Scott, C., and, 4:177–178
 sleepiness or sleeping during analysis, in *Holding and Interpretation*, 4:323, 332–333, 344, 345–346, 349, 389, 396, 407, 422, 423, 426–427, 428, 430, 432–433, 435, 444, 446, 450, 451–452, 455, 467, 468; 5:470
 sleeplessness, 2:85; 8:323, 366
 'Sleep Refusal in Children' (1968), 8:**323–325**

therapeutic consultation and, 10:371, 377, 406, 411, 412
true and false self and, 7:29
unconsciousness of a fit and, 4:177
Slesinger, Bernard, 7:380
Slovenko, Ralph, 7:248*n*i
smallpox
 popular urticaria mistaken for, 1:345
 vaccination against, 1:86; 2:218
smiling, 5:116–117
Smirnoff, Victor, letter to (1958), 5:**385–388**
'Smith' (1913), 1:**31–33**
smoking
 by patient, 4:418–419, 420; 8:370
 by prisoners, 6:274–276
smouldering rheumatism, 1:196, 220–223, 226
'The Snag' (1921), 1:**65–66**
snake, symbolism of, 10:35, 68, 120
social anthropology and study of infancy, 9:43–45
'Social Aspects of Autism' (1966), 7:**345–347**
social health, 8:65, 69–70
socialization, 6:470, 491
social sense, development of, 6:345
Social Services Act (1971), 8:49
social structure, 2:88
social unrest and memory of dependence, 3:339*n*iii
social work
 'Behaviour Therapy' (letter to *Child Care News*; 1969), 9:**63–65**
 'Child Psychiatry, Social Work, and Alternative Care' (1970), 9:**171–174**
 Family Welfare Association social work, 8:58–59
 as field of study for Association for Child Psychology and Psychiatry, 8:56–57
 hospital social workers, 8:58
 professional, 6:201; 7:37. *See also* psychiatric social workers
Société Psychoanalytique de Paris, 6:45
society
 'The Mother's Contribution to Society' (1957), 5:13, **293–296**
 responsibility in child development, 4:254–255
 unconscious reactions to insanity in, 3:75
Society for Autistic Children (now National Autistic Society), 7:345, 349, 361–362, 363
Society for Psychosomatic Research, 5:9; 6:117; 7:67; 9:95
Society of Analytical Psychology, 9:169
sociology of knowledge, 9:391–394
Soddy, Kenneth, 7:365–366
 Clinical Child Psychiatry (1960; reviewed 1961), 6:**223**
 letter to (1959), 5:**465**

Solnit, Albert, 8:8
Solomon, Joseph C., 'Fixed Idea as an Internalized Transitional Object' (1962), 9:263
soma. *See* psyche-soma
'Some Principles of Child Analysis' (1969), 9:**51**
'Some Psychological Aspects of Juvenile Delinquency' (1946), 3:**43–48**, 322*n*1
'Some Thoughts on the Meaning of the Word Democracy' (1950), 3:195*n*i, 197, 199, 405*n*1, **407–421**; 7:126*n*i; 8:143*n*i; 11:86*n*4
Soper, Philip, 8:388*n*iii
the soul, 9:28; 11:76–77
  breath and, 2:366; 11:183
  as inner world, 3:263, 324
  relation to body/soma, 3:322, 279; 6:257; 8:270
spanking. *See* corporal punishment
Sparks, Richard F., 7:369
spastic diplegia, 6:391*n*i
spasticity, 1:91–92, 190–191, 292, 304
spatula game, 1: lxiii, 5, 8, 138, 188, 190, 273, 310, 425–431; 2:10–11, 16, 122–126, 132–138; 3:285–288, 304; 8:309–310
Spearman, Charles, 10:5
The Spectator, 8:124
  letter to (1954), 4:**181–182**
speech and speaking. *See also* communication; deafness
  anxiety and, 1:331, 334, 335
  hysterical mutism, 1:270, 334
  incessant talking, 1:334
  lateness in, 1:329–330, 331, 335
  'Speech Disorders', from *Clinical Notes* (1931), 1:**329–336**
  Stein, Leopold, *The Infancy of Speech and the Speech of Infancy* (1949; reviewed 1950), 3:**363–364**
  stuttering, 1:332–334, 335; 2:149–150. *See also* '"Bob" aet 6 Years'
  value of speech to the child, 1:330–331
Spence, James, 3:130, 139*n*1; 5:5
  Paediatrics and Psychiatry (1948), 11:129
Spence, Marjorie
  letter to (November 23, 1967), 8:**199–200**
  letter to (November 27, 1967), 8:**201–202**
Spillius, Elizabeth Bott, 6:235*n*i
spina bifida, 9:235–243
spinal cord, birth injuries to, 1:295
spiritualism, 2:163*n*4
Spitz, René A., 3:157–158, 473–474, 492; 4:37, 188; 5:5, 255*n*i, 255–256; 6:283; 8:300
  'Autoerotism' (1949), 3:461
  'Hospitalism' (1945), 11:101*n*1
  'Relevancy of direct infant observation' (1950), 3:461
split-off male and female elements in men and women

age constancy of other-sex part, 9:310
'Answers to comments on "The split-off male and female elements"' (1972), 9:14, 15, **149–154**
appropriate terminology for, 7:329*n*3
being and doing, 9:13–15, 150–151, 153, 314–316
bisexuality and, 7:317, 321, 323, 371; 9:308–309, 310–311
breast and identity, 9:313–314
clinical example, 7:318–323
clinical observations, 9:305–308
contrasting male and female elements, 7:327–328
creativity and, 9:13–15, 305–317
dissociation in, 7:321, 322, 328; 9:308–309
environmental factors, 7:326–327
in genital phase of development, 11:69–72
good-enough mothering and, 7:326
homosexuality and, 7:318, 323; 9:151, 310–311
impotence and, 7:323
issues in treating, 9:309–311
Jungian anima/animus and, 9:14, 169
mother-child relationship and, 7:194–195
object-relating and, 7:324–326; 9:311–313
projective identification difficulties and, 9:330, 331–332, 334
'The Split-off Male and Female Elements to Be Found in Men and Women' (1966/1971), 6:519; 7:8–9, **319–332**; 9:13–14, 15, 169, 169*n*ii, 317*n*7, 355
stealing and, 7:329; 9:317
as theoretical approach, 9:152–154
transference/countertransference and, 9:152
unified personality with capacity to identify with opposite sex versus, 7:371–372
in women versus men, 9:311, 317*n*11, 330
split/splitting. *See also* personality split; schizophrenia
  as defence, 4:154, 206
  defined, 4:109–110, 11:154
  of the ego, 4:131, 134
  in environmental-individual set-up, 4:41–43
  failure in initial contact with reality and, 11:125–126
  loss of capacity for concern leading to, 6:355
  mechanisms, 5:252
  of object, 6:388*n*1
  as reverse of integration, 6:415
Spock, Benjamin, 7:83, 335
  Baby and Child Care (1955), 4:117; 7:17, 113
  letter to (1962), 6:**289–293**
spoiling, 5:74; 10:304
'Spoken Comments on Obsessional Neurosis and Frankie' (1965), 7:**197–201**
spontaneity, in first year of life, 5:327–328
spoon game, 3:285–288, 304. *See also* spatula game

sports, DWW's enjoyment of, 1: lviii, 37, 51
spurious pregnancy, 1:193–194
squiggle game
    Ada case not using, 10:308
    Albert playing with DWW, 10:233, 233–251, 235–240, 242–251
    Alfred playing with DWW, 10:165–181, 166–179, 181
    Ashton playing with DWW, 10:214–228, 215–225, 227–228
    birth control and, 9:104–105
    Bob playing with DWW, 10:114–136, 115–131, 133–136, 140
    Cecil playing with DWW, 10:347–359, 347–360, 363–364
    Charles playing with DWW, 10:192–209, 192–211, 211
    child using his/her own squiggle, 10:181
    DWW's first reference to, 10:29nii
    DWW's use of, 10:11–13, 29
    ego support and, 10:42
    Eliza playing with DWW, 10:84–108, 84–109
    found objects and waifs in, 9:373
    Hesta playing with DWW, 10:254–264, 254–272, 269–272
    Iiro playing with DWW, 10:37–53, 38–53
    'Interrelating Apart from Instinctual Drive and in Terms of Cross-identifications' (1971), 9:321–323
    Jason playing with DWW, 10:455–465, 455–469, 479–488, 479–492
    Mark playing with DWW, 10:372–378, 372–379, 380–387, 381–387, 388–398, 388–398
    Milton playing with DWW, 10:277–287, 278–287
    mother's madness as ego-alien factor and, 9:141–145; 9:142–144; 9:146
    in paediatric consultations, 1:8
    Patrick playing with DWW, 7:281–288
    Peter playing with DWW, 10:406, 407
    physical deformity or difference, children with, 9:226, 230, 237–238, 280
    in *Psychoanalytic Explorations*, 10:3
    purpose of, 10:29
    Robert playing with DWW, 10:144–152, 144–153
    Robin playing with DWW, 10:58–67, 58–81, 69–81
    Ruth playing with DWW, 10:421–439, 422–437, 530–531
    Sakari playing with DWW (1961), 6:241–257
    'The Squiggle Game' (1968), 8:18n5, 100, 207, 319, 320, **415–440**; 10:3, 29nii
    in 'String', 6:136
    in *Therapeutic Consultations*, 8:8
    transitional object pathology and, 9:280
    uncertainty, capacity to tolerate, 10:16
St. *See entries at* Saint

stability of external objects, DWW's theory of, 2:197
stage of concern
    aggression and, 3:5, 3:335–336
    in child development, 3:402–403; 4:187; 6:17
    'The Development of the Capacity for Concern' (1962), 6:16–17, **351–356**
    guilt versus, 6:351
    Klein's concept of depressive position and, 6:16
    pre-concern, 2:366
    primitive behaviour and, 2:15
    scope of concept of, 4:14, 16; 6:351–352
stammer. *See* '"Alfred" aet 10 Years'; stuttering
standard analysis, 11:8–9
Standing Conference of Organisations of Social Workers, 9:179nii
Standing Conference of Societies Registered for Adoption, 5:67
Standley, D. W., 5:119
Stanislavski, Konstantin, 5:364
Stapleton, Thomas, 5:437–438, 475–476
    letter to (1954), 4:**267–268**
    letter to (1955), 5:**25**
    letter from (1954), 4:267–268nii
State medicine. *See* National Health Service
State services for children, 2:288
statistics, use of, 4:111–112; 6:220–221
stealing
    adolescents, psychotherapeutic interviews with, 7:57–58
    as antisocial behaviour, 3:46, 52–53, 55, 79, 239, 241–242; 5:153–154; 8:93, 95, 97; 10:17, 303, 305, 346, 360–363, 366n1, 370, 393, 399–401, 403–404, 406, 407, 412, 419, 421, 436, 438, 445, 446, 452, 454, 478, 486, 530, 532
    as belief in something good, 3:52, 55; 8:17n2
    Child Department consultations regarding, 2:150, 154
    child's lack of understanding of, 3:239, 242, 319–320
    delinquency and, 2:73–74
    dissociation and, 7:245, 251–273. *See also* dissociation
    guilt sense, loss and recovery of, 5:146–147
    'The Impulse to Steal' (1949), 3:**319–322**
    'The Management of a Case of Compulsive Thieving', 4:97ni
    masturbation and, 7:257, 260, 265; 10:313
    'Meet to Be Stolen From' (ca. 1939–1945), 2:16–17, **141–142**
    motivations for, 2:198–199; 8:93
    psychological significance of, 3:46, 242, 314–315, 320, 336nii, 371, 451; 5:104, 150–151, 153–154; 10:17–18, 304
    residential therapy and recovery of child, 9:205
    sexual desire and, 3:107

stealing (*Cont.*)
  shopping, compulsive, 5:156
  split-off male and female elements in men and women and, 7:329; 9:317
  'Stealing and Telling Lies' (1949), 3:**313–317**
  transitional object, exaggerated addiction to, 9:112
  trauma after birth of sibling leading to, 7:181
Steele, G. D. F., 3:467
Stein, Leopold, *The Infancy of Speech and the Speech of Infancy* (1949; reviewed 1950), 3:**363–364**
Steiner, J., 2:9, 14
  The Freud-Klein Controversies 1941–45 (1991), 5:7
Steiner, Riccardo (ed.), *The Freud-Klein Controversies, 1941–45*, 7:377*n*i, 380
Stengel, Professor, 7:407
Stephen, Leslie, 7:409
stepparents
  'For Stepparents' (1955), 5:**55–59**
  nastiness of some stepchildren, 5:58–59
  Thomson, Helen, *The Successful Step-Parent* (1966; reviewed 1967), 8:**89–90**
  unsuccess story, value of, 5:57–59
  'Unsuccess Story: Myself as Step-Mother, by a Listener in Despair' (*Woman's Hour* radio broadcast; 1955), 5:55
  the wicked stepmother, 5:55–57
Sterba, Dr, 9:151
Sterling, W., 1:81, 88
Stevenson, Olive, 5:77, 77*n*2, 412; 6:64; 9:262
  The First Treasured Possession (preface; 1954), 4:**297–299**
Stewart, Alice, 5:468
  'Maternal Care and the Welfare State' (1959), 5:467*n*i
Stewart, Ann, 4:118
Stewart, C. M., 3:113
Stewart, Sheila, *A Home from Home* (1967; reviewed 1967), 8:**105–106**
Stierlin, Helm
  Conflict and Reconciliation, 9:91
  letter to (1969), 9:**91–92**
Still, G. F., 2:49, 57; 7:380
  Common Disorders and Diseases of Childhood (1927), 1:237, 238*nn*3–4
Still, Robert, 8:263*n*i
Stiner, O., 1:86, 87, 88
Stoddart, W. H. B., 5:392
Stokes, Adrian
  'Form in Art' (1955), 5:33*n*i
  Imago group and, 8:263*n*i
  Smooth and Rough (1951), 4:61, 61*n*iii; 5:33
Stolkind, E., 1:96, 142
Stone, G. K., *The Principles of Clinical Pathology in practice* (with G. Bourne; 1929), 1:197*n*1

Stone, L. Joseph, letter to (1968), 8:**319–320**, 413; 10:29*n*ii
Stone, Marjorie, letter to (1949), 3:**183–184**
Storr, Charles Anthony
  Human Aggression (reviewed 1968), 8:**321–322**, 329, 329*n*i
  letter to (1965), 7:**215**
story-telling
  adoption, telling children about, 5:21–22
  the wicked stepmother, 5:55–57
Strachey, Alix, 1:11; 5:392; 7:407, 408; 8:124–127
Strachey, James, 1: lviii, 10, 11–12, 13; 4:53; 5:251, 392; 6:326, 327; 7:407, 408, 409, 410, 429; 8:40, 124–126, 125; 9:60, 356; 10:7, 9; 11:189
  Letters of James and Alix Strachey (Meisel & Kendrick, eds. 1986), 8:124*n*i
  letter to (1951), 3:**435–436**
  obituary (1969), 8:**123–127**; 10:9
  Standard Edition of the Complete Psychological Works of Sigmund Freud (Strachey, ed. 1966), 1: lxxviii; 8:123, 126
Strachey, Lytton, 7:409; 8:126–127
Strachey, St Loe, 8:124
'Strength Out of Misery' (1964), 6:461
streptococcal infection, 1:120, 220–221, 288
stress
  as environmental issue, 9:126–127
  as internal process, 9:124–126
  parental dealing with, 9:124–127
'String: A Technique of Communication' (1960), 3:447; 5:519*n*i, 522*n*i; 6:**135–139**, 318*n*i; 9:265, 279–284, 288*n*3
'Struggling Through the Doldrums' (1963), 6:**423–432**, 493; 7:51*n*i, 399*n*ii; 9:101*n*i.
  See also 'Adolescence: Struggling Through the Doldrums' (1961)
'A Study on Envy and Gratitude' (1956), 5:**131–132**; 9:47
Stungo, E., 3:35, 36
stuttering, 1:332–334, 335; 2:149–150
subacute rheumatic fever, 1:205, 226, 230; 2:54–62, 63*n*1
subjective object
  creative illusion and, 9:7–11
  methodological approach of DWW to child development and, 3:6–7; 8:349; 10:8, 10, 18
  mother-infant mutuality and, 9:132–134
  prefiguring in comparison of thumb-sucking and infant gaze, 2:317*n*iii
  psychoanalyst as, 10:30, 140, 299
  survival of, 9:10
sublimation, 9:12
Suez Emergency (1956), 5:6
suffering
  meaning of, 4:12
  psychotherapy and, 6:449

relief from, 4:182, 208
suicide
    adolescents and, 6:195, 431, 494; 8:68; 9:344, 346
    analyst affected by, 8:405; 9:27, 177
    anorexia representing suicidal impulse, 7:455
    'Berlin Wall' within self and, 9:117
    child psychosis and, 3:353
    destruction and, 9:373
    erotic asphyxiation versus, 3:215
    failure of psychoanalysis resulting in, 4:61, 73
    hysteria and, 7:403, 404
    inner world, child's management of, 3:338
    loss of creativity and, 9:302
    as murder, 3:333
    precipitating factors of, 9:290–291
    right to commit, 3:468
    shock therapy for relief from suicidal thoughts, 2:268
    suicidal dreams, 6:334
    suicidal wishes, 2:213–214; 8:222
    true self and, 6:10
    violence and, 9:55
sulking, 6:466
Sullivan, Arthur, 7:77niv
Sullivan, Ellie Ragland, 6:46ni
sulphanilamide, 2:255–256
'*Sum, I Am*' (1968), 8:14, **267–274**
summer diarrhoea, 9:99–100
superego
    in child development, 2:387
    'Comments on Joseph Sandler's "On the Concept of the Superego"' (1960), 6:14–15, **127–133**
    guilt and, 5:136, 138–139
    in *The Piggle*, 11:252nX, 253n4, 305
    restatement of Freud's instinct theory and, 11:79–80
    sadistic superego, 6:128
'Support for Normal Parents' (radio broadcast 1943–44), 2:21niii, 12:9 (1945), 2:**287–289**
surveys, DWW refusing to participate in, 6:111–112, 421–422. *See also* questionnaires
Susan (young girl who lived with Winnicotts), 2:19
suspended animation, in manic defence, 1:363–364
suspicious attitude, 2:189–190
Sussex Postgraduate Federation, The Geigy Bequest Lecture (1968), 8:221
Sutherland, G. A., 1:96, 100, 139, 167, 185n1; 5:361ni
Sutherland, John, 6:235ni
Sutherland, Miriam, 3:161
Suttee, 8:35, 41
Swallow, Nigel, 5:77
sweating and skin diseases, 1:461–462

'symbiosis', concept of, 8:44
symbiotic relationship, infant's determination to outgrow, 6:292
symbolism
    of atom bomb, 7:152
    Blessed Sacrament, for Catholics versus Protestants, 9:270
    Bowlby's 'On 'Separation Anxiety'' and, 5:499
    child's acceptance of, 7:132
    of deprivation, 7:269–270, 270
    fertility symbols, 7:269–272, 270
    Lacan on, 6:45
    in manic defence, 1:365–366
    professional attitude compared to, 5:508
    satisfaction in play and, 9:375, 376
    symbol formation, 6:63; 8:299, 447–450
    symbolic realisation, concept of, 5:523–524; 6:164, 169, 231, 348–349
    'Thinking and Symbol-Formation' (1968), 1: lxxi; 8:6, **441–444**
    transitional objects and, 3:456; 4:164; 5:410; 9:270, 286
sympathy
    for being ill, 1:334, 348
    mother's, for child's illness, 1:400
    in practicing medicine, 1:70–71, 217
    in practicing psychoanalysis, 1:53
'Symptoms Suggesting Post-Encephalitis' (1929), 1:**131–132**
'Symptom Tolerance in Paediatrics' (1953), 4:**77–95**; 8:320; 10:29nii
syndactele/syndactyly, 9:226–227, 233; 10:37, 41, 515
syphilis
    aortic regurgitation and, 1:214
    circumcision and, 2:26
    congenital, 1:92, 173, 293, 296
    gonorrhoea versus, 1:4
    epiphysitis and, 1:296
    hemiplegia, syphilitic, 1:92
    neuro-syphilis, 1:293
    prophylactic treatment of newborns for, 1:68
    syphilophobia, 1:461
systolic murmur, 1:214, 231–232
systolic thrills, 1:209
Szasz, Thomas
    letter to (1959), 5:**503**
    questionnaire from, 5:503ni

Mrs T., letter to (1968), 8:**327–328**
taboos
    adolescence and, 5:189, 190, 191, 192
    adopted children and taboo on sex experience in the home, 5:70
tachycardia, 1:271
Tagore, Rabindranath, 'On the Seashore', 7:429
Tahta, Dikran, 8:267, 267ni

'Tailpiece to *Playing and Reality*' (1971), 9:**349**
'Taking Children's Temperatures' (letter to the *British Medical Journal*; 1949), 3:**181–182**
Talking to parents (Winnicott, C., Bollas, C., Davis, M., & Shepherd, R., eds.), 6:31
tantrums, 2:284, 286
   in normal children, 3:396
   in sensitive children, 5:91
T.A.T. (Thematic Apperception Test), 8:415
Tavistock Clinic, 1:17; 3:327, 438; 5:162–163, 263, 307, 401; 6:299, 306; 12:4
Tavistock Publications, 4:225; 5:479–480; 8:144*n*ii
Tavistock Research Seminar, 7:417
Taylor, Alice. *See also* Winnicott, Alice, 3:195*n*ii, 197*n*i, 383–384; 8:399*n*ii
Taylor, J. M., 1:364
Taylor, Pauline, 8:399
TB. *See* tuberculosis
'The Teacher, the Parent and the Doctor' (1936), 1:17, **375–387**. *See also* school and teaching
teachers. *See* nursery schools; schools and teaching
   and depressive position, 11:85
   resistance to concept of Oedipal complex, 11:60–61
team approach to psycho-therapy, 2:180–181
teamwork and casework, 5:490–491; 6:19–20
teasing, 10:475
teething, 2:85–86
telepathy, 1:35
television
   'The Child, the Family and the Young Offender' (UK Government Home Office White Paper), 7:203
   DWW on talking to mothers on, 7:84
   sponsored television (letter to *The Times*, 1954), 4:**259**
temper, in *Holding and Interpretation*, 4:423. *See also* anger
temperature
   factors regulating, 1:195–201
   'Taking Children's Temperatures' (letter to the *British Medical Journal*; 1949), 3:**181–182**
temper tantrums. *See* tantrums
Temple, William, 6:214
'A Tendency in Therapeutics' (1944), 2:207*n*i, **255–259**
Tensing Norgay, 7:262
terrors, child experiencing, 2:160. *See also* night terrors
theft. *See* stealing
'Their Standards and Yours'
   paper (1945), 2:**277–280**
   radio broadcast (1944), 2:21*n*iii, 277

Thematic Apperception Test (T.A.T.), 8:415
'Theoretical Statement of the Field of Child Psychiatry' (1958), 5:**421–429**
theory of mind, 3:247–250
'The Theory of the Parent-Infant Relationship' (1960), 6:3–9, 115, **141–158**, 359, 363; 8:184*n*i, 218*n*1, 232*n*ii; 9:301, 304; 10:518
'The Theory of the Parent-Infant Relationship: Contributions to Discussion', 6:**363–365**, 369
'The Theory of the Parent-Infant Relationship: Further Remarks', 6:359, **359–361**
therapeutic consultations
   adolescents, psychotherapeutic interviews with, 7:52–65
   antisocial behaviour, 10:303–515. *See also* antisocial behaviour
   'A Child Psychiatry Case Illustrating Delayed Reaction to Loss' (1965), 7:**281–306**
   contact with child as critical element, 10:519–520
   dissociation in case of compulsive stealing, 7:251–273
   'Dissociation Revealed in a Therapeutic Consultation' (1966), 7:12, **245–273**; 10:307
   'The Exploitation of the First Interview with a Child: A Study of the Dangers and the Potential Value of Such Procedure' (lecture; 1968), 8:349
   first interview, importance of, 6:439; 8:349–354, 413; 10:8, 9, 11, 29, 519, 522–523
   'First Interview with Child May Start Resumption of Maturation' (1968) (report quoting DWW), 8:**349–354**
   focus of DWW on, 7:10–13; 10:7–11
   interpretation facilitating therapy, 10:9, 299
   'Interrelating Apart from Instinctual Drive and in Terms of Cross-identifications' (1971), 9:320–328
   patient, not therapist, as responsible for structuring consultation, 10:449*n*1
   psychoanalysis distinguished, 7:273–274, 277; 8:413; 10: 298, 518
   results from, 10:32–33, 521
   techniques for, 7:252, 275–277; 8:349, 353–354. *See also* squiggle game
   Therapeutic Consultations in Child Psychiatry (1971), 1: lxi, 8; 6:237, 241; 7:149, 251*n*ii; 8:8, 311, 349, 417*n*iv; 9:139*n*5, 336*n*2; 10:3, 4, 8, 13–14, 19, 37, 57, 83, 113, 141, 157, 165, 233, 253, 275, 307, 335, 369, 403, 419, 441, 451, 453, 495
   trauma and the family, 7:169–170, 177–179, 183–184

'The Value of the Therapeutic Consultation' (1968), 7:11, 13, **273–278**
therapists
    analogy of analyst-patient to mother-infant relationship, 8:12, 15
    caseload of child psychiatrist versus psychoanalyst, 10:369
    communication between analyst and patient, 5:81. *See also* communication
    description of work of, 8:6
    despair suffered by, 6:72
    differences among, 6:288
    envy of, by patient, 6:316
    father-substitute, psychoanalyst as, 4:284, 303, 366, 405
    goals for, 6:285–288
    good analyst, destruction of, 6:269, 317
    good-enough analyst, 6:322–323, 335; 8:6; 10:8
    interaction with psychoanalyst producing fantasies, 3:121–122
    limitation on power of, 6:153
    mental health of, 1: lxv; 6:19;
    mother-substitute, psychoanalyst as, 4:414, 427, 456, 473
    multidisciplinary teams, benefits of, 6:19–20
    need for training of child analysts, 2:162–163
    professional standards of, 4:98–99; 5:505–511; 6:203
    'The Psycho-analyst and Child Psychiatry: A Matter of Economics' (1962), 6:**357–358**
    punctuality of psychoanalyst, 4:211; 6:19, 203
    reliability of, 6:142; 8:316–317
    retaliation on, 8:360
    sick parents as, for their own children, 5:520–522
    split between teacher and analyst, 6:269–270
    as subjective object, 10:30, 140, 299
    survival of, 8:409–410
    training of, 4:119–120, 228; 5:7–8; 6:177–178, 197; 8:335–336; 10:27, 369, 521–522
    transference and. *See* transference
    trust of patient in, 8:255, 350, 356, 413. *See also* trust
Thiel, J. H., 7:407
thinking
    cataloguing, 7:141–142
    creativity and, 7:142, 144
    fantasy versus, 7:143
    as mother-substitute, 7:142–144
    'New Light on Children's Thinking' (1965), 7:7, **139–144**
    'Thinking and Symbol-Formation' (1968), 1: lxxi; 8:6, **449–452**

'Thinking and the Unconscious' (1945), 2:**341–342**
uses of word, 7:139–140
'This Feminism' (1986), 5:294*n*i; 7:5, **103–111**, 126*n*i
Thomas, A., S. Chess, S., and H. G. Birch, *Your Child Is a Person* (1960; reviewed by DWW 1966), 7:**415**
Thomas, Dr, 1:123
Thomas, Ruth, 5:261
Thomas, William, 'Primitive behaviour' (1937), 1:441
Thompson (nominee for BPAS Scientific Secretary), 5:347
Thompson, Clara, 8:320*n*ii
Thomson, Helen, *The Successful Step-Parent* (1966; reviewed 1967), 8:**89–90**
Thomson, John, 1:253*n*1
    The clinical study and treatment of sick children (1925), 1:237, 238*n*2
Thorner, Hans
    'Cause and Reason: A Psychoanalytic Contribution to the Understanding of Psychosomatic Phenomena' (1966), 7:341, 343–344
    letter to (1966), 7:**341**, 343*n*i
thrashings. *See* corporal punishment
threadworms, 1:171, 319
'The Threat to Freedom' (1969), 9:**83–87**
thrill
    pre-systolic, 1:209, 232
    systolic, 1:209, 217
throat. *See* nose and throat
Through Paediatrics to Psycho-Analysis (1975), 9:265; 11:190
Thucydides, 1:39
thumb-sucking
    age of child and, 5:251
    fantasy and, 4:275
    interpretation of, 4:307, 337
    personal pattern, development of, 9:268
    as primitive retaliation, 2:367–368
    representing breast or bottle, 2:317, 318
    therapeutic consultation and, 10:337, 339–344, 354, 361, 366
    as transitional object, 3:452, 454; 4:162, 165–166, 298; 5:101–102; 6:290; 10:337
tics or habit-spasms, 1:136, 246–247, 250
time, in therapy sessions
    first interview, importance of, 6:439; 8:349–354, 413; 10:8, 9, 11, 29, 519, 522–523
    'Notes on the Time Factor in Treatment' (1961), 6:**225–227**; 8:269*n*iv
    patient's awareness of, 2:361; 4:211, 306
    punctuality of patient, 4:306, 324, 334, 415–416; 6:19, 203

The Times, 1:398
  'I Qant Stand It' (letter; 1957), 5:**219**
  letter of Archbishop of Canterbury Lord Fisher
    to (1966), 7:449
  letters of DWW to (1954), 4:**259**, **279–280**
  letters of DWW to (1966), 7:**315**, **339**,
    365–366, 369
  letter of Robert Graves to (1966), 7:315–316*n*i
  'Maladjusted Children: Damaging Effect of
    Delay' (letter; 1950), 3:**361–362**
  on nationalisation of medical profession
    (DWW letter; 1946), 3:**39**; 5:8, 10
  on nationalisation of medical profession (J.
    R. Sandy letter; 1948), 3:141
  'Neglected Children' (letter; 1950), 3:**349–350**
  'Nursery Schools: A Definition of Functions'
    (letter; 1951), 3:**471–472**
  'Nursery Schools Essential' (letter; 1959), 5:**461**
  'Punishment and Crime: A Psychologist's View'
    (letter; 1949), 3:**237–238**, 239, 241, 359, 359*n*i
  refusal to publish letter from Bowlby and
    Durbin on evacuation of children, 2:6
timid children
  parents need to adjust to, 2:155
  WWII's effect on, 2:98
tincture of stramonium, 1:287–288
tiredness
  of mothers, 6:74
  of patient, 4:324. *See also* sleep
Tizard, David, 9:24
Tizard, J. Peter M., 1: lxix*n*iii, 19
  letter to (1956), 5:**175–178**
tobacco. *See* smoking
Tod, Robert J. N., 1:6; 3:327
  Disturbed Children (1968), DWW preface to,
    8:10, **261–262**; 9:99
  letter to (1969), 9:**99–100**
toddlers. *See* pre-school children
toilet training, 1:393; 3:282–283; 8:293–294; 10:336
tonsils, tonsillitis, and tonsillectomies
  convulsions and fits, 1:303
  heart murmur and, 1:213
  medical histories, taking, 1:174, 176
  micturition disturbances and, 1:316, 318
  'The Nose and Throat', from *Clinical Notes*
    (1931), 1:**203–205**
  pathological sleeping following, 1:149
  rheumatic fever and, 1:124, 205, 221, 240
  Robertson, Joyce, 'A Mother's Observations
    on the Tonsillectomy of Her Four-year-old
    Daughter', 5:317, 531
Topeka (Kansas) Psychoanalytic Society, 6:351
Torrie, Margaret
  Cruse Clubs founded by, 8:277
  letter to (September 4, 1967), 8:**147–148**, 277
  letter to (September 5, 1967), 8:**149–150**, 277
  The Widow's Child (foreword by DWW; 1964),
    7:**99**; 8:147, 277
total behaviour, described, 2:88, 91
total happenings, 3:287–288
totalitarianism, 2:115
'Towards an Objective Study of Human Nature'
  (1945), 2:**381–388**; 4:53*n*i; 8:10
'Towards a Theory of Psychotherapy: The Link
  with Playing' (1967), 8:12
town planning, 1:31–33, 68
toys used in diagnosing and treating children,
  1:374*n*7; 4:281
training
  of child care workers, social workers, health
    visitors, probation officers, 5:339–344
  in child psychiatry, 6:299–307; 7:419–422
  of children, 3:299
  of hostel staff, 3:89–90
  of medical professionals, 5:403
  of psychoanalysts, 4:119–120, 228; 5:7–8;
    6:177–178, 197; 10:27, 369
'Training for Child Psychiatry' (1962), 6:**299–307**
'Training for Child Psychiatry: The Paediatric
  Department of Psychology' (1996). *See* 'The
  Paediatric Department of Psychology' (1961)
Tramer, Moritz, 10:5
*Transactions of the Ophthalmological Society of the
  United Kingdom*, 2:313
transference. *See also* countertransference;
    neurosis
  in children, 7:219; 10:31
  'Clinical Varieties of Transference' (1955),
    1: lxxii; 5:*16*; 5:**61–65**; 6:467*n*2
  delusional, 6:341, 515; 7:173–174, 176, 177, 234,
    240; 8:4, 46
  dependence and, 6:145, 334
  depressive position in, 4:193
  destructiveness of, 8:331, 361, 376
  homosexual aspect of, 4:285–286
  hysteria and, 7:403–404
  infantile state of psychotic patient in, 4:71
  maternal and paternal versions of, 5:129
  negative, 3:233; 4:211; 5:65; 6:267; 7:210
  oral qualities in, 4:203, 225, 236
  in *The Piggle*, 11:310–314
  positive transference, 6:269
  primitive emotional development and, 2:358
  projections of patient, analyst's acceptance of,
    7:343–344; 8:374–375
  psychoanalytical use of, 5:353–354; 6:152, 198,
    203, 365; 8:356
  repetition of original failure situation in,
    1: lxxii–lxxiii; 6:7
  responsible agents as aspects of, 7:73

shock therapy and, 2:266–2687
split-off male and female elements in men and women and, 9:152
therapeutic consultation and, 10:517
transference neurosis, 4:304; 5:62, 64, 133*n*i, 446, 482, 506–510; 6:412; 7:179, 252, 274
use of term, 5:506
transitional objects and phenomena
abnormalities associated with, 3:450–451
addiction to, 5:250, 406, 410, 419; 9:112, 283–284
adolescents, psychotherapeutic interviews with, 7:57
adult patient, analysis of, 9:284–288
affectionate behaviour and, 5:117, 385
age of child and, 5:250–251; 9:268
aggression, correlation with DWW's conception of, 3:9–10
animals using, 5:251
application of theory, 9:278–279
auto-erotism and allo-erotism, 3:448, 455, 456, 459, 461
breastfeeding and, 9:271, 273
British monarchy and, 9:182–183, 185
characteristics of, 3:450; 5:409–410
children, obtaining information from, 9:272
clinical observations, 3:448, 451–455; 4:164–166; 5:410–412; 9:112, 270–273; 9:272; 9:279–287
'Comforters' (*British Medical Journal* letter; 1955), 5:12, 77
cultural experience and, 7:430–431, 432; 8:263
defined, 3:448; 6:320; 9:359–360
degenerate forms of, 9:360
depressive position and, 3:457–458
deprivation and, 3:378–380; 10:17
direct child observation in psychoanalysis, 5:249, 250–254; 10:155
DWW's theory of, 1: lxix–lxx; 3:448–451; 8:45–46; 9:266; 10:17
encouraging children to say 'ta' for, 5:102–103, 116
evacuated children and, 2:332*n*ii
examples, availability of, 4:167, 298–299
experiencing and, 5:388
faeces and, 9:273, 280, 287
family and, 7:3920–392
'The Fate of the Transitional Object' (1959), 5:12, **523–528**; 11:136*n*iii
feeding and, 5:116–117, 118
fetishes and, 9:273
'First Experiments in Independence' (1955), 5:12, **101–105**
first not-me possession, 4:160–161; 5:406–410; 9:266–267
in first year of life, 5:329–330
gender and, 4:163; 9:269

good-enough mother and, 9:274
hair-pulling by infant and, 8:327–328, 337
hallucination and, 5:409, 523
handkerchiefs of DWW as, 9:40
human nature and, 9:267
illusion and disillusionment, 5:413–418; 9:273–278; *9:276*
importance in DWW's thought, 5:12; 6:64; 8:47
infant development and, 3:405
inherent paradox, 8:265, 358
instinct tensions and quiet states, 3:457
introjection and projection, 3:456
Klein's birthday book, possible article for, 3:381
Klein's concept of internal object and, 4:167–168; 5:244, 413; 9:273
literature review, 3:458–461
loss of meaning over time, 9:269–270
Me and *Not-Me*, 9:265, 266
medical histories, taking, 9:272
methodological approach of DWW to child development and, 3:6–7; 4:297–298
mother as, 9:360
mother-child relationship and, 1: lxx
'The Niffle' (probably before 1961; published 1996), 9:**383–387**
pattern of, 3:448–450; 4:162
in *Peanuts* cartoon, 5:109
personal pattern, development of, 4:162–163; 5:407–409; 9:267–269
in *The Piggle*, 11:209
play and, 8:301–302
Playing and Reality (1971), introduction to, 9:**261–263**
pleasure-pain principle, 9:274
primary narcissism and, 3:10–11, 11
primitive emotional development and, 2:15, 365
psychology of stealing and, 3:451
psychopathology and, 9:279–284
reality and, 9:267, 273, 274
as resting place of illusion, 5:387
reviews by DWW and, 7:16
separation and, 9:281–283, 285–288
special qualities of infant-object relationship, 9:269–270
split-off male and female elements in men and women and, 7:326
'String' (1960/1965), 9:265, 279–284, 288*n*3
symbolism and, 3:456; 4:164; 5:410; 9:270, 286
theoretical approaches to, 3:455–458; 4:167–172; 5:413–418; 6:290–291; 9:273–278; *9:276*
theoretical first feed and, 4:38, 40*f*
therapeutic consultation and, 10:75, 210–211, 280, 337, 475–476
thumb-sucking and. *See* thumb-sucking

transitional objects and phenomena (*Cont.*)
　'Transitional Objects and Transitional Phenomena' (1951; presentation notes), 1: lxix–lxx; 3:435, **447–461**; 5:12, 405; 6:169; 7:438*n*1; 9:265
　'Transitional Objects and Transitional Phenomena' (1953 version), 4:**159–174**, 189, 297; 5:77, 81, 405; 8:11, 110*n*i; 9:261, 265; 10:156*n*1
　'Transitional Objects and Transitional Phenomena' (1958 version), 2:139*n*9; 5:385–388, **405–420**, 519*n*i; 6:157*n*14, 230, 289, 435, 467*n*1; 7:187*n*6; 9:265
　'Transitional Objects and Transitional Phenomena' (1971 version), 1: lxxii, lxxvi; 5:405; 6:312*n*i; 8:110*n*i; 9:7, 8, **265–288**
　'Transitional Objects and Transitional Phenomena' (French translation), 6:46
　typical use of, 4:165–164; 8:13–14
　value of, 11:123–126
　'What Do We Know About Babies as Cloth Suckers?' (1956), 5:12, **115–118**
　words or sounds for, 9:269
transitivity, 2:15
'The Transmission of Theory and Technique, My Own in Particular' (1968), 8:35, 335*n*i. *See also* 'D. W. W. on D. W. W.'
Tranströmer, Tomas, *The Truth Barrier* (1978), 9:10
trauma and the family
　clinical observations, 7:171–177, 178–184, 180–183
　'The Concept of Trauma in Relation to the Development of the Individual Within the Family' (1965), 7:**169–187**
　evacuation of children during WWII and, 10:18
　functioning of family and, 7:169–170, 177–178, 182–184, 186–187
　good-enough families, 7:170–171
　mother's absence as triggering event, 7:431
　nature of trauma, 7:184–186
　protection from trauma, family providing, 7:169, 179, 186–187
　Reality Principle and disillusioning process, 7:184, 185
　staging of minute traumata by patient, 7:173–174
　therapeutic consultations and, 7:169–170, 177–179, 183–184
　trauma, defined, 8:66
treatment. *See also* leucotomy; shock therapy
　antisocial behaviour, 5:157–158
　anxiety, 1:275–276
　asthma, 2:126–129
　castration, as medical treatment, 3:479

cosmetic medical treatments, 1:70
delinquent children, magistrate's role requiring knowledge of treatment methods, 2:233–236
encephalitis, 1:285–288
infections, 2:255–259, 294
medical and surgical, 1:69–70
neurosis, 5:168
'On In-Patient Treatment for Rheumatic Fever and Chorea' (ca. 1923–1931), 1:**161–163**
papular urticaria, calamine lotion as treatment for, 1:327, 344
salt in water treatment for adenoids, 1:203–204
syphilis, prophylactic treatment of newborns for, 1:68
TB, prophylactic treatment for, 1:68, 69
'Treatment of Mental Disease by Induction of Fits', 2:207*n*i, **211–216**
'The Tree' (1963), 6:20, **499–500**
triangular relationship (*see also* Oedipus Complex), 2:187; 4:251–252, 320, 323, 354, 360, 400, 453
'A Tribute on the Occasion of Willi Hoffer's Seventieth Birthday' (1967), 8:**107–113**
Trilling, Lionel, 8:223
trio of women in myths and dreams, 11:5, 74
'Trips into Partisanship', 8:**191–193**
Trotter, Wilfred, 5:389
Trowell, Judith, 1:l, lii, liv
true and false self
　aetiology of false self, 6:163–164; 8:73–74
　Bion's views on the neurotic part of the personality and, 5:86
　in borderline cases, 7:305–306
　classification of psychiatric disorders and, 5:445, 453–454, 458; 10:529
　clinical application, 6:169
　communication and, 6:440–441
　'The Concept of the False Self' (1964), 6:159; 7:**27–31**
　creative illusion and, 9:7–8
　defined, 9:359
　degrees of false self, 6:168–169
　destruction of false self, 6:416
　DWW's personal contribution on, 6:160, 361
　'Ego Distortion in Terms of True and False Self' (1960), 3:4, 14; 6:9–10, **159–171**
　example of false self, 6:161–163
　failure in initial contact with reality and, 11:125–126
　false-self defence, 6:392
　girls versus boys, and revelation of false self, 6:69
　group influences on maladjusted children and, 5:44, 50
　guilt, problem of, 7:442

history of concept, 6:159–160
in *Holding and Interpretation: Fragment of an Analysis* (1955), 4:337, 414, 418, 421
isolation of individual and, 6:149
latent neurosis/psychosis and, 4:42; 5:426
mind allowing for false self, 6:15, 163
mother's recognition of true self, 6:11, 92, 164–166
normal equivalent of false self, 6:168
potential to develop false self, 8:5, 270
primary maternal preoccupation and, 5:188; 6:13
psychoanalysis of false self, 6:169–171, 416, 486
psychotic illness designed to protect true self, 4:2140
regression and false self, 4:203, 204
shift from false to true self, 4:214–215, 224; 6:167–169
splitting and, 11:154
transference and, 5:60–61
Trüper, Johannes, 10:5
trust
  'The Building Up of Trust' (1969), 9:**121–128**
  child's development of, 6:378; 10:529
  good-enough parenting and, 9:122
  of patient in analyst, 6:203; 8:255, 350, 356, 413; 10:214
truth, as scientific aim of psychoanalysis, 2:145–146; 4:8
tuberculosis (TB)
  anxiety and, 1:257
  encephalitis and poliomyelitis, differential diagnosis of, 1:288
  intracranial, 1:119, 290
  medical histories, taking, 1:173, 176
  meningitis, tuberculous, 1:119, 192, 282–284
  peritonitis, tuberculous, 1:191
  physical examinations and, 1:191–192
  pre-tubercular children, 1:171, 266
  prophylactic treatment and, 1:68, 69
  renal, 1:318
  rheumatic fever, differential diagnosis of, 1:228, 233n2
  temperatures and medical charts, 1:201
Tuckett, David, 6:235ni
twins
  adult psychiatric issues stemming from infant treatment of, 3:133–134, 175
  Bion, 'The Imaginary Twin' (1950), 3:433ni
  birth memories of, 3:214
  identical twins, differences between, 7:439
  maternal love for one child and hatred for the other, 1:279–280n4
  transitional objects and, 3:452

'Twins' (published & radio broadcast 1945), 2:21niii, **343–347**
two, theme of, 7:207–211
'Two Adopted Children' (1954), 4:**139–149**
two-body relationship, 4:57, 252; 6:5
'Two Cases of Post-Encephalitic Hyperpnoea' (1926), 1:**95–97**
'Two Further Clinical Examples' (undated, probably 1970), 9:225, **235–245**
'Two Notes on the Use of Silence' (1963), 6:**513–517**
Tyson, Alan, 7:407, 409
Tyson, R. L., 8:16

ulcer, gastric, as psychosomatic disorder, 11:177–176
uncertainty, 2:79–80
the unconscious
  anxiety and, 1:256–259, 262, 268, 269, 270–271, 273n4, 275, 277, 279–280n4
  arthritis and, 1:243n2
  British monarchy and, 9:182, 183
  central nervous system disease and, 1:281, 286, 290n1
  Controversial Discussions on, 1: lxiv
  convulsions and fits, 1:307
  delinquent children and, 1:354–355, 433, 434, 435; 3:43–44, 54
  'Development of the Theme of the Mother's Unconscious as Discovered in Psycho-Analytic Practice' (1969), 9:**75–78**
  DWW's engagement with, 1: lxi, lviii, lix–lx, lxiii, lxxii, 6, 10
  in DWW's integration of paediatrics and psychoanalysis, 1:14, 15, 16
  eating disorders and, 1:414, 417, 422
  enuresis and, 1:141, 144, 147, 389, 390, 392, 393
  environmental and infant development, 1: lxv
  family's existence, 6:120
  fears, unconscious, 1:262
  S. Freud on importance of, 3:43, 54; 4:107
  general acceptance of psychoanalysis and concept of, 7:425–426
  heart conditions and, 1:213
  homosexuality, unconscious, 5:30
  importance for doctors of understanding force of, 1:451
  infancy and childhood, adult memory of, 3:101
  influencing, 2:109–113
  instinct theory and, 11:82–83
  Jung on, 7:120–122
  in Kanner's *Child Psychiatry*, 1:440
  'Knowing and Not Knowing' (undated; first published 1989), 9:**367–368**
  manic defence and, 1:359, 360–363, 365
  masturbation and, 1:324

the unconscious (*Cont.*)
   mental defect and, 1:300–301
   micturition disturbances and, 1:319, 321
   neurosis and, 5:165, 166
   the only child and, 1:103
   papular urticaria and, 1:344, 346, 350, 352
   parental love-hate relationship with children, 1:277, 278–279*n*4
   in pre-school children, 1:398, 400, 404, 407, 408, 409
   psychoanalysis and, 11:79, 82
   psyche-soma and, 1: lxxi
   psycho-neurosis and, 6:410
   repressed unconscious, 3:101–102, 208; 4:107; 6:410; 9:355; 11:82, 155
   school, effects on home life of, 1:444
   shyness and, 1:446, 447
   skin changes and, 1:450–459
   society's unconscious reactions to insanity, 3:75
   speech disorders and, 1:334
   teachers, parents, and doctors, interrelationship of, 1:377–382, 384–386
   'Thinking and the Unconscious' (1945), 2:**341–342**
   'The Unconscious' (1953), 4:**107–108**
   'The Unconscious' (1966), 1: lix, lx; 7:15, **425–426**
   unconscious co-operation, 6:286
   war, value of, 7:152
unconsciousness (physical), 3:210–211
the unexpected, child learning to deal with, 6:40–41
unintegration. *See also* disintegration; integration
   ACPP and use of term, 8:51
   chaos and, 11:153–154
   defences against, 4:38
   dissociation and, 2:363; 6:233–234
   face-masks, use of, and, 2:227
   holding infant in unintegrated state, 4:252–253
   lack of anxiety at regression to unintegrated state, 4:58
   mother-child relationship and, 6:90
   opposed to disintegration (*see* disintegration)
   primary, 2:14, 361–363, 366; 6:233
   progress from/regression into, 11:117*n*2, 133–136, 149
   psychosis and, 2:318; 4:43, 43*f*, 52, 56–57, 197
   sense of self and, 8:179*n*2
   squint and, 2:318
   the unconscious and, 4:108
United Kingdom. *See entries at* Britain *and* British
United Nations programme for the welfare of homeless children, 3:438
United States
   American Association of Psychiatric Clinics for Children, 8:349; 10:253

American Psychoanalytic Association, 5:391
American Psychopathological Association, 5:391
comparison of British and American psychoanalytical approaches, 8:13
DWW on, 3:352, 418; 4:238–239
illness and hospitalisation of DWW while in New York (1968), 8:3, 12, 18*n*8, 379–391, 397; 9:3, 23–24, 29, 39, 41
letter to American Correspondent (1969), 9:**29–31**
speaking tours of DWW in, 8:12. *See also* specific cities
unit status
   depressive position and, 11:91–102
   dramatisation of chaos after achievement of, 11:144
   'Establishment of Unit Status' (Part III of *Human Nature*; 1988), 11:**89–114**
   hypochondriacal anxiety and, 11:113–114
   in infant emotional development, 11:89
   inner world of the child, development of, 11:103–106
   'Integration' (from *Human Nature*; 1988), 11:**133–137**
   material presented by patients in analysis and, 11:107–111
   Me and *Not-Me*, 11:90
   in *The Piggle*, 11:233*n*XVIII
University College Hospital, 6:223
unthinkable anxiety, 9:29–30, 95, 138, 386
untidiness as irksome to mothers, 6:73–77
urban planning, 1:31–33, 68
urinary erotism, 3:108
urticaria, papular. *See* papular urticaria
urticarial rash, 1:193
Urwick, Desmond and Isobel Alison, 1:60
'The Use of an Object and Relating Through Identifications' (1968), 3:4, 18; 4:7, 10; 8:3, 5, 6, 12, 14–15, 243, **352–361**, 362, 398, 401, 403, 403*nv*
   on the analytic encounter, 11:9
   'Comments on My Paper "The Use of an Object"' (1989), 6:17; 8:15, 249, 390*n*iii, **393–395**; 9:33
   creativity, DWW on, 9:5
   cross-identifications and, 9:335
   'D. W. W's notes for the Vienna Congress 1971' (Appendix I), 8:**363–364**
   'Further Clinical Illustration (1968), 8:**369–377**
   instinct theory and, 11:86*n*6
   letter to Anna Freud (1969) about, 9:35–36
   mistakes made by analysts and, 9:26*n*i
   presented at New York Psychoanalytic Society, 9:3, 36

on primitive emotional development, 11:15, 102n6
  theme of, 9:355–356
'The Use of an Object in the Context of *Moses and Monotheism*' (1969), 6:6, 16, 17, 507; 8:249, 355; 9:33, **33–38**, 36, 38n6; 10:12
  creativity, DWW on, 9:9, 15
  notes anticipating, 7:163
'The Use of the Word "Use"' (1968), 8:**249–251**, 355; 9:8:355, 33

vaccination
  compulsory, 2:217–218
  against smallpox, 1:86; 2:218
vagina
  development of child's ideas about, 11:3, 69, 7, 74, 282
  excitement or stimulation of, 4:342, 7:105
value in emotional development, concept of, 11:89
'The Value of Depression' (1963), 6:15, **461–467**
'The Value of the Therapeutic Consultation' (1968), 7:11, 13, **273–278**; 8:319
values. *See* morality and ethics
van der Leeuw, P. J., 7:407, 410
Vanderpol, Maurice, 8:30
van der Waals, Herman Gijsbert, letters to (1959), 5:**477–478**
van Gogh, Vincent, 3:138
van Ophuijsen, J. H. W., 'On the Origin of the Feeling of Persecution', 11:102nn7–8
'Varicella Encephalitis and Vaccinia Encephalitis' (with Nancy Gibbs; 1926), 1:7, **75–90**
  chicken pox, cases complicated by, 1:79–81
  Dutch cases, 1:78–79, 84–87
  measles encephalitis, 1:88–89
  relationship between, 1:87, 88
  vaccinia encephalitis, 1:83–87
  varicella encephalitis, 1:75–83
'Varieties of Psychotherapy' (1961), 6:19, **197–204**
'Various Types of Psycho-Therapy Material' (from *Human Nature*; 1988), 10:15; 11:**107–111**
vaso-motor instability, 1:269
venereal disease, 6:190–191, 196n1, 426
venesection, 1:212, 217, 218
vengeance. *See* revenge
Versailles Treaty, War Guilt Clause in, 2:142
vertigo, 4:55–56, 58
viability, of foetus, 7:451
Victoria (Queen), 9:186
Vietnam, changing situation in, 5:6
Villa 21, Shenley Psychiatric Hospital, St Albans, 9:55, 9:55nii
violence
  coping with violent patients, 9:54–55
  'Death and Murder in the Adolescent Process' (1969), 9:337, **342–348**, 348n2

differentiated from aggression, 7:129
virtue. *See* morality and ethics
vision. *See* blindness; eyes
visiting children in hospital
  changing attitudes toward, 5:5
  emotional development, importance to, 11:171
  foundations of mental health and, 3:438
  'Visiting Children in Hospital' (1952), 3:**441–445**
Voices, 8:320, 413
Volkov, Peggy, 9:179
vomiting
  anxiety and, 1:257, 265, 266–267
  chorea and, 1:139
  cyclical or recurrent, 1:257, 264, 267, 418
  differential diagnosis of hysterical vomiting from vomiting due to intra-cranial tumour, 1:281
  eating disorders and, 1:418, 422
  encephalitis and, 1:80–81, 82, 86
  fear of, 1:265, 380
  hysterical, 1:281, 418
  intracranial tumour and, 1:281, 289, 290
  micturition disturbances and, 1:320
  speech disorders and, 1:333

Waddington, K., 1:4niii
Waddington, Mary, 6:105
Walker, Kenneth, 2:25–27
'Walking', from *Clinical Notes* (1931), 1:**291–297**
Wallace, Alfred, 7:17
Wallace Heaton (retailer), 8:389
Wallbridge, David, and Madeleine Davis, *Boundary and Space: An Introduction to the Work of D. W. Winnicott*, 9:255n1
Wallon, Henri, 6:371
war. *See also* World War I; World War II
  causes of, 2:115–116
  democracy at, 3:419–420
  unconscious value of, 7:152
wardens. *See* hostels
Ware, M., 7:407
Warlock, Peter, 9:117n1
Warner, E. C., 1:238
Wassermann reaction, 1:144, 293
Watson, J. A. F., *The Child and the Magistrate* (1950; reviewed 1951), 3:**431–432**
weaning
  age of, 4:186
  antisocial behaviour and, 6:13
  babies beginning to feel sorry and, 8:131–136
  child's needs and, 4:1584
  depression and, 6:13
  depressive position and, 4:36, 186, 202
  difficulties in, 5:279; 10:370, 399–400

weaning (*Cont.*)
    illusion-disillusionment and, 3:306; 4:37, 170–171, 200*n*8; 5:417
    good experience in, 3:303–306; 5:419*n*6; 6:354
    in *Holding and Interpretation*, 5:419*n*6
    inability to wean, 7:185
    of Juliet in *Romeo and Juliet*, 3:187–189
    mother's depression and, 10:370
    mother's preoccupation with infant and, 6:88
    self-weaning, 6:354
    transitional objects and, 3:451, 452, 453; 9:271, 277
    'Weaning' (1949), 3:**303–306**; 7:187*n*1, 187*n*4; 8:131; 11:102*n*9
'The Wearing of Masks in the Nursing of Premature and Older Infants' (abstract; 1943), 2:**227**
Weber, F. Parkes, 1:111, 112
Weissman, Philip, 5:364
Welfare Centres, 3:273
'The Welfare of Children in Hospital', 5:544*n*ii
West End Hospital for Nervous Diseases, 5:400
Westmacott, Irene, 'Psychiatric Social Work in a Paediatric Setting' (1961), 6:185*n*1
West Sussex County Council Children's Committee, 6:225
wetting the bed. *See* enuresis
Weymouth, E. S., 5:390
Wharton-Smith, 1:82, 88
'What About Father?'
    paper (1945), 2:**271–275**
    radio broadcast (1944), 2:21*n*iii, 271
'What Do We Know About Babies as Cloth Suckers?' (1956), 5:12, **115–118**
'What Do We Mean by a Normal Child?'
    paper (1946), 2:**281–286**; 7:148*n*i
    radio broadcast (1944), 2:21*n*iii, 12:9
'What Irks?' (1960), 6:**73–86**
'What Is Psychoanalysis?' (1952 reissue). *See* 'Towards an Objective Study of Human Nature' (1945)
'What Is Worthwhile in Medicine' (ca. 1917–1923), 1:**67–71**
Wheelis, A., 6:443–444
'Where Angels Fear to Tread' (1958), 5:**339–344**
'Where the Food Goes' (1949), 3:**277–280**
White, J. Stanley, 1:59, 60
Whitehead, A. N., 3:121
WHO. *See* World Health Organization
whole experiences, 2:135–136
wholeness, sense of, 4:187, 202
whooping cough, 1:119
'Why Children Play' (1942), 1: lxxvii; 2:**167–170**; 8:11
'Why Courts Must Act Swiftly' (1966), 7:**349–363**
'Why Do Babies Cry?'
    (radio broadcast 1944), 2:21*n*iii, 237; 8:137
    paper (1944), 1: lxvi
    paper (1945), 2:**237–245**
'Winnicott's Wisdom' (1967), 8:**137–142**
wickedness, 6:379, 386–387, 429
Wickes, Frances G.
    chapter in Harms, Ernest (ed.), *Handbook of Child Guidance* (1947; reviewed 1949), 3:235
    The Inner World of Man: With Psychological Drawings and Paintings (1938/1950; reviewed 1951), 3:**463**; 6:443
widows, children of, 7:99
Wigley, Dr, 1:462
Wilde, Oscar
    'The Ballad of Reading Gaol' (1898), 7:133
    'The Importance of Being Earnest' (1895), 9:196
Wilkinson, Agnes, letter to (1969), 9:**57–58**, 337
William Alanson White Institute (New York), 8:320
Williams, Norma, 8:405, 405*n*ii
Williams, Pearse, 5:438, 475
Williams, Vaughan, IV Symphony, 9:112
Williamson, B., 1:185*n*1
Willmott, P., *Family and Kinship in East London* (1957; Young co-author), 6:122
Wills, David, 2:7, 8, 17, 103, 291; 9:199, 200–201
Wills, Doris M., 7:376
Wills, Ruth, 2:103, 291; 9:199
Wilson, A. Tommy M., letter to (1959), 5:**479–480**
Wilson, Ambrose Cyril, 2:261–262, 266–268
    'Deprivation of Initiative' (1948), 5:399
    'Homosexuality' (1946), 5:399
    'An Individual Point of View on Shock Therapy' (1943), 2:261, 269*n*n1–2
    obituary (1958), 5:**399–400**
    'The Rôle of Fixation in Perversion and Masturbation' (1947), 5:399
Wilson, Ambrose John, 5:399
Wilson, Dr, 3:227
Wilson, Kinnier, 1:305
Winnicott, Alice (née Taylor; first wife), 1: lviii, 11, 13*n*vi, 167; 2:18; 3:195*n*ii, 197*n*i, 383–384; 5:9; 8:399*n*ii; 12:305
Winnicott, Clare (née Britton; second wife)
    archiving and publication of DWW's work, 1: xlvii–xlix; 5:10, 12:xlix
    'Casework Techniques in the Child Care Services', 6:6
    at celebration of publication of S. Freud's *Standard Edition*, 7:407
    Child Care and Social Work (1964), 5:492*n*1, 492*n*3
    cited by DWW, 5:97
    Coles, Joyce, correspondence with, while DWW in NYC hospital (November & December

1968), 8:379, 379nni–ii, 381, 385, 387, 387nii, 389, 389nii, 399ni, 399niii, 403, 406nv
collaborating with DWW, 1: lix, lxx; 2:103ni; 12:306
contribution to Tod's *Disturbed Children* (1968), 9:99
Curtis Commission (Home Office Committee on Children's Homes), evidence given to, 2:4–5, 369–370; 5:72ni
'D. W. W.: A reflection' (afterword) 1:27, 29, 12:**295–309**
on date of 'Fear of Breakdown', 6:523
on DWW, 1: lviii–lix, 18; 2:19; 5:9; 6:6; 12:295–309
on DWW's death, 9:3, 12:284–285, 297–298
on DWW and Nemon's statue of Freud, 9:18, 12:4, 12:15n4
on DWW's career, 10:7; 12:305–306
on DWW's early family life, 6:20; 12:298–304
on 'The Use of an Object and Relating Through Identifications' (1968), 8:14
evacuated children in Oxford, work with, 2:8–9; 5:5
The Family and Individual Development dedicated to, 7:309
on Finnish Psychoanalytic Society and DWW, 7:84; 8:8
flu suffered by, 9:255
hostel work of, 2:8–9, 332nii, 373; 5:439
knowledge of *The Piggle*, 11:189
mentioned in DWW's letters to other correspondents, 5:217, 221; 7:343; 9:39, 40, 111
letter to (1950), 3:**331**
Mrs. Winnicott in *The Piggle*, 11:237, 238, 253n2
New York City illness and hospitalisation of DWW, 8:3, 12, 18n8, 379nni–ii, 379–391, 397, 399, 405–406
occupation therapy, use of, 3:266
photograph with DWW, 7:20
preface to *Human Nature*, 11:**25**, 12:liv
preface to *The Piggle*, 11:**187–188**, 190
'The Problem of Homeless Children' (with DWW; 1944), 2:291ni, **299–311**; 3:27n1
'Residential Management as Treatment for Difficult Children' (with Winnicott; 1947), 3:27n1, **77–93**
social work and, 5:9; 6:418
transitional objects and, 9:40; 12:308
Winnicott, Donald Woods (DWW in this index), 1: lvii–lxxix, 3–19
1911–1923, 1:27–71
1926–1930, 1:73–163
1931, 1:165–336. *See also* Clinical Notes on Disorders of Childhood
1932–1939, 1:337–465
1939, 2:25–75
1940, 2:77–99
1941, 2:101–142
1942, 2:143–174
1943, 2:175–230
1944, 2:231–319
1945, 2:321–395
1946, 3:23–55
1947, 3:59–113
1948, 3:117–176
1949, 3:179–328
1950, 3:331–427
1951, 3:431–493
1952, 4:19–67
1953, 4:69–174
1954, 4:175–299
1955, 4:301–474; 5:19–110
1956, 5:115–193
1957, 5:197–302
1958, 5:305–429
1959, 5:433–545
1960, 6:29–171
1961, 6:173–279
1962, 6:281–395
1963, 6:397–531
1964, 7:27–135
1965, 7:139–312
1966, 7:315–460
1967, 8:1–218
1968, 8:219–444
1969, 9:23–164
1970, 9:167–252
1971, 9:255–356
'An Allotted Spanner in the Works,' (ca. 1966–67), 7:**459**; 7:**460**
biography, 1: lvii–lix; 12:li–lii, 298–304
adaptation of technique by, 11:187–188, 191–192
age affecting work with children and adolescents, 9:171
analysis as approached by, 11:8–11, 191–192
archiving and publication of works, 1: xlvii–l
BBC broadcasts by. *See* BBC broadcasts
British Psychoanalytical Society (BPAS), role in. *See* British Psychoanalytical Society
challenge of unexpected in life of, 10:7; 12:305, 306–307
character and personality, writings revealing, 7:3, 14–18; 12:li–lii
chronological arrangement and reading of works of, 1: lx–lxi, lxxviii; 12:l
chronology/timeline, 1:467–472; 2:397–401; 3:495–501; 4:475–481; 5:547–552; 7:461–467; 8:445–450; 9:397–403; 10:535–541; 11:319–324
clinical work, insights for. *See* clinical observations
on consultations, 7:10–13

Winnicott, Donald Woods (DWW in this index) (*Cont.*)
contemporaries' work with children and, 1:17–18
on creativity, 1: lxv–lxxvi; 9:3–15
death, preparation for, 1:xlix; 8:381, 383; 9:3, 351–353; 12:l, lii, lv, 297–298, 309
on death of friends in WWI, 7:459, 9:175, 210–211, 255, 351, 12:lv
disintegration and dissociation, interest in, 7:8–10
drawings by, 12:*279–288*
'D. W. W.: A Reflection' (Clare Winnicott), 12:**295–309**
'D. W. W. on D. W. W.', 8: **35–47**
early life, 8:245–246; 9:352–353; 12:298–304
early paediatric experience and practice, 1: lviii, 6–9; 4:228; 12:305
early writings of, 1: lxi–lxiii; 12:liv–lv
as English writer and international author, 1: xlviii–xlix; 12:li
failure, feelings of, 5:480–481; 8:13, 357
A. Freud-Klein controversy and, 4: 241–243; 5:6–8, 10–11, 12, 19–20, 33, 87; 6:331; 8:42
health as conceived by, 11:5, 11–14
heart condition, 1: lx; 3:221*n*ii, 383; 5:9, 365; 9:3, 23–34, 189; 10:3
illness and hospitalisation while in New York (1968), 8:3, 12, 18*n*8, 379–391, 397; 9:3, 23–24, 29, 39, 41
images and photographs of, 1:*ii, 21–24*; 3:*20*; 4:*17*; 5:*16*; 6:*24–27*; 7:*20–23*; 8:*21–30*; 9:*18–20*
independence in thinking, 7:3, 14–15, 17–18; 8:39, 161
influences on, 5:7; 8:4–5, 35–47; 12:305. See also Freud; Klein; Melanie; Sigmund; 'D.W.W. on D.W.W.'
integration of psychoanalysis and paediatrics, 1:12–17; 4:228; 6:19–20, 183–184, 310–311, 490; 8:81; 12:li–lii
interpsychic processes, awareness of, 3:7–9
jargon and technical language, avoiding use of, 7:14, 341
lay readers, writing for, 1: xlviii, xlix; 2:13, 12:li, 8
at Market End House, 2:103*n*i
marriage to Clare Britton, 1: lviii–lix, 18; 5:9; 12:308
medical education, 1: lviii, 3–6, 18, 65–71; 7:333; 12:304–305
medical profession, early interest in, 1:29–30; 8:40
National Health Service, opinion of, 2:18, 235; 3:35, 37, 139; 5:8–9
natural childbirth movement and, 5:12–13, 239, 305; 10:138

nonspecialised audiences, interest in communicating with, 7:14–15, 83, 125–126; 8:43; 12:8
Paddington Green Children's Hospital, role at. *See* Paddington Green Children's Hospital
pedagogy as means of developing and communicating ideas, 11:3–4, 25
personal experience influencing theories of, 5:4–6; 6:20; 12:305
pet mice as child, 9:106
plan of DWW's working space at 87 Chester Square, London, 11:*186*
presidencies of societies, 5:9; 12:li
psychoanalytical education, 1:10–12, 53–55; 2:179; 6:180; 8:40–41; 12:305
publication of *Collected Works*, 1: xlvii–l, lx–lxi, lxxviii–lxxix; 5:3; 12:xlix
publications during lifetime, 1: lix, lx–lxi; 4:225; 5:3; 12:xlix, liii, 5–6
recognition of work of, 1:18–19; 2:5
religion and, 4:245; 12:li, 301
retirement of, 1:xvi; 6:3, 9, 19, 270–271; 9:99
separation and divorce from first wife, 3:195*n*ii, 197*n*i; 5:9
signatures of, 12:*289–293*
surveys, refusing to participate in, 6:111–112, 421–422. *See also* questionnaires
theories of, 1: lix–lxi, lxv–lxxi; 8:15–17, 43–47; 11:14–18
Training Committee, British Psychoanalytical Society, 4:1879–1840, 243; 8:334
United States, speaking tours in, 8:12. *See also specific cities*
varied clinical experience of, 5:301; 12:li
World War II work during, 2:3–4, 5; 6:181; 8:5, 42; 10:18
writing style of, 1: xlvii, lix–lxi; 5:11–12; 7:3, 4–8, 10–14; 9:4
Winnicott, Elizabeth (mother), 1: lviii, **27, 35, 37, 43, 49, 51**; 12:298–302
Winnicott, Sir John Frederick (father), 1: lviii, 27, 29, **35, 37, 43, 51**; 5:9; 9:352–353; 12:301, 304
Winnicott, Kathleen (sister), 1:27, **35, 37, 43, 51**; 12:298–302
Winnicott Trust, The, 1: xlviii–xlix, li–lii, 12:xlix
Winnicott, Violet (sister), 1: lix, lx, 10, 27, **35, 37, 43, 51, 53–55**; 12:298–302
Winnicott on the child (2002), 6:31
Winnicott Publications Committee
preface to *The Piggle*, 11:**187–188**
publication of *The Piggle* (1977) by, 11:3
'Winnicott's Axiom' (1963), 6:523, 537*n*ii
'Winnicott's Wisdom', 12:lvi
'Hobgoblins and Good Habits' (1967), 8:**151–155**

'How a Baby Begins to Feel Sorry and to Make
  Amends' (1967), 8:**131–136**
'The Meaning of Mother Love' (1967), 8:**117–120**
'Why Do Babies Cry?' (1967), 8:**137–142**
Winnie the Pooh, 7:353, 9:261
Winton, Professor, 7:407
Wisdom, John, 1: lxviii; 7:95*n*i, 190; 8:263*n*i
  letter to (1964), 7:17, **95–97**
wish fulfilment, 6:15, 132
withdrawal. *See also* regression
  adolescents, psychotherapeutic interviews with,
    7:52, 54
  'Case Notes for a Psychoanalytic
    Seminar: Withdrawal, Regression, Male
    Identification' (1965), 7:**239–242**
  defined, 11:159
  fantasy belonging to, in *Holding and
    Interpretation*, 4:308, 309
  'Notes on Withdrawal and Regression'
    (1989), 7:6
  regression distinguished, 7:6–7, 240
  'Withdrawal and Regression' (from *Human
    Nature*; 1988), 11:**159–160**
  'Withdrawal and Regression' (read 1954 & 1955;
    published 1955), 1: lxxiii; 4:**283–289**; 5:253*n*i;
    6:157*n*7, 170; 10:367*n*8
Wolf, Elizabeth, 1:lii
Wolf, Katherine M., 4:118
Wolfenden Report (Departmental Committee
  on Homosexual Offences and Prostitution),
  4:267*n*i; 5:27
Wolff, Heinz, 8:206
Wolff, Megan, 12:xlix
Wolff, Werner, *The Personality of the Preschool
  Child: The Child's Search for His Self* (1947;
  reviewed 1948), 3:**159–160**
women
  fear of, 3:416–417, 421*n*4; 5:294–295; 7:126–127
  three, in myth and dreams, 11:74*n*5
Woodhead, Barbara, 6:181–182, 184
Woolf, Leonard, 7:409; 8:125
Woolf, Virginia, 7:409
  Albee, Edward, *Who's Afraid of Virginia Woolf?*
    (1962), 9:220
  The Waves (1931), 9:40
'wool-gathering', 4:173*n*4
Wordsworth, William
  I Wandered Lonely as a Cloud (1802/
    1807), 9:216
  Ode: Intimations of Immortality (1807), 3:100*n*i;
    4:410; 6:310, 313
work and play, relationship between, 7:413–414
work, capacity for, in depressive position,
  11:94, 171
workhouses, 1:409*n*iii

*The World Biennial of Psychiatry and
  Psychotherapy* (Arieti, ed.), 10:521
World Federation for Mental Health, 5:203; 8:319
World Health Organization (WHO)
  Conference (Geneva 1953), 4:229
  Congress (Stockholm 1954), 4:229
  Expert Committee on Mental Health,
    3:437–439
'The World in Small Doses' (1949), 3:**293–297**;
  7:187*n*3
World Medicine (journal), 9:59
World War I
  cousin of DWW killed in, 5:4
  DWW on death of friends in, 7:459, 9:175,
    210–211, 255, 351, 12:lv
  DWW in, 1:xvi, 3–4; 2:5; 5:5; 12:304
  Jones, Ernest, in, 5:391–392
  shell shock, 1:53; 3:327*n*i
World War II. *See also* death; 'Discussion of War
    Aims' (1940); evacuation of children
  aftermath of, 5:6
  bombings and air raids, 3:454; 7:384
  children in children's homes during. *See* greed;
    guilt; hate and hatred; hostels
  'Children in the War' (published 1940 & radio
    broadcast 1939), 2:5, **95–99**
  effect on antisocial behaviour and crime, 3:410
  'Discussion of War Aims' (1940), 2:16–17, **87–94**
  DWW working during, 2:3–4, 5; 6:181; 8:5,
    42; 10:18
  A. Freud during, 9:94
  homeless children as result of, 2:299–311
  inability of people to discuss opinions on,
    2:79–80
  'Meet to Be Stolen From' (ca. 1939–1945),
    2:16–17, 141–142
  Nazis, Nazism, and treatment of Jews, 1:xxii,
    17, 408, 463; 2:89–90, 93; 3:35; 5:7, 394–395,
    535–536; 9:94
  nephew of DWW killed in, 5:4
  Oxfordshire Evacuation Scheme, 1: lix, 18;
    8:42; 12:306
  paediatric nutrition initiatives during, 5:5; 12:11
  prisoners of war and refugees, 3:226
  Tavistock Clinic and, 3:327*n*i
  vanquished enemy, recommendations for,
    2:93–94
Worster-Drought, C. C., 1:118, 142; 5:400
Wride, Dr, 6:107; 7:408
Wright, Ken, 1: lxxvii
Wulff, M., 4:297; 5:413, 417; 6:64
  'Fetishism and Object Choice in Early
    Childhood' (1946), 3:458; 4:40, 167, 175–176,
    177*n*7; 5:419*n*5; 8:301; 9:273
Wyllie, W. G., 1:172*n*1

Yale Child Study Centre, 8:8
Yates, Sybil, 1:18
'Yes, but How Do We Know It's True?' (1950), 3:**423–427**
Yorke, Clifford, 6:235*n*i
Young, Lady Aurelia, 12:16*n*10
Young, M., *Family and Kinship in East London* (1957; Willmott co-author), 6:122
Young, Mr and Mrs, letter to (1960), 6:**111–112**
Young, Robert, 5:399
Young-Bruehl, Elisabeth, 1: xlix; 12:xlix
'The Young Child at Home and at School' (lecture 1962), 6:377. *See also* 'Morals and Education'
Young Children (1949), 3:307

'Young Children and Other People' (1949), 3:**307–312**; 8:159
Younghusband, Dame Eileen, 7:407
Your Child (unserialised weekly childcare encyclopedia), 9:247, 249
'Youth Will Not Sleep' (1964), 7:**79–81**; 8:269*n*iv

Zetzel, Elizabeth, 5:318; 6:293, 293*n*ii, 340–341; 8:12, 391
  'Additional Notes Upon a Case of Obsessional Neurosis' (1966), 7:198
  'Current Concepts of Transference' (1956), 6:339–340
Ziman, Edmund, *Jealousy in Children* (reviewed 1951), 3:**469**